Cardiovascular-Kidney-Metabolic Syndrome

Mariana Floria • Daniela Maria Tanase
Editors

Cardiovascular-Kidney-Metabolic Syndrome

Springer

Editors
Mariana Floria
Grigore T. Popa University of Medicine and Pharmacy
Iași, Romania

Daniela Maria Tanase
Saint Spiridon Emergency Hospital
Iași, Romania

ISBN 978-3-032-11444-0 ISBN 978-3-032-11445-7 (eBook)
https://doi.org/10.1007/978-3-032-11445-7

This Springer imprint is published by the registered company Springer Nature Switzerland AG
The registered company address is: Gewerbestrasse 11, 6330 Cham, Switzerland

Contents

Chapter 1
Introduction

Mariana Floria and Daniela Maria Tanase

Cardiovascular-kidney-metabolic syndrome emerged as a critical concept in modern medicine, reflecting the complex interrelationship between cardiovascular disease, chronic kidney disease, and metabolic disorders such as diabetes and obesity. In recent decades, the global burden of chronic disease has risen dramatically. Cardiovascular disease remains the leading cause of death worldwide, while diabetes and obesity have reached epidemic levels. Similarly, chronic kidney disease, often a silent contributor, is a critical risk amplifier in both cardiovascular and metabolic contexts. Collectively, these overlapping pathologies that define CKM syndrome underscore the complex pathophysiology and progression toward organ failure. The prolonged but progressive nature of this syndrome demands a unified, multidisciplinary approach to diagnosis, treatment, and long-term management.

This book provides a comprehensive exploration of CKM syndrome from its evolution to its current integrative model, identifying key risk factors and demographic trends. The global surge in metabolic disorders driven by sedentary lifestyles, dietary changes, and population aging is a major public health concern and has a determinant role in the onset and progression of CKM syndrome. The insidious progression is marked by subclinical inflammation, neurohormonal dysregulation, endothelial dysfunction, oxidative stress, and insulin resistance, which coexist and exacerbate one another, shifting the paradigm from organ-specific to systemic approaches. Ongoing research on the genetic and molecular basis sheds light on

M. Floria · D. M. Tanase (✉)
Grigore T. Popa University of Medicine and Pharmacy, Iasi, Romania

Saint Spiridon Emergency Hospital, Iasi, Romania
e-mail: daniela.tanase@umfiasi.ro

M. Floria, D. M. Tanase (eds.), *Cardiovascular-Kidney-Metabolic Syndrome*,
https://doi.org/10.1007/978-3-032-11445-7_1

inherited and acquired drivers in parallel with environmental and behavioral factors in CKM syndrome.

In addressing prevention and treatment, current knowledge advocates for comprehensive strategies beyond organ-specific interventions. Effective management requires a holistic approach that integrates lifestyle modification, pharmacological therapies, and patient education within a coordinated multidisciplinary team.

Ultimately, this book is designed for clinicians and healthcare professionals seeking a thorough understanding of current knowledge on CKM syndrome to improve patient outcomes. Emphasis is placed on early identification, risk stratification, personalized treatment, and the ability to recognize CKM syndrome as it will be a cornerstone of modern healthcare.

Chapter 2
The Evolution of Cardiovascular-Kidney-Metabolic Syndrome

Stefan Iliescu, Paula Cristina Morariu, Mariana Floria, and Adrian Covic

Cardio-Renal Syndrome

Short History

Homage to thee, O my heart! Homage to thee, O my kidneys! [1]

The connection between the heart and the kidneys long precedes the birth of modern medicine, starting in Ancient Egypt, where the first written text that mentions the two organs in parallel was published as early as 1600–1240 BC. This link is more clearly defined in the Bible, where the kidneys, referred to as "reins," were thought to be linked with desires, not unlike the heart. Together, they were the organs that God examined to pass judgement: "Examine me, O Lord, and prove me; try my reins and my heart" (Psalm 26:2) [2].

The first references to pathology seem to come from ancient China. In the Five Element Theory, the heart represents fire, while the kidneys are linked with water. Shen Jinao states in his *Compendium of Honoring Life* that "before the heart fire can harmoniously blend with the kidney water, however, the kidney water must be sufficient. Otherwise the heart fire will flare out of control, and all kinds of heart and kidney ailments will arise." These *ailments* Shen Junao refers to seem to be the first documented description of cardio-renal syndrome called "heart and kidney failing

S. Iliescu · P. C. Morariu (✉) · M. Floria
Grigore T. Popa University of Medicine and Pharmacy, Iasi, Romania

Saint Spiridon Emergency Hospital, Iasi, Romania

A. Covic
Grigore T. Popa University of Medicine and Pharmacy, Iasi, Romania

Dr. C.I Parhon Clinical Hospital, Iasi, Romania

M. Floria, D. M. Tanase (eds.), *Cardiovascular-Kidney-Metabolic Syndrome*,
https://doi.org/10.1007/978-3-032-11445-7_2

to link" manifesting as palpitations, oliguria or nicturia, restlessness, and dizziness [2].

In the Western world, Gentile da Foligno is considered to be the first cardio-nephrologist. He noticed the link between heart disease and differences in urinary color and output. A few centuries later, in the 1800s, Bright and Traube were among the first to report that patients with chronic kidney disease (CKD) often exhibited cardiac hypertrophy [2].

The first definition of cardio-renal syndrome was proposed in 1914 by Alfred Stengel, an American surgeon who wrote: "The clinician encounters many cases [...] in which evidences of cardiac weakness [...] are associated with signs of failure of renal function or urinary indications of renal disease. When this combination of symptoms is of such character that the observer cannot readily assign to either the cardiovascular system or to the kidneys the preponderance of responsibility, the term 'cardio-renal disease' is often employed." Stengel also proposed a three-way classification: (1) primary heart condition with secondary kidney disease; (2) primary vascular condition with secondary heart and kidney disease; (3) primary renal dysfunction with secondary cardiac disease [3].

Definition and Classification

In 2004, the National Heart, Lung, and Blood Institute developed the first formal definition of cardio-renal syndrome that stated, "In heart failure, it is the result of interactions between the kidneys and other circulatory compartments that increase circulating volume and symptoms of heart failure and disease progression are exacerbated. At its extreme, cardio-renal dysregulation leads to what is termed 'cardio-renal syndrome' in which therapy to relieve congestive symptoms of heart failure is limited by further decline in renal function" [4]. The need for this initiative came from the observation that patients hospitalized for decompensated heart failure who presented worsening renal function had worse outcomes. Moreover, this group of patients seemed to be excluded from major clinical trials [4].

Four years later, Acute Dialysis Quality Initiative (ADQI) published a consensus in which they proposed a classification of cardio-renal syndrome based on the primary insult site (cardiac or renal) and the nature (acute or chronic) [5]. Therefore, five different subtypes were defined (Fig. 2.1).

- Type 1, acute cardio-renal syndrome, is defined as an acute deterioration of heart function that leads to kidney injury. Worsening renal function is a relatively common complication of acutely decompensated heart failure or acute coronary syndromes and is associated with higher mortality rates [5].
- Type 2, chronic cardio-renal syndrome, in which chronic cardiac dysfunction promotes kidney injury, appears in almost two-thirds of patients hospitalized for congestive heart failure. The first two subtypes are interconnected as patients seem to frequently transition between them [5].

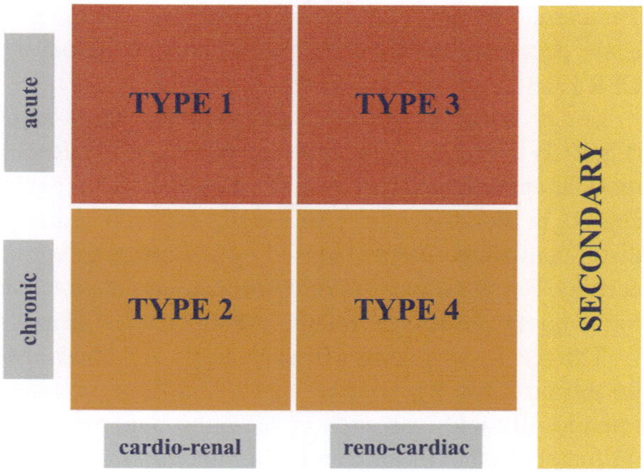

Fig. 2.1 Cardio-renal syndrome classification

- Type 3, acute reno-cardiac syndrome, is defined as an acute deterioration of renal function that leads to acute cardiac injury or dysfunction. Due to the multiple causes and pathophysiological mechanisms involved in acute kidney injury (AKI), it is difficult to estimate clinical outcomes or its epidemiology [5].
- Type 4, chronic reno-cardiac syndrome, where CKD is responsible for cardiac dysfunction, is well documented. In predialysis CKD patients, the prevalence of cardiovascular disease correlates with the severity of the renal dysfunction [5].
- Type 5 or secondary cardio-renal syndrome refers to a systemic condition that simultaneously affects both the heart and the kidneys. This subtype includes clinical scenarios where although there is no primary cardiac or renal dysfunction, a systemic disease such as diabetes mellitus, amyloidosis, or systemic lupus erythematosus involves both organs [5].

Pathophysiology of Cardio-Renal Interactions

At its most basic level, cardio-renal syndrome refers to the interplay between the heart and the kidneys where the dysfunction of one system leads to the dysfunction of the other. This maladaptive relationship is influenced by numerous factors, such as hemodynamic and metabolic alterations, neurohormonal activation, and the pro-inflammatory status present in this group of patients. Although the specific pathophysiological pathways differ in importance based on the subtype (acute versus chronic), the underlying mechanisms are frequently overlapping.

Being a low-resistance circuit, the kidneys receive a disproportionately large percentage of the cardiac output (25%). Furthermore, kidneys have an extremely high degree of sensitivity to hypoxia-induced lesions because of the low oxygen tension in the outer medulla and the low resistance nature of the renal vascular system [6].

The classic theory is that a rapid decrease in CO, as seen in cardiogenic shock or acute decompensated heart failure, leads to kidney hypoperfusion and a drop in GFR [7, 8].

Lower renal blood flow activates the renin-angiotensin-aldosterone system (Fig. 2.2) in order to restore tissue perfusion [6]. Renin is secreted by the juxtaglomerular apparatus in response to changes in renal perfusion (sensed by mechanoreceptors in the afferent arteriole wall), reduced sodium and chloride delivery to the distal convoluted tubule (sensed by the macula densa), and increased sympathetic activity. Renin cleaves angiotensinogen into angiotensin I, which is further cleaved into angiotensin II by the angiotensin converting enzyme (ACE).

The rise in angiotensin II levels leads to sodium reabsorption by its direct effect on the proximal convoluted tubule and through aldosterone secretion, free water retention through vasopressin secretion, and vasoconstriction [9]. These changes ultimately lead to sodium and water retention, an increase in preload, and worsening pump failure [6].

Adequate renal blood flow and consequently glomerular filtration rate are dependent on the difference between arterial and venous pressures [6].

Because ofe renal autoregulatory mechanisms, renal blood flow seems to be relatively stable when cardiac output is slightly reduced and starts to drop only after mean arterial pressure falls below 70 mmHg [10]. A post hoc analysis of the Evaluation Study of Congestive Heart Failure and Pulmonary Artery Catheter Effectiveness trial (ESCAPE) trial, which included 575 patients who underwent pulmonary artery catheterization, found no statistically significant association between cardiac index and renal function [11]. In another analysis of the same trial, Nohria et al. found right atrial pressure to be the only hemodynamic parameter associated with baseline kidney dysfunction [12]. The Acute Decompensated Heart Failure (ADHERE) National Registry showed no difference in increasing in creatinine levels in patients with acute heart failure with preserved or reduced ejection fraction [6].

Based on the same equation, elevated central venous pressure leads to renal venous hypertension with an increased renal resistance and a decline in the filtration

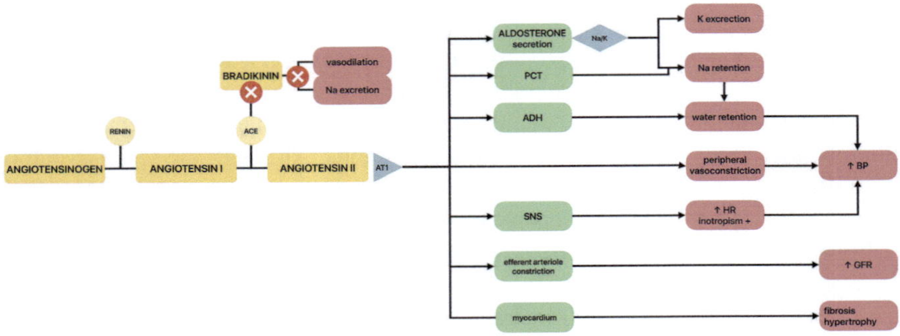

Fig. 2.2 Renin-angiotensin-aldosterone system

rate [6]. The consequent increase in renal interstitial pressure may promote a hypoxic state of the renal parenchyma, which further declines kidney function [13]. In 2009, Mullens et al. observed in 145 ADHF patients that venous congestion was the most important predictor for worsening renal function. This effect referred to both higher venous pressure at admission ($p < 0.001$) and insufficient reduction after intensive management ($p = 0.04$). In contrast, the cardiac index was stable between the two groups [13]. Another factor that influences this mechanism seems to be the increase of intraabdominal pressure caused by ascites or abdominal organ edema. The same investigators found a strong correlation ($p = 0.009$) between renal dysfunction and abdominal pressure values above 8 mmHg [14].

Besides the hemodynamic factors that are involved in the pathophysiology of cardio-renal syndrome, there are several other pathways that seem to weigh at least the same. Kidney disease and heart failure involve chronic inflammatory processes. Proinflammatory molecules are important biomarkers as they are involved in tissue lesions in both organs [8]. Tumor necrosis factor a (TNF-a) and interleukins 1 and 6 (IL-1, IL-6) have been shown to rise in kidney disease and have a known cardiodepressant effect [6, 15]. TNF-a and IL-6 promote the accumulation of monocyte chemotactic factors in the renal interstitium, increasing the inflammatory cells. Furthermore, TNF-a alone causes mesangial cells apoptosis, further damaging kidney function [8]. Oxidative stress is another pathway involved in kidney and cardiac dysfunction. Reactive oxygen species (ROS) have been linked with type 1 cardio-renal syndrome. Higher ROS levels are involved in cardiac dysfunction, inhibiting contractility, ionic transport, and calcium homeostasis. At the renal level, nitric oxide (which in normal conditions promotes vasodilation) is now responsible for vasoconstriction and vascular and renal dysfunction [16].

Oxidative stress is also increased by the accumulation of uremic toxins and ultimately leads to cardiac and renal fibrosis [8]. Fibroblast growth factor 23 (FGF-23) normally regulates calcium and vitamin D metabolism, and its levels seem to be increased in CKD. Chronically elevated levels of FGF-23 have been shown to play a causal role in left ventricular hypertrophy [17].

Clinical Relevance of Cardio-Renal Syndrome

Cardio-renal syndrome should not be perceived only as a pathophysiological model of heart–kidney interactions, but rather as a major clinical syndrome that worsens the outcomes of the affected patients and complicates management.

Cardiovascular mortality is responsible for 25% of the deaths of patients with normal kidney function, but this percentage rises to almost 50% in patients with CKD stages 4 and 5. Moreover, the association of cardiovascular disease seems to increase the rate of hospitalization in CKD patients [18]. The Chronic Renal Insufficiency Cohort (CRIC) study followed a total of 3314 participants for a median of 10 years in order to compare the incidence, risk factors, and outcomes of heart failure with preserved or reduced ejection fraction in CKD patients with a median estimated glomerular function rate (eGFR) of 44.7 mL/min/1.73m^2. The results showed a higher incidence of HFpEF (8.6% vs 6.7% per 1000 person-year) [19]. In the EMPEROR Preserved trial that included almost 6000 patients, almost 50% of them had an eGFR under 60 mL/min/1.73m^2 [20].

This association also has major prognostic implications. In a retrospective cohort study of over 7500 patients with incident CKD, Yu et al. showed an increase in 1-year mortality in patients with heart failure, the greatest risk being for patients with reduced ejection fraction [18]. A report from the ADHERE database showed more than half of patients with acutely decompensated heart failure had at least moderate kidney dysfunction, defined as an eGFR under 60 mL/min/1.73 m^2. In-hospital mortality rates increased up to 7.6% in patients with severe kidney dysfunction compared with 1.9% in those with normal renal function. Similarly, the loss in eGFR was associated with a rise in inotrope and diuretic use and a decline in renin-angiotensin-aldosterone system (RAAS) inhibitors [21].

Diagnosis

Due to the complex interplay between cardiac and renal dysfunction, the timely diagnosis of cardio-renal syndrome represents a challenge in the context of prognosticating the disease and identifying high-risk patients that require intensive management. Clinical examination, biomarkers assessment, imaging techniques, and invasive monitoring are all essential tools in identifying and monitoring cardiorenal syndrome. The aim of these diagnosis strategies is to simultaneously assess both cardiac and renal parameters [6].

A thorough clinical history is essential in identifying and assessing comorbidities such as hypertension, diabetes mellitus, CKD and coronary artery disease. These comorbid associations influence both the pathophysiology of cardio-renal syndrome (CRS) and outcomes and are a vital part of understanding the individual risk factors of the patients [22].

The clinical exam should focus on identifying common findings in cardiac and renal diseases, such as a decrease in exercise tolerance, fatigue, dyspnea, edema, and signs of fluid overload [22].

Biomarkers

In the wide clinical spectrum of cardio-renal dysfunction, cardiac and renal biomarkers provide discrimination between phenotypes and offer valuable insights about outcomes [6]. Their purpose has been divided into three main components: (1) providing prognostic insights; (2) differentiating between the different CRS subtypes; and (3) identifying patients most likely to respond to CRS-specific therapy [23].

Markers of myocardial injury (troponin) and stretch (B-type natriuretic peptide) are routinely assessed in clinical practice. Both these cardiac biomarkers have an integral role in the management of acute coronary syndromes and heart failure. The European Society of Cardiology (ESC) recommends their use with a class I of recommendation, level of evidence B [24, 25].

Independent of myocardial ischemia, high troponin levels have been associated with an increased risk of mortality in both ADHF and CKD [22, 26]. In a prospective study of 4726 patients with suspected acute myocardial infarction, patients with kidney disease were more likely to have elevated troponin levels, diminishing the specificity for type 1 myocardial infarction. However, irrespective of the presence of coronary obstruction, these patients had a twofold heightened risk of cardiac events at 1 year [27].

CKD patients present with elevated levels of BNP compared with patients with acute heart failure and normal renal function. This difference seems to be caused by both increased natriuretic peptide production as a result of volume overload and reduced kidney clearance [22].

If cardiac markers are routinely used and their role in patient management is clearly specified, the same cannot be fully stated about biomarkers of renal dysfunction. While the hope is to be able to use them in order to identify patients most likely to benefit from CRS-specific treatment, at the moment most of the renal biomarkers' role is in prognostication [22].

The time difference between the initial renal insult and the changes in serum creatinine or urinary output creates a significant delay in diagnosing AKI, thus giving rise to the need to identify at-risk patients [6].

In the first stages of glomerular damage, albumin is excreted into the renal tubules. Additionally, in cases of tubular injury, albumin reabsorption is inhibited, resulting in albuminuria. An analysis of the 2310 patients included in the CHARM trial (Candesartan in Heart Failure: Assessment of Reduction in Mortality and Morbidity) reported abnormal levels of urinary albumin per creatinine ratio (UACR) in 41% of the participants irrespective of ejection fraction. Albuminuria was associated with an increased risk for all-cause mortality (HR 1.62 for microalbuminuria vs. normoalbuminuria and 1.76 for macroalbuminuria vs. normoalbuminuria) and for the composite outcome of cardiovascular mortality and heart failure admission (HR 1.43 for microalbuminuria vs. normoalbuminuria and 1.62 for macroalbuminuria vs. normoalbuminuria) [28]. A post hoc analysis of GISSI-HF trial (Gruppo Italiano per lo Studio della Sopravvivenza nella Insufficienza Cardiaca–Heart Failure) showed similar results. Mortality seems to increase proportionally with UACR, and the difference starts being statistically significant even at UACR values that are considered to be within normal range (15–30 mg/g) [29]. Although albuminuria offers important prognostic information, it lacks specificity. Without means to determine the exact etiology of urinary albumin in patients with comorbid diabetes or hypertension, its diagnostic value is limited [23].

Cystatin C (CysC), a cysteine proteinase produced by all nucleated cells at a constant rate, is freely filtered, completely reabsorbed, and not secreted by the kidneys [22, 23]. Its role in early detection of AKI seems to outperform serum creatinine [22]. A study using the data from the PREVEND trial (Prevention of Renal and Vascular End-Stage Disease) cohort found a statistically significant association between high levels of CysC and new onset HFpEF (HR 1.45, CI 1.03–2.04, $p = 0.033$) [30]. Additionally, a cross-sectional study on almost 400 Chinese participants showed a significant correlation between CysC levels, NYHA class, and diastolic dysfunction (E/A ratio) [31]. In a study on 480 participants with acute heart failure, Lassus et al. showed that together with NT-proBNP, CysC elevation is associated with increased mortality at 1 year (40.4% vs. 12.6% in patients with normal values for both biomarkers) [32].

Neutrophil gelatinase-associated lipocalin (NGAL) is a protein found in neutrophil granules. It is filtered by the glomerulus, but almost completely reabsorbed by the proximal convoluted tubule [23]. In a study on 2070 patients with chronic heart failure, Streng et al. found a significant increase in NGAL values in HFpEF compared to HFrEF patients (58.1 ug/gCr vs. 28.1 ug/gCr, $p < 0.001$) [33]. In acutely decompensated heart failure, NGAL showed positive correlation with the risk of developing AKI or death [34].

N-Acetyl-ß-D-Glucosaminidase (NAG) is a lysosomal protein. Its increased urinary levels are indicative of proximal tubular injury [23]. In another substudy of the GISSI-HF trial, Damman et al. showed statistical correlation between higher NAG values and a combined endpoint of death or heart failure hospitalization. This effect seems to be independent of eGFR [35]. However, in a more recent study on 319 consecutive patients with HFpEF and CKD who were hospitalized for acute heart failure, high NAG values were not found to be a relevant predictor of heart failure–related events (defined as progressive heart failure leading to hospitalization or resulting in death) [36].

Kidney injury molecule–1 (KIM-1) is a transmembrane glycoprotein that is secreted into urine in cases of ischemia or hypoxia [22]. Heart failure patients seem to have elevated levels of KIM-1 despite normal renal function. Similar to NAG, KIM-1 levels seem to rise with the decline in ejection fraction and the progression of NYHA class [23].

Imaging

As seen from pathophysiology, the two main pillars of cardio-renal dysfunction are congestion and decreased cardiac output. Echography is an essential tool for the assessment of both.

Cardiac output is measured by multiplying stroke volume with heart rate. Noninvasive echocardiographic estimation of stroke volume is the product of left ventricular outflow tract diameter and velocity time integral of the pulsed wave Doppler signal in the left ventricular outflow tract. Although this measurement is influenced by significant aortic regurgitation (in which case it cannot be done) and the variable shape of the outflow tract, it offers relatively accurate values [37].

Left ventricular ejection fraction has implications in both risk stratification and treatment. However, subclinical systolic dysfunction and heart failure can appear independent of left ventricular ejection fraction values. Global longitudinal strain (GLS) seems to be a more reliable indicator of systolic dysfunction in these patients. Although reduced GLS is associated with a lower eGFR and worse outcomes, currently there is scarce evidence that using GLS clinical scenarios improves outcomes [38].

Diastolic dysfunction seems to be associated with lower eGFR, and patients with CKD who have the criteria for diastolic dysfunction exhibit a faster decline in renal function [39]. The left atrium dilates in response to left ventricle pressure or volume overload. Prolonged high pressure in the left atrium will eventually lead to pulmonary hypertension and consequently right atrial hypertension with systemic venous congestion [38]. Left atrial enlargement is linked to worse cardiovascular and renal outcomes [40]. The role of left atrial strain rate in CKD patients has been evaluated in a few studies. A prospective trial on 243 patients with stage 3/4 CKD showed LASr as the only independent predictor of death from cardiovascular causes and MACE [41]. Kadappu et al. followed 60 patients with an eGFR between 30 and 59 mL/min/1.73 sm for 60 months. They showed that left atrial global strain, left atrial volume index, and left ventricular strain rate were independent predictors of MACE (defined as death, cardiovascular events, and end-stage renal failure) [42].

Being in continuity with the right atrium, the inferior vena cava (IVC) and its collapsibility are reliable indicators of right atrial pressures. A dilated IVC (over 21 mm) with an inspiratory collapse under 50% suggests high right atrial pressures and systemic congestion and seems to be associated with worse cardiovascular outcomes [38, 43].

When IVC measurements are not possible, the internal jugular vein (IJV) can be scanned. Moreover, nephrologists frequently perform vascular ultrasound when inserting dialysis catheters. Correct evaluation of the IJV should be performed with the patient lying down with the head elevated at a 45-degree angle, and the probe should be positioned as to not compress the vein. The ratio between IJV diameter during Valsalva maneuver and during rest is usually decreased (lower than 4) in congested patients [38].

Renal venous flow can also be used to assess congestion. The examination should use pulsed wave Doppler of the interlobar veins during an end-expiratory breath hold. In euvolemic patients, the normal renal venous flow is continuous [44]. However, as congestion worsens, the signal first becomes biphasic (with systolic and diastolic peaks), and then in severe congestion, it becomes monophasic (with only the diastolic peak) [38]. Puzzovivo et al. studied some 338 patients with stable CKD for a median follow-up of 38 months. They showed that both biphasic and monophasic patterns of the RVF are associated with a composite outcome consisting of death and/or heart transplant and/or heart failure hospitalization [45].

The pulsed wave Doppler exam of the hepatic venous waveform is also associated with higher right atrial pressures and poorer outcomes. While in normal subjects the systolic wave has a higher amplitude than the diastolic wave (S > D), in congested patients the ratio changes or even the reversal of the S wave can be seen [38].

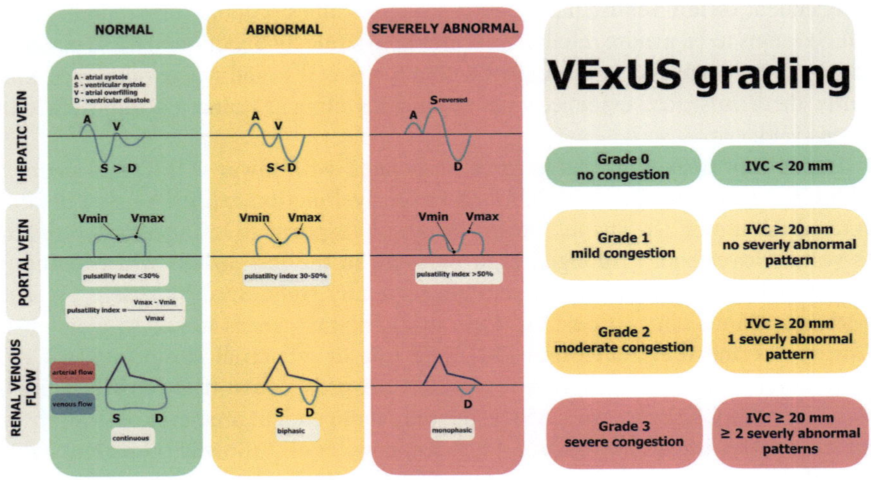

Fig. 2.3 Venous excess ultrasound grading system [38]

Portal vein flow is usually continuous. However, as congestion worsens, the waveform becomes more pulsatile. A portal flow pulsatility index (the difference between the maximal and minimal velocities divided by the maximal velocity) under 30% is considered to be normal, while values that exceed 50% are associated with high right atrial pressures and right ventricle dysfunction [38].

The venous excess ultrasound grading system (VExUS) (Fig. 2.3) includes evaluation of the inferior vena cava, renal venous flow, hepatic venous waveform, and portal vein flow. A score of 0 (IVC less than 20 mm) excludes the presence of congestion. Grade 1 congestion refers to the presence of a dilated IVC but with no severely abnormal patterns. Moderate congestion (grade 2) is defined as dilated IVC with one severely abnormal pattern, while grade 3 (severe congestion) mandates the presence of at least two severely abnormal patterns [38]. In a study on 290 patients with acute heart failure, the VExUS score improved prediction of in-hospital mortality (odds ratio, 8.03; 95% CI [2.25–28.61], $P = 0.001$) [46]. In a recent randomized clinical trial, 140 patients were randomized to decongestion with using either VExUS or usual clinical evaluation. The results show that there was no difference in the rates of improvement in kidney function; however; VExUS improved the odds of achieving decongestion [47].

Management

Due to the complex heart–kidney interaction, the management of cardio-renal syndrome is a challenge. An individualized approach involving both cardiologists and nephrologists is mandatory in order to improve outcomes.

As fluid retention is a major part of the pathophysiology of cardio-renal syndrome, diuretics represent an important pillar in the management of these patients. Congestion and increased central venous pressure had been associated with higher mortality, but paradoxically, decongestive treatment seems to offer no benefits on short- or long-term mortality [6, 48].

The European Society of Cardiology guidelines for the diagnosis and treatment of acute and chronic heart failure offer a practical algorithm on how decongestive therapies could be used. This approach implies doubling the dose every 12 hours until reaching adequate diuresis (over 100–150 mL/h) or sodium excretion (urinary Na over 50–70 mEq/L). If these criteria are not met with the maximum dose of loop-diuretic, the ESC suggests adding another diuretic [25].

A temporary increase in serum creatinine levels is to be expected in patients receiving diuretics. This increase is a marker of hemodynamic changes rather than of kidney injury [22]. Moreover, studies have shown that the combination of diuretics and RAAS inhibitors increases natriuresis and urinary output without significantly worsening renal function [49, 50].

Diuretic resistance is the main challenge in congestion management. It refers to the gradually diminishing effect of the drugs. Diuretics' pharmacological properties and the breaking phenomenon and tubular remodeling all play a role in the development of diuretic resistance. Because loop diuretics are protein bound, hypoalbuminemia decreases the availability of the drugs. Both CKD and HF influence diuretic response. CKD decreases the secretion of the drug into the tubular lumen, while uremic toxins can inhibit drug transport across tubular cells. Similarly, heart failure limits the maximal effect by increasing proximal tubular reabsorption of sodium (through RAAS activation) [6].

The breaking phenomenon is defined as the diminished diuretic efficiency noticed with each successive dose. Although the mechanism is unclear, it is thought that increased proximal and distal sodium reabsorption plays an important role [6].

In patients who do not respond to diuretic treatment, ultrafiltration (UF) can be used as a decongestive measure. However, clinical trials failed to show a clear benefit, especially in patients with HFpEF [22].

The Ultrafiltration Versus Intravenous Diuretics for Patients Hospitalized for Acute Decompensated Heart Failure (UNLOAD) trial randomized 200 patients to either ultrafiltration or intravenous diuretics. After 48 hours, both weight and fluid loss were significantly higher in the UF group. Although the study failed to show a benefit of ultrafiltration regarding dyspnea, the authors found significantly greater freedom from rehospitalization in the UF group [51].

In contrast, the CARESS-HF trial showed that UF was associated with a statistically significant increase in serum creatinine with no difference in weight loss [52]. It is important to mention that both trials included mainly patients with a reduced ejection fraction. More than 70% of the participants in UNLOAD trial had an LVEF under 40%, while the median ejection fraction was 30–35% in CARESS-HF.

Although angiotensin converting enzyme inhibitors (ACEi) and angiotensin II receptor blockers (ARB) have undisputable effects in the management of both HFrEF and CKD, their benefit in patients with preserved LVEF is not as well defined [22]. A retrospective analysis of 1340 patients with HFpEF and CKD showed the benefit of ACEi/ARBs on mortality in patients with an eGFR under 45 mL/min/1.73 m^2 [53]. In a post hoc analysis of the SOLVD (Study of Left Ventricular Dysfunction) trial, Khan et al. showed that enalapril reduced the risk for all-cause mortality in patients with a low eGFR and was not associated with a negative impact on kidney function [54].

Angiotensin receptor neprilysin inhibitors are a class I recommendation for the management of heart failure with preserved ejection fraction. However, in patients with preserved ejection fraction, the European Guidelines and AHA guidelines offer a 2b recommendation [25, 55, 56]. In a recent pooled analysis of two major ARNI trials (PARAGLIDE-HF and PARAGON-HF), sacubitril/valsartan significantly reduced the number of cardiovascular or renal events [57].

Mineralocorticoid receptor antagonists are one of the main pillars of HFrEF treatment. In CKD patients, they have been associated with a slower decline in kidney function [22]. Finerenone is a new nonsteroidal mineralocorticoid receptor antagonist that seems to offer cardio-renal protection. Two large randomized control studies (FIGARO-DKD and FIDELIO-DKD) showed significantly improved cardiovascular outcomes in patients with diabetic kidney disease [58, 59]. Hyperkaliemia is a common side effect that limits the usage of mineralocorticoid receptor antagonists. The dosage should be reduced or even stopped at a potassium level of over 5 mEq/L [22].

With multiple studies showing improvement of cardiovascular and renal outcomes, sodium-glucose transporter 2 inhibitors (SGLT2i) are recommended in both CKD regardless of the presence of diabetes or the LVEF [22, 56]. In a meta-analysis of four large studies on SGLT1 inhibitors (EMPA-REG OUTCOME, CANVAS, CREDENCE, and DECLARE-TIMI), Neuen et al. showed that this drug class reduced the risk of acute kidney injury, dialysis, transplantation, or death due to kidney disease [60].

In conclusion, the CRS represents the complex interaction between cardiac and renal dysfunction, creating significant challenges in both diagnosis and management. Being able to understand the distinct subtypes of CRS leads to a more targeted therapeutic approach, while emerging pharmacological agents, such as SGLT2 inhibitors, offer encouraging results in mitigating both cardiac and renal deterioration. Despite these advances, managing CRS requires a careful balance between optimizing cardiac output and preserving renal function, emphasizing the need for multidisciplinary care. Ongoing research into the pathophysiology and treatment of CRS will continue to influence clinical practice, with the goal of improving patient prognosis and their quality of life.

Cardio-Metabolic Syndrome

Background

Cardio-metabolic syndrome (CMS) encompasses a cluster of metabolic disturbances that collectively elevate the risk of cardiovascular disease (CVD) and type 2 diabetes mellitus (T2DM). This condition arises from a combination of metabolic dysregulation—including insulin resistance, hypertension, hyperlipidemia, and visceral obesity—alongside genetic, environmental, and behavioral factors. Key features of CMS include insulin resistance, abdominal obesity (reflected by a high body mass index and/or increased waist circumference), elevated serum triglycerides, reduced high-density protein (HDL) cholesterol levels, and hypertension. These interrelated abnormalities contribute to the development and progression of CVD and T2DM [61–63].

Recent epidemiological data demonstrate significant variations in CMS prevalence across North America and Europe, with notable association with demographic and socioeconomic factors. Analysis of the 2011–2018 National Health and Nutrition Examination Survey (NHANES) reveals a concerning increase in CMS prevalence in the United States from 37.6% to 41.8%, with elevated blood glucose levels identified as a primary contributing factor. These findings indicate a disproportionate disease burden among populations with lower educational attainment, highlighting the influence of socioeconomic determinants on metabolic health outcomes. In Canada, population studies estimate CMS prevalence at 41.9%. The data reveal significant gender disparities, with male subjects demonstrating higher susceptibility to CMS development, while female subjects exhibit greater association with material deprivation indicators. The Mexican population presents a distinct epidemiological pattern, with prevalence rates of 28.9% in male and 44.4% in female participants, characterized by particularly high rates of abdominal obesity and dyslipidemia among women [64].

European cohort studies provide additional insights into diagnostic and demographic variations. The MORGAM Project's analysis of 26 cohorts demonstrates substantial differences in prevalence rates depending on diagnostic criteria, the National Cholesterol Education Program Adult Treatment Panel III (NCEP ATP III) classification yielding higher estimates (19.9% male, 32.1% female) compared to the International Diabetes Federation (IDF) standards (9.7% male, 29.5% female) [64].

Asia's CMS epidemic reveals striking regional variations. Japan shows an 11.9–17.9% prevalence in men depending on diagnostic criteria. South Korea's overall rate rose from 27% to 33% (2001–2020), with men's prevalence jumping to 40% while women's slightly declined—a paradox tied to changing diets and activity levels. China reports a 19.4% overall prevalence, but men are twice as affected as women (31% vs. 17%). A meta-analysis indicates a CMS prevalence of 32.4% across 29 African nations, demonstrating significant regional heterogeneity. Notably, HIV-positive populations exhibit distinct metabolic profiles, with a 21%

prevalence characterized by dyslipidemia (47.3% with low HDL-cholesterol) rather than conventional obesity patterns [64].

Over the past 20 years, there has been significant debate regarding the most accurate terminology to describe the cardiovascular and metabolic risks associated with metabolic syndrome. In 1988, Reaven first described "Syndrome X," linking insulin resistance, hypertension, dyslipidemia, and obesity to increased cardiovascular risk. The World Health Organization (WHO) later introduced "metabolic syndrome," sparking debate about whether insulin resistance or obesity was a primary driver. Subsequent definitions emphasized different aspects: By the early 2000s, the NCEP ATP III guidelines highlighted abdominal obesity and inflammation, while the European Group for the Study of Insulin Resistance (EGIR) focused on insulin resistance, renaming it "insulin resistance syndrome." Over time, alternative terms emerged, including "dysmetabolic syndrome" and "cardio-metabolic syndrome," with some experts emphasizing visceral fat accumulation. Medical coding has also evolved, transitioning from "dysmetabolic syndrome X" to the current "metabolic syndrome" (Classification of Diseases—10) [65–67].

This syndrome represents a chronic and progressive condition marked by interconnected metabolic abnormalities that collectively increase the risk of atherosclerotic cardiovascular disease (ASCVD) and T2DM. Rather than simply being a collection of separate risk factors, it contributes to a distinct clinical entity with its own pathophysiology. Research confirms that the syndrome independently predicts cardiovascular risk and mortality even after accounting for its individual components, with one analysis showing a 54% increased risk of ASCVD or death [67, 68]. The diagnostic framework for CMS focuses on core metabolic disturbances while recognizing that additional biomarkers may contribute to residual cardiovascular risk. This comprehensive view underscores that CMS represents more than just the sum of its parts, reflecting complex underlying metabolic dysfunction with significant clinical implications [67].

The exact mechanisms behind the development of CMS remain unclear, but multiorgan insulin resistance—a hallmark of the condition—is believed to play a key role. Insulin resistance not only increases the risk of T2DM but also contributes to hypertension by promoting vasoconstriction and enhancing sodium reabsorption in the kidneys. A major driver of insulin resistance is dysfunctional adipose tissue metabolism, particularly abnormal fatty acid release and altered adipokine signaling. When excess fatty acids enter the bloodstream, they interfere with insulin's ability to stimulate glucose uptake in muscles and inhibit glucose production in the liver. Additionally, chronic low-grade inflammation, triggered by cytokine secretion from adipocytes and adipose tissue macrophages, further exacerbates insulin resistance. Elevated free fatty acids also impact lipid metabolism by stimulating the liver to produce more very low-density lipoprotein (VLDL), triglycerides, contributing to dyslipidemia—a common feature of CMS. Together, these metabolic disruptions create a vicious cycle that worsens insulin resistance and accelerates cardiovascular and metabolic disease progression [61, 69].

Cardio-Metabolic Syndrome: Definitions and Clinical Components

Cardio-metabolic syndrome encompasses insulin resistance, hypertension, dyslipidemia, and visceral adiposity, influenced by genetic predisposition, environmental factors, and lifestyle behaviors. Among various diagnostic criteria, the National Cholesterol Education Program Adult Treatment Panel III (NCEP ATP III) guidelines remain the most clinically utilized:

1. *NCEP ATP III, 2005*—diagnosis requires =3 of the following:
   - Fasting plasma glucose =100 mg/dL (or treated hyperglycemia)
   - Waist circumference = 102 cm (men) or 88 cm (women)
   - HDL cholesterol <40 mg/dL (men) or < 50 mg/dL (women) (or treated)
   - Triglycerides =150 mg/dL (or treated)
   - Blood pressure = 130/85 mmHg (or treated hypertension) [70].
2. *IDF (International Diabetes Federation), 2005*—mandatory criteria: Ethnicity-specific central obesity (e.g., European men =94 cm, women =80 cm; South Asian men =90 cm, women =80 cm), plus =2 of the following:
   - Fasting plasma glucose =100 mg/dL (or diagnosed diabetes)
   - HDL cholesterol <40 mg/dL (men) or < 50 mg/dL (women) (or treated)
   - Triglycerides =150 mg/dL (or treated)
   - Blood pressure: = 130/85 mmHg (or treated) [71]
3. *EGIR, 1999*—required criteria: Insulin resistance (top 25% of fasting insulin levels) or impaired fasting glucose (110–125 mg/dL), plus =2 of the following:
   - Obesity: Waist circumference = 94 cm (men) or = 80 cm (women)
   - HDL cholesterol <40 mg/dL
   - Triglycerides =180 mg/dL (or treated)
   - Blood pressure = 140/90 mmHg (or treated) [69]
4. *American Association of Clinical Endocrinology (AACE, 2003, Updated 2020)*—focuses more on clinical judgment based on risk factors rather than strict cutoffs. Key considerations:
   - Overweight/obesity patterns: body mass index (BMI) = 25 kg/m2)
   - Dysglycemia (fasting glucose 110–126 mg/dL, 2-hour post 75 g glucose test >140 mg/dL)
   - Hypertension (blood pressure = 130/85 mmHg or antihypertensive therapy)
   - Dyslipidemia (triglycerides =150 mg/dL, HDL cholesterol <40 mg/dL in men or < 50 mg/dL in women)
   - Family history of metabolic disease
   - Additional risk factors (e.g., polycystic ovary syndrome, metabolic-associated fatty liver disease, CVD history) [72]

Obesity and Metabolic Dysregulation

Obesity, defined by a BMI = 30 kg/m^2, reflects excessive adipose tissue accumulation. Current clinical guidelines of the American Association of Endocrinology emphasize additional anthropometric measures, including waist circumference and waist-to-heigh ratio, for comprehensive assessment. Notably, ethnic variations exist in fat distribution patterns—the Asian population demonstrates heightened visceral adiposity at lower BMI compared to other ethnic groups. Global epidemiological data reveal alarming prevalence rates, with 39% of adults overweight and 13% meeting obesity criteria as of 2016 [63, 73].

The metabolic consequences of obesity extend beyond simple weight metrics. Epicardial adipose tissue, a visceral fat depot surrounding cardiac structures, has emerged as a significant contributor to cardiovascular pathology. EAT secretes pro-inflammatory mediators, including cytokines and chemokines, promoting coronary artery disease through local and systemic effects. Furthermore, EAT-derived free fatty acids disrupt cardiac electrophysiology, increasing arrhythmia risk while contributing to myocardial fibrosis and ventricular remodeling [74, 75].

Dyslipidemia and Atherogenic Risk

Characterized by elevated total cholesterol, LDL-cholesterol, or triglycerides, dyslipidemia affects approximately 12% of US adults with total cholesterol >240 mg/dL, while 17% demonstrate suboptimal HDL levels (< 40 mg/dL). Statins remain first-line therapy, offering both lipid-lowering benefits and pleiotropic anti-inflammatory effects that reduce cardiovascular events [74, 76].

Hypertension Pathophysiology and Management

Affecting over one billion adults globally, hypertension (defined as BP = 130/80 mmHg) arises from multifactorial mechanisms, including vascular stiffness, sodium retention, and neurohormonal dysregulation. Current American College of Cardiology/American Heart Association (ACC/AHA) 2017 guidelines recommend pharmacologic intervention at this threshold, with therapeutic options including RAAS inhibitors, calcium channel blockers, and thiazide diuretics tailored to individual patient profiles [63].

Insulin Resistance

Most individuals with CMS exhibit insulin resistance, which demonstrates strong correlations with other metabolic abnormalities and CVD risk. While these associations led to the alternative designation "insulin resistance syndrome," the precise mechanisms linking insulin resistance to cardiovascular risk factors remain incompletely understood. This uncertainty prompted ATP III to categorize insulin resistance as an emerging risk factor rather than a definitive diagnostic criterion. Chronic insulin resistance often progresses to impaired glucose tolerance, and when advancing to overt diabetes, hyperglycemia becomes an established independent cardiovascular risk factor [77].

Chronic Inflammation

A state of low-grade systemic inflammation, typically evidenced by elevated C-reactive protein (CRP) levels, frequently accompanies CMS. Adipose tissue dysfunction plays a central role in this process, as hypertrophied adipocytes secrete proinflammatory cytokines that stimulate hepatic CRP production. This inflammatory state contributes to endothelial dysfunction and atherogenesis [77].

Prothrombotic State

CMS commonly presents with coagulation abnormalities, particularly increased levels of plasminogen activator inhibitor-1 (PAI-1) and fibrinogen. These hemostatic alterations create a thrombogenic environment that predisposes to vascular events. Notably, fibrinogen shares with CRP the characteristic of being an acute-phase reactant, suggesting common inflammatory pathways underlying both the prothrombotic and proinflammatory states observed in CMS [77].

From Cardio-Renal Syndrome and Cardio-Metabolic Syndrome to Cardio-Kidney-Metabolic Syndrome

The global population is aging rapidly, demanding stronger efforts in disease prevention and treatment. CVD remains the world's leading cause of death. While mortality has declined in older adults, rates among younger populations remain stagnant, emphasizing the urgent need for early prevention through education, healthier lifestyles, and risk factor reduction. Obesity, T2DM, CVD, and CKD pose significant health challenges worldwide. From 1990 to 2019, cases of CVD and CKD nearly doubled, rising from 271 million to 523 million. Once treated as distinct disorders, these diseases are now recognized as interconnected, sharing common pathways that drive their progression. Cardio-renal syndrome highlights the bidirectional link between heart and kidney function, often leading to organ failure. Similarly, CMS increases the risk of CVD and T2DM. CMS is also tied to CKD, creating a vicious cycle where dysfunction in one system worsens another [78, 79].

This complex interplay led the American Heart Association (AHA) to define cardiovascular-kidney-metabolic (CKM) syndrome in 2023. CKM syndrome stems from dysfunctional fat accumulation and requires a staged approach for prevention and management. Poor CKM health drives morbidity and early mortality, making integrated intervention crucial. CKM syndrome affects nearly every major organ system, contributing to: kidney failure, cognitive decline, metabolic dysfunction-associated steatotic liver disease (MASLD), obstructive sleep apnea, and increased cancer risk. However, its most significant impact lies in the disproportionate burden of CVD, including coronary artery disease, stroke, heart failure, peripheral artery disease, and arrhythmias. The rising prevalence of obesity and diabetes has intensified CKM-related health disparities [79–81].

CKM syndrome imposes staggering healthcare costs, with obesity-related conditions accounting for half a trillion dollars annually in direct medical expenses and $1.2 trillion in lost productivity. More critically, it drastically reduces life expectancy:

1. Severe obesity (BMI = 40 kg/m2) shortens median survival by 8–10 years.
2. Diabetes reduces lifespan by 13–14 years compared to nondiabetic individuals.
3. Advanced CKD (eGFR between 15 and 29 mL/min/1.73 m2) is associated with a > 20-year decrease in life expectancy, with CVD being a leading cause of death.
4. The synergistic effects of diabetes and CKD elevate 10-year mortality to 31.3%, far exceeding the risks of either condition alone [78].

Establishing a clear framework for identifying patients with or at risk for CKM syndrome represents a critical foundation for effective diagnosis and management. Unlike a disease diagnosis, CKM syndrome represents a constellation of interrelated signs and symptoms stemming from shared pathophysiological mechanisms. This conceptualization recognizes the intricate relationship between various contributing elements and the progressive nature of CKM-related conditions, ranging from initial metabolic disturbance to end-stage organ impairment. This encompasses:

1. At-risk individuals with metabolic disorders and/or CKD but without established CVD
2. Patients with existing CVD exacerbated by metabolic and/or kidney dysfunction [79, 80]

For public health communication purposes, a simplified conceptualization was proposed: CKM syndrome is characterized by the interconnected relationship between CVD, renal dysfunction, metabolic disorders, and adiposity, through which adverse health outcomes are collectively exacerbated. This tiered definitional approach effectively balances the need for clinical accuracy with public health messaging requirements, while highlighting both the pathophysiological complexity of this multisystem disorder and the importance of addressing modifiable social determinants of health [79, 80].

Kidney function and cardiovascular health are closely linked, as those with reduced kidney function face a higher risk of CVD, with the risk increasing as kidney impairment worsens. Because of this relationship, predicting a decline in kidney function or kidney failure has significant implications for cardiovascular health.

Additionally, certain cardiovascular medications can help slow kidney function decline, highlighting the importance of risk-based strategies to protect both kidney and heart health. Existing risk prediction models for kidney function decline can guide clinical decisions and improve patient selection for future prevention trials, particularly for individuals at different stages of CKM syndrome [78, 81, 82].

Pathophysiology of Cardiovascular-Kidney-Metabolic Syndrome

The pathophysiology of CKM syndrome involves a complex interplay among cardiovascular, renal, and metabolic dysfunctions. A principal contributor to this pathophysiology is dysfunctional adipose tissue, which serves as an endocrine organ that drives metabolic perturbations, including hypertension, dyslipidemia (particularly hypertriglyceridemia), insulin resistance, and CKD. The chronic accumulation of these metabolic and hemodynamic disturbances promotes the development of subclinical coronary atherosclerosis, detectable via coronary artery calcification and early echocardiographic or functional imaging abnormalities. Parallel to these cardiovascular changes, a progressive decline in renal function occurs, further amplifying the risk of overt cardiovascular events, end-stage renal disease, and associated morbidity and mortality. The bidirectional interplay between metabolic dysfunction, cardiovascular pathology, and renal impairment defines the progressive nature of CKM syndrome [78–80].

The heart and kidneys engage in a bidirectional pathological relationship, perpetuating a self-sustaining cycle of dysfunction through hemodynamic alterations and maladaptive neurohormonal activation. A key mediator of this process is the overactivation of mineralocorticoid receptors, which upregulates NADPH oxidase, proinflammatory cytokines, and fibrotic mediators, driving progressive tissue injury in both organs. Renal manifestations include glomerular damage, proteinuria, tubular dysfunction, and diminished renal perfusion due to impaired microcirculation. Concurrently, the cardiovascular system exhibits deleterious remodeling, characterized by endothelial dysfunction, increased arterial stiffness, myocardial hypertrophy, ventricular fibrosis, and reduced coronary flow, ultimately predisposing to ischemic injury [79, 80].

Inflammation is the body's defense mechanism against injury or disease, where the immune system identifies and reacts to harmful stimuli to restore balance. Chronic inflammation can contribute to various disorders. Persistent inflammation is closely linked to cardiovascular and metabolic diseases, as well as CKD, often alongside oxidative stress. It also promotes arterial stiffness and serves as an independent risk factor for cardiovascular conditions. Chronic inflammation and oxidative stress can create a pro-fibrotic, proinflammatory state, disrupting insulin signaling and endothelial function [78, 81, 82]. Key mechanisms include:

- Endoplasmic reticulum stress, linked to cardiomyocyte apoptosis, atherosclerosis, and diabetic kidney disease progression.
- Redox imbalance, where excessive reactive oxygen species and reactive nitrogen species impair smooth muscle relaxation, platelet function, and metabolic signaling.

- Adipose tissue dysfunction, particularly perivascular and perirenal fat deposits, which secrete proinflammatory cytokines, exacerbating vascular and renal damage. Perivascular and perirenal adipose tissue can affect cardiovascular and renal structures, serving as early indicators of metabolic-induced cardio-renal dysfunction. Perivascular adipose tissue alters immune cell activity and proinflammatory cytokine release, potentially leading to vascular damage, systemic inflammation, and RAAS activation [78, 81, 82].

A chronic, low-grade inflammatory state is associated with aging, which increases susceptibility to CVD, CKD, and CMS. This condition is tied to heightened activity of the RAAS, altered vascular smooth muscle tone, and oxidative stress, all of which contribute to arterial inflammation and organ damage. CMS patients often exhibit increased left ventricular stiffness, a consequence of vascular aging and systemic inflammation [82]. Beyond systemic effects, inflammation also impacts surrounding tissues and organs. For instance, adipose tissue dysfunction plays a key role in CKM development. Perivascular and perirenal adipose tissue can affect cardiovascular and renal structures, serving as early indicators of metabolic-induced cardio-renal dysfunction. Furthermore, many CKM risk factors stem from abnormal adipose tissue accumulation or dysfunction [82].

Hyperinsulinemia exacerbates adipose tissue inflammation and stimulates RAAS, resulting in vasoconstriction. Inflammation also disrupts insulin signaling, promoting insulin resistance, which impairs endothelial function and contributes to cardiovascular stiffness. Additionally, insulin resistance is implicated in obesity-related heart failure [78, 82].

RAAS, a hormonal system regulating blood pressure, can be triggered by inflammatory cytokines, hyperinsulinemia, leptin-mediated sympathetic nervous system activation, and chronic inflammation. Overactivation of RAAS leads to hypertension, vascular and cardiac hypertrophy, arterial stiffness, and impaired cardiac function. RAAS also modulates autophagy, a critical process for cellular homeostasis, with dysregulation linked to CRS. Inflammation-induced endothelial dysfunction can further disrupt RAAS activity [78, 82].

Cardiovascular-Kidney-Metabolic Syndrome: Risk Stratification and Therapeutic Implications

The AHA's 2023 presidential advisory established a novel framework for CKM syndrome, recognizing the complex interplay between cardiovascular, metabolic, and kidney diseases. This classification system identifies four progressive stages (0–4), each requiring distinct management strategies:

- Stage 0 represents individuals without current risk factors, focusing on primordial prevention through "Life's Essential 8"—a set of evidence-based lifestyle measures, including physical activity, smoking cessation, good sleep habits, and metabolic health optimization.

- Stage 1 includes patients with early metabolic derangements (abdominal obesity, prediabetes). Management emphasizes intensive lifestyle modification to prevent disease progression.
- Stage 2 encompasses established metabolic disease (T2DM, hypertension, dyslipidemia) or early kidney dysfunction, requiring aggressive risk factor control to avert cardiovascular and renal complications.
- Stage 3 involves subclinical CVD in high-risk patients.
- Stage 4 is characterized by symptomatic cardiovascular disease, with substages accounting for kidney failure presence [79, 80].

The advisory identifies risk-enhancing factors:

- Demographic: South Asian ancestry, low socioeconomic status.
- Genetic: Variants in metabolic pathways (ENPP1, AP2A2) showing ethnic-specific associations.
- Clinical: Sleep disorders, mental health conditions, inflammatory diseases.
- Sex-specific: Adverse pregnancy outcomes, polycystic ovary syndrome, premature menopause [78].

The complex interplay between metabolic, cardiovascular, and renal health demands innovative prevention approaches. Three key pillars emerge from current evidence that offer the most promising path forward in addressing the growing burden of CKM syndrome:

1. Standardized screening protocols for early detection. Regular assessment of metabolic parameters—including BMI, blood glucose, blood pressure, and lipid profiles—should be complemented by routine kidney function evaluation, particularly in high-risk groups. Notably, universal glycemic screening regardless of body weight promotes health equity in diabetes prevention [78–80].
2. Emerging research underscores the importance of early-life interventions. The developmental origins of CKM risk highlight promising opportunities for prevention, though optimal strategies for maternal and pediatric interventions require further investigation. This life-course perspective is particularly relevant given the rising prevalence of childhood metabolic disorders [78–80].
3. Addressing social determinants of health represents an underutilized yet critical component of prevention. Preliminary evidence suggests that integrating social needs assessment with clinical care may enhance outcomes, though more robust studies are needed to quantify these benefits [78–80].

The complex pathophysiology of CKM syndrome necessitates a paradigm shift toward integrated multidisciplinary care models. These collaborative frameworks synergize expertise across cardiology, nephrology, endocrinology, and health professions to optimize patient outcomes through comprehensive therapeutic strategies. Successful implementation requires establishment of standardized protocols incorporating several critical components: unified electronic health record systems facilitating seamless information exchange, structured interdisciplinary case conferences for complex patient management, and evidence-based treatment algorithms that incorporate novel pharmacotherapies with pleiotropic benefits. Of particular importance are sodium-glucose co-transporter 2 inhibitors and glucagon-like peptide-1 receptor agonists, which demonstrate robust cardio-renal protection while simultaneously addressing metabolic dysfunction [79–81].

By addressing the shared mechanisms underlying cardiovascular, renal, and metabolic dysfunction, multidisciplinary approaches have the potential to significantly reduce the substantial morbidity, mortality, and economic burden with this increasingly prevalent syndrome.

Learning Objectives

- Understanding the maladaptive interplay between the heart and the kidneys that ultimately leads to cardiorenal syndrome
- Understanding the complex pathophysiological mechanisms that form the basis of CMS
- Recognizing the similarities between cardio-renal and cardio-metabolic syndromes
- Explaining the way two distinct pathological entities converged into cardiovascular-kidney metabolic syndrome

Recognizing the common management options with emphasis on the multidisciplinary approach

Key Reading

- *Cardio-renal syndrome* refers to the interplay between the heart and the kidneys where the dysfunction of one system leads to the dysfunction of the other. This maladaptive relationship is influenced by numerous factors, such as hemodynamic and metabolic alterations, neurohormonal activation, and the proinflammatory status that is present in this group of patients.
- *Cardio-metabolic syndrome* encompasses a cluster of metabolic disturbances that collectively elevate the risk of cardiovascular disease and type 2 diabetes mellitus, including insulin resistance, abdominal obesity (high body mass index and/or increased waist circumference), elevated serum triglycerides, reduced HDL-cholesterol levels, and hypertension.
- *Cardiovascular-kidney-metabolic syndrome* is characterized by the interconnected relationship between cardiovascular disease, renal dysfunction, metabolic disorders, and adiposity, through which adverse health outcomes are collectively exacerbated.
- *Key pathophysiological mechanisms* involved in CKM syndrome development include dysfunctional adipose tissue, oxidative stress, chronic inflammation, hyperinsulinemia, and RAAS activation.

References

1. Budge E, Budge E. The Egyptian book of the dead [Internet]. 1967 [cited 2025 Apr 14]. Available from: https://zoraweb.com/files/zw/books/Egyptian-Book-of-the-Dead%20.pdf
2. Salam AM, Carr AS. From "heart and reins" to clinical syndromes: origin and evolution of cardio-renal disease. Heart Views [Internet]. 2021 [cited 2025 Apr 14];22(1):80. Available from: https://pmc.ncbi.nlm.nih.gov/articles/PMC8254159/. https://doi.org/10.4103/HEARTVIEWS.HEARTVIEWS_210_20
3. Stengel A. Cardiorenal disease: the clinical determination of cardiovascular and renal responsibility, respectively, in its disturbances. JAMA [Internet]. 1914 [cited 2025 Apr 14];LXIII(17):1463–1469. Available from: https://jamanetwork.com/journals/jama/fullarticle/437695. https://doi.org/10.1001/jama.1914.02570170031008.
4. Cardio-renal connections in heart failure and cardiovascular disease. NHLBI, NIH. [cited 2025 Apr 15]; Available from: https://www.nhlbi.nih.gov/events/2004/cardio-renal-connections-heart-failure-and-cardiovascular-disease
5. Ronco C, McCullough P, Anker SD, Anand I, Aspromonte N, Bagshaw SM, et al. Cardio-renal syndromes: report from the consensus conference of the Acute Dialysis Quality Initiative. Eur Heart J [Internet]. 2009 [cited 2025 Apr 15];31(6):703. Available from: https://pmc.ncbi.nlm.nih.gov/articles/PMC2838681/. https://doi.org/10.1093/eurheartj/ehp507.
6. Rangaswami J, Bhalla V, Blair JEA, Chang TI, Costa S, Lentine KL, et al. Cardiorenal syndrome: classification, pathophysiology, diagnosis, and treatment strategies: a scientific statement from the American Heart Association. Circulation [Internet]. 2019 [cited 2025 Apr 23];139(16):E840–E878. Available from: https://www.ahajournals.org/doi/10.1161/CIR.0000000000000664. https://doi.org/10.1161/cir.0000000000000664.
7. Di Lullo L, Bellasi A, Barbera V, Russo D, Russo L, Di Iorio B, et al. Pathophysiology of the cardio-renal syndromes types 1–5: an uptodate. Indian Heart J. 2017;69(2):255–65. https://doi.org/10.1016/j.ihj.2017.01.005.
8. Prastaro M, Nardi E, Paolillo S, Santoro C, Parlati ALM, Gargiulo P, et al. Cardiorenal syndrome: Pathophysiology as a key to the therapeutic approach in an under-diagnosed disease. J Clin Ultrasound [Internet]. 2022 Oct 1 [cited 2025 Apr 23];50(8):1110–1124. Available from: https://onlinelibrary.wiley.com/doi/full/10.1002/jcu.23265. https://doi.org/10.1002/jcu.23265.
9. Fountain JH, Kaur J, Lappin SL. Physiology, renin angiotensin system. StatPearls [Internet]. 2023. [cited 2025 May 1]; Available from: https://www.ncbi.nlm.nih.gov/books/NBK470410/
10. Thind GS, Loehrke M, Wilt JL. Acute cardiorenal syndrome: Mechanisms and clinical implications. Cleve Clin J Med [Internet]. 2018 [cited 2025 Apr 23];85(3):231–239. Available from: https://www.ccjm.org/content/85/3/231. https://doi.org/10.3949/ccjm.85a.17019.
11. Hanberg JS, Sury K, Perry Wilson F, Brisco MA, Ahmad T, Ter Maaten JM, et al. Reduced cardiac index is not the dominant driver of renal dysfunction in heart failure. J Am Coll Cardiol [Internet]. 2016 [cited 2025 Apr 23];67(19):2199–2208. Available from: https://www.jacc.org/doi/10.1016/j.jacc.2016.02.058. doi: https://doi.org/10.1016/j.jacc.2016.02.058.
12. Nohria A, Hasselblad V, Stebbins A, Pauly DF, Fonarow GC, Shah M, et al. Cardiorenal interactions: insights from the ESCAPE trial. J Am Coll Cardiol. 2008;51(13):1268–74. https://doi.org/10.1016/j.jacc.2007.08.072.
13. Mullens W, Abrahams Z, Francis GS, Sokos G, Taylor DO, Starling RC, et al. Importance of venous congestion for worsening of renal function in advanced decompensated heart failure. J Am Coll Cardiol [Internet]. 2009 [cited 2025 May 1];53(7):589–596. Available from: https://www.jacc.org/doi/10.1016/j.jacc.2008.05.068. doi: https://doi.org/10.1016/j.jacc.2008.05.068.
14. Mullens W, Abrahams Z, Skouri HN, Francis GS, Taylor DO, Starling RC, et al. Elevated intra-abdominal pressure in acute decompensated heart failure: a potential contributor to worsening renal function? J Am Coll Cardiol [Internet]. 2008 [cited 2025 May 1];51(3):300–306. Available from: https://www.jacc.org/doi/10.1016/j.jacc.2007.09.043. https://doi.org/10.1016/j.jacc.2007.09.043.

15. Kadatane SP, Satariano M, Massey M, Mongan K, Raina R. The role of inflammation in CKD. Cells [Internet]. 2023 [cited 2025 May 1];12(12):1581. Available from: https://pmc.ncbi.nlm.nih.gov/articles/PMC10296717/. https://doi.org/10.3390/cells12121581.
16. Virzì GM, Clementi A, De Cal M, Brocca A, Day S, Pastori S, et al. Oxidative stress: dual pathway induction in cardiorenal syndrome type 1 pathogenesis. Oxid Med Cell Longev [Internet]. 2015 [cited 2025 May 1];2015(1):391790. Available from: https://onlinelibrary.wiley.com/doi/full/10.1155/2015/391790. doi: https://doi.org/10.1155/2015/391790.
17. Faul C, Amaral AP, Oskouei B, Hu MC, Sloan A, Isakova T, et al. FGF23 induces left ventricular hypertrophy. J Clin Invest [Internet]. 2011 [cited 2025 May 1];121(11):4393. Available from: https://pmc.ncbi.nlm.nih.gov/articles/PMC3204831/. https://doi.org/10.1172/jci46122.
18. Yu AS, Pak KJ, Zhou H, Shaw SF, Shi J, Broder BI, et al. All-cause and cardiovascular-related mortality in ckd patients with and without heart failure: a population-based cohort study in Kaiser Permanente Southern California. Kidney Med [Internet]. 2023 [cited 2025 May 2];5(5):100624. Available from: https://pmc.ncbi.nlm.nih.gov/articles/PMC10151415/. https://doi.org/10.1016/j.xkme.2023.100624.
19. Bansal N, Zelnick L, Go A, Anderson A, Christenson R, Deo R, et al. Cardiac biomarkers and risk of incident heart failure in CKD: The CRIC (Chronic Renal Insufficiency Cohort) Study. J Am Heart Assoc [Internet] 2019 [cited 2025 May 2];8(21). Available from: https://www.ahajournals.org/doi/10.1161/JAHA.119.012336. https://doi.org/10.1161/jaha.119.012336.
20. Anker SD, Butler J, Filippatos G, Ferreira JP, Bocchi E, Böhm M, et al. Empagliflozin in heart failure with a preserved ejection fraction. N Engl J Med [Internet] 2021 [cited 2025 May 2];385(16):1451–1461. Available from: https://www.nejm.org/doi/full/10.1056/NEJMoa2107038. https://doi.org/10.1056/nejmoa2107038.
21. Heywood JT, Fonarow GC, Costanzo MR, Mathur VS, Wigneswaran JR, Wynne J. High prevalence of renal dysfunction and its impact on outcome in 118,465 patients hospitalized with acute decompensated heart failure: a report from the ADHERE database. J Card Fail [Internet] 2007 [cited 2025 May 2];13(6):422–430. Available from: https://onlinejcf.com/action/showFullText?pii=S1071916407001030. https://doi.org/10.1016/j.cardfail.2007.03.011.
22. Khandait H, Sodhi SS, Khandekar N, Bhattad VB. Cardiorenal syndrome in heart failure with preserved ejection fraction: insights into pathophysiology and recent advances. Cardiorenal Med [Internet]. 2025 [cited 2025 May 4];15(1):41–60. Available from: https://doi.org/10.1159/000542633.
23. Brisco MA, Testani JM. Novel renal biomarkers to assess cardiorenal syndrome. Curr Heart Fail Rep [Internet]. 2014 [cited 2025 May 4];11(4):485–99. Available from: https://link.springer.com/article/10.1007/s11897-014-0226-4. https://doi.org/10.1007/s11897-014-0226-4.
24. Byrne RA, Rossello X, Coughlan JJ, Barbato E, Berry C, Chieffo A, et al. 2023 ESC Guidelines for the management of acute coronary syndromes: developed by the task force on the management of acute coronary syndromes of the European Society of Cardiology (ESC). Eur Heart J [Internet]. 2023 [cited 2025 May 4];44(38):3720–826. Available from:. https://doi.org/10.1093/eurheartj/ehad191.
25. McDonagh TA, Metra M, Adamo M, Baumbach A, Böhm M, Burri H, et al. 2021 ESC Guidelines for the diagnosis and treatment of acute and chronic heart failure: Developed by the Task Force for the diagnosis and treatment of acute and chronic heart failure of the European Society of Cardiology (ESC) With the special contribution of the Heart Failure Association (HFA) of the ESC. Eur Heart J [Internet] 2021 [cited 2025 May 4];42(36):3599–3726. Available from: https://doi.org/10.1093/eurheartj/ehab368
26. Banerjee D, Perrett C, Banerjee A. Troponins, acute coronary syndrome and renal disease: from AKI through end-stage kidney disease. Eur Cardiol Rev [Internet]. 2019 [cited 2025 May 4];14(3):187. Available from: https://pmc.ncbi.nlm.nih.gov/articles/PMC6950405/. https://doi.org/10.15420/ecr.2019.28.2
27. Miller-Hodges E, Anand A, Shah ASV, Chapman AR, Gallacher P, Lee KK, et al. High-sensitivity cardiac troponin and the risk stratification of patients with renal impairment presenting with suspected acute coronary syndrome. Circulation [Internet]. 2018 [cited 2025 May

4];137(5):425–435. Available from: https://pmc.ncbi.nlm.nih.gov/articles/PMC5793996/. https://doi.org/10.1161/circulationaha.117.030320.
28. Jackson CE, Solomon SD, Gerstein HC, Zetterstrand S, Olofsson B, Michelson EL, et al. Albuminuria in chronic heart failure: prevalence and prognostic importance. Lancet [Internet] 2009 [cited 2025 May 4];374(9689):543–550. Available from: https://www.thelancet.com/action/showFullText?pii=S0140673609613787. https://doi.org/10.1016/s0140-6736(09)61378-7.
29. Masson S, Latini R, Milani V, Moretti L, Rossi MG, Carbonieri E, et al. Prevalence and prognostic value of elevated urinary albumin excretion in patients with chronic heart failure data from the GISSI-heart failure trial. Circ Heart Fail [Internet] 2010 [cited 2025 May 4];3(1):65–72. Available from: https://www.ahajournals.org/doi/10.1161/CIRCHEARTFAILURE.109.881805. https://doi.org/10.1161/circheartfailure.109.881805.
30. Brouwers FP, De Boer RA, Van Der Harst P, Voors AA, Gansevoort RT, Bakker SJ, et al. Incidence and epidemiology of new onset heart failure with preserved vs. reduced ejection fraction in a community-based cohort: 11-year follow-up of PREVEND. Eur Heart J [Internet] 2013 [cited 2025 May 4];34(19):1424–1431. Available from: https://pubmed.ncbi.nlm.nih.gov/23470495/. https://doi.org/10.1093/eurheartj/eht066.
31. Xu CC, Fu GX, Liu QQ, Zhong Y. Association between cystatin C and heart failure with preserved ejection fraction in elderly Chinese patients. Z Gerontol Geriatr [Internet] 2018 [cited 2025 May 4];51(1):92–97. Available from: https://pubmed.ncbi.nlm.nih.gov/27206415/. https://doi.org/10.1007/s00391-016-1058-5.
32. Lassus J, Harjola VP, Sund R, Siirilä-Waris K, Melin J, Peuhkurinen K, et al. Prognostic value of cystatin C in acute heart failure in relation to other markers of renal function and NT-proBNP. Eur Heart J [Internet]. 2007 [cited 2025 May 4];28(15):1841–1847. Available from: https://pubmed.ncbi.nlm.nih.gov/17289743/. https://doi.org/10.1093/eurheartj/ehl507.
33. Streng KW, Hillege HL, ter Maaten JM, van Veldhuisen DJ, Dickstein K, Samani NJ, et al. Urinary marker profiles in heart failure with reduced versus preserved ejection fraction. J Cardiovasc Transl Res [Internet]. 2023 [cited 2025 May 4];17(1):3. Available from: https://pmc.ncbi.nlm.nih.gov/articles/PMC10896953/. https://doi.org/10.1007/s12265-023-10356-y.
34. Macdonald S, Arendts G, Nagree Y, Xu XF. Neutrophil Gelatinase-Associated Lipocalin (NGAL) predicts renal injury in acute decompensated cardiac failure: a prospective observational study. BMC Cardiovasc Disord [Internet]. 2012 [cited 2025 May 4];12. Available from: https://pubmed.ncbi.nlm.nih.gov/22340728/. https://doi.org/10.1186/1471-2261-12-8.
35. Damman K, Masson S, Hillege HL, Maggioni AP, Voors AA, Opasich C, et al. Clinical outcome of renal tubular damage in chronic heart failure. Eur Heart J [Internet]. 2011 [cited 2025 May 4];32(21):2705–2712. Available from: https://pubmed.ncbi.nlm.nih.gov/21666249/. https://doi.org/10.1093/eurheartj/ehr190.
36. Otaki Y, Watanabe T, Shimizu M, Tachibana S, Sato J, Kobayashi Y, et al. Renal tubular damage and clinical outcome in heart failure with preserved ejection fraction and CKD. ESC Heart Fail [Internet]. 2023 [cited 2025 May 4];10(4):2458. Available from: https://pmc.ncbi.nlm.nih.gov/articles/PMC10375165/. https://doi.org/10.1002/ehf2.14378.
37. Beigel R, Cercek B, Siegel RJ, Hamilton MA. Echo-Doppler hemodynamics: an important management tool for today's heart failure care. Circulation [Internet] 2015 [cited 2025 May 13];131(11):1031–1034. Available from: https://www.ahajournals.org/doi/10.1161/CIRCULATIONAHA.114.011424. https://doi.org/10.1161/circulationaha.114.011424.
38. Ei Khin HH, Cuthbert JJ, Koratala A, Aquaro GD, Pugliese NR, Gargani L, et al. Imaging of congestion in cardio-renal syndrome. Curr Heart Fail Rep 2025 22:1 [Internet]. 2025 [cited 2025 May 13];22(1):1–11. Available from: https://link.springer.com/article/10.1007/s11897-025-00695-z. https://doi.org/10.1007/s11897-025-00695-z.
39. Borrelli S, De Nicola L, Garofalo C, Paoletti E, Lucà S, Chiodini P, et al. Prevalence and renal prognosis of left ventricular diastolic dysfunction in non-dialysis CKD patients with preserved systolic function. J Hypertens [Internet] 2022 [cited 2025 May 13];40(4):723–731.

Available from: https://pubmed.ncbi.nlm.nih.gov/34939994/. https://doi.org/10.1097/hjh.0000000000003069.
40. Paoletti E, Zoccali C. A look at the upper heart chamber: the left atrium in CKD. Nephrol Dial Transplant [Internet] 2014 [cited 2025 May 13];29(10):1847–53. Available from: https://doi.org/10.1093/ndt/gft482
41. Gan GCH, Kadappu KK, Bhat A, Fernandez F, Gu KH, Cai L, et al. Left atrial strain is the best predictor of adverse cardiovascular outcomes in patients with CKD. J Am Soc Echocardiogr [Internet]. 2021 [cited 2025 May 13];34(2):166–175. Available from: https://pubmed.ncbi.nlm.nih.gov/33223356/. https://doi.org/10.1016/j.echo.2020.09.015.
42. Kadappu K, Cai L, Xuan W, French J, Thomas L. Left atrial strain an early marker of future adverse cardiovascular events in CKD. J Am Coll Cardiol [Internet] 2016 [cited 2025 May 13];67(13):1704. Available from: https://www.jacc.org/doi/10.1016/S0735-1097(16)31705-3. https://doi.org/10.1016/S0735-1097(16)31705-3.
43. Iaconelli A, Cuthbert J, Kazmi S, Maffia P, Clark AL, Cleland JGF, et al. Inferior vena cava diameter is associated with prognosis in patients with chronic heart failure independent of tricuspid regurgitation velocity. Clin Res Cardiol [Internet] 2023 [cited 2025 May 13];112(8):1077–1086. Available from: https://pubmed.ncbi.nlm.nih.gov/36894788/. https://doi.org/10.1007/s00392-023-02178-4.
44. Assavapokee T, Rola P, Assavapokee N, Koratala A. Decoding VExUS: a practical guide for excelling in point-of-care ultrasound assessment of venous congestion. 16srl; 2024. https://doi.org/10.1186/s13089-024-00396-z, Ultrasound J.
45. Puzzovivo A, Monitillo F, Guida P, Leone M, Rizzo C, Grande D, et al. Renal venous pattern: a new parameter for predicting prognosis in heart failure outpatients. J Cardiovasc Dev Dis [Internet]. 2018 [cited 2025 May 13];5(4):52. Available from: https://pmc.ncbi.nlm.nih.gov/articles/PMC6306853/. https://doi.org/10.3390/jcdd5040052.
46. Anastasiou V, Peteinidou E, Moysidis D V., Daios S, Gogos C, Liatsos AC, et al. Multiorgan congestion assessment by venous excess ultrasound score in acute heart failure. J Am Soc Echocardiogr [Internet] 2024 [cited 2025 May 13];37(10):923–933. Available from: https://onlinejase.com/action/showFullText?pii=S0894731724002347. https://doi.org/10.1016/j.echo.2024.05.011.
47. Islas-Rodríguez JP, Miranda-Aquino T, Romero-González G, Rio JH Del, Camacho-Guerrero JR, Covarrubias-Villa S, et al. Effect on kidney function recovery guiding decongestion with VExUS in patients with cardiorenal syndrome 1: a randomized control trial. Cardiorenal Med [Internet] 2024 [cited 2025 May 13];14(1):1–11. Available from: https://pubmed.ncbi.nlm.nih.gov/38061346/. https://doi.org/10.1159/000535641.
48. Damman K, van Deursen VM, Navis G, Voors AA, van Veldhuisen DJ, Hillege HL. Increased central venous pressure is associated with impaired renal function and mortality in a broad spectrum of patients with cardiovascular disease. J Am Coll Cardiol [Internet]. 2009 [cited 2025 May 13];53(7):582–588. Available from: https://pubmed.ncbi.nlm.nih.gov/19215832/. https://doi.org/10.1016/j.jacc.2008.08.080.
49. Kula AJ, Hanberg JS, Wilson FP, Brisco MA, Bellumkonda L, Jacoby D, et al. Influence of titration of neurohormonal antagonists and blood pressure reduction on renal function and decongestion in decompensated heart failure. Circ Heart Fail [Internet]. 2016 [cited 2025 May 13];9(1). Available from: https://pubmed.ncbi.nlm.nih.gov/26699390/. https://doi.org/10.1161/circheartfailure.115.002333.
50. Chen HH, Redfield MM, Nordstrom LJ, Cataliotti A, Burnett JC. Angiotensin II AT1 receptor antagonism prevents detrimental renal actions of acute diuretic therapy in human heart failure. Am J Physiol Renal Physiol 2003 [cited 2025 May 13];284(5 53–5). Available from: https://journals.physiology.org/doi/10.1152/ajprenal.00337.2002. https://doi.org/10.1152/ajprenal.00337.2002.
51. Costanzo MR, Guglin ME, Saltzberg MT, Jessup ML, Bart BA, Teerlink JR, et al. Ultrafiltration versus intravenous diuretics for patients hospitalized for acute decompensated heart failure. J

Am Coll Cardiol [Internet]. 2007 [cited 2025 May 13];49(6):675–683. Available from: https://pubmed.ncbi.nlm.nih.gov/17291932/. https://doi.org/10.1016/j.jacc.2006.07.073.
52. Bart BA, Goldsmith SR, Lee KL, Givertz MM, O'Connor CM, Bull DA, et al. Ultrafiltration in decompensated heart failure with cardiorenal syndrome. N Engl J Med [Internet]. 2012 [cited 2025 May 13];367(24):2296–2304. Available from: https://pubmed.ncbi.nlm.nih.gov/23131078/. https://doi.org/10.1056/nejmoa1210357.
53. Ahmed A, Rich MW, Zile M, Sanders PW, Patel K, Zhang Y, et al. Renin-angiotensin inhibition in diastolic heart failure and CKD. Am J Med [Internet]. 2013 [cited 2025 May 13];126(2):150–161. Available from: https://pubmed.ncbi.nlm.nih.gov/23331442/. https://doi.org/10.1016/j.amjmed.2012.06.031.
54. Khan NA, Ma I, Thompson CR, Humphries K, Salem DN, Sarnak MJ, et al. Kidney function and mortality among patients with left ventricular systolic dysfunction. J Am Soc Nephrol [Internet] 2006 [cited 2025 May 13];17(1):244–53. Available from: https://pubmed.ncbi.nlm.nih.gov/16291840/. https://doi.org/10.1681/asn.2005030270.
55. Heidenreich PA, Bozkurt B, Aguilar D, Allen LA, Byun JJ, Colvin MM, et al. 2022 AHA/ACC/HFSA guideline for the management of heart failure: a report of the American College of Cardiology/American Heart Association Joint Committee on Clinical Practice Guidelines. Circulation [Internet]. 2022 [cited 2025 May 13];145(18):E895–1032. Available from: www.ahajournals.org/journal/circ. https://doi.org/10.1161/cir.0000000000001063.
56. McDonagh TA, Metra M, Adamo M, Gardner RS, Baumbach A, Böhm M, et al. 2023 Focused Update of the 2021 ESC Guidelines for the diagnosis and treatment of acute and chronic heart failure: Developed by the task force for the diagnosis and treatment of acute and chronic heart failure of the European Society of Cardiology (ESC) With the special contribution of the Heart Failure Association (HFA) of the ESC. Eur Heart J [Internet] 2023 [cited 2025 May 13];44(37):3627–3639. Available from: https://doi.org/10.1093/eurheartj/ehad195
57. Vaduganathan M, Mentz RJ, Claggett BL, Miao ZM, Kulac IJ, Ward JH, et al. Sacubitril/valsartan in heart failure with mildly reduced or preserved ejection fraction: a pre-specified participant-level pooled analysis of PARAGLIDE-HF and PARAGON-HF. Eur Heart J [Internet]. 2023 [cited 2025 May 13];44(31):2982–2993. Available from: https://pubmed.ncbi.nlm.nih.gov/37210743/. https://doi.org/10.1093/eurheartj/ehad344.
58. Pitt B, Filippatos G, Agarwal R, Anker SD, Bakris GL, Rossing P, et al. Cardiovascular events with finerenone in kidney disease and type 2 diabetes. N Engl J Med [Internet]. 2021 [cited 2025 May 13];385(24):2252–2263. Available from: https://pubmed.ncbi.nlm.nih.gov/34449181/. https://doi.org/10.1056/nejmoa2110956.
59. Bakris GL, Agarwal R, Anker SD, Pitt B, Ruilope LM, Rossing P, et al. Effect of finerenone on ckd outcomes in type 2 diabetes. N Engl J Med [Internet]. 2020 [cited 2025 May 13];383(23):2219–2229. Available from: https://pubmed.ncbi.nlm.nih.gov/33264825/. https://doi.org/10.1056/nejmoa2025845.
60. Neuen BL, Young T, Heerspink HJL, Neal B, Perkovic V, Billot L, et al. SGLT2 inhibitors for the prevention of kidney failure in patients with type 2 diabetes: a systematic review and meta-analysis. Lancet Diabetes Endocrinol [Internet] 2019 [cited 2025 May 13];7(11):845–854. Available from: https://pubmed.ncbi.nlm.nih.gov/31495651/. https://doi.org/10.1016/s2213-8587(19)30256-6.
61. Kirk EP, Klein S. Pathogenesis and pathophysiology of the cardiometabolic syndrome. J Clin Hypertens. 2009;11(12):761–5. https://doi.org/10.1111/j.1559-4572.2009.00054.x.
62. Cho DH, Choi J, Gwon JG. Metabolic syndrome and the risk of COVID-19 infection: a nationwide population-based case-control study. Nutr Metab Cardiovasc Dis. 2021 Aug;31(9):2596–604. https://doi.org/10.1016/j.numecd.2021.05.016.
63. Dey S, Rzechorzek W, Aronow W. Cardiometabolic syndrome and COVID-19: pathophysiological aspects. In: Features, transmission, detection, and case studies in COVID-19. Elsevier; 2024. p. 321–32. https://doi.org/10.1016/B978-0-323-95646-8.00008-1.
64. Neeland IJ, Lim S, Tchernof A, Gastaldelli A, Rangaswami J, Ndumele CE, et al. Metabolic syndrome Nat Rev Dis Primers 2024;10(1):77. https://doi.org/10.1038/s41572-024-00563-5.

65. Comment on the provisional report from the WHO consultation. Diabet Med. 1999;16(5):442–3. https://doi.org/10.1046/j.1464-5491.1999.00059.x.
66. Reaven GM. Role of insulin resistance in human disease. Diabetes. 1988;37(12):1595–607. https://doi.org/10.1146/annurev.me.44.020193.001005.
67. Sperling LS, Mechanick JI, Neeland IJ, Herrick CJ, Després JP, Ndumele CE, et al. The cardiometabolic health alliance. J Am Coll Cardiol. 2015;66(9):1050–67. https://doi.org/10.1016/j.jacc.2015.06.1328.
68. Gami AS, Witt BJ, Howard DE, Erwin PJ, Gami LA, Somers VK, et al. Metabolic syndrome and risk of incident cardiovascular events and death. J Am Coll Cardiol. 2007;49(4):403–14. https://doi.org/10.1016/j.jacc.2006.09.032.
69. Alberti KGMM, Eckel RH, Grundy SM, Zimmet PZ, Cleeman JI, Donato KA, et al. Harmonizing the metabolic syndrome: a joint interim statement of the international diabetes federation task force on epidemiology and prevention; national heart, lung, and blood institute; American heart association; world heart federation; international atherosclerosis society; and international association for the study of obesity. Circulation [Internet]. 2009 [cited 2025 May 15];120(16):1640–1645. Available from: https://www.ahajournals.org/doi/10.1161/CIRCULATIONAHA.109.192644. https://doi.org/10.1161/circulationaha.109.192644.
70. Expert Panel on Detection E and T of HBC in A. Executive summary of the third report of the National Cholesterol Education Program (NCEP) Expert Panel on Detection, Evaluation, and Treatment of High Blood Cholesterol in Adults (Adult Treatment Panel III). JAMA. 2001;285(19):2486–97. https://doi.org/10.1001/jama.285.19.2486.
71. Rodríguez-Ortiz D, Reyes-Pérez A, León P, Sánchez H, Mosti M, Aguilar-Salinas CA, et al. Assessment of two different diagnostic guidelines criteria (National Cholesterol Education Adult Treatment Panel III [ATP III] and International Diabetes Federation [IDF]) for the evaluation of metabolic syndrome remission in a longitudinal cohort of patients undergoing Roux-en-Y gastric bypass. Surgery. 2016 Apr;159(4):1121–8. https://doi.org/10.1016/j.surg.2015.11.015.
72. Bloomgarden ZT. American Association of Clinical Endocrinologists (AACE) consensus conference on the insulin resistance syndrome. Diabetes Care. 2003;26(4):1297–303. https://doi.org/10.2337/diacare.26.4.1297.
73. Ruiz-García A, Arranz-Martínez E, Morales-Cobos LE, García-Álvarez JC, Iturmendi-Martínez N, Rivera-Teijido M. Tasas de prevalencia de sobrepeso y obesidad y sus asociaciones con factores cardiometabólicos y renales. Estudio SIMETAP-OB. Clínica e Investigación en Arteriosclerosis. 2022;34(6):291–302. https://www.elsevier.es/es-revista-clinica-e-investigacion-arteriosclerosis-15-articulo-tasas-prevalencia-sobrepeso-obesidad-sus-S0214916822000389
74. Mechanick JI, Rosenson RS, Pinney SP, Mancini DM, Narula J, Fuster V. Coronavirus and Cardiometabolic Syndrome. J Am Coll Cardiol. 2020;76(17):2024–35. https://doi.org/10.1016/j.jacc.2020.07.069.
75. Dutour A, Achard V, Sell H, Naour N, Collart F, Gaborit B, et al. Secretory type II phospholipase A2 is produced and secreted by epicardial adipose tissue and overexpressed in patients with coronary artery disease. J Clin Endocrinol Metab. 2010;95(2):963–7. https://doi.org/10.1210/jc.2009-1222.
76. Tsao CW, Aday AW, Almarzooq ZI, Alonso A, Beaton AZ, Bittencourt MS, et al. Heart disease and stroke statistics—2022 update: a report from the American Heart Association. Circulation. 2022;145(8) https://doi.org/10.1161/cir.0000000000001052.
77. Grundy SM, Brewer HB, Cleeman JI, Smith SC, Lenfant C. Definition of metabolic syndrome. Arterioscler Thromb Vasc Biol. 2004;24(2) https://doi.org/10.1161/01.cir.0000111245.75752.c6.
78. Sebastian SA, Padda I, Johal G. Cardiovascular-kidney-metabolic (CKM) syndrome: a state-of-the-art review. Curr Probl Cardiol. 2024;49(2):102344. https://doi.org/10.1016/j.cpcardiol.2023.102344.

79. Ndumele CE, Rangaswami J, Chow SL, Neeland IJ, Tuttle KR, Khan SS, et al. Cardiovascular-kidney-metabolic health: a presidential advisory from the American Heart Association. Circulation. 2023;148(20):1606–35. https://doi.org/10.1161/cir.0000000000001184.
80. Ndumele CE, Neeland IJ, Tuttle KR, Chow SL, Mathew RO, Khan SS, et al. A synopsis of the evidence for the science and clinical management of cardiovascular-kidney-metabolic (CKM) syndrome: a scientific statement from the American Heart Association. Circulation. 2023;148(20):1636–64. https://doi.org/10.1161/CIR.0000000000001186.
81. Mutruc V, Bologa C, Șorodoc V, Ceasovschih A, Morărașu BC, Șorodoc L, et al. Cardiovascular–kidney–metabolic syndrome: a new paradigm in clinical medicine or going back to basics? J Clin Med. 2025;14(8):2833. https://doi.org/10.3390/jcm14082833.
82. Kittelson KS, Junior AG, Fillmore N, da Silva GR. Cardiovascular-kidney-metabolic syndrome—an integrative review. Prog Cardiovasc Dis. 2024;87:26–36. https://doi.org/10.1016/j.pcad.2024.10.012.

Chapter 3
Epidemiology and Risk Factors in Cardiovascular-Kidney-Metabolic Syndrome

Stefan Iliescu, Alexandru Florinel Oancea, Mariana Floria, and Adrian Covic

Introduction

After formally defining cardiovascular-kidney-metabolic syndrome as "a systemic disorder characterized by pathophysiological interactions among metabolic risk factors, chronic kidney disease (CKD), and the cardiovascular system leading to multiorgan dysfunction", the American Heart Association offered a staging framework in order to better underscore the progressive nature of this disorder. The authors defined four stages ranging from 0 (no CKM risk factors) to 4 (clinical cardiovascular disease, further classified into 4a (without CKD) and 4b (with CKD) [1].

Similarly, the European Atherosclerosis Society developed a consensus regarding systemic metabolic disorders. In order to help risk prediction, the authors developed a three-stage classification system (Table 3.1) [2].

S. Iliescu · A. F. Oancea (✉) · M. Floria
Grigore T. Popa University of Medicine and Pharmacy, Iasi, Romania

Saint Spiridon Emergency Hospital, Iasi, Romania
e-mail: alexandru.oancea@umfiasi.ro

A. Covic
Grigore T. Popa University of Medicine and Pharmacy, Iasi, Romania

Dr. C.I Parhon Clinical Hospital, Iasi, Romania

M. Floria, D. M. Tanase (eds.), *Cardiovascular-Kidney-Metabolic Syndrome*,
https://doi.org/10.1007/978-3-032-11445-7_3

Table 3.1 Stages of systemic metabolic disorder [2]

Stage	Description
Stage 1	1. Insulin resistance/prediabetes. or 2. Overweight/dysfunctional adipose tissue + *at least one of the following:* (a) Liver steatosis. (b) Hypertension. (c) Atherogenic dyslipidemia.
Stage 2	Type 2 diabetes mellitus *or* asymptomatic diastolic dysfunction *or* MASH *or* albuminuria *or* G1–2 CKD *or* subclinical atherosclerosis (no events)
Stage 3	Symptomatic HFpEF *or* liver failure *or* G3–5 CKD *or* clinical atherosclerosis (with events)

Epidemiology in CKM Syndrome

According to the American Heart Association's report on heart disease and stroke statistics, in 2021 cardiovascular disease was the leading cause of death in 19.5 million people, an increase of over 6 million compared to 1990. The main driver behind these numbers seems to be ischemic heart disease, followed by stroke and hypertensive heart disease, all of which have seen an increase in the last 30 years. The most incriminated risk factors seem to be high systolic blood pressure, dietary risks, and ambient pollution. Other important risk factors mentioned include high plasma glucose, high body mass index, high low-density lipoprotein cholesterol (LDL-C), and kidney dysfunction, each accounting for more than 5 million deaths in 2021. The same report states that 46.7% of US adults had hypertension, 10.6% had diagnosed diabetes, and 46.4% had prediabetes. The prevalence of obesity was 41.8% compared to 19.7% in children. There were some sex differences in the prevalence of severe obesity (6.6% in males and 11.7% in females) [3].

United States

Using data from NHANES (National Health and Nutrition Examination Study), Ostrominski et al. developed a cohort study on 11.607 US adults in order to better evaluate the overlap between cardiac, renal, and metabolic disease. Their results showed that more than a quarter of the participants had at least one CKM condition. Chronic kidney disease seemed to be the most prevalent (13.9%), followed by diabetes mellitus and cardiovascular disease (13.3% and 8.6%, respectively). Following temporal trends, the authors noticed an increase in the number of people that had at least one CKM comorbidity from 21.2 in 1999 to 26.3% in 2020 [4].

A similarly designed study, but using AHA's (American Heart Association) staging for CKM syndrome, was published in 2024. Their results show that 90% of the participants met the criteria for CKM stage 1 or higher, while 15% had advanced stages. Older, male, and black participants were more likely to have advanced stages. Alarmingly, only 18.2% of the participants between 20 and 44 years had stage 0. The prevalence remained relatively stable during the study period. A possible reason for this finding seems to be the simultaneous improvement and worsening of the prevalence of specific risk factors. Although the authors incorporated physical examination and a number of laboratory measurements, they lacked specific tests that would have better estimated the prevalence of stages 3 and 4. Thus, these stages might be underestimated in the study [5].

Social determinants of health (SDOH) are nonmedical risk factors that indicate health equity. They include income, education, housing, employment, food security, and access to medical resources. A cross-sectional study using data from NHANES published in 2024 showed that unfavorable SDOH were associated with higher stages of CKM. Unemployment, low income, and food insecurity were the most important factors. Interestingly, women who were unmarried, living alone, or living in a rented space had a higher prevalence of advanced stages of CKM. This association was not statistically significant in men [6].

Asia and Europe

A large-scale Korean study showed slightly different results in the South Asian population. The most prevalent stages were 2 and 1. From the beginning of the analysis in 2011, an increasing trend of advanced stages was noticed, particularly in vulnerable groups as well as in males, older adults, obese participants, smokers, and drinkers. Participants with a lower educational status and lower income had a higher prevalence of advanced stages. However, the same cannot be stated regarding the region of residence. Urban residents had a slightly higher prevalence of stage 0 (22.7% vs. 19.8% for rural residents), while for the other stages the differences were minimal (stage 1: 25.7% vs. 25.1%; stage 2: 41.7% vs. 44.9%; stage 3: 7.2% vs. 7.3%; stage 4: 2.7% vs. 2.9%). This study revealed some notable differences between the Korean and US population. There has been a higher proportion of stage 0 CKM (21.1% vs 10.6%). Moreover, the authors noticed an increase in the prevalence of stages 3 and 4 during the study period (attributing it to the growing burden of CVD), while in the US population the prevalence remained stable [7].

In Europe, a subanalysis on 1691 participants in the Rotterdam Study showed that 83% of them were classified as CKM stage 3. Over a median follow-up period of 10.3 years, cardiovascular events were not reported in participants classified as stage 0 or 1, but they occurred in 1.8% of those at stage 2 and in 17% of individuals at stage 3 [8].

A single center retrospective analysis of electronic medical records in Belgium included 1333 patients with heart failure with mild reduced left ventricular ejection fraction (40–50%) and reduced left ventricular ejection fraction (<50%) ejection fraction. Their results show that the presence of type 2 diabetes mellitus (T2DM) or CKD is significantly associated with mortality and a composite outcome of mortality and readmission for heart failure [9].

Using data from COMEGEN (COoperativa di MEdicina GENerale), a primary care database from Italy, Trimarco et al. published a cohort study where they focused on the differences in CKM syndrome epidemiology before and during the COVID-19 pandemic. The total cohort included 81,051 patients (32,650 from the 2017–2019 period and 48,401 from the 2020–2022 period). Before 2020, only one CKM condition was seen in 20% of the participants, two CKM conditions were present in 10.8% of the population, while only 3.3% had all three comorbidities. The authors noted an increase in all three categories in the post-COVID cohort (27% for 1 out of 3; 13.8% for 2 out of 3; and 4% for all three). Conversely, the percentage of participants without comorbidities decreased from 66% to 56%. It seems that during the pandemic, the prevalence increased for all CKM risk factors (21% vs 70% for prediabetes, 69% vs. 80% for dyslipidemia, 33% vs. 56% for hypertension, 16% vs. 24% for obesity). Although many factors can contribute to these temporal changes (such as acute or chronic complications of COVID-19 infection), this study offers insights into the epidemiology of CKM syndrome in Europe where data is still scarce [10].

In conclusion, CKM syndrome is a highly prevalent disease. Irrespective of age, a high proportion of individuals can be classified into a CKM stage higher than 1. Moreover, vulnerable populations are more likely to have advanced stages. This data shows the importance of a multidisciplinary approach in both preventing and mitigating the consequences of CKM syndrome.

Risk Factors in Cardiovascular-Kidney-Metabolic Syndrome

The CKM syndrome shows how metabolic, cardiovascular, and renal homeostasis deteriorate in an interconnected manner through a complex network of common risk factors. The American Heart Association made an announcement on it, and according to that, the following main risk factors contribute to the development and progression of CKM syndrome [11, 12]: obesity and dysfunctional adipose tissue, T2DM, hypertension, dyslipidemia, chronic inflammation and oxidative stress, renin-angiotensin-aldosterone system (RAAS), genetic and epigenetic factors, behavioral- and sex-specific risk factors, and early-life and in-utero factors.

Obesity and Dysfunctional Adipose Tissue

Obesity, particularly characterized by visceral adiposity and dysfunctional adipose tissue, serves as an initial and critical driver in the cascade leading to CKM. Adipose tissue dysfunction induces chronic low-grade inflammation, oxidative stress, insulin resistance, and activation of the renin-angiotensin-aldosterone system (RAAS), all of which synergistically contribute to endothelial dysfunction, hypertension, and glomerular damage, which may lead to CKM syndrome.

Dysfunctional adipose tissue releases a spectrum of proinflammatory cytokines, adipokines, and free fatty acids, all of which contribute to insulin resistance, oxidative stress, chronic inflammation, and direct tissue damage in metabolic, cardiovascular, and renal systems. Visceral adiposity is particularly harmful compared to subcutaneous fat as it is associated with increased secretion of interleukin-6 (IL-6), tumor necrosis factor-α (TNF-α), and resistin, which affect insulin signaling pathways and promote systemic inflammation by activating signaling pathways, such as c-Jun N-terminal kinase (JNK) and the nuclear factor-kappa B (NF-κB), leading to phosphorylation of insulin receptor substrate proteins on serine residues instead of tyrosine residues, impairing insulin response; this disruption of insulin signaling is essential for the pathophysiology of CKM syndrome. Moreover, this chronic inflammatory state promotes endothelial dysfunction, increased oxidative stress and vascular injury, which are critical factors in the progression of both CKD and cardiovascular disease. In addition, the inflammatory environment exacerbates the decline in renal function by promoting fibrosis and glomerular injury, thereby accelerating the progression of CKD [13–15].

In addition to the systemic metabolic disorders induced by obesity, ectopic lipid accumulation in nonadipose tissues, particularly in the heart and kidneys, plays a key role in organ dysfunction and the progression of cardio-renal diseases. When the storage capacity of adipose tissue is exceeded, lipids are stored in organs where they should not physiologically accumulate, a phenomenon known as lipotoxicity. In the heart, the latter is generated by the accumulation of saturated fatty acids and is characterized by:

- Mitochondrial dysfunction: Excess fatty acids disrupt mitochondrial function, leading to increased reactive oxygen species (ROS) production and impaired ATP synthesis [16].
- Endoplasmic reticulum stress: Accumulated lipids cause endoplasmic reticulum stress, triggering apoptotic pathways and contributing to cardiomyocyte apoptosis [17].
- Inflammatory responses: Lipid-induced activation of inflammatory signaling pathways exacerbates cardiac remodeling and dysfunction [16].

Similarly, in the kidneys, lipid accumulation results in:

- Podocyte injury: Lipid deposits damage podocytes, essential for glomerular filtration, leading to proteinuria [18].
- Tubulointerstitial fibrosis: Lipids promote fibrotic changes in the renal interstitium, compromising reabsorption function [19].
- Inflammation and oxidative stress: Similar to the heart, lipid accumulation in the kidneys promotes inflammatory responses and oxidative stress, further damaging renal tissues [20].

Finally, adipose tissue dysfunction also alters secretion patterns of beneficial adipokines like adiponectin, a hormone that enhances insulin sensitivity and possesses anti-inflammatory properties. In obesity, adiponectin levels decrease, exacerbating insulin resistance and vascular damage. Furthermore, obesity-induced activation of the RAAS and sympathetic nervous system contributes to hypertension and glomerular injury, essential steps in CKM syndrome progression. Mitochondrial dysfunction within adipocytes leads to impaired oxidative phosphorylation and enhanced reactive oxygen species (ROS) production, promoting endothelial dysfunction and atherosclerosis, leading to CKM syndrome [21, 22].

Type 2 Diabetes Mellitus

Hyperglycemia and insulin resistance are crucial mechanisms linking diabetes to kidney and cardiovascular damage. Type 2 diabetes mellitus is a central driver of CKM syndrome, tightly interwoven with obesity and adipose tissue dysfunction. It is characterized by hyperglycemia resulting from insulin resistance and progressive pancreatic β-cell failure. Chronic hyperglycemia initiates a cascade of pathogenic mechanisms detrimental to cardiovascular and renal health. At the molecular level, hyperglycemia induces the overproduction of mitochondrial superoxide, leading to oxidative stress and endothelial dysfunction. This oxidative environment activates harmful pathways such as the polyol pathway, protein kinase C activation, hexosamine pathway flux, and formation of advanced glycation end products. Advanced glycation end products cross-link collagen and elastin fibers, increasing vascular stiffness and promoting glomerulosclerosis [12].

Furthermore, in the context of CKM syndrome, hyperglycemia plays an essential role in creating and maintaining a proinflammatory environment. Elevated glucose levels stimulate the uptake of various proinflammatory chemokines as well as adhesion molecules such as intercellular adhesion molecule-1 and vascular cell adhesion molecule-1. These molecules collectively promote endothelial dysfunction, increase leukocyte recruitment, and facilitate vascular inflammation, thereby accelerating atherogenesis. In addition, persistent hyperglycemia induces glomerular and tubular damage via similar inflammatory pathways, contributing to the development and progression of diabetic kidney disease. Chronic activation of these inflammatory cascades not only exacerbates cardiovascular and renal damage but also establishes a vicious cycle that is central to the pathophysiology of CKM syndrome [23].

Epidemiologically, people with T2DM are two to four times more at risk of developing cardiovascular disease than people without diabetes. T2DM is also the leading cause of end-stage kidney disease (ESKD) worldwide. Cohort studies have shown that 24% of initial clinical events in diabetics without previous cardiovascular or kidney disease are heart failure events, while 36% are related to the onset of CKD [24, 25].

Therapeutic strategies for T2DM in the context of CKM syndrome have evolved considerably. Sodium-glucose co-transporter-2 inhibitors (SGLT2i) and Glucagon-Like Peptide-1 receptor agonists (GLP-1 Ras) have emerged as first-line treatments due to their proven benefits in reducing cardiovascular mortality, hospitalizations for heart failure, and progression of renal disease. Importantly, the optimal management of T2DM requires a holistic approach that addresses all components of the metabolic syndrome, including blood pressure control, lipid-lowering therapies, weight reduction, and promotion of physical activity. Screening for albuminuria and routine estimation of glomerular filtration rate are essential steps for early detection of diabetic kidney disease and timely intervention [26].

Hypertension and Dyslipidemia

Hypertension and dyslipidemia are pivotal modifiable risk factors that contribute significantly to the initiation and progression of CKM syndrome. On one hand, hypertension exerts deleterious effects on both cardiovascular and renal systems. Elevated blood pressure induces endothelial dysfunction, promotes arterial stiffness, and accelerates atherosclerosis, thereby increasing the risk of CVD. In the kidneys, hypertension leads to glomerular hyperfiltration and subsequent nephron loss, culminating in CKD progression. The activation of the RAAS in hypertension further exacerbates these effects by promoting inflammation and fibrosis in both cardiac and renal tissues [27]. On the other hand, dyslipidemia, characterized by elevated LDL-C, triglycerides, and reduced high-density lipoprotein cholesterol (HDL-C), is a well-established risk factor for atherosclerotic cardiovascular disease. Abnormal lipid profiles contribute to endothelial dysfunction, oxidative stress, and inflammation, which are central to CKM syndrome pathogenesis. In the kidneys, lipid accumulation can lead to glomerulosclerosis and tubulointerstitial fibrosis, further advancing CKD [28].

The coexistence of hypertension and dyslipidemia amplifies the risk of CKM syndrome. Both conditions synergistically exacerbate endothelial dysfunction, promote a proinflammatory state, and accelerate atherogenesis. This combination increases the likelihood of cardiovascular events and accelerates renal function decline. The pathophysiology underlying the contribution of hypertension and dyslipidemia to CKM syndrome involves several interconnected mechanisms:

- Endothelial dysfunction: Both conditions impair endothelial nitric oxide production, leading to vasoconstriction and increased vascular resistance [29].
- Inflammation: Elevated blood pressure and abnormal lipid levels promote the release of proinflammatory cytokines, contributing to vascular and renal inflammation [30].
- Oxidative stress: An imbalance between reactive oxygen species production and antioxidant defenses damages vascular and renal tissues [31].
- Insulin resistance: Hypertension and dyslipidemia are associated with insulin resistance, further linking metabolic disturbances to CKM syndrome [32].

Early identification and management of high blood pressure and dyslipidemia are essential to prevent progression of CKM syndrome. Lifestyle modifications, including dietary changes, regular physical activity, and weight management, are fundamental. Pharmacologic interventions, antihypertensive agents such as ACE inhibitors or ARB (Angiotensin Receptor Blockers) and lipid-lowering therapies such as statins, are essential for achieving target blood pressure and lipid values [1, 33].

Chronic Inflammation and Oxidative Stress

Persistent low-grade inflammation and increased production of ROS amplify endothelial dysfunction, fibrosis, and organ damage, creating a vicious cycle across metabolic, cardiovascular, and renal systems.

Chronic inflammation in CKM syndrome is predominantly driven by metabolic abnormalities such as obesity, insulin resistance, and dyslipidemia. Expansion of adipose tissue, particularly visceral fat accumulation, leads to deregulated adipokine secretion and a proinflammatory state characterized by increased levels of cytokines, including TNF-α, IL-6 (as mentioned before), and monocyte chemoattractant protein-1. This inflammatory environment impairs insulin signaling, enhances endothelial dysfunction, and promotes atherosclerotic plaque formation. In addition, in patients with chronic kidney disease, the proinflammatory environment is perpetuated due to decreased renal clearance of inflammatory mediators, leading to further vascular and metabolic complications [34, 35].

Oxidative stress, resulting from an imbalance between ROS production and antioxidant defense mechanisms, plays a parallel and amplifying role. Hyperglycemia, common in metabolic syndrome and diabetes, favors mitochondrial dysfunction and excessive ROS generation. Oxidative stress not only directly harms cellular components but also activates key inflammatory pathways, in particular through NF-κB signaling axis. This activation leads to a further increase in adhesion molecules, cytokines, and pro-thrombotic factors, fueling vascular injury, glomerulosclerosis, and cardiac remodeling [34, 36].

Importantly, oxidative stress and inflammation reinforce each other, forming a damaging feedback loop. ROS production triggers inflammatory responses, while inflammatory cytokines, such as TNF-α, increase ROS production by activating NADPH oxidase and mitochondrial pathways. This cycle accelerates endothelial dysfunction, arterial stiffness, and myocardial fibrosis, central features of the progression of CKM syndrome. Recent clinical studies have highlighted the prognostic role of biomarkers of inflammation (such as CRP, IL-6) and oxidative stress (such as oxidized LDL-C, F2-isoprostanes) in predicting cardiovascular events, renal decline, and mortality in patients with diabetes, CKD, and heart failure. High levels of high-sensitivity CRP, for example, are independently associated with adverse cardiovascular outcomes in a wide range of populations, while higher levels of F2-isoprostanes are correlated with severity of renal dysfunction [37, 38].

In summary, chronic inflammation and oxidative stress are not just byproducts, but fundamental factors in the pathophysiology of CKM syndrome. Understanding and targeting these processes are critical strategies for modifying disease progression and improving outcomes across the interconnected spectrum of cardiovascular, renal, and metabolic diseases.

Renin-Angiotensin-Aldosterone System Activation

The RAAS plays an essential role in regulating blood pressure, fluid balance, and electrolyte homeostasis. However, when deregulated, chronic activation of the RAAS emerges as a central pathologic mechanism contributing to the development and progression of CKM syndrome. Persistent activation of this hormonal cascade links metabolic dysfunction to kidney damage and cardiovascular disease, creating a self-perpetuating cycle that leads to multiorgan damage [39].

In the context of CKM, RAAS activation is often triggered by hyperglycemia, insulin resistance, obesity, and low nephron count. These stimuli lead to increased renin secretion, increased levels of angiotensin II (Ang II), and increased aldosterone production. Ang II is a potent vasoconstrictor that promotes hypertension, a fundamental factor in heart and kidney damage. In addition, Ang II exerts proinflammatory, pro-oxidative, and profibrotic effects through its interaction with angiotensin type 1 receptors (AT1R), leading to endothelial dysfunction, vascular remodeling, myocardial hypertrophy, and glomerulosclerosis (Fig. 3.1) [40].

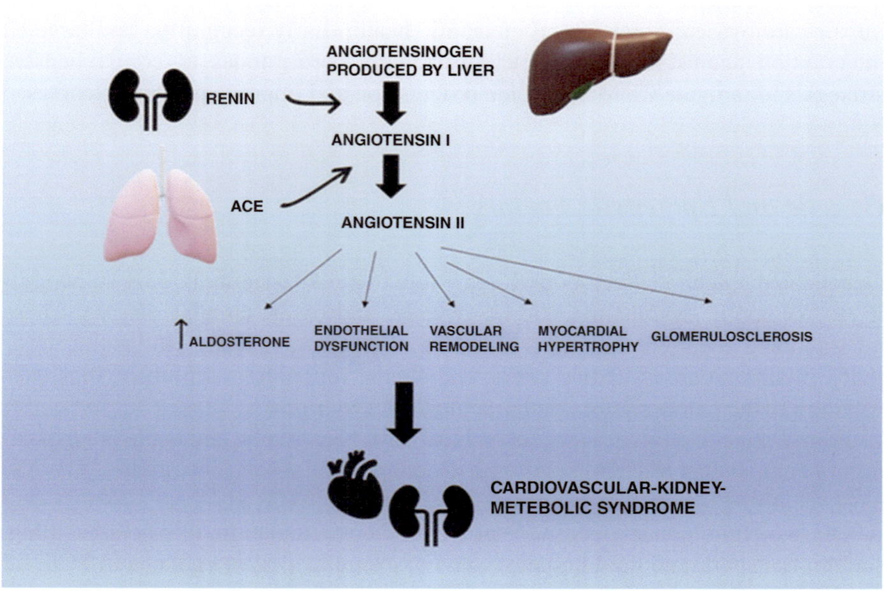

Fig. 3.1 Renin-angiotensin-aldosterone system promoting the genesis of Cardiovascular-Kidney-Metabolic syndrome

Beyond its hemodynamic actions, RAAS activation has significant direct cellular effects. Ang II stimulates the production of reactive oxygen species (ROS) by activating NADPH oxidase, thereby inducing oxidative stress and enhancing inflammatory signaling cascades. At the same time, aldosterone promotes sodium retention, vascular stiffness, and fibrosis in the heart and kidneys by activating mineralocorticoid receptors. These pathological processes are aggravated in the context of metabolic diseases, in which obesity and insulin resistance sensitize tissues to RAAS overactivation, even in the absence of overt hypertension [40].

Clinical evidence emphasizes the centrality of RAAS activation in CKM syndrome. Elevated plasma aldosterone concentrations are associated with increased risks of heart failure, myocardial infarction, and progression of chronic kidney disease. Furthermore, polymorphisms in RAAS-related genes have been linked to susceptibility to hypertension, diabetic nephropathy, and cardiovascular events in different populations. Pharmacologic blockade of the RAAS pathway with ACE inhibitors, ARBs, and mineralocorticoid receptor antagonists (MRAs) has demonstrated significant reductions in cardiovascular morbidity, mortality, and progression of renal disease in several high-risk groups. The protective benefits observed with RAAS inhibition extend beyond blood pressure control, highlighting the contribution of nonhemodynamic effects, such as anti-inflammatory, antioxidative, and antifibrotic actions. Recent clinical trials have also explored the synergistic potential of combining RAAS inhibitors with newer agents, such as SGLT2 inhibitors and nonsteroidal mineralocorticoid receptor antagonists, offering promising strategies to more effectively target the multifactorial pathophysiology of CKM syndrome [41–43].

In conclusion, persistent activation of the RAAS is a fundamental driver of the interconnected pathologies that define CKM syndrome. It promotes a deleterious milieu of hypertension, oxidative stress, inflammation, and fibrosis that collectively impair cardiovascular, renal, and metabolic health. Early recognition and targeted intervention against RAAS overactivity remain cornerstones of comprehensive strategies to mitigate CKM syndrome progression and improve patient outcomes.

Genetic and Epigenetic Factors

Genetic and epigenetic factors play a key role in modulating individual vulnerability to metabolic dysfunction, kidney disease, and cardiovascular disease. These inherited and acquired alterations affect cellular pathways related to insulin sensitivity, inflammation, oxidative stress, endothelial function, and fibrosis, thus contributing to the pathophysiologic basis of CKM syndrome.

From a genetic point of view, several loci have been implicated in the predisposition to components of CKM syndrome. Genome-wide association studies (GWAS) have identified variants in genes such as TCF7L2, FTO, SLC2A9, UMOD, and APOE, which influence glucose metabolism, fat accumulation, uric acid handling, sodium transport, and lipid homeostasis. For example, polymorphisms in TCF7L2 have been consistently associated with impaired insulin secretion and increased risk of type 2 diabetes, while variants in UMOD affect renal sodium reabsorption and susceptibility to hypertension. These genetic variants may act independently or synergistically to increase risk, particularly in individuals with adverse environmental or lifestyle exposures (Table 3.2) [47, 54].

In addition to inherited variations in DNA sequence, epigenetic modifications—heritable changes in gene expression without changes in DNA sequence—are increasingly recognized as central contributors to CKM syndrome. These include DNA methylation, histone modifications, and noncoding RNA regulation, which together orchestrate the transcriptional landscape of key metabolic, renal, and vascular tissues. In patients with diabetes or obesity, hyperglycemia and lipid accumulation can induce epigenetic reprogramming of immune and endothelial cells, leading to persistent proinflammatory phenotypes even after metabolic normalization—a phenomenon termed "metabolic memory" [55, 56].

Table 3.2 Genes Involved in CKM syndrome: Roles, variants, and clinical implications

Gene	Biological role	Variant(s)/ mutation(s)	Consequences in CKM syndrome	Reference
TCF7L2	Transcription factor in Wnt signaling, regulates insulin secretion	rs7903146 (C > T)	Increased risk of T2DM due to β-cell dysfunction	Grant SF et al., 2006 [44]
FTO	Regulates appetite and energy balance	rs9939609 (T > A)	Obesity, insulin resistance, and T2DM risk	Frayling TM et al., 2007 [45]
SLC2A9	Urate transporter in renal tubules	rs7442295, rs16890979	Hyperuricemia, renal dysfunction, CV risk	Vitart V et al., 2008 [46]
UMOD	Regulates sodium handling and kidney function	rs4293393 (G > A)	Increased hypertension and CKD risk	Köttgen A et al., 2010 [47]
APOE	Cholesterol transport and lipid metabolism	ε2, ε3, ε4 (focus on ε2)	Dyslipidemia, atherosclerosis, CVD	Heidemann et al., 2021 [48]
ACE	Catalyzes angiotensin I to II, regulates BP via RAAS	Insertion/Deletion (I/D) polymorphism	D allele: higher ACE activity → hypertension, diabetic nephropathy	Rigat B et al., 1990 [49]
PPARG	Adipocyte differentiation, lipid and glucose metabolism	Pro12Ala (rs1801282)	Altered insulin sensitivity, risk of T2DM	Deeb SS et al., 1998 [50]
KCNJ11	ATP-sensitive potassium channel in β-cells	E23K (rs5219)	Reduced insulin secretion, elevated T2DM risk	Gloyn AL et al., 2003 [51]
NPHS2	Podocyte integrity and glomerular filtration	R229Q (rs61747728)	Proteinuria, CKD in diabetics	Zhou et al., 2022 [52]
ADIPOQ	Produces adiponectin, regulates insulin sensitivity and inflammation	rs266729, rs2241766	Low adiponectin: metabolic syndrome, insulin resistance, CV complications	de Oliveira et al., 2015 [53]

One of the best characterized epigenetic modifications is DNA methylation of promoter regions in genes that regulate oxidative stress and inflammation. For example, PPARGC1A hypermethylation impairs mitochondrial biogenesis and antioxidant responses, whereas hypomethylation of proinflammatory genes such as TNF and IL6 enhances their expression in vascular and renal tissues. Similarly, dysregulated microRNAs, such as miR-21, miR-155, and miR-29, modulate fibrosis, endothelial dysfunction, and insulin signaling in both the heart and kidney, influencing disease progression. Emerging studies also suggest that prenatal and early-life exposures may lead to long-lasting epigenetic changes that predispose individuals to CKM syndrome later in life. Nutritional status during fetal development, maternal diabetes, and exposure to environmental toxins have all been associated with altered DNA methylation patterns and increased incidence of metabolic and cardiovascular disorders in offspring [57, 58].

Epigenetic mechanisms also offer a promising avenue for therapeutic intervention. Lifestyle modifications, such as diet, exercise, and weight loss, have been shown to reverse some maladaptive epigenetic changes. In addition, certain pharmacological agents, including histone deacetylase (HDAC) inhibitors and SGLT2 inhibitors, may exert beneficial effects by modulating gene expression via epigenetic pathways. The integration of genomic and epigenomic profiling into clinical practice may enable future personalized risk assessment and precision prevention strategies for CKM syndrome [59].

In summary, genetic and epigenetic factors contribute significantly to the onset and progression of CKM syndrome. Their influence on metabolic regulation, renal function, and cardiovascular integrity emphasizes the importance of understanding inherited and acquired molecular changes in disease susceptibility. Future research aimed at unraveling these complex interactions has the potential to transform prevention and treatment paradigms for this multifaceted syndrome.

Behavioral Risk Factors

Behavioral risk factors play a pivotal role in the development and progression of CKM syndrome. While genetic predisposition and molecular mechanisms form the biological substrate of the disease, lifestyle-related behaviors significantly influence its trajectory. These modifiable factors, including diet, physical activity, substance use, sleep patterns, and psychosocial stress, act through multiple interconnected pathways to exacerbate metabolic dysregulation, endothelial dysfunction, inflammation, and organ damage.

Firstly, dietary habits are among the most influential behavioral factors in CKM syndrome. Diets high in saturated fats, trans fats, and sodium promote weight gain, dyslipidemia, insulin resistance, and hypertension, all of which are central features of CKM syndrome. In contrast, dietary patterns such as the mediterranean or DASH diets—rich in fruits, vegetables, whole grains, legumes, nuts, and unsaturated fats—have been associated with improved insulin sensitivity, blood pressure regulation, and cardiovascular outcomes. Nutritional excess or deficiency directly affects the metabolic milieu, influencing systemic inflammation, oxidative stress, and vascular function [60, 61].

Secondly, physical inactivity represents another cornerstone behavioral risk. Sedentary behavior contributes to visceral adiposity, reduced muscle mass, and impaired glucose and lipid metabolism. A lack of regular physical activity diminishes endothelial function and increases sympathetic nervous system activity, favoring hypertension and metabolic imbalance. Exercise has been shown to enhance insulin sensitivity, promote lipid oxidation, reduce systemic inflammation, and improve renal and cardiovascular hemodynamics, offering a protective effect against CKM syndrome [62].

Then tobacco use remains a well-established modifiable risk factor with systemic effects across all three domains of CKM syndrome. Cigarette smoke contains numerous pro-oxidative and proinflammatory compounds that damage vascular endothelium, accelerate atherosclerosis, and impair renal function. Smoking also increases sympathetic tone and activates the RAAS, promoting hypertension and glomerular injury. Chronic tobacco exposure is strongly associated with increased incidence of chronic kidney disease, coronary artery disease, and metabolic syndrome. Alcohol consumption has a complex relationship with cardiometabolic health; while moderate alcohol intake may confer some cardiovascular benefits in certain populations, excessive or chronic consumption is clearly associated with detrimental outcomes. High alcohol intake contributes to hepatic insulin resistance, increases triglyceride levels, elevates blood pressure, and may directly impair myocardial structure and function [30].

Not least, sleep quality and duration are emerging as critical factors in CKM syndrome. Chronic sleep deprivation and poor sleep quality disrupt circadian rhythms, alter hormonal regulation of appetite and glucose metabolism, and increase sympathetic nervous system activity. Sleep disorders such as obstructive sleep apnea are independently associated with hypertension, insulin resistance, and increased risk of chronic kidney disease. Inadequate sleep is also linked to increased oxidative stress and inflammatory cytokine production, compounding cardiometabolic risk [63].

Finally, chronic psychological stress is another significant, yet often underappreciated, behavioral factor. Prolonged exposure to stress activates the hypothalamic-pituitary-adrenal axis and increases cortisol secretion, which in turn impairs glucose metabolism, raises blood pressure, and promotes central fat accumulation. Stress-induced behaviors, such as emotional eating, smoking, and alcohol consumption, further aggravate the risk of CKM syndrome. Inflammation and autonomic dysregulation linked to chronic stress have direct effects on both cardiovascular and renal systems [64].

Sex-Specific Risk Factors

Sex-specific risk factors significantly influence the incidence, course, and outcome of CKM syndrome. Biological differences between men and women, including hormonal profiles, body composition, and gene expression, contribute to distinct pathophysiological responses. In addition to these biological determinants, sex- and gender-specific socio-cultural and behavioral factors further modulate disease susceptibility and clinical manifestation [65].

CVD, a core component of CKM syndrome, shows notable sex differences. Premenopausal women generally have a lower incidence of CVD than men of the same age, a protection largely attributed to the cardiometabolic benefits of endogenous estrogens. Estrogens exert vasodilatory effects via nitric oxide pathways and favorably modulate lipid profiles by increasing HDL-C. However, this protective effect diminishes after menopause, leading to a sharp increase in cardiovascular risk. Postmenopausal women often show atypical symptoms and are more likely to suffer from HFpEF, a phenotype increasingly associated with metabolic dysfunction [66].

Renal pathophysiology also varies by gender. In general, men are at higher risk of developing CKD at an older age, partly due to differences in glomerular structure, renal hemodynamics, and testosterone-related pathways that favor fibrosis. However, women with CKD often progress more rapidly to end-stage renal disease (ESRD), particularly in the context of diabetes and hypertension. Female sex hormones appear to provide initial nephroprotection but may become harmful in advanced stages of kidney disease. In addition, gender-related barriers such as delayed diagnosis and limited access to specialized care may further worsen outcomes in women [67].

Metabolic regulation and obesity-related comorbidities are also influenced by gender. Women typically accumulate subcutaneous fat, which is less metabolically damaging than the visceral adiposity more common in men. Despite this, women with central obesity, particularly at postmenopause, have a disproportionately higher risk of insulin resistance and T2DM. In addition, conditions such as polycystic ovary syndrome (PCOS) uniquely predispose women to early-onset metabolic abnormalities, including dyslipidemia, impaired glucose tolerance, and increased cardiovascular risk. Sex hormones directly modulate insulin sensitivity and glucose metabolism. Estrogen enhances insulin action, while androgens in excess, as seen in PCOS, promote insulin resistance. In men, declining testosterone levels with aging are associated with increased visceral fat, reduced insulin sensitivity, and increased cardiometabolic risk. These hormonal influences emphasize the importance of considering sex-specific endocrine profiles in stratifying CKM risk [68].

Pregnancy-related complications, such as gestational diabetes mellitus (GDM) and preeclampsia, serve as early indicators of increased risk of CKM in women. Women with a history of these complications are more likely to develop hypertension, T2DM, and CKD later in life. These conditions share common pathophysiologic pathways with CKM syndrome, including endothelial dysfunction and chronic inflammation [69].

In addition to biological differences, psychosocial and behavioral factors determined by gender norms have an impact on CKD risk. Women are more likely to experience psychosocial stress, caregiving burdens, and economic disadvantage, all of which contribute to suboptimal self-care and limited access to preventive healthcare. In contrast, men often engage in riskier behaviors, such as smoking and excessive alcohol consumption, which further aggravate their risk profile. In clinical practice, sex differences are often overlooked, leading to underdiagnosis and undertreatment of women. Cardiovascular symptoms in women may be misattributed to noncardiac causes, and clinical trials have historically underrepresented women, leading to evidence gaps. Recognition of sex-specific phenotypes and incorporation of sex-disaggregated data into research and clinical guidelines are imperative to advance personalized care in CKM syndrome.

Early-Life and In-Utero Factors

Factors in early life and intrauterine life are increasingly recognized as key contributors to the development of CKM syndrome. The developmental origins of health and disease (DOHaD) hypothesis posits that environmental exposures during critical periods of fetal and early postnatal life can induce permanent physiological and metabolic changes that influence susceptibility to disease throughout life. These early exposures can lead to structural and functional programming of viscera such as the heart, kidneys, pancreas, and vascular system, thereby setting the stage for future cardiometabolic risk [70].

One of the most studied in-utero risk factors is maternal undernutrition. Inadequate maternal nutrition during pregnancy may lead to intrauterine growth restriction (IUGR), resulting in low birth weight, which may be associated with impaired nephron development, reduced renal reserve, endothelial dysfunction, and insulin resistance. People born with low birth weight are more likely to develop hypertension, CKD, and T2DM in adulthood. This association is thought to result from fetal adaptations to nutrient deficiency that prioritize immediate survival but compromise long-term health [71].

On the other hand, maternal supranutritional status and GDM also pose significant risks. The fetus of mothers with GDM is exposed to intrauterine hyperglycemia, leading to hyperinsulinemia and fetal adiposity. These metabolic disorders predispose the child to obesity, impaired glucose tolerance, and insulin resistance from an early age. In addition, maternal obesity has been associated with increased systemic inflammation and oxidative stress during pregnancy, further influencing the metabolic programming of offspring [72].

Prenatal exposure to glucocorticoids (either due to maternal stress or medical treatment) may also have long-lasting effects on CKM risk. Glucocorticoids modulate the expression of genes involved in glucose metabolism, renal sodium handling, and vascular tone. Excessive fetal exposure may lead to a heightened hypothalamic-pituitary-adrenal (HPA) axis response, predisposing the individual to hypertension and metabolic syndrome later in life. Epigenetic modifications provide a mechanistic link between early-life exposures and long-term disease risk. DNA methylation, histone modifications, and microRNA expression can be altered by in-utero conditions and early nutrition, leading to persistent changes in gene expression without altering the genetic code. For example, altered methylation of genes involved in insulin signaling and lipid metabolism has been identified in offspring exposed to maternal obesity or undernutrition. These epigenetic marks can remain stable over time, influencing disease risk well into adulthood [73].

Infections and inflammation during pregnancy, such as maternal urinary tract infections or preeclampsia, have also been linked to adverse cardiometabolic outcomes in offspring. These conditions may impair placental perfusion and fetal nutrient delivery, triggering compensatory mechanisms that promote altered vascular development and metabolic dysfunction [74].

Then postnatal factors, including early feeding practices and rapid weight gain during infancy, can compound prenatal risk. Breastfeeding has been associated with a reduced risk of obesity, hypertension, and T2DM, whereas early introduction of high-calorie formula and rapid catch-up growth in LBW (Low Birth Weight) infants may accelerate metabolic dysregulation. These findings emphasize the importance of early nutrition in modulating CKM risk [75].

Moreover, environmental exposures in early life, such as tobacco smoke, air pollution, and endocrine-disrupting chemicals, also contribute to cardiometabolic programming. These agents can interfere with hormonal signaling and oxidative balance, affecting organ development and immune function. Children exposed to secondhand smoke or pollutants have shown increased markers of systemic inflammation and vascular stiffness, which are early predictors of CKM-related conditions [76].

Learning Objectives

- Understand the epidemiological trends and global burden of CKM syndrome
- Identify and describe the major modifiable and nonmodifiable risk factors contributing to CKM syndrome
- Explain the interrelated pathophysiological mechanisms linking obesity, type 2 diabetes, hypertension, and chronic kidney disease
- Analyze the role of chronic inflammation, oxidative stress, and RAAS activation in CKM progression
- Evaluate the influence of genetic, epigenetic, behavioral, and sex-specific factors in CKM syndrome development
- Recognize the significance of early-life and in-utero exposures in shaping long-term cardiometabolic risk

Key Reading

- *CKM syndrome* represents the convergence of cardiovascular, kidney, and metabolic disorders, with overlapping risk factors and pathophysiological mechanisms.
- *Obesity and adipose tissue dysfunction* are primary drivers of CKM syndrome, promoting inflammation, oxidative stress, and insulin resistance that affect both cardiovascular and renal systems.
- *Type 2 diabetes mellitus* plays a central role through chronic hyperglycemia and insulin resistance, contributing to vascular and glomerular injury.
- *Hypertension and dyslipidemia* act synergistically to exacerbate endothelial dysfunction, inflammation, and organ damage.
- *Chronic inflammation and oxidative stress* form a self-reinforcing loop that accelerates endothelial injury, fibrosis, and CKM progression.
- *Activation of the RAAS* promotes vasoconstriction, fluid retention, and fibrosis, directly linking metabolic dysfunction to cardiovascular and renal damage.
- *Genetic and epigenetic factors* modulate individual susceptibility, influencing pathways related to metabolism, inflammation, and organ resilience.
- *Behavioral risk factors* such as unhealthy diet, physical inactivity, smoking, poor sleep, and stress significantly increase CKM risk.
- *Sex-specific differences* affect disease incidence, symptoms, and outcomes due to hormonal, structural, and behavioral disparities.
- *Early-life and in-utero exposures*, including maternal nutrition and fetal growth patterns, have long-term impacts on cardiometabolic health through developmental programming.

References

1. Ndumele CE, Rangaswami J, Chow SL, Neeland IJ, Tuttle KR, Khan SS, et al. Cardiovascular-kidney-metabolic health: a presidential advisory from the American Heart Association. Circulation. 2023;148(20):1606–35. https://doi.org/10.1161/CIR.0000000000001184.
2. Romeo S, Vidal-Puig A, Husain M, Ahima R, Arca M, Bhatt DL, et al. Clinical staging to guide management of metabolic disorders and their sequelae: a European Atherosclerosis Society consensus statement. Eur Heart J. 2025:ehaf314. https://doi.org/10.1093/eurheartj/ehaf314.
3. Martin SS, Aday AW, Allen NB, Almarzooq ZI, Anderson CAM, Arora P, et al. 2025 Heart disease and stroke statistics: a report of US and Global Data From the American Heart Association. Circulation [Internet]. 2025 [cited 2025 May 15];151(8). Available from: https://doi.org/10.1161/CIR.0000000000001303.
4. Ostrominski JW, Arnold SV, Butler J, Fonarow GC, Hirsch JS, Palli SR, et al. Prevalence and overlap of cardiac, renal, and metabolic conditions in US adults, 1999-2020. JAMA Cardiol. 2023;8(11):1050. https://doi.org/10.1001/jamacardio.2023.3241.
5. Aggarwal R, Ostrominski JW, Vaduganathan M. Prevalence of cardiovascular-kidney-metabolic syndrome stages in US adults, 2011-2020. JAMA. 2024;331(21):1858. https://doi.org/10.1001/jama.2024.6892.

6. Zhu R, Wang R, He J, Wang L, Chen H, Niu X, et al. Prevalence of cardiovascular-kidney-metabolic syndrome stages by social determinants of health. JAMA Netw Open. 2024;7(11):e2445309. https://doi.org/10.1001/jamanetworkopen.2024.45309.
7. Yim Y, Lee JE, Son Y, Kim S, Lee H, Lee S, et al. Long-term trends in the prevalence of cardiovascular-kidney-metabolic syndrome in South Korea, 2011–2021: a representative longitudinal serial study. Lancet Reg Health West Pac. 2025;55:101474. https://doi.org/10.1016/j.lanwpc.2025.101474.
8. Shah N, Huang X, Yang S, Allen NB, Chaker L, Bos D, et al. Defining high risk in the cardiovascular-kidney-metabolic syndrome and associated cardiovascular disease outcomes. Eur Heart J. 2024 Oct 28;45(Supplement_1):ehae666.2686. https://doi.org/10.1093/eurheartj/ehae666.2686.
9. Beles M, Masuy I, Verstreken S, Bartunek J, Dierckx R, Heggermont W, et al. Cardio–renal–metabolic syndrome: clinical features and dapagliflozin eligibility in a real-world heart failure cohort. ESC Heart Failure. 2023;10(4):2269–80. https://doi.org/10.1002/ehf2.14381.
10. Trimarco V, Izzo R, Pacella D, Virginia Manzi M, Trama U, Lembo M, et al. Increased prevalence of cardiovascular-kidney-metabolic syndrome during COVID-19: a propensity score-matched study. Diabetes Res Clin Pract. 2024 Dec;218:111926. https://doi.org/10.1016/j.diabres.2024.111926.
11. Correction to: Cardiovascular-kidney-metabolic health: a presidential advisory from the American Heart Association. Circulation [Internet]. 2024 [cited 2025 Apr 27];149(13). Available from: https://doi.org/10.1161/CIR.0000000000001241.
12. Sebastian SA, Padda I, Johal G. Cardiovascular-kidney-metabolic (CKM) syndrome: a state-of-the-art review. Curr Probl Cardiol. 2024 Feb;49(2):102344. https://doi.org/10.1016/j.cpcardiol.2023.102344.
13. Hotamisligil GS. Inflammation and metabolic disorders. Nature. 2006;444(7121):860–7. https://doi.org/10.1038/nature05485.
14. Steppan CM, Bailey ST, Bhat S, Brown EJ, Banerjee RR, Wright CM, et al. The hormone resistin links obesity to diabetes. Nature. 2001 Jan;409(6818):307–12. https://doi.org/10.1038/35053000.
15. Mihai S, Codrici E, Popescu ID, Enciu AM, Albulescu L, Necula LG, et al. Inflammation-related mechanisms in chronic kidney Disease prediction, progression, and outcome. J Immunol Res. 2018;2018:2180373. https://doi.org/10.1155/2018/2180373.
16. Sletten AC, Peterson LR, Schaffer JE. Manifestations and mechanisms of myocardial lipotoxicity in obesity. J Intern Med. 2018;284(5):478–91. https://doi.org/10.1111/joim.12728.
17. Drosatos K, Schulze PC. Cardiac lipotoxicity: molecular pathways and therapeutic implications. Curr Heart Fail Rep. 2013;10(2):109–21. https://doi.org/10.1007/s11897-013-0133-0.
18. Ren L, Cui H, Wang Y, Ju F, Cai Y, Gang X, et al. The role of lipotoxicity in kidney disease: from molecular mechanisms to therapeutic prospects. Biomed Pharmacother. 2023;161:114465. https://doi.org/10.1016/j.biopha.2023.114465.
19. Bobulescu IA. Renal lipid metabolism and lipotoxicity. Curr Opin Nephrol Hypertens. 2010;19(4):393–402. https://doi.org/10.1097/mnh.0b013e32833aa4ac.
20. Ge M, Fontanesi F, Merscher S, Fornoni A. The vicious cycle of renal lipotoxicity and mitochondrial dysfunction. Front Physiol. 2020;11:732. https://doi.org/10.3389/fphys.2020.00732.
21. Shargorodsky M, Boaz M, Goldberg Y, Matas Z, Gavish D, Fux A, et al. Adiponectin and vascular properties in obese patients: is it a novel biomarker of early atherosclerosis? Int J Obes (Lond). 2009;33(5):553–8. https://doi.org/10.1038/ijo.2009.37.
22. Thethi T, Kamiyama M, Kobori H. The link between the renin-angiotensin-aldosterone system and renal injury in obesity and the metabolic syndrome. Curr Hypertens Rep. 2012;14(2):160–9. https://doi.org/10.1007/s11906-012-0245-z.
23. Ferdinand KC. An overview of cardiovascular-kidney-metabolic syndrome. Am J Manag Care. 2024;30(10 Suppl):S181–8. https://doi.org/10.37765/ajmc.2024.89670.

24. The Emerging Risk Factors Collaboration. Diabetes mellitus, fasting blood glucose concentration, and risk of vascular disease: a collaborative meta-analysis of 102 prospective studies. Lancet. 2010;375(9733):2215–22. https://doi.org/10.1016/S0140-6736(10)60484-9.
25. Guo FS, Dou JH, Wang JX, Guo C, Wu RY, Sun XL, et al. Association of the stress hyperglycemia ratio for all-cause and cardiovascular mortality in population with cardiovascular-kidney-metabolic syndrome stages 0–4: evidence from a large cohort study. Diabetol Metab Syndr. 2025;17(1):109. https://doi.org/10.1186/s13098-025-01671-2.
26. Laaksonen DE. Metabolic syndrome and development of diabetes mellitus: application and validation of recently suggested definitions of the metabolic syndrome in a prospective cohort study. Am J Epidemiol. 2002;156(11):1070–7. https://doi.org/10.1093/aje/kwf145.
27. Ndumele CE, Neeland IJ, Tuttle KR, Chow SL, Mathew RO, Khan SS, et al. A synopsis of the evidence for the science and clinical management of cardiovascular-kidney-metabolic (CKM) syndrome: a scientific statement from the American Heart Association. Circulation. 2023;148(20):1636–64. https://doi.org/10.1161/CIR.0000000000001186.
28. Massy ZA, Drueke TB. Combination of cardiovascular, kidney, and metabolic diseases in a syndrome named cardiovascular-kidney-metabolic, with new risk prediction equations. Kidney Int Rep. 2024 Sep;9(9):2608–18. https://doi.org/10.1016/j.ekir.2024.05.033.
29. Gallo G, Savoia C. New insights into endothelial dysfunction in cardiometabolic diseases: potential mechanisms and clinical implications. IJMS. 2024;25(5):2973. https://doi.org/10.3390/ijms25052973.
30. Gao C, Gao S, Zhao R, Shen P, Zhu X, Yang Y, et al. Association between systemic immune-inflammation index and cardiovascular-kidney-metabolic syndrome. Sci Rep. 2024;14(1):19151. https://doi.org/10.1038/s41598-024-69819-0.
31. Rubattu S, Mennuni S, Testa M, Mennuni M, Pierelli G, Pagliaro B, et al. Pathogenesis of chronic cardiorenal syndrome: is there a role for oxidative stress? IJMS. 2013;14(11):23011–32. https://doi.org/10.3390/ijms141123011.
32. Zhang K, Li J, Li Y, Yan K, Zhao X. Abstract 4140042: impact of inflammatory and insulin resistance biomarkers on long-term risks in coronary heart disease patients with cardiovascular-kidney-metabolic syndrome. Circulation. 2024;150(Suppl_1):A4140042. https://doi.org/10.1161/circ.150.suppl_1.4140042.
33. Kadowaki T, Maegawa H, Watada H, Yabe D, Node K, Murohara T, et al. Interconnection between cardiovascular, renal and metabolic disorders: a narrative review with a focus on Japan. Diabetes Obes Metab. 2022;24(12):2283–96. https://doi.org/10.1111/dom.14829.
34. Furman D, Campisi J, Verdin E, Carrera-Bastos P, Targ S, Franceschi C, et al. Chronic inflammation in the etiology of disease across the life span. Nat Med. 2019;25(12):1822–32. https://doi.org/10.1038/s41591-019-0675-0.
35. Libby P. Inflammation and cardiovascular disease mechanisms. Am J Clin Nutr. 2006;83(2):456S–60S. https://doi.org/10.1093/ajcn/83.2.456s.
36. Navarro-González JF, Mora-Fernández C. The role of inflammatory cytokines in diabetic nephropathy. J Am Soc Nephrol. 2008;19(3):433–42. https://doi.org/10.1681/asn.2007091048.
37. Duni A, Liakopoulos V, Rapsomanikis KP, Dounousi E. Chronic kidney disease and disproportionally increased cardiovascular damage: does oxidative stress explain the burden? Morishita R, editor. Oxid Med Cell Longev. 2017;2017(1):9036450. https://doi.org/10.1155/2017/9036450.
38. Ridker PM, Cannon CP, Morrow D, Rifai N, Rose LM, McCabe CH, et al. C-reactive protein levels and outcomes after statin therapy. N Engl J Med. 2005;352(1):20–8. https://doi.org/10.1056/nejmoa042378.
39. Fyhrquist F, Saijonmaa O. Renin-angiotensin system revisited. J Intern Med. 2008;264(3):224–36. https://doi.org/10.1111/j.1365-2796.2008.01981.x.
40. Paul M, Poyan Mehr A, Kreutz R. Physiology of local renin-angiotensin systems. Physiol Rev. 2006;86(3):747–803. https://doi.org/10.1152/physrev.00036.2005.
41. Bakris GL, Agarwal R, Anker SD, Pitt B, Ruilope LM, Rossing P, et al. Effect of finerenone on chronic kidney disease outcomes in type 2 diabetes. N Engl J Med. 2020;383(23):2219–29. https://doi.org/10.1056/nejmoa2025845.

42. Effects of an angiotensin-converting–enzyme inhibitor, ramipril, on cardiovascular events in high-risk patients. N Engl J Med. 2000;342(3):145–53. https://doi.org/10.1056/nejm200001203420301.
43. Patel VB, Zhong JC, Grant MB, Oudit GY. Role of the ACE2/angiotensin 1–7 axis of the renin–angiotensin system in heart failure. Circ Res. 2016;118(8):1313–26. https://doi.org/10.1161/CIRCRESAHA.116.307708.
44. Grant SFA, Thorleifsson G, Reynisdottir I, Benediktsson R, Manolescu A, Sainz J, et al. Variant of transcription factor 7-like 2 (TCF7L2) gene confers risk of type 2 diabetes. Nat Genet. 2006;38(3):320–3. https://doi.org/10.1038/ng1732.
45. Frayling TM, Timpson NJ, Weedon MN, Zeggini E, Freathy RM, Lindgren CM, et al. A common variant in the FTO gene is associated with body mass index and predisposes to childhood and adult obesity. Science. 2007;316(5826):889–94. https://doi.org/10.1126/science.1141634.
46. Vitart V, Rudan I, Hayward C, Gray NK, Floyd J, Palmer CN, et al. SLC2A9 is a newly identified urate transporter influencing serum urate concentration, urate excretion and gout. Nat Genet. 2008;40(4):437–42. https://doi.org/10.1038/ng.106.
47. Köttgen A, Pattaro C, Böger CA, Fuchsberger C, Olden M, Glazer NL, et al. New loci associated with kidney function and chronic kidney disease. Nat Genet. 2010;42(5):376–84. https://doi.org/10.1038/ng.568.
48. Heidemann BE, Wolters FJ, Kavousi M, Gruppen EG, Dullaart RP, Marais AD, et al. Adiposity and the development of dyslipidemia in APOE ε2 homozygous subjects: a longitudinal analysis in two population-based cohorts. Atherosclerosis. 2021;325:57–62. https://doi.org/10.1016/j.atherosclerosis.2021.04.001.
49. Rigat B, Hubert C, Alhenc-Gelas F, Cambien F, Corvol P, Soubrier F. An insertion/deletion polymorphism in the angiotensin I-converting enzyme gene accounting for half the variance of serum enzyme levels. J Clin Invest. 1990;86(4):1343–6. https://doi.org/10.1172/jci114844.
50. Deeb SS, Fajas L, Nemoto M, Pihlajamäki J, Mykkänen L, Kuusisto J, et al. A Pro12Ala substitution in PPARγ2 associated with decreased receptor activity, lower body mass index and improved insulin sensitivity. Nat Genet. 1998;20(3):284–7. https://doi.org/10.1038/3099.
51. Gloyn AL, Weedon MN, Owen KR, Turner MJ, Knight BA, Hitman G, et al. Large-scale association studies of variants in genes encoding the pancreatic β-cell KATP channel subunits Kir6.2 (KCNJ11) and SUR1 (ABCC8) confirm that the KCNJ11 E23K variant is associated with type 2 diabetes. Diabetes. 2003;52(2):568–72. https://doi.org/10.2337/diabetes.52.2.568.
52. Zhou Q, Weng Q, Zhang X, Liu Y, Tong J, Hao X, et al. Association between NPHS2 p.R229Q and focal segmental glomerular sclerosis/steroid-resistant nephrotic syndrome. Front Med. 2022;9:937122. https://doi.org/10.3389/fmed.2022.937122.
53. De Oliveira R, Moraes TI, Cerda A, Hirata MH, Fajardo CM, Sousa MC, et al. ADIPOQ and IL6 variants are associated with a pro-inflammatory status in obeses with cardiometabolic dysfunction. Diabetol Metab Syndr. 2015;7(1):34. https://doi.org/10.1186/s13098-015-0027-2.
54. Mahajan A, Taliun D, Thurner M, Robertson NR, Torres JM, Rayner NW, et al. Fine-mapping type 2 diabetes loci to single-variant resolution using high-density imputation and islet-specific epigenome maps. Nat Genet. 2018;50(11):1505–13. https://doi.org/10.1038/s41588-018-0241-6.
55. The international consortium for blood pressure genome-wide association studies. Genetic variants in novel pathways influence blood pressure and cardiovascular disease risk. Nature. 2011;478(7367):103–9. https://doi.org/10.1038/nature10405.
56. Small EM, Olson EN. Pervasive roles of microRNAs in cardiovascular biology. Nature. 2011;469(7330):336–42. https://doi.org/10.1038/nature09783.
57. Greco CM, Condorelli G. Epigenetic modifications and noncoding RNAs in cardiac hypertrophy and failure. Nat Rev Cardiol. 2015;12(8):488–97. https://doi.org/10.1038/nrcardio.2015.71.
58. Aagaard-Tillery KM, Grove K, Bishop J, Ke X, Fu Q, McKnight R, et al. Developmental origins of disease and determinants of chromatin structure: maternal diet modifies the primate fetal epigenome. J Mol Endocrinol. 2008;41(2):91–102. https://doi.org/10.1677/jme-08-0025.

59. Gluckman PD, Hanson MA. Developmental origins of disease paradigm: a mechanistic and evolutionary perspective. Pediatr Res. 2004;56(3):311–7. https://doi.org/10.1203/01.pdr.0000135998.08025.fb.
60. Mozaffarian D, Benjamin EJ, Go AS, Arnett DK, Blaha MJ, Cushman M, et al. Heart disease and stroke statistics—2016 update: a report From the American Heart Association. Circulation [Internet]. 2016 [cited 2025 Apr 29];133(4). Available from: https://doi.org/10.1161/cir.0000000000000350.
61. Gherasim A, Arhire LI, Niţă O, Popa AD, Graur M, Mihalache L. The relationship between lifestyle components and dietary patterns. Proc Nutr Soc. 2020;79(3):311–23. https://doi.org/10.1017/s0029665120006898.
62. Tremblay MS, Warburton DER, Janssen I, Paterson DH, Latimer AE, Rhodes RE, et al. New Canadian physical activity guidelines. Appl Physiol Nutr Metab. 2011;36(1):36–46. https://doi.org/10.1139/h11-009.
63. St-Onge MP, Grandner MA, Brown D, Conroy MB, Jean-Louis G, Coons M, et al. Sleep duration and quality: impact on lifestyle behaviors and cardiometabolic health: a scientific statement from the American Heart Association. Circulation [Internet]. 2016 [cited 2025 Apr 29];134(18). Available from: https://doi.org/10.1161/cir.0000000000000444.
64. Satyjeet F, Naz S, Kumar V, Aung NH, Bansari K, Irfan S, et al. Psychological stress as a risk factor for cardiovascular disease: a case-control study. Cureus [Internet]. 2020 [cited 2025 Apr 29]; Available from: https://www.cureus.com/articles/42459-psychological-stress-as-a-risk-factor-for-cardiovascular-disease-a-case-control-study. https://doi.org/10.7759/cureus.10757.
65. Regitz-Zagrosek V. Sex and gender differences in health: Science & Society Series on sex and science. EMBO Rep. 2012 Jul;13(7):596–603. https://doi.org/10.1038/embor.2012.87.
66. Maas AHEM, Appelman YEA. Gender differences in coronary heart disease. Neth Heart J. 2010 Nov;18(12):598–603. https://doi.org/10.1007/s12471-010-0841-y.
67. Neugarten J, Golestaneh L. Gender and the prevalence and progression of renal disease. Adv Chronic Kidney Dis. 2013;20(5):390–5. https://doi.org/10.1053/j.ackd.2013.05.004.
68. Varlamov O, Bethea CL, Roberts CT. Sex-specific differences in lipid and glucose metabolism. Front Endocrinol [Internet] 2015 [cited 2025 May 8];5. Available from: https://doi.org/10.3389/fendo.2014.00241.
69. Peters SAE, Woodward M. Sex differences in the burden and complications of diabetes. Curr Diab Rep. 2018;18(6):33. https://doi.org/10.1007/s11892-018-1005-5.
70. Barker DJP. The developmental origins of adult disease. J Am Coll Nutr. 2004;23(suppl 6):588S–95S. https://doi.org/10.1080/07315724.2004.10719428.
71. Simmons RA. Developmental origins of adult disease. Pediatr Clin North Am. 2009;56(3):449–66. https://doi.org/10.1016/j.pcl.2009.03.004.
72. Godfrey KM, Reynolds RM, Prescott SL, Nyirenda M, Jaddoe VWV, Eriksson JG, et al. Influence of maternal obesity on the long-term health of offspring. Lancet Diabetes Endocrinol. 2017;5(1):53–64. https://doi.org/10.1016/s2213-8587(16)30107-3.
73. Dodic M, Moritz K, Wintour EM. Prenatal exposure to glucocorticoids and adult disease. Arch Physiol Biochem. 2003;111(1):61–9. https://doi.org/10.1076/apab.111.1.61.15144.
74. Kumar M, Saadaoui M, Al Khodor S. Infections and pregnancy: effects on maternal and child health. Front Cell Infect Microbiol. 2022;12:873253. https://doi.org/10.3389/fcimb.2022.873253.
75. Lindholm A, Bergman S, Alm B, Bremander A, Dahlgren J, Roswall J, et al. Nutrition- and feeding practice-related risk factors for rapid weight gain during the first year of life: a population-based birth cohort study. BMC Pediatr. 2020;20(1):507. https://doi.org/10.1186/s12887-020-02391-4.
76. Braun JM. Early-life exposure to EDCs: role in childhood obesity and neurodevelopment. Nat Rev Endocrinol. 2017;13(3):161–73. https://doi.org/10.1038/nrendo.2016.186.

Chapter 4
Genetic and Molecular Aspects of Cardiovascular-Kidney-Metabolic Syndrome

Cristina Rusu, Monica Cristina Pânzaru, and Irina Nucă

Introduction

The American Heart Association characterizes cardiovascular-kidney-metabolic (CKM) syndrome as a medical concern resulting from the interconnections among cardiovascular disease (CVD), chronic kidney disease (CKD), and metabolic syndrome, most commonly with type 2 diabetes mellitus and obesity [1]. Cardiovascular, renal, and metabolic illnesses are major contributors to global morbidity and mortality.

Metabolic factors such as hypertension, insulin resistance, dyslipidemia, and obesity frequently co-occur and accelerate each other's progression. Lifestyle and environmental factors are important; nonetheless, genetic and molecular substrates are crucial to illness susceptibility and pathogenesis [1, 2].

C. Rusu · M. C. Pânzaru
Grigore T. Popa University of Medicine and Pharmacy, Iasi, Romania

Regional Genetics Center of St. Maria Children's Clinical Hospital, Iasi, Romania
e-mail: monica.panzaru@umfiasi.ro

I. Nucă (✉)
Grigore T. Popa University of Medicine and Pharmacy, Iasi, Romania
e-mail: irina.resmerita@umfiasi.ro

M. Floria, D. M. Tanase (eds.), *Cardiovascular-Kidney-Metabolic Syndrome*,
https://doi.org/10.1007/978-3-032-11445-7_4

Metabolic Syndrome

Metabolic syndrome (MetS) is a group of metabolic features that significantly increase the risk of CVD and diabetes. This pathology has been recognized for a long time, but its importance as a public health issue has only lately been brought to attention, with prevalence increasing across all age demographics [3].

The patient's phenotype at the moment of diagnosis can differ significantly even among affected members of the same family. This heterogeneity results in difficulty for genetic research that is based on a clearly clinical phenotype for relevance of the results.

As a polygenic condition, type 2 diabetes is known to be genetically determined by more than 800 susceptibility loci [4]. The majority of genetic studies has used GWAS-identified common variants with low penetrance. Such risk alleles have little effect on disease risk alone, but polygenic scores may enhance risk prediction [5, 6]. Studies indicate that East Asians are more likely to develop type 2 diabetes than Europeans with similar body mass index or waist circumference, suggesting a genetic predisposition to insulin resistance or diabetes. Although most susceptibility loci for type 2 diabetes have been discovered in European GWAS, non-European-specific loci may still exist (Table 4.1) [7].

Central obesity is caused by a complex interaction of hereditary and environmental variables [8]. Genetic studies have revealed how certain genetic variables affect energy homeostasis, especially the control of appetite [9, 10]. Multiple studies have highlighted important genes (Table 4.2) as key contributors, improved our

Table 4.1 Genes involved in type 2 diabetes, chromosomal locus, and effect

Gene	Locus	Effect
TCF7L2	10q25.2–q25.3	Regulator of insulin secretion and β-cell function
FTO	16q12.2	Affect adipocyte differentiation and appetite regulation
PPARG	3p25.2	Regulator of adipogenesis; mutations reduce insulin sensitivity
KCNJ11	11p15.1	Controls β-cell membrane potential and insulin secretion
ABCC8	11p15.1	Regulator of ATP-sensitive potassium channels of β-cells; variants linked to impaired insulin release
SLC30A8	8q24.11	Regulates zinc accumulation in insulin granules in β-cells; essential for proper insulin crystallization
IRS1	2q36.3	Mediates insulin signal transduction; variants lead to insulin resistance
HHEX	10q23.33	Involved in pancreatic islet development; variants affect β-cell function and insulin secretion
CDKAL1	6p22.3	Inhibits proinsulin processing; strongly linked to β-cell dysfunction
MTNR1B	11q21	Impacts circadian regulation of insulin secretion; variants impair glucose tolerance

Table 4.2 Frequent genes associated with obesity and metabolic syndrome

Gene	Locus	Effect
FTO	16q12.2	Regulation of energy intake
MC4R	18q21.3	Impairs satiety signaling
LEP	7q31.3	Regulator of leptin production
LEPR	1p31	Disrupts leptin signaling;
POMC	2p23.3	Affects melanocortin pathway; associated with severe obesity when deficient
SH2B1	16p11.2	Insulin and leptin signaling; variants linked to BMI increase
NEGR1	1p31.1	Implicated in neuronal growth and body weight regulation
BDNF	11p14.1	Regulator of brain function and appetite; low expression linked to obesity
TMEM18	2p25.3	Possibly involved in energy homeostasis

understanding of its molecular foundation, and created new options for prevention and treatment [9]. The fat mass and obesity-associated (*FTO*) gene variations were found to be a major risk factor for obesity in the general population and severe juvenile obesity. The earliest intron of *FTO* had the strongest connection with single-nucleotide SNPs. Appetite modulation helps *FTO* gene mutations affect energy balance by increasing energy consumption and a preference for high-calorie foods [11–15].

Cardio-Renal Syndrome

Studies have estimated a heritability of the glomerular filtration rate between 6% and 30% in the general population, and several loci have been reported to be associated with kidney function: *UMOD, CUBN, OAF, CACNA1S, RPL3L, CERS2*, and *C9* [16, 17] The strongest risk gene is *UMOD*, which encodes uromodulin, the most abundant protein in normal urine [18]. Uromodulin plays a variety of physiological roles, including the regulation of the renal outer medullary potassium channel, modulation of the sodium-potassium-chloride cotransporter, and control of the Na^+/Cl^- cotransporter in the early distal convoluted tubule. It also contributes to calcium homeostasis through transient receptor potential cation channels TRPV5 and TRPV6 and magnesium balance via the TRPM6 channel. Additionally, uromodulin regulates blood pressure and protects against kidney stone formation. Pathogenic variants in UMOD are associated with autosomal-dominant tubulo-interstitial kidney disease [19].

CUBN is a gene locus associated with albuminuria. Elevated urinary albumin-to-creatinine ratio (UACR) is a hallmark of kidney dysfunction and predicts poor clinical outcomes: end-stage kidney disease, cardiovascular disease, and mortality. Genetic variants associated with UACR have been reported in many other genes,

Table 4.3 Genes involved in diabetic kidney disease, chromosomal locus, and effect

Gene	Locus	Effect
ABCG2	*4q22*	Involved in uric acid transport
AFF3	*2q11.2*	Associated with autoimmune conditions
AGER (RAGE)	*6p21.3*	Contributes to oxidative stress and inflammation
AUH	*9q22.31*	Regulator of leucine metabolism
CERS2	*1q21.3*	Regulator of ceramide synthesis; implicated in diabetes and kidney function
CDCA7	*2q31*	Regulator of glomerular function
CNDP1	18q22.3	Encodes carnosinase 1 (CN1) polymorphism 5 L–5 L is associated with protection against diabetic nephropathy
ELMO1	7p14.1	Implicated in diabetic nephropathy; elevated ELMO1 expression increases oxidative stress and kidney damage

including *HBB, NR3C2, COL4A4, OAF, PRKC1, TGFB1*, *MUC1*, and *CYP1A1*. *NR3C2* encodes a key factor of the renin–angiotensin–aldosterone system and links this pathway to albuminuria [20]. Some genes, like *CUBN*, *COL4A4, and MUC1*, are also associated with monogenic kidney disorders (e.g., chronic proteinuria, Alport syndrome, and tubulointerstitial kidney disease, autosomal dominant). While pathogenic, deleterious variants can lead to monogenic disorders, hypomorphic and/or regulatory variants can have a milder effect but a higher frequency in the general population. Polygenic risk scores (PRS) combine the effects of many genetic variants and may increase prediction accuracy [21].

Also, the identification of individuals at increased risk of ESKD is challenging. Rapid decline in creatinine-based eGFR is associated with increased ESKD risk (5- and 12-fold). A GWAS meta-analysis reported significant variants for rapid kidney function decline in *UMOD-PDILT*, *PRKAG2*, *WDR72*, and *OR2S2* [22].

In African populations, polymorphisms in *APOL1* gene are associated with the risk of CKD development [23].

Genetic variations have a significant role in susceptibility to diabetic kidney disease. SNPs in genes associated with oxidative stress (e.g., *SOD1/2*, *PPARG*, *GPX1*, *CYBA*, *MT2A*), metabolism (e.g., *SPP1*, *BGLAP*, *MGP*, *CYP24A1*, *HSD11B1*, *ABCG8*), the renin-angiotensin-aldosterone system (e.g., *ACE2*, *AGTR2, RENBP*), immune function (e.g., *ML2*), transcription regulation (e.g., *EP300*), and transmembrane channels (e.g., *AQP11*) have been linked to an increased risk of CKD progression in patients with diabetes [24]. Other genes associated with susceptibility or resistance to diabetic kidney disease are *ABCG2, AFF3, AGER,, AUH, CARS, CERS2, CDCA7/SP3, CHN2, CNDP1, ELMO1, ERBB4, FRMD3, GCKR, GLRA3, KNG1, LIMK2, MMP9, NMUR2, MSRB3/HMGA2, MYH9, PVT1, RAET1L, RGMA/MCTP2, RPS12, SASH1, SCAF8/CNKSR3, SHROOM3, SLC12A3, SORBS1, TMPO, UMOD,* and *ZMIZ1* (Table 4.3) [25]. Chronic hyperglycemia promotes inflammation, oxidative stress, immune cell infiltration, lipid peroxidation, DNA damage, and fibrosis.

Kidney Metabolic Syndrome

Epigenetic factors, including abnormal DNA methylation, histone modifications, and changes in microRNA expression (and consequently gene transcription silencing), contribute to kidney dysfunctions (e.g., transforming growth factor-beta1 signaling regulates the expression of some microRNAs, such as miR-21, miR-132, and miR-433, that play a pathological role in kidney diseases). Hypermethylation of RASAL1 has been associated with fibroblast activation and fibrogenesis in the fibrotic kidneys [26].

Table 4.4 Genes associated with kidney disease, chromosomal locus, and effect

Gene	Locus	Effect
APOL1	22q12.3	Apolipoprotein L1—susceptibility to focal segmental glomerulosclerosis in African Americans
C9	5p13.1	Key component of the membrane attack complex—associated with membrane disruption
CACNA1S	1q32.1	L-type voltage-dependent calcium channel—leading to muscle weakness and kidney dysfunction
CERS2	1q21.3	Very-long-chain ceramides signaling molecules—associated with albuminuria, CKD, DKD
COL4A4	2q36.3	Alpha chains of the heterotrimeric type IV collagen—component of basement membranes, hematuria and Alport syndrome
CUBN	10p13	Dysfunction of cubilin coexpressed with megalin (megalin-mediated endocytosis) in renal proximal tubules—low molecular weight proteinuria
HBB	11p15.4	Abnormal hemoglobin—vaso-occlusion, ischemia-reperfusion, and hemolysis-induced renal injury
MUC1	1q22	Transmembrane mucin expressed on the apical borders of secretory epithelial cells—tubulointerstitial kidney disease
NR3C2	4q31.23	Nuclear receptor acts as a ligand-dependent transcription factor and mediates the effects of mineralocorticoids on the distal parts of the nephron
OAF	11q13.1	Regulator of tubular uptake of albumin
PRKAG2	7q36.1	Regulator of cellular energy homeostasis
PTH1R	3p21.31	Bone and kidney signaling and calcium metabolism
RPL3L	16p13.3	Encodes a ribosomal protein-like protein specific to skeletal and cardiac muscle
PRKC1	3q26.2	Involved in cell survival, polarity, and insulin signaling pathways
TGFB1	19q13.2	Key role in kidney disease, vascular remodeling, and insulin resistance
UMOD	16p12.3	Associated with CKD and hypertension via tubular salt handling and immune modulation
WDR72	15q21.3	Associated with distal renal tubular acidosis and enamel defects
WIPF3	20q13.12	Actin cytoskeleton regulator

Table 4.5 Genes associated with cardio-renal dysfunction, chromosomal locus, and their effect

Gene	Locus	Effect
NOS3	1q32.1	Activation pathway of angiotensinogen—regulator of blood pressure and electrolyte balance
EDN1	6p24.1	Regulator of vascular tone, blood pressure, and contributes to endothelial dysfunction.
INS	11p15.5	Regulation of carbohydrate, fat, and protein metabolism; mutations affect insulin secretion and insulin resistance
TGFB1	19q13.2	Involved in fibrosis, inflammation, and insulin resistance.
EGFR	7p11.2	Cellular proliferation, differentiation, and survival; dysregulation linked to obesity-related metabolic disorders
CCL2	17q12	Mediates the initiation and amplification of inflammatory responses, especially in adipose tissue, vascular inflammation, and insulin resistance. It is linked to metabolic syndrome and cardiovascular disease by promoting monocyte infiltration into vascular endothelium and adipose tissue
SERPINE1	7q22.1	Contributes to prothrombotic state in MetS
TIMP2	17q25.3	Inhibits matrix metalloproteinases, involved in vascular integrity and tissue repair. Altered activity affects cardiovascular remodeling
MPO	17q22	Key role in oxidative stress and inflammation in vascular and metabolic disorders
REN	1q32.1	Regulator of blood pressure and fluid balance. Polymorphisms are linked to hypertension and insulin resistance
CRP	1q23.2	Mediator of systemic inflammation in obesity and MetS
ACE	17q23.3	Involved in blood pressure regulation, endothelial dysfunction, and vascular inflammation

Monogenic disorders (e.g., ADPKD, Alport syndrome, autosomal-dominant tubulointerstitial kidney disease) are responsible for 10–15% of adults, and the majority of pediatric patients who need KRT (Table 4.4).

Neurohormonal factors like the autonomic nervous system, the renin-angiotensin-aldosterone system (RAAS), arginine vasopressin (AVP), and endothelin-1 (ET-1) have major roles in hemodynamic stability and cardio-renal dysfunction. The genes associated with cardio-renal dysfunction are involved in protease binding, regulation of blood vessel diameter, advanced glycation endproducts (AGE-RAGE) signaling pathway in diabetic complications, and HIF-1 signaling pathway [27, 28] (Table 4.5).

Learning Objectives

- Understand the genetic basis of CKM syndrome
- Evaluate the influence of genetic and epigenetic factors in CKM syndrome development
- Explain the role of genetic testing in patients with metabolic syndrome, CKD, and CVD
- Identify common genetic variants associated with CKM syndrome, and explain their role in pathogenesis
- Explain the intrafamilial phenotypic variability
- Analyze the role of polygenic scores in risk prediction
- Recognize the circumstances that arouse suspicion of a monogenic disease

Key Reading

- *CKM syndrome components*—metabolic syndrome, CKD, and CVD—are interconnected through shared molecular and pathophysiological pathways.
- Inflammation, endothelial dysfunction, renin-angiotensin-aldosterone system, dysregulation of adipokines, insulin resistance, and mitochondrial dysfunction enhance *the risk of disease progression.*
- *Genetic and epigenetic factors* modulate susceptibility to CKM syndrome and related phenotypes.
- *Many susceptibility loci have been identified for each component*, but further large studies are necessary to establish the key genetic factors linking these entities.
- *Epigenetic factors* involve DNA methylation, histone modification, and non-coding RNA regulation.
- *Some genetic variants have a mild effect*, but polygenic risk scores combine the effects of many polymorphisms and may increase prediction accuracy.
- *Screening for CKM should begin early*, and identification of genetic variants associated with high risk is mandatory.
- Despite the rarity of monogenic disorders, taken together, *a nonnegligible percentage of patients with CKM have a purely genetic disease* (e.g., MODY, ADPKD, Alport syndrome).

Genetic testing in the context of CKM syndrome aims to assess risk, guide prevention, and help inform treatment decisions. In present, for cardiovascular disease the common genes tested are *APOE*, *PCSK9*, *LDLR*, *LPA*, which are involved in cholesterol metabolism, familial hypercholesterolemia, risk stratification; for chronic kidney disease the most common gene tested are *UMOD*, *APOL1,* and *SLC7A9*, which are predictive in hereditary nephropathies and progressive CKD; for type 2 diabetes the most common tested genes are *TCF7L2*, *PPARG*, *FTO*, *KCNJ11*; and for obesity/metabolic syndrome the most common tested genes are *TCF7L2*, *PPARG*, *FTO*, *KCNJ11*. Genetic testing in CKM is useful in order to identify high-risk individuals earlier, personalize lifestyle recommendations or treatment choices, and inform family members of their hereditary risk.

References

1. Ndumele CE, Rangaswami J, Chow SL, Neeland IJ, Tuttle KR, Khan SS, et al. Cardiovascular-kidney-metabolic health: a presidential advisory from the American Heart Association. Circulation. 2023;148(20):1606–35. https://doi.org/10.1161/CIR.0000000000001184.
2. Bansal N, Weiner D, Sarnak M. Cardiovascular-kidney-metabolic health syndrome: what does the American Heart Association framework mean for nephrology? J Am Soc Nephrol. 2024;35(5):649–52. https://doi.org/10.1681/ASN.0000000000000323.
3. Falkner B, Cossrow ND. Prevalence of metabolic syndrome and obesity-associated hypertension in the racial ethnic minorities of the United States. Curr Hypertens Rep. 2014;16(7):449. https://doi.org/10.1007/s11906-014-0449-5.
4. Imamura M, Maeda S. Genetic studies of type 2 diabetes, and microvascular complications of diabetes. Diabetol Int. 2024;15(4):699–706. https://doi.org/10.1007/s13340-024-00727-4.
5. Chan JC, Malik V, Jia W, Kadowaki T, Yajnik CS, Yoon KH, et al. Diabetes in Asia: epidemiology, risk factors, and pathophysiology. JAMA. 2009;301(20):2129–40. https://doi.org/10.1001/jama.2009.726.
6. Huxley R, James WP, Barzi F, Patel JV, Lear SA, Suriyawongpaisal P, et al. Ethnic comparisons of the cross-sectional relationships between measures of body size with diabetes and hypertension. Obes Rev. 2008;9(Suppl 1):53–61. https://doi.org/10.1111/j.1467-789X.2007.00439.x.
7. Cho YS, Chen CH, Hu C, Long J, Ong RT, Sim X, et al. Meta-analysis of genome-wide association studies identifies eight new loci for type 2 diabetes in east Asians. Nat Genet. 2011;44(1):67–72. https://doi.org/10.1038/ng.1019.
8. Lister NB, Baur LA, Felix JF, Hill AJ, Marcus C, Reinehr T, et al. Child and adolescent obesity. Nat Rev Dis Primers. 2023;9(1):24. https://doi.org/10.1038/s41572-023-00435-4.
9. Vourdoumpa A, Paltoglou G, Charmandari E. The genetic basis of childhood obesity: a systematic review. Nutrients. 2023;15(6) https://doi.org/10.3390/nu15061416.
10. Littleton SH, Berkowitz RI, Grant SFA. Genetic determinants of childhood obesity. Mol Diagn Ther. 2020;24(6):653–63. https://doi.org/10.1007/s40291-020-00496-1.
11. Dina C, Meyre D, Gallina S, Durand E, Korner A, Jacobson P, et al. Variation in FTO contributes to childhood obesity and severe adult obesity. Nat Genet. 2007;39(6):724–6. https://doi.org/10.1038/ng2048.
12. Wardle J, Llewellyn C, Sanderson S, Plomin R. The FTO gene and measured food intake in children. Int J Obes (Lond). 2009;33(1):42–5. https://doi.org/10.1038/ijo.2008.174.

13. Frayling TM, Timpson NJ, Weedon MN, Zeggini E, Freathy RM, Lindgren CM, et al. A common variant in the FTO gene is associated with body mass index and predisposes to childhood and adult obesity. Science. 2007;316(5826):889–94. https://doi.org/10.1126/science.1141634.
14. Ipekoglu G, Ari E, Aydogdu A, Korkmaz F, Celik H, Ozturk F, et al. Genetic insights into endurance athlete status: a meta-analysis of ACVR1B, AGT, FTO, IL-6, and NRF2 gene polymorphisms. J Biol Methods. 2024;11(3):e99010021. https://doi.org/10.14440/jbm.2024.0013.
15. Sharma T, Badaruddoza B. Genetic association of FTO gene polymorphisms with obesity and its related phenotypes: a case-control study. J Cardiovasc Thorac Res. 2024;16(2):102–12. https://doi.org/10.34172/jcvtr.33038.
16. Torra R, Furlano M, Ortiz A, Ars E. Genetic kidney diseases as an underrecognized cause of chronic kidney disease: the key role of international registry reports. Clin Kidney J. 2021;14(8):1879–85. https://doi.org/10.1093/ckj/sfab056.
17. Tin A, Kottgen A. Genome-wide association studies of CKD and related traits. Clin J Am Soc Nephrol. 2020;15(11):1643–56. https://doi.org/10.2215/CJN.00020120.
18. Kottgen A, Pattaro C. The CKDGen Consortium: ten years of insights into the genetic basis of kidney function. Kidney Int. 2020;97(2):236–42. https://doi.org/10.1016/j.kint.2019.10.027.
19. Thielemans R, Speeckaert R, Delrue C, De Bruyne S, Oyaert M, Speeckaert MM. Unveiling the hidden power of uromodulin: a promising potential biomarker for kidney diseases. Diagnostics (Basel). 2023;13(19) https://doi.org/10.3390/diagnostics13193077.
20. Smith SB, Parisien M, Bair E, Belfer I, Chabot-Dore AJ, Gris P, et al. Genome-wide association reveals contribution of MRAS to painful temporomandibular disorder in males. Pain. 2019;160(3):579–91. https://doi.org/10.1097/j.pain.0000000000001438.
21. Wuttke M, Li Y, Li M, Sieber KB, Feitosa MF, Gorski M, et al. A catalog of genetic loci associated with kidney function from analyses of a million individuals. Nat Genet. 2019;51(6):957–72. https://doi.org/10.1038/s41588-019-0407-x.
22. Gorski M, Jung B, Li Y, Matias-Garcia PR, Wuttke M, Coassin S, et al. Meta-analysis uncovers genome-wide significant variants for rapid kidney function decline. Kidney Int. 2021;99(4):926–39. https://doi.org/10.1016/j.kint.2020.09.030.
23. Kanji Z, Powe CE, Wenger JB, Huang C, Ankers E, Sullivan DA, et al. Genetic variation in APOL1 associates with younger age at hemodialysis initiation. J Am Soc Nephrol. 2011;22(11):2091–7. https://doi.org/10.1681/ASN.2010121234.
24. Mira FS, Oliveiros B, Carreira IM, Alves R, Ribeiro IP. Genetic variants related to increased CKD progression-a systematic review. Biology (Basel). 2025;14(1) https://doi.org/10.3390/biology14010068.
25. Gu HF. Genetic and epigenetic studies in diabetic kidney disease. Front Genet. 2019;10:507. https://doi.org/10.3389/fgene.2019.00507.
26. Chung AC, Lan HY. MicroRNAs in renal fibrosis. Front Physiol. 2015;6:50. https://doi.org/10.3389/fphys.2015.00050.
27. Ahmed MM, Tazyeen S, Alam A, Farooqui A, Ali R, Imam N, et al. Deciphering key genes in cardio-renal syndrome using network analysis. Bioinformation. 2021;17(1):86–100. https://doi.org/10.6026/97320630017086.
28. Wang Z, Nakayama T. Inflammation, a link between obesity and cardiovascular disease. Mediators Inflamm. 2010;2010:535918. https://doi.org/10.1155/2010/535918.

Chapter 5
Pathophysiology and Mechanisms of Cardiovascular-Kidney-Metabolic Syndrome

Lidia Iuliana Graur and Laura Mihalache

Introduction

Health and well-being should be viewed as a continuum. They are relative concepts that refer to processes that involve a range of situations, from optimal health to illness/disability or death. The continuum postulates a holistic approach that includes the assessment/knowledge of physical, mental, emotional, and spiritual health, as well as the biological, family, and social environment influences. Holistic framing in this health continuum includes awareness of the need for appropriate preventive strategies, early detection, and treatment of risk factors that trigger diseases [1]. For several decades, the concept of cardiovascular continuum [2] has been used to explain the evolution of coronary pathology, from risk factors to the clinical stage of atherosclerotic disease and to death. Numerous epidemiological, observational, and interventional clinical studies, as well as fundamental/experimental research, have led to a better understanding of the evolution of pathogenic processes in the cardiovascular continuum [3, 4]. Screening methods, the application of new markers of disease progression, and appropriate preventive and curative therapies (control of risk factors and innovative medications) have favorably influenced the prognosis of cardiovascular disease (CVD) and have brought real progress in the knowledge of the underlying pathophysiology. Let us recall only the concept of atherosclerosis as an inflammatory disease [5]. In addition to the already known risk factors, CVD is the adverse result of the synergistic impact of several metabolic processes/conditions, such as insulin resistance (IR), glucose metabolism disorder, abdominal

L. I. Graur (✉) · L. Mihalache
Grigore T. Popa University of Medicine and Pharmacy, Iasi, Romania

Saint Spiridon Emergency Hospital, Iasi, Romania
e-mail: lidia.graur@umfiasi.ro

M. Floria, D. M. Tanase (eds.), *Cardiovascular-Kidney-Metabolic Syndrome*,
https://doi.org/10.1007/978-3-032-11445-7_5

obesity, or dyslipidemia. One can speak of a cardiometabolic continuum. Knowledge and interruption of the chain of events in this continuum could lead to the prevention or slowing down of the development of many pathologies [6].

Although the constellation of metabolic (diabetogenic) and atherogenic (multiple cardiovascular pathologies) abnormalities has benefited from the attention of specialists, it is Reaven's merit to unite them in a physiopathological entity. An illustrious physiologist, the discoverer of the insulin suppression test [7], Reaven managed to elegantly demonstrate that insulin resistance/compensatory hyperinsulinemia can lead to glucose intolerance, hypertriglyceridemia/hypoHDLcholesterolemia, and hypertension in nondiabetic individuals, which, having the same substrate (insulin resistance), can be united under the umbrella of a syndrome. Insulin resistance is not only a fundamental defect/risk factor but is the cause of the increased prevalence of type 2 diabetes mellitus (T2DM) and a major determinant of cardiovascular disease (CVD) [8]. Numerous studies followed that confirmed the proposed basic associations, but added new criteria and markers related to insulin resistance. Research has shown that excess adipose tissue, especially ectopic/dysfunctional adiposity, plays an important role in the development of the syndrome, increases the risk of multiorgan damage, and contributes to increased mortality rates [9]. Initially called syndrome X or insulin resistance syndrome, it became known as metabolic syndrome (MetS) and has gained wide recognition. MetS has proven to be a useful concept from a multifactorial pathophysiological, clinical, epidemiological, and public health point of view. It has been confirmed by the World Health Organization (WHO) [10], European Group for the Study of Insulin Resistance (EGIR) [11], National Cholesterol Education Program (NCEP) [12], and International Diabetes Federation (IDF) [13], the criteria being harmonized in 2009 in a more comprehensive definition [9]. Considered more as having an educational and research purpose and less as a diagnostic or therapeutic tool, maintaining the concept of MetS can become extremely beneficial for population-based preventive measures [14]. A specific diagnostic code has been assigned to the metabolic syndrome (ICD-9: 277.7) even though there is still controversy whether it can be considered a disease [15] or just a tool for cardiovascular risk stratification [16, 17]. The definition of metabolic syndrome no longer has specific conditions imposed today (insulin resistance/T2DM or abdominal obesity) but only the fulfillment of at least three of five criteria [18]. Even the establishment of visceral adiposity by measuring waist circumference has specific thresholds for different populations [19]. The identified MetS components can predict morbidity and mortality rates from cardiovascular disease [20] through the greater number of features of the syndrome or by association with the severity of each feature, increasing the risk burden [21, 22]. Some studies show that it is unusual for patients to have only one component of the syndrome: For example, only 6.4% of people in an outpatient registry had only T2DM [23]. The question remains whether insulin resistance or dysfunctional adipose tissue is causal in the development of the syndrome/cardiometabolic risk since not all people with obesity develop diabetes or people without obesity can have insulin resistance, develop elements of the syndrome, and have increased cardiovascular morbidity and mortality [24]. There is discussion about subtypes of

MetS in which the severity is given by the prominence of arterial hypertension, chronic hyperglycemia, or their association [25]. Components of MetS have been used as population screening: hypertriglyceridemic waist [26] or hypertensive waist [27], later confirmed as clinical predictors of severity [28]. The initial framework has been expanded as cardiometabolic syndrome (CMS), which includes a wide range of interconnected risk factors, but which are dependent on environmental (including social environment) and behavioral factors (sedentary lifestyle, unhealthy diets, smoking) on a background of genetic/epigenetic susceptibility [29]. Its characteristics are abdominal/visceral obesity, dysglycemia, atherogenic dyslipidemia (excessive release of free fatty acids in plasma, hypertriglyceridemia, increased apolipoprotein B and reduced HDL-chol), hypertension and proinflammatory (elevated high sensitivity C-reactive protein, inflammatory cytokines, decrease in adiponectin plasma levels), and prothrombotic (fibrinolytic factors—PAI-1, etc., clotting factors—fibrinogen, etc.) states [30].

Prevalent pathologies that separately represent major public health problems, which are due to homeostatic disturbances, can be grouped together as cardiorenal syndrome (CRS) [31], cardiovascular-renal-hepatic-metabolic syndrome [32], and from 2023, cardiovascular-renal metabolic syndrome (CKM) [33–35]. Most arguments regarding the association of these conditions/pathologies come from cross-sectional studies, which cannot definitely argue causality, but more and more cohort or interventional research is able to demonstrate significant pathogenic overlaps that allow us today to present them together [36]. Metabolic dysfunction is the pathophysiological basis of the cardiovascular and renal bidirectional interactions, and renal damage aggravates cardiovascular risk factors and precipitates the evolution of CVD toward heart failure. CKM also originates in excess and/or dysfunction of visceral adipose tissue, which aggravates insulin resistance, with proinflammatory and prooxidative effects, and endothelial dysfunction [32, 37], and especially in the complex and individualized interaction between metabolic, cardiovascular, and renal risk factors [33].

Cardiovascular-Kidney-Metabolic Syndrome: Pathophysiology and Mechanisms

The components of the metabolic syndrome are considered both risk factors and pathogens, active contributors to the progression of cardiovascular and renal diseases. Thus, obesity and diabetes mellitus, but also chronic kidney disease, are major risk factors for atherosclerotic cardiovascular pathology. The current metabolic syndrome, in its existing variants, attests to the interconnection of the components and constitutes a challenge for risk prediction, early diagnosis, and holistic and multidisciplinary therapy [34]. The CKM syndrome includes people who do not yet have clinical cardiovascular disease, but have traditional risk factors (through the presence of metabolic dysfunction, chronic kidney disease, or both) and patients with existing cardiovascular disease that is related to metabolic risk factors or chronic kidney disease. In addition to the risk inherent to each of the CKM conditions, there are several biological and environmental risk factors that, when interconnected, aggravate the progression of the disease. It is estimated that 1 in 3 people have risk factors that contribute to cardiovascular disease, metabolic disorders, and/or kidney disease [33]. Patients who have all three conditions (cardio-reno-metabolic) are at the highest risk of primary events [22].

If obesity is considered the central element, then insulin resistance, atherogenic dyslipidemia, hypertension, and hyperglycemia can be considered major risk factors (they can directly cause cardiovascular and kidney damage), and the prothrombotic state and proinflammatory states can be called emerging risk factors [38, 39].

The pathogenesis of CKM involves the complex and continuous interaction of metabolic, inflammatory, neurohormonal, and hemodynamic pathways that maintain the severity and self-reinforcing disease process [40–43]. This vicious cycle of disease progression includes reciprocal and asymmetric involvement of each organ. For example, renal dysfunction can overload the heart through hypertension and fluid retention [44], and cardiovascular dysfunction leads to reduced renal perfusion and worsening glomerular damage [45]. All of these occur against the background of metabolic disorders that intervene in all systems. Chronic kidney disease increases cardiovascular risk, the most common cause of mortality in these patients being heart failure and atherosclerotic coronary heart disease [46]. Chronic kidney disease induces disorders of bone metabolism, often with the consequence of vascular calcification and exacerbation of cardiovascular morbidity [47]. Microalbuminuria is a valuable indicator of metabolic syndrome, systemic endothelial dysfunction, a predictor of cardiovascular risk but also an early marker of chronic kidney disease. Metabolic syndrome is an independent risk factor for the development of chronic kidney disease and amplifies the adverse effects of diabetes mellitus [42].

The Relationship Between Obesity–T2DM– Cardiovascular and Renal Damage

Insulin Resistance

Resistance to insulin-stimulated glucose absorption has been considered the central element in the pathophysiology of the metabolic syndrome, and historically the syndrome was defined around this defect in insulin action. According to the WHO, insulin resistance was evidenced by the presence of impaired glucose tolerance, impaired fasting glucose, type 2 diabetes or other evidence of it such as euglycemic clamp studies [10]. In addition to this mandatory requirement (demonstration of IR), two additional criteria had to be met, from the following four: obesity, dyslipidemia, hypertension, and microalbuminuria. According to the EGIR definition, hyperinsulinemia had to be demonstrated: plasma insulin >75th percentile [11]. In this classification and in subsequent ones, the presence of dysglycemia implied insulin resistance (patients with T2DM could be hyper-, normo-, or hypoinsulinemic at the time of diagnosis). Insulin resistance (IR) can be due to a genetic predisposition or can be acquired. Severe obesity is a major risk factor for insulin resistance, the development of T2DM [48], and all other components of the cardiovascular-renal-metabolic syndrome (CKM) [49].

Physiologically, a sudden increase in blood glucose triggers insulin secretion from pancreatic β cells, which promotes cellular glucose uptake and utilization. In individuals with insulin resistance, tissues are less sensitive to this acute increase in insulin, resulting in higher serum glucose levels and hyperinsulinemia. Impaired insulin secretion, signaling pathways, and defects in insulin receptors may contribute to insulin resistance. These abnormalities result in impaired glucose metabolism, fat deposition, cardiotoxicity, and chronic inflammation. Insulin resistance (IR) can be defined as a state in which normal amounts of insulin produce a reduced/subnormal biological response in insulin-targeting tissues [50]. The insulin signaling system is responsible for controlling energy homeostasis by regulating metabolism and growth. The diminished biological response to endogenous/exogenous insulin refers to the ineffectiveness of the hormone on carbohydrate, lipid, and protein metabolism, as well as on cell growth and differentiation, DNA synthesis, and regulation of gene transcription [51]. There are two known pathways of insulin signaling. In the dominant pathway, insulin bound to its receptor activates an intrinsic tyrosine protein kinase, autophosphorylates the receptor, and acts on a group of proteins known as insulin receptor substrates (IRS). In skeletal muscle, insulin binds to insulin receptor tyrosine kinase (IRTK) and activates insulin receptor substrate-1 (IRS-1), which recruits phosphatidylinositol-3-OH kinase (PI3K) and activates Akt. The Akt protein is a serine/threonine kinase that stimulates an effector of PI3-K that promotes glucose uptake by translocating storage vesicles to the plasma membrane via glucose transporter type 4 (GLUT4) [52]. Insulin stimulates glycogen synthesis by inhibiting glycogen synthase kinase 3 (GSK3) and inactivating glycogen phosphorylase. In the liver, Akt decreases gluconeogenesis by suppressing the expression of gluconeogenic genes mediated by forkhead box O1 (FOXO1). Insulin increases glycogen synthesis and hepatic de novo lipogenesis by upregulating sterol regulatory element-binding protein 1c (SREBP-1c). In white adipose tissue, insulin suppresses lipolysis, which in turn suppresses hepatic glucose production by reducing gluconeogenic substrates. Insulin promotes glucose transport, lipogenesis, and adipogenesis [53].

The alternative pathway ("ras/MAP-kinase") is also a serine-protein kinase cascade. Mitogen-activated protein kinase (MAPK) includes three isoforms that work sequentially for vital signal transduction, differentiation and proliferation/cell growth, and protein synthesis [50]. Maintaining activation of the PKC-MAPK pathway, mediated by excessive diacylglycerol (DAG) production and oxidative stress, leads to the development of multiple pathologies related to insulin resistance [54]. Chronic hyperglycemia, increasing the influx of glucose into cells, leads to the production of mitochondrial superoxide, which results in the exacerbation of oxidative stress [55]. Increased production of reactive oxygen species (ROS) causes tissue damage by activating the polyol pathway, hexosamine, activation of protein kinase C (PKC), and the formation of advanced glycation end products (AGEs). These (AGEs) produce cross-linking of matrix proteins, endothelial dysfunction, with stiffening of target tissues/organs [56].

Obesity—Chronic Inflammation—Atherogenic Dyslipidemia—Endothelial Dysfunction

Many of the chronic noncommunicable diseases are recognized as chronic inflammatory conditions in which the triggering factor is not well defined, but which do not involve infections or tissue damage. This group includes obesity, T2DM [57], metabolic syndrome, atherosclerosis, neurodegenerative diseases, cancer, but also aging [58]. It is a disorder of the appropriate coordination through negative feedback of the inflammatory response, a specific chronic deficiency of the regulation of oxidative events, that is, the constant creation of a prooxidative cellular environment, triggering and stabilizing in turn a subclinical systemic proinflammatory state [59]. Called "OxInflammation," this dysfunction induces a decrease in the adaptive/homeostatic capacities of the body with metabolic consequences and multiple pathologies [60].

Obesity is seen as the result of a positive energy balance, but fats are not distributed uniformly as triglycerides accumulate. Intra-abdominal lipid storage has been associated with adverse effects. Visceral fat is defined as adipose tissue located within the peritoneal cavity—in the parietal peritoneum and transversalis fascia, excluding the spine and paraspinal muscles [61]. Without using a "gold standard" for assessing regional fat distribution in human studies, most studies have shown a strong association between visceral fat, insulin resistance, and the risk of metabolic and cardiovascular complications [62]. Insulin resistance generally increases with increasing BMI; however, there is a wide range of insulin sensitivities at the same level of body fat due to the distribution/dysfunction of adipose tissue [63, 64], or the biology itself [65]. Epidemiological studies have shown that obesity increases the risk of T2DM eightfold and that there is an inverse correlation between plasma fatty acid concentrations and insulin sensitivity [66]. Most people with T2DM are overweight or obese, with predominantly abdominal adiposity. Due to the strong association between obesity and diabetes, the term "diabesity" has been proposed, suggesting a causal link between these pathologies [67]. Insulin resistance, adipose tissue dysfunction, and chronic inflammation have been proposed as core components of the pathogenesis of CKM syndrome [68]. It is accepted that excessive caloric intake and sedentary lifestyle initially lead to fat accumulation in the subcutaneous tissue and subsequently in other tissue compartments, such as the liver, pancreas, skeletal muscle, perivascular, and pericardium [69]. This ectopic fat accumulation increases tissue insulin resistance, while pancreatic fat accumulation causes β-cell dysfunction [70]. The progression from obesity-related insulin resistance to T2DM involves a failure of pancreatic β-cells to compensate for insulin resistance, leading to chronic hyperglycemia, oxidative stress, chronic low-grade/subclinical inflammation, and immune activation, observed in visceral obesity and exacerbated during the development of related metabolic disorders [71]. It is generally accepted that decreased insulin sensitivity precedes clinical diabetes by up to 15 years [72]. Even minimal abnormalities in blood glucose (dysglycemia in prediabetes) have been shown to be associated with inflammatory processes, as well as complications of T2DM [73]. Chronic inflammation has also been associated with comorbidities of T2DM, such as atherosclerosis and coagulation disorders, CVD, kidney disease, and cancers [74]. Although chronic inflammation is the main cause of the development of cardiometabolic pathologies, inflammatory markers are not specific (CRP), are not routinely measured (IL-6), or are difficult to assess in clinical routine (genetic predisposition, sedentary lifestyle, energy-dense food intake) [75].

Advances in research into adipocyte biology have placed adipose tissue at the epicenter of the metabolic disease pandemic. Adipocytes store excess calories in the form of triglycerides (triacylglycerols –TAG), mediate the balance between lipolysis and lipogenesis, release hormones (with auto-, para-, or endocrine action), and have the capacity to secrete numerous effectors (exosomes, microRNAs, complement factors, lipids, inflammatory cytokines) that elicit local and/or systemic metabolic responses. Adipocytes are insulin-sensitive cells that stimulate glucose uptake and modulate lipid metabolism by increasing the accumulation and decreasing the breakdown of TAGs [76]. Leptin, a hormone derived from adipocytes [77], plays a role in regulating body weight at a central level ("adipostate") but also peripherally by acting on glucose metabolism and immunity [78, 79].

Adipose tissue retains the ability to expand/adapt to caloric excess through hypertrophy (increase in adipocyte size) or hyperplasia/adipogenesis (increase in adipocyte number), or both. Cardiometabolic health depends on the mechanisms of adipose tissue expansion. Deficient expansion causes ectopic fat accumulation and "lipotoxicity" in nonadipose tissues, the development of inflammation and fibrosis [80]. An abundance of "small" adipocytes, with a limited capacity to expand/accumulate lipids, has been correlated with an increased number of components of the metabolic syndrome [81, 82]. As adipose tissue expandability reaches its limit, there is a strong association between adipocyte size and death. Proinflammatory macrophages surround dead cells and remove debris from the affected area by producing inflammatory cytokines. In individuals with obesity, cytokine production becomes chronic and impairs insulin signaling and exacerbates inflammation and the vicious cycle of adipose tissue dysfunction [83].

Hypertrophied and dysfunctional adipose tissue causes the release of reactive oxygen species (ROS) and proinflammatory cytokines. Excess free fatty acids (FFAs) become ectopic fats, generating lipotoxicity [84]. Thus, cellular organelles (mitochondria, endoplasmic reticulum, lysosomes) are affected, and inflammation is amplified, which becomes systemic. This chronic subclinical inflammation maintains changes in insulin signaling and the occurrence of dysglycemia [85].

Experimental and clinical studies have established that insulin-sensitive tissues are predilection sites for the development of inflammation in individuals with obesity and T2DM. Macrophage infiltration into these tissues (adipose, hepatic, muscle) and cytokine release is observed in animal models of obesity and diabetes, as well as in obese human individuals with metabolic syndrome [86, 87]. These cells, by releasing proinflammatory cytokines, act in an autocrine and paracrine manner to exacerbate insulin resistance by affecting insulin signaling in peripheral tissues through activation of the c-JUN N-terminal kinase (JNK) and nuclear factor-kappa B (NF-kB) pathways [88].

Obesity and metabolic syndrome (including CKM) are positively associated with inflammatory biomarker levels, which are predictive of insulin resistance, T2DM incidence, and CVD [89, 90]. Upregulation of genes encoding inflammatory factors and overproduction of cytokines and chemokines in excess adipose tissue have been confirmed [87]. Reduction of insulin resistance through weight loss has been accompanied by a decrease in the expression of proinflammatory genes [91, 92]. Hypertrophic adipocytes themselves produce cytokines and chemokines, which are chemical mediators that control cells involved in immune responses. However, it has been shown that macrophages recruited to dysfunctional adipose tissue play a crucial role in the production of proinflammatory cytokines, an action correlated with the degree of obesity, insulin resistance, and other biomarkers of inflammation [93]. Several data have indicated that proinflammatory cytokines, including interleukin 6 (IL-6) and tumor necrosis factor alpha (TNF-α), are elevated in subjects with T2DM, predicting endothelial dysfunction and subsequent development of atherosclerosis [94, 95]. C-reactive protein (CRP) is considered to be the link between inflammation and atherosclerosis, being a predictor of cardiovascular events and the development of acute coronary syndromes [96]. Elevated levels of CRP and fibrinogen and reduced levels of adiponectin can be used for early diagnosis of T2DM and may predict chronic complications of the disease [97]. Hyperglycemia appears to activate the immune system/macrophage-monocytes and stimulate the production of cytokines and acute phase proteins that are involved in decreasing endothelium-dependent vasodilation through a mechanism involving superoxide anion [74]. In subjects with T2DM, inflammation appears to be more closely related to abdominal obesity than to glycemic control [98, 99]. Visceral (but not subcutaneous) adipose tissue has been linked to markers of systemic inflammation that are associated with vascular wall remodeling [100]. Immune system activation is closely linked to the incidence and progression of obesity to insulin resistance and related pathologies, and both adaptive and innate immunity are implicated in subclinical inflammation [85]. Proinflammatory cytokines, chemokines, and other indirect markers of inflammation, such as fibrinogen, sialic acid, and PAI-1, may be considered predictors of T2DM [101, 102]. Recruitment of B and T cells precedes macrophage infiltration of adipose tissue. Macrophages are divided into two distinct subtypes, M1 and M2, based on their functions. M1 macrophages, the "classically activated" phenotype, originating from the bone marrow, predominate in obesity, secrete proinflammatory cytokines (IL-1b, IL-6, TNF-α), and induce insulin resistance. The M2 phenotype, "alternatively activated macrophages," is predominantly found in the adipose tissue of nonobese individuals and secretes anti-inflammatory cytokines (e.g., IL-10) that would maintain insulin sensitivity [86]. In addition to the infiltration of adipose tissue with macrophages, obesity causes a switch from the M2 to the M1 phenotype, correlating with insulin resistance [103]. The switch in macrophage phenotype from the predominantly anti-inflammatory M2 type to increased proportions of proinflammatory M1 type macrophages plays a crucial role in the initiation and amplification of inflammation in the islets of Langerhans but also in other organs such as the liver, skeletal muscle, kidney, and even the nervous system [89, 104]. Inflammation has been demonstrated in pancreatic islets of patients with T2DM by early macrophage infiltration together with increased levels of proinflammatory cytokines and chemokines, the presence of amyloid deposits, fibrosis, and increased β-cell death [57]. This local inflammation/macrophage infiltration, together with increased levels of proinflammatory cytokines and chemokines, through β-cell apoptosis, leads to decreased islet mass and function. Inflammasome/IL-1beta signaling is mediated by amyloid polypeptides, free fatty acids (FFA), and endocannabinoids [105]. Dysfunctional fat through the production of adipokines regulates the interaction between metabolism and vascular function/endothelial dysfunction. The renin-angiotensin system is activated in adipose tissue, leading to hypertension and increased insulin resistance. In addition to proinflammatory cytokines, free fatty acids (FFAs) and bioactive lipid intermediates released in excess from visceral fat act synergistically to affect the PI3K-Akt pathway and increase oxidative stress [106].

A future therapeutic target for treating obesity and metabolic complications may be browning of white adipose tissue. Brown adipose tissue, through the release of irisin, may have a positive effect on cardiometabolic health, enhance pancreatic beta cell protection and insulin secretion, reduce de novo lipogenesis and hepatic inflammation, increase glucose and fatty acid uptake in skeletal muscle, and improve cardiomyocyte oxygenation [107].

In epidemiological studies, the link between obesity and its secondary complications cannot be generated by a single pathophysiological hypothesis. Three hypotheses have been proposed:

- The "inflammation hypothesis" is based on the idea that obesity is a state of chronic subclinical inflammation, also called "metainflammation," in which macrophages infiltrated into adipose tissue can be considered a reservoir of proinflammatory molecules that exert pathological changes in insulin-sensitive tissues (including β cells) [108], such as tumor necrosis factor alpha (TNF-α), TNF-Like Weak Inducer of Apoptosis, Monocyte Chemotactic Protein-1, Interleukin-6 (IL-6), and Toll-like-4 (TLR-4). Inflammation alone cannot explain how obesity affects insulin sensitivity because not all overweight or obese individuals will become diabetic [109].
- The "lipid overflow hypothesis," also known as the "adipose tissue expandability hypothesis," aims to demonstrate that obesity leads to the increase of "ectopic" lipid deposits due to the limited capacity of subcutaneous adipose tissue to store excess energy. Lipid components and potentially harmful metabolites can exert

cytotoxic effects on peripheral cells by inhibiting insulin signal transduction [110–112].
- The "adipokine hypothesis" refers to the main characteristic of white adipose tissue as an endocrine organ. As this organ expands, more adipocyte-derived factors (TNF-α, IL-1β, IL-6, and MCP-1, but also leptin, adiponectin, resistin, Retinol Binding Protein 4, visfatin, and Retinol Binding Protein 4) with auto-para or endocrine action will be formed. This dysfunctional secretion will have repercussions on insulin-sensitive organs, including pancreatic β cells [113, 114].

Visceral obesity contributes to/is associated with atherogenic dyslipidemia by increasing insulin resistance. Impaired insulin signaling increases lipolysis and free fatty acid (FFA) levels. These serve as substrates for triglyceride synthesis and by interfering with apoB production lead to an increase in very low-density lipoproteins (VLDL). Insulin resistance, in addition to increasing production, also decreases VLDL clearance by regulating lipoprotein lipase activity. VLDL is metabolized into residual lipoproteins and small dense LDL, both of which can promote the formation of atherosclerotic plaques. Triglycerides from VLDL are transferred to HDL-chol, which is thus readily removed from the circulation (by the action of hepatic lipase), decreasing reverse cholesterol transport. Key features of atherogenic dyslipidemia are elevated plasma TG levels, low HDL cholesterol levels, and an increase in small dense LDL [115]. Both insulin resistance and free fatty acids play a major role in the pathogenesis of hypertension, dyslipidemia, and the prothrombotic state [116]. Endothelial dysfunction occurs when the endothelium can no longer use its normal physiological and protective mechanisms (production of vasoactive substances, including nitric oxide, prostacyclin, and endothelins). Several cardiovascular risk factors, including insulin resistance, lead to endothelial dysfunction, which constitutes the final pathway in the pathogenesis of atherosclerosis. We discuss a "maladapted endothelial phenotype" characterized by reduced nitric oxide (NO) bioavailability, increased oxidative stress, increased expression of proinflammatory and prothrombotic factors, and abnormal vasoreactivity [117]. The balance between the nitric oxide (NO)-dependent vasodilator and endothelin-1-dependent vasoconstrictor actions of insulin is regulated in the vascular endothelium by phosphatidylinositol 3-kinase (PI3K)-dependent and mitogen-activated protein kinase (MAPK)-dependent signaling, respectively. Dysfunction can occur when normal endothelial responses are impaired by oxidative stress, hyperglycemia, advanced glycation end products, free fatty acids (FFA), inflammatory cytokines, or adipokines. Insulin resistance causes an imbalance between NO production and endothelin-1 secretion. Visceral adiposity causes endothelial dysfunction through the effects of adipokines that modulate endothelial function and eNOS phosphorylation. Some may be protective (adiponectin, omentin), while others may be detrimental (leptin, resistin, FABP4) [118].

Neurohormonal Activation

The main pathogenic feature in the progression of CKM syndrome is neurohormonal activation/overactivation, that is, the dynamic interaction between the renin-angiotensin-aldosterone system (RAAS) and the sympathetic nervous system (SNS) that initiates and maintains a cascade of negative effects [119]. The renin-angiotensin-aldosterone system (RAAS) is important in the humoral regulation of central and peripheral hemodynamics. The RAAS has a significant role in maintaining homeostasis of cardiovascular function and water and mineral balance, as well as in the regulation of blood pressure and renal blood flow. The RAAS is involved in target organ damage in patients with hypertension. Overactivation of the renin-angiotensin-aldosterone system (RAAS) is the element that accentuates metabolic disorders and the central mechanism of the development and progression of renal and cardiac dysfunction [120]. Under physiological conditions, RAAS activity is determined by plasma renin activity, which is also the most reliable marker of its activity. Angiotensin II (Ang II), which is considered to be the most important effector of the RAAS, would be a better index, but it is difficult to determine due to its very short half-life. When reninemia increases, angiotensinogen (produced by the liver) is hydrolyzed to angiotensin I (Ang I), which stimulates the secretion of epinephrine and norepinephrine [121]. Under the action of angiotensin-converting enzymes (ACEs) (produced by the lungs), Ang I is converted to angiotensin II (Ang II). Ang II-stimulated AT2R promotes nitric oxide production and counteracts inflammation. Ang II-stimulated AT1R regulates several physiological processes, including vasoconstriction, ventricular hypertrophy, generation of reactive oxygen species (ROS), inflammation, atherosclerosis, and aldosterone synthesis. Aldosterone can increase sodium retention and potassium excretion in the kidney, resulting in fluid overload, hypertension, increased glomerular pressure, and increased mechanical load on the heart, with deterioration of renal and cardiac function. Aldosterone exerts physiological and pathological effects through activation of the mineralocorticoid receptor (MR). Activation of the MR can induce cardiac, vascular, and renal inflammation and fibrosis, and may increase susceptibility to cardiac arrhythmias through sympathetic excitation. Aldosterone can increase ROS production, induce mitochondrial and adrenergic receptor dysfunction, and coronary vasoconstriction, which can lead to heart failure (HF). Furthermore, aldosterone stimulates epidermal growth factor receptor activation via the MR, which regulates the renin-angiotensin-aldosterone system (RAAS) and ultimately modulates cardiovascular physiology [122].

As myocardial performance and cardiac output decrease, tissue hypoperfusion occurs, leading to increases in afterload, preload, and heart rate. Although initially compensatory, these can create hemodynamic stress for the already damaged heart, which is compounded by the activation of neurohormonal systems that promote structural remodeling.

Simultaneously with overactivation of the RAAS, the sympathetic nervous system releases excess norepinephrine that binds to adrenergic receptors (present in the heart, blood vessels, and kidneys) [123].

Prolonged activation of β-adrenergic receptors on cardiomyocytes has long-term deleterious effects. In the heart, this results in compensatory increases in heart rate and inotropism that over time become maladaptive, disrupting excitation-contraction coupling, promoting arrhythmias, ventricular hypertrophy, and heart failure [124]. In addition, SNS stimulation increases renin release, aggravating overactivation of the RAAS. In the vessels, norepinephrine reduces the bioavailability of nitric oxide, promoting endothelial dysfunction and contributing to the development of hypertension [125].

In the kidney, sympathetic activation reduces renal perfusion by vasoconstriction of the afferent arteriole and leads to renal failure (decreased glomerular filtration rate, GFR) [126, 127].

In CKM syndrome, overworked RAAS and SNS contribute to persistent fluid retention and hypertension. The chronic increase in natriuretic peptides, determined by continuous volume overload, leads to downregulation of their receptors, reducing their efficacy and diminishing their protective actions [128]. This further increases sodium and fluid retention, worsening the pressure on the cardiovascular and renal systems. Furthermore, these neurohormonal disorders lead to overproduction of ROS and proinflammatory cytokines, increasing oxidative stress and inflammation [129].

Hemodynamic Abnormalities

Hemodynamic abnormalities lead to cardiac and renal function disorders through the combination of metabolic, biochemical, mechanical, and neurohormonal factors, with hypertension as a central element [130]. Hypertension is found in all classifications/classifications of metabolic syndromes with organic damage (from the cardiovascular, renal, hepatic, cerebral continuum, etc.). They are defined as a combination of neurohormonal overload, renal damage, and endothelial dysfunction. The renin-angiotensin-aldosterone system (RAAS) through angiotensin II increases vascular resistance. Ang II acts on AT1 receptors in smooth muscle cells, causing calcium influx through L-type calcium channels that amplify muscle contraction, accentuating vasoconstriction [131, 132]. Hypertension constantly overloads the heart, leading to cardiac remodeling, diastolic dysfunction, left ventricular hypertrophy, and heart failure [133]. In the kidneys, hypertension increases intraglomerular pressure, leading to glomerulosclerosis (reducing renal filtration capacity) and progressive renal damage [134]. Angiotensin II induces vasoconstriction on the efferent arteriole, maintaining glomerular filtration in the short term, but increasing mechanical stress on the glomerular capillaries and accelerating the loss of functional nephrons [135, 136]. Albuminuria/proteinuria develops as a result of glomerular dysfunction, which is also used as a biomarker.

On the other hand, the water and sodium retention characteristic of renal damage (RAAS and SNS activation) leads to volume overload [137], which accentuates cardiac dysfunction/failure. A vicious circle is entered in which tissue/renal hypoperfusion compensatorily increases RAAS and SNS activity [35, 138]. Due to reduced perfusion, hypoxic injury of renal tubular cells occurs with the release of damage-associated molecular patterns (DAMPS) that activate inflammatory pathways and contribute to chronic renal injury [139]. In diabetic kidney disease, dysregulation of metabolic, inflammatory, and hemodynamic pathways explains renal damage (hyperfiltration → fibrosis) but also the evolution toward CVD [140]. ROS, AGEs/RAGE levels are increased and the PKC pathway is activated. Hyperglycemia, AGEs, and glomerular hypertension can increase TGF-β (transforming growth factor) expression [141]. Intestinal dysbiosis generated by excess dietary lipids and AGEs accentuates inflammation via the NF-κB pathway and macrophage accumulation by upregulating the mineralocorticoid receptor and TGF-β. Hemodynamic abnormalities are further exacerbated by endothelial dysfunction generated by oxidative stress, reduced endothelial nitric oxide (eNOS) bioavailability, vasoconstriction, increased vascular resistance, and further increase in arterial pressure [142, 143].

Fibrosis

The culmination and irreversible point of the pathological continuum within the CKM syndrome is fibrosis, defined as excessive accumulation of extracellular matrix components (ECM) and impaired degradation of these components (collagen, fibronectin) leading to permanent scarring, loss of normal tissue architecture, organ dysfunction, and end-stage injury [144]. Endogenous triggers are released from damaged cells and facilitate inflammation that is primarily mediated by macrophages. In the myocardium, fibrosis is a hallmark of heart failure and is primarily mediated by cardiac fibroblasts activated by signaling molecules such as transforming growth factor-beta (TGF-β) and angiotensin II [145]. Angiotensin II, through interaction with AT1 receptors, activates downstream kinases such as mitogen-activated protein kinases (MAPK) and protein kinase C (PKC), which further amplify fibroblast activation.

Diastolic dysfunction occurs due to interstitial and perivascular fibrosis that increases myocardial stiffness and decreases ventricular compliance [146, 147]. Similar mechanisms have been described in the kidney, leading to tubular epithelial cell damage and apoptosis, the release of damage-associated molecular patterns (DAMPS) that activate fibroblasts and recruit immune cells [148]. Macrophages infiltrate the interstitium, secreting mediators such as TGF-β, platelet-derived growth factor (PDGF), and connective tissue growth factor (CTGF). These cytokines and growth factors stimulate the differentiation of fibroblasts and myofibroblasts that secrete large amounts of collagen types I and III, leading to tubulointerstitial fibrosis and glomerulosclerosis. Progressive scarring of renal tissue reduces nephron function, promoting the decline in glomerular filtration rate (GFR) and the development of end-stage renal disease [149]. Fibrosis is exacerbated by oxidative stress, which perpetuates a proinflammatory and profibrotic environment [150]. In endothelial cells, ROS contribute to endothelial-mesenchymal transition (EndMT), a process in which endothelial cells lose their normal phenotype and acquire fibroblast-like properties, further increasing the number of ECM-producing cells [151]. Metabolic factors also contribute significantly to fibrosis. Insulin resistance, with its corollary hyperinsulinemia, increases the formation of insulin-like growth factor 1 (IGF-1), which promotes connective tissue growth and fibrosis. Obesity, through leptin secretion and maintenance of inflammatory factors, induces intrarenal expression of transforming growth factor-beta (TGF-β) and synthesis of type IV collagen. Adiponectin deficiency is linked to vascular intimal thickening and smooth muscle cell proliferation, leading to increased glomerular volume (podocyte hypertrophy and mesangial matrix growth) [152]. Hyperglycemia accelerates the production of AGEs that are capable of inducing fibrosis processes. Dyslipidemia contributes to the profibrotic environment, as lipid accumulation in nonadipose tissues, such as the myocardium and kidney, induces lipotoxicity, with the release of proinflammatory cytokines and growth factors that promote fibroblast activation [153, 154]. In advanced stages of CKM, fibrosis becomes self-sustaining; stiff, scarred tissue disrupts mechanosensitive signaling pathways. In the heart, increased stiffness impairs conduction pathways leading to arrhythmias, and in the kidney, capillary networks are encased in scars, aggravating hypoxia and ischemic injury [155]. All of these perpetuate a vicious cycle of progressive fibrosis and multiorgan failure, underscoring the importance of early intervention strategies.

All of these interconnected synergistic pathologies can also be integrated into a continuum of disease progression, increased cardiovascular and renal complications, and mortality [156]. Timely diagnostic and therapeutic interventions based on knowledge of the pathophysiology can stop the progression of these diseases or even reverse the poor prognosis.

Conclusions

Metabolic diseases (obesity and type 2 diabetes mellitus) and chronic kidney disease are major risk factors for atherosclerotic cardiovascular diseases. Metabolic syndrome, cardiovascular diseases, and kidney diseases have been shown to have a common pathophysiology, underlying excess/dysfunctional adipose tissue, which mutually influences their evolution and prognosis. Being chronic pathologies with increasing prevalence, which maintain a high overall mortality, they impose diagnostic and therapeutic challenges. The development of a conceptual framework of the cardiovascular-renal-metabolic syndrome (CKM) was done to develop risk prediction tools, early diagnostic biomarkers, and a holistic, integrated clinical framework with an emphasis on coherent multidisciplinary therapeutic approaches. CKM syndrome is a complex condition in which dysfunctions of the cardiovascular, renal, and metabolic systems interact and worsen each other, creating a vicious self-reinforcing cycle of multiorgan damage. The pathophysiological basis is mainly given by insulin resistance, chronic inflammation, oxidative stress, activation of the renin-angiotensin-aldosterone system (RAAS), and neurohormonal dysfunction. The pathophysiology and progressive trajectory of CKM syndrome must be understood on a continuum of evolution from risk factors to irreversible lesions. Knowledge of each evolutionary step, understanding the overlap of conditions, and identification of biological factors underline the need for integrated knowledge that allows personalized interventions in the complex interactions between cardiovascular, renal, and metabolic health. Deepening the mechanisms (cellular and molecular) that underlie CKM syndrome is important for the development of innovative therapies.

Learning Objectives

- What are the elements of pathophysiology and the mechanisms of cardiovascular-kidney-metabolic syndrome.
- What is the relationship between obesity, type 2 diabetes mellitus, and cardiovascular and renal damage?

Key Reading

- *Obesity, type 2 diabetes mellitus, and chronic kidney disease* are major risk factors for atherosclerotic cardiovascular diseases.
- *Metabolic syndrome, cardiovascular diseases, and kidney diseases* have a common pathophysiology, underlying excess/dysfunctional adipose tissue.
- *The new concept of cardiovascular-renal-metabolic syndrome* helped develop risk prediction tools, early diagnostic biomarkers and a holistic, integrated clinical framework with an emphasis on coherent multidisciplinary therapeutic approaches.

References

1. Caron RM, Noel K, Reed RN, Sibel J, Smith HJ. Health promotion, health protection, and disease prevention: challenges and opportunities in a dynamic landscape. AJPM Focus. 2023;3:100167. https://doi.org/10.1016/j.focus.2023.100167.
2. Dzau V, Braunwald E. Resolved and unresolved issues in the prevention and treatment of coronary artery disease: a workshop consensus statement. Am Heart J. 1991;121:1244–63. https://doi.org/10.1016/0002-8703(91)90694-d.
3. Dzau VJ, Antman EM, Black HR, Hayes DL, Manson JE, Plutzky J, et al. The cardiovascular disease continuum validated: clinical evidence of improved patient outcomes: part I: pathophysiology and clinical trial evidence (risk factors through stable coronary artery disease). Circulation. 2006;114:2850–70. https://doi.org/10.1161/CIRCULATIONAHA.106.655688.

4. Chrysant SG. A new paradigm in the treatment of the cardiovascular disease continuum: focus on prevention. Hippokratia. 2011;15:7–11.
5. Ross R. Atherosclerosis—An inflammatory disease. N Engl J Med. 1999;340:115–26. https://doi.org/10.1056/NEJM199901143400207.
6. Arocha Rodulfo JI. Approach to the cardiometabolic continuum. Narrative description. Clin Invest Arterioscler. 2021;33:158–67. https://doi.org/10.1016/j.arteri.2020.10.003.
7. Shen SW, Reaven GM, Farquhar JW. Comparison of impedance to insulin-mediated glucose uptake in Normal subjects and in subjects with latent diabetes. J Clin Invest. 1970;49:2151–60. https://doi.org/10.1172/JCI106433.
8. Reaven GM. Banting Lecture 1988. Role of insulin resistance in human disease. Diabetes. 1988;37:1595–607. https://doi.org/10.2337/diab.37.12.1595.
9. Alberti KG, Eckel RH, Grundy SM, et al. Harmonizing the metabolic syndrome: a joint interim statement of the International Diabetes Federation Task Force on Epidemiology and Prevention; National Heart, Lung, and Blood Institute; American Heart Association; World Heart Federation; International Atherosclerosis Society; and International Association for the Study of Obesity. Circulation. 2009;120:1640–5. https://doi.org/10.1161/CIRCULATIONAHA.109.192644.
10. World Health Organization Definition, diagnosis and classification of diabetes mellitus and its complications: report of a WHO consultation. Part 1, diagnosis and classification of diabetes mellitus. World health Organization 1999. Available online: https://iris.who.int/handle/10665/66040.
11. Balkau B, Charles MA. Comment on the provisional report from the WHO consultation. European Group for the Study of Insulin Resistance (EGIR). Diabet Med. 1999;16:442–3. https://doi.org/10.1046/j.1464-5491.1999.00059.x.
12. Expert Panel on Detection, Evaluation, and Treatment of High Blood Cholesterol in Adults. Executive summary of the third report of the National Cholesterol Education Program (NCEP) expert panel on detection, evaluation, and treatment of high blood cholesterol in adults (adult treatment panel III). JAMA. 2001;285:2486–97. https://doi.org/10.1001/jama.285.19.2486.
13. Alberti KG, Zimmet P, Shaw J. Metabolic syndrome—a new world-wide definition. A consensus statement from the international diabetes federation. Diabet Med. 2006;23:469–80. https://doi.org/10.1111/j.1464-5491.2006.01858.x.
14. Grundy SM. Adipose tissue and metabolic syndrome: too much, too little or neither. Eur J Clin Invest. 2015;45:1209–17. https://doi.org/10.1111/eci.12519.
15. Huang PL. A comprehensive definition for metabolic syndrome. Dis Model Mech. 2009;2:231–7. https://doi.org/10.1242/dmm.001180.
16. Won KB, Chang HJ, Kim HC, Jeon K, Lee H, Shin S, et al. Differential impact of metabolic syndrome on subclinical atherosclerosis according to the presence of diabetes. Cardiovasc Diabetol. 2013;12:41. https://doi.org/10.1186/1475-2840-12-41.
17. Lakka HM, Laaksonen DE, Lakka TA, Niskanen LK, Kumpusalo E, Tuomilehto J, Salonen JT. The metabolic syndrome and total and cardiovascular disease mortality in middle-aged men. JAMA. 2002;288:2709–16. https://doi.org/10.1001/jama.288.21.2709.
18. Peterseim CM, Jabbour K, Kamath Mulki A. Metabolic syndrome: an updated review on diagnosis and treatment for primary care clinicians. J Prim Care Community Health. 2024;15:21501319241309168. https://doi.org/10.1177/21501319241309168.
19. Ross R, Neeland IJ, Yamashita S, Shai I, Seidell J, Magni P, Santos RD, et al. Waist circumference as a vital sign in clinical practice: a consensus statement from the IAS and ICCR working group on visceral obesity. Nat Rev Endocrinol. 2020;16:177–89. https://doi.org/10.1038/s41574-019-0310-7.
20. Di Pietro P, Izzo C, Carrizzo A. Editorial: the role of metabolic syndrome and disorders in cardiovascular disease. Front Endocrinol (Lausanne). 2023;14:1327394. https://doi.org/10.3389/fendo.2023.1327394.
21. Cubeddu LX, Hoffmann IS. Metabolic syndrome: An all or none or a continuum load of risk? Metab Syndr Relat Disord. 2012;10:14–9. https://doi.org/10.1089/met.2011.0058.

22. Ostrominski JW, Thierer J, Claggett BL, Miao ZM, Desai AS, Jhund PS, et al. Cardio-renal-metabolic overlap, outcomes, and Dapagliflozin in heart failure with mildly reduced or preserved ejection fraction. JACC Heart Fail. 2023;11:1491–503. https://doi.org/10.1016/j.jchf.2023.05.015.
23. Arnold SV, Kosiborod M, Wang J, Fenici P, Gannedahl G, LoCasale RJ. Burden of cardio-renal-metabolic conditions in adults with type 2 diabetes within the diabetes collaborative registry. Diabetes Obes Metab. 2018;20:2000–3. https://doi.org/10.1111/dom.13303.
24. Shi TH, Wang B, Natarajan S. The influence of metabolic syndrome in predicting mortality risk among US adults: importance of metabolic syndrome even in adults with Normal weight. Prev Chronic Dis. 2020;17:E36. https://doi.org/10.5888/pcd17.200020.
25. Li S, Wen CP, Tu H, Wang S, Li X, Xu A, et al. Metabolic syndrome including both elevated blood pressure and elevated fasting plasma glucose is associated with higher mortality risk: a prospective study. Diabetol Metab Syndr. 2025;17:72. https://doi.org/10.1186/s13098-025-01628-5.
26. Lemieux I, Pascot A, Couillard C, Lamarche B, Tchernof A, Alméras N, et al. Hypertriglyceridemic waist: a marker of the Atherogenic metabolic triad (hyperinsulinemia; Hyperapolipoprotein B; small, dense LDL) in men? Circulation. 2000;102:179–84. https://doi.org/10.1161/01.cir.102.2.179.
27. Nita C, Rusu A, Hancu N, Roman G, Bala C. Hypertensive waist and lipid accumulation product as predictors of metabolic syndrome. Metab Syndr Relat Disord. 2018;16:505–6. https://doi.org/10.1089/met.2018.0098.
28. Rabiee Rad M, Ghasempour Dabaghi G, Sadri H, Darouei B, Amani-Beni R, Mazaheri-Tehrani S. Triglyceride glucose-waist circumference as a predictor of mortality and subtypes of cardiovascular disease: a systematic review and meta-analysis. Diabetol Metab Syndr. 2025;17:59. https://doi.org/10.1186/s13098-025-01616-9.
29. Ferdinand KC, Rodriguez F, Nasser SA, Caballero AE, Puckrein GA, Zangeneh F, et al. Cardiorenal metabolic syndrome and cardiometabolic risks in minority populations. Cardiorenal Med. 2014;4:1–11. https://doi.org/10.1159/000357236.
30. Castro JP, El-Atat FA, McFarlane SI, Aneja A, Sowers JR. Cardiometabolic syndrome: pathophysiology and treatment. Curr Hypertens Rep. 2003;5:393–401. https://doi.org/10.1007/s11906-003-0085-y.
31. Rangaswami J, Bhalla V, Blair JEA, Chang TI, Costa S, Lentine KL, et al. Cardiorenal syndrome: classification, pathophysiology, diagnosis, and treatment strategies: a scientific statement from the American Heart Association. Circulation. 2019;139:e840–78. https://doi.org/10.1161/CIR.0000000000000664.
32. Theodorakis N, Nikolaou M. From cardiovascular-kidney-metabolic syndrome to cardiovascular-renal-hepatic-metabolic syndrome: proposing an expanded framework. Biomolecules. 2025;15:213. https://doi.org/10.3390/biom15020213.
33. Ndumele CE, Neeland IJ, Tuttle KR, Chow SL, Mathew RO, Khan SS, et al. A synopsis of the evidence for the science and clinical management of cardiovascular-kidney-metabolic (CKM) syndrome: a scientific statement from the American Heart Association. Circulation. 2023;148:1636–64. https://doi.org/10.1161/CIR.0000000000001186.
34. Sebastian SA, Padda I, Johal G. Cardiovascular-kidney-metabolic (CKM) syndrome: a state-of-the-art review. Curr Probl Cardiol. 2024;49:102344. https://doi.org/10.1016/j.cpcardiol.2023.102344.
35. Kittelson KS, Junior AG, Fillmore N, da Silva Gomes R. Cardiovascular-kidney-metabolic syndrome—An integrative review. Prog Cardiovasc Dis. 2024;87:26–36. https://doi.org/10.1016/j.pcad.2024.10.012.
36. Kirk EP, Klein S. Pathogenesis and pathophysiology of the cardiometabolic syndrome. J Clin Hypertens (Greenwich). 2009;11:761–5. https://doi.org/10.1111/j.1559-4572.2009.00054.x.
37. Rana MN, Neeland IJ. Adipose tissue inflammation and cardiovascular disease: an update. Curr Diab Rep. 2022;22:27–37. https://doi.org/10.1007/s11892-021-01446-9.

38. Raimundo M, Lopes JA. Metabolic syndrome, chronic kidney disease, and cardiovascular disease: a dynamic and life-threatening triad. Cardiol Res Pract. 2011;2011:747861. https://doi.org/10.4061/2011/747861.
39. Ye Z, Liu EH, Higgins JP, Keavney BD, Lowe GD, Collins R, Danesh J. Seven haemostatic gene polymorphisms in coronary disease: meta-analysis of 66,155 cases and 91,307 controls. Lancet. 2006;367:651–8. https://doi.org/10.1016/S0140-6736(06)68263-9.
40. Tain YL, Hsu CN. The renin-angiotensin system and cardiovascular-kidney-metabolic syndrome: focus on early-life programming. Int J Mol Sci. 2024;25:3298. https://doi.org/10.3390/ijms25063298.
41. Zhu R, Wang R, He J, Wang L, Chen H, Wang Y, et al. Associations of cardiovascular-kidney-metabolic syndrome stages with premature mortality and the role of social determinants of health. J Nutr Health Aging. 2025;29:100504. https://doi.org/10.1016/j.jnha.2025.100504.
42. Ferdinand KC. An overview of cardiovascular-kidney-metabolic syndrome. Am J Manag Care. 2024;30(10 Suppl):S181–8. https://doi.org/10.37765/ajmc.2024.89670.
43. Tuttle KR, Agarwal R, Alpers CE, Bakris GL, Brosius FC, Kolkhof P, Uribarri J. Molecular mechanisms and therapeutic targets for diabetic kidney disease. Kidney Int. 2022;102:248–60. https://doi.org/10.1016/j.kint.2022.05.012.
44. Claudel SE, Verma A. Cardiovascular-kidney-metabolic syndrome: a step toward multi-disciplinary and inclusive care. Cell Metab. 2023;35:2104–6. https://doi.org/10.1016/j.cmet.2023.10.015.
45. Kanbay M, Guldan M, Ozbek L, Copur S, Covic AS, Covic A. Exploring the nexus: the place of kidney diseases within the cardiovascular-kidney-metabolic syndrome spectrum. Eur J Intern Med. 2024;127:1–14. https://doi.org/10.1016/j.ejim.2024.07.014.
46. Chen J, Budoff MJ, Reilly MP, Yang W, Rosas SE, Rahman M, et al. Coronary artery calcification and risk of cardiovascular disease and death among patients with chronic kidney disease. JAMA Cardiol. 2017;2:635–43. https://doi.org/10.1001/jamacardio.2017.0363.
47. Covic A, Vervloet M, Massy ZA, Torres PU, Goldsmith D, Brandenburg V, et al. Bone and mineral disorders in chronic kidney disease: implications for cardiovascular health and ageing in the general population. Lancet Diabetes Endocrinol. 2018;6:319–31. https://doi.org/10.1016/S2213-8587(17)30310-8.
48. Kahn SE, Hull RL, Utzschneider KM. Mechanisms linking obesity to insulin resistance and type 2 diabetes. Nature. 2006;444:840–6. https://doi.org/10.1038/nature05482.
49. Kosmas CE, Bousvarou MD, Kostara CE, Papakonstantinou EJ, Salamou E, Guzman E. Insulin resistance and cardiovascular disease. J Int Med Res. 2023;51:03000605231164548. https://doi.org/10.1177/03000605231164548.
50. Lee SH, Park SY, Choi CS. Insulin resistance: from mechanisms to therapeutic strategies. Diabetes Metab J. 2022;46:15–37. https://doi.org/10.4093/dmj.2021.0280.
51. Cheng Z, Tseng Y, White MF. Insulin signaling meets mitochondria in metabolism. Trends Endocrinol Metab. 2010;21:589–98. https://doi.org/10.1016/j.tem.2010.06.005.
52. Farese RV, Sajan MP, Standaert ML. Insulin-sensitive protein kinases (atypical protein kinase C and protein kinase B/Akt): actions and defects in obesity and type II diabetes. Exp Biol Med (Maywood). 2005;230:593–605. https://doi.org/10.1177/153537020523000901.
53. Beale EG. Insulin signaling and insulin resistance. J Invest Med. 2013;61:11–4. https://doi.org/10.2310/JIM.0b013e3182746f95.
54. Trappanese DM, Sivilich S, Ets HK, Kako F, Autieri MV, Moreland RS. Regulation of mitogen-activated protein kinase by protein kinase C and mitogen-activated protein kinase phosphatase-1 in vascular smooth muscle. Am J Physiol Cell Physiol. 2016;310:C921–30. https://doi.org/10.1152/ajpcell.00311.2015.
55. Forbes JM, Cooper ME. Mechanisms of diabetic complications. Physiol Rev. 2013;93:137–88. https://doi.org/10.1152/physrev.00045.2011.
56. Kadowaki T, Maegawa H, Watada H, Yabe D, Node K, Murohara T, Wada J. Interconnection between cardiovascular, renal and metabolic disorders: a narrative review with a focus on Japan. Diabetes Obes Metab. 2022;24:2283–96. https://doi.org/10.1111/dom.14829.

57. Donath MY, Shoelson SE. Type 2 diabetes as an inflammatory disease. Nat Rev Immunol. 2011;11:98–107. https://doi.org/10.1038/nri2925.
58. Monti D, Ostan R, Borelli V, Castellani G, Franceschi C. Inflammaging and human longevity in the omics era. Mech Ageing Dev. 2017;165(Pt B):129–38. https://doi.org/10.1016/j.mad.2016.12.008.
59. Wenzel P, Kossmann S, Münzel T, Daiber A. Redox regulation of cardiovascular inflammation—immunomodulatory function of mitochondrial and Nox-derived reactive oxygen and nitrogen species. Free Radic Biol Med. 2017;109:48–60. https://doi.org/10.1016/j.freeradbiomed.2017.01.027.
60. Valacchi G, Virgili F, Cervellati C, Pecorelli A. OxInflammation: from subclinical condition to pathological biomarker. Front Physiol. 2018;9:858. https://doi.org/10.3389/fphys.2018.00858.
61. Thomas EL, Fitzpatrick JA, Malik SJ, Taylor-Robinson SD, Bell JD. Whole body fat: content and distribution. Prog Nucl Magn Reson Spectrosc. 2013;73:56–80. https://doi.org/10.1016/j.pnmrs.2013.04.001.
62. Huang JC, Huang YC, Lu CH, Chuang YS, Chien HH, Lin CI, et al. Exploring the relationship between visceral fat and coronary artery calcification risk using metabolic score for visceral fat (METS-VF). Life (Basel). 2024;14:1399. https://doi.org/10.3390/life14111399.
63. Bogardus C, Lillioja S, Mott DM, Hollenbeck C, Reaven G. Relationship between degree of obesity and in vivo insulin action in man. Am J Physiol. 1985;248(3 Pt 1):E286–91. https://doi.org/10.1152/ajpendo.1985.248.3.E286.
64. Arneth B. Mechanisms of insulin resistance in patients with obesity. Endocrine. 2024;5:153–65. https://doi.org/10.3390/endocrines5020011.
65. Yaghootkar H, Whitcher B, Bell JD, Thomas EL. Ethnic differences in adiposity and diabetes risk—insights from genetic studies. J Intern Med. 2020;288:271–83. https://doi.org/10.1111/joim.13082.
66. Neeland IJ, Turer AT, Ayers CR, Powell-Wiley TM, Vega GL, Farzaneh-Far R, et al. Dysfunctional adiposity and the risk of prediabetes and type 2 diabetes in obese adults. JAMA. 2012;308:1150–9. https://doi.org/10.1001/2012.jama.11132.
67. Farag YM, Gaballa MR. Diabesity: an overview of a rising epidemic. Nephrol Dial Transplant. 2011;26:28–35. https://doi.org/10.1093/ndt/gfq576.
68. Guess J, Beltran TH, Choi YS. Prediction of metabolic syndrome in U.S. adults using homeostasis model assessment-insulin resistance. Metab Syndr Relat Disord. 2023;21:156–62. https://doi.org/10.1089/met.2022.0097.
69. Sattar N, Gill JM. Type 2 diabetes as a disease of ectopic fat? BMC Med. 2014;12:123. https://doi.org/10.1186/s12916-014-0123-4.
70. Taylor R. Pathogenesis of type 2 diabetes: tracing the reverse route from cure to cause. Diabetologia. 2008;51:1781–9. https://doi.org/10.1007/s00125-008-1116-7.
71. Esser N, Legrand-Poels S, Piette J, Scheen AJ, Paquot N. Inflammation as a link between obesity, metabolic syndrome and type 2 diabetes. Diabetes Res Clin Pract. 2014;105:141–50. https://doi.org/10.1016/j.diabres.2014.04.006.
72. Tabák AG, Jokela M, Akbaraly TN, Brunner EJ, Kivimäki M, Witte DR. Trajectories of glycaemia, insulin sensitivity, and insulin secretion before diagnosis of type 2 diabetes: an analysis from the Whitehall II study. Lancet. 2009;373:2215–21. https://doi.org/10.1016/S0140-6736(09)60619-X.
73. Hanna-Moussa A, Gardner MJ, Kurukulasuriya LR, Sowers JR. Dysglycemia/prediabetes and cardiovascular risk factors. Rev Cardiovasc Med. 2009;10:202–8. https://doi.org/10.3909/ricm0474.
74. Galicia-Garcia U, Benito-Vicente A, Jebari S, Larrea-Sebal A, Siddiqi H, Uribe KB, et al. Pathophysiology of type 2 diabetes mellitus. Int J Mol Sci. 2020;21:6275. https://doi.org/10.3390/ijms21176275.
75. Ellulu MS, Samouda H. Clinical and biological risk factors associated with inflammation in patients with type 2 diabetes mellitus. BMC Endocr Disord. 2022;22:16. https://doi.org/10.1186/s12902-021-00925-0.

76. Carobbio S, Pellegrinelli V, Vidal-Puig A. Adipose tissue function and expandability as determinants of lipotoxicity and the metabolic syndrome. Adv Exp Med Biol. 2017;960:161–96. https://doi.org/10.1007/978-3-319-48382-5_7.
77. Zhang Y, Proenca R, Maffei M, Barone M, Leopold L, Friedman JM. Positional cloning of the mouse obese gene and its human homologue. Nature. 1994;372:425–32. https://doi.org/10.1038/372425a0.
78. La Cava A, Matarese G. The weight of leptin in immunity. Nat Rev Immunol. 2004;4:371–9. https://doi.org/10.1038/nri1350.
79. Erichsen JM, Fadel JR, Reagan LP. Peripheral versus central insulin and leptin resistance: role in metabolic disorders, cognition, and neuropsychiatric diseases. Neuropharmacology. 2022;203:108877. https://doi.org/10.1016/j.neuropharm.2021.108877.
80. Virtue S, Vidal-Puig A. Adipose tissue expandability, lipotoxicity and the metabolic syndrome—an allostatic perspective. Biochim Biophys Acta. 2010;1801:338–49. https://doi.org/10.1016/j.bbalip.2009.12.006.
81. McLaughlin T, Lamendola C, Coghlan N, Liu TC, Lerner K, Sherman A, Cushman SW. Subcutaneous adipose cell size and distribution: relationship to insulin resistance and body fat. Obesity (Silver Spring). 2014;22:673–80. https://doi.org/10.1002/oby.20209.
82. White UA, Fitch MD, Beyl RA, Hellerstein MK, Ravussin E. Association of in vivo adipose tissue cellular kinetics with markers of metabolic health in humans. J Clin Endocrinol Metab. 2017;102:2171–8. https://doi.org/10.1210/jc.2016-4000.
83. Crewe C, An YA, Scherer PE. The ominous triad of adipose tissue dysfunction: inflammation, fibrosis, and impaired angiogenesis. J Clin Invest. 2017;127:74–82. https://doi.org/10.1172/JCI88883.
84. Nakamura M. Lipotoxicity as a therapeutic target in obesity and diabetic cardiomyopathy. J Pharm Pharm Sci. 2024;27:12568. https://doi.org/10.3389/jpps.2024.12568.
85. Ahmed B, Sultana R, Greene MW. Adipose tissue and insulin resistance in obese. Biomed Pharmacother. 2021;137:111315. https://doi.org/10.1016/j.biopha.2021.111315.
86. Chawla A, Nguyen KD, Goh YP. Macrophage-mediated inflammation in metabolic disease. Nat Rev Immunol. 2011;11:738–49. https://doi.org/10.1038/nri3071.
87. Ouchi N, Parker JL, Lugus JJ, Walsh K. Adipokines in inflammation and metabolic disease. Nat Rev Immunol. 2011;11:85–97. https://doi.org/10.1038/nri2921.
88. Wu H, Ballantyne CM. Metabolic inflammation and insulin resistance in obesity. Circ Res. 2020;126:1549–64. https://doi.org/10.1161/CIRCRESAHA.119.315896.
89. Tsalamandris S, Antonopoulos AS, Oikonomou E, Papamikroulis GA, Vogiatzi G, Papaioannou S, et al. The role of inflammation in diabetes: current concepts and future perspectives. Eur Cardiol. 2019;14:50–9. https://doi.org/10.15420/ecr.2018.33.1.
90. Lempesis IG, Georgakopoulou VE. Physiopathological mechanisms related to inflammation in obesity and type 2 diabetes mellitus. World J Exp Med. 2023;13:7–16. https://doi.org/10.5493/wjem.v13.i3.7.
91. Bianchi VE. Weight loss is a critical factor to reduce inflammation. Clin Nutr ESPEN. 2018;28:21–35. https://doi.org/10.1016/j.clnesp.2018.08.007.
92. Klejbuk K, Strączkowski M. Impact of weight loss on the expression of negative regulators of nuclear FactorκB (NLRP12, NLRC3, and NLRX1) in subcutaneous adipose tissue. Pol Arch Intern Med. 2024;134:16721. https://doi.org/10.20452/pamw.16721.
93. Jiang N, Li Y, Shu T, Wang J. Cytokines and inflammation in Adipogenesis: An updated review. Front Med. 2019;13:314–29. https://doi.org/10.1007/s11684-018-0625-0.
94. Kajitani N, Shikata K, Nakamura A, Nakatou T, Hiramatsu M, Makino H. Microinflammation is a common risk factor for progression of nephropathy and atherosclerosis in Japanese patients with type 2 diabetes. Diabetes Res Clin Pract. 2010;88:171–6. https://doi.org/10.1016/j.diabres.2010.01.012.
95. Jung UJ, Choi MS. Obesity and its metabolic complications: the role of adipokines and the relationship between obesity, inflammation, insulin resistance, dyslipidemia and nonalcoholic fatty liver disease. Int J Mol Sci. 2014;15:6184–223. https://doi.org/10.3390/ijms15046184.

96. Balducci S, Zanuso S, Nicolucci A, Fernando F, Cavallo S, Cardelli P, et al. Anti-inflammatory effect of exercise training in subjects with type 2 diabetes and the metabolic syndrome is dependent on exercise modalities and independent of weight loss. Nutr Metab Cardiovasc Dis. 2010;20:608–17. https://doi.org/10.1016/j.numecd.2009.04.015.
97. Swellam M, Sayed Mahmoud M, Abdel-Fatah Ali A. Clinical implications of adiponectin and inflammatory biomarkers in type 2 diabetes mellitus. Dis Markers. 2009;27:269–78. https://doi.org/10.3233/DMA-2009-0672.
98. Hansen D, Dendale P, Beelen M, Jonkers RA, Mullens A, Corluy L, et al. Plasma adipokine and inflammatory marker concentrations are altered in obese, as opposed to non-obese, type 2 diabetes patients. Eur J Appl Physiol. 2010;109:397–404. https://doi.org/10.1007/s00421-010-1362-5.
99. Rohm TV, Meier DT, Olefsky JM, Donath MY. Inflammation in obesity, diabetes, and related disorders. Immunity. 2022;55:31–55. https://doi.org/10.1016/j.immuni.2021.12.013.
100. Lee YJ, Kim JJ, Kim J, Cho DW, Won JY. The correlation between waist circumference and the pro-inflammatory adipokines in diabetic retinopathy of type 2 diabetes patients. Int J Mol Sci. 2023;24:2036. https://doi.org/10.3390/ijms24032036.
101. Phillips CM, Perry IJ. Does inflammation determine metabolic health status in obese and nonobese adults? J Clin Endocrinol Metab. 2013;98:E1610–9. https://doi.org/10.1210/jc.2013-2038.
102. Wang X, Bao W, Liu J, Ouyang YY, Wang D, Rong S, et al. Inflammatory markers and risk of type 2 diabetes: a systematic review and meta-analysis. Diabetes Care. 2013;36:166–75. https://doi.org/10.2337/dc12-0702.
103. Guria S, Hoory A, Das S, Chattopadhyay D, Mukherjee S. Adipose tissue macrophages and their role in obesity-associated insulin resistance: an overview of the complex dynamics at play. Biosci Rep. 2023;43:BSR20220200. https://doi.org/10.1042/BSR20220200.
104. Kunz HE, Hart CR, Gries KJ, Parvizi M, Laurenti M, Dalla Man C, et al. Adipose tissue macrophage populations and inflammation are associated with systemic inflammation and insulin resistance in obesity. Am J Physiol Endocrinol Metab. 2021;321:E105–21. https://doi.org/10.1152/ajpendo.00070.2021.
105. Westwell-Roper CY, Ehses JA, Verchere CB. Resident macrophages mediate islet amyloid polypeptide-induced islet IL-1β production and β-cell dysfunction. Diabetes. 2014;63:1698–711. https://doi.org/10.2337/db13-0863.
106. Manna P, Jain SK. Obesity, oxidative stress, adipose tissue dysfunction, and the associated health risks: causes and therapeutic strategies. Metab Syndr Relat Disord. 2015;13:423–44. https://doi.org/10.1089/met.2015.0095.
107. Arhire LI, Mihalache L, Covasa M. Irisin: a hope in understanding and managing obesity and metabolic syndrome. Front Endocrinol (Lausanne). 2019;10:524. https://doi.org/10.3389/fendo.2019.00524.
108. Gregor MF, Hotamisligil GS. Inflammatory mechanisms in obesity. Annu Rev Immunol. 2011;29:415–45. https://doi.org/10.1146/annurev-immunol-031210-101322.
109. Burhans MS, Hagman DK, Kuzma JN, Schmidt KA, Kratz M. Contribution of adipose tissue inflammation to the development of type 2 diabetes mellitus. Compr Physiol. 2018;9:1–58. https://doi.org/10.1002/cphy.c170040.
110. Tan CY, Vidal-Puig A. Adipose tissue expandability: the metabolic problems of obesity may arise from the inability to become more obese. Biochem Soc Trans. 2008;36:935–40. https://doi.org/10.1042/BST0360935.
111. Mittendorfer B. Origins of metabolic complications in obesity: adipose tissue and free fatty acid trafficking. Curr Opin Clin Nutr Metab Care. 2011;14:535–41. https://doi.org/10.1097/MCO.0b013e32834ad8b6.
112. Korac A, Srdic-Galic B, Kalezic A, Stancic A, Otasevic V, Korac B, Jankovic A. Adipokine signatures of subcutaneous and visceral abdominal fat in normal-weight and obese women with different metabolic profiles. Arch Med Sci. 2021;17:323–36. https://doi.org/10.5114/aoms/92118.

113. Virtue S, Vidal-Puig A. It's not how fat you are, it's what you do with it that counts. PLoS Biol. 2008;6:e237. https://doi.org/10.1371/journal.pbio.0060237.
114. Hayden MR. Overview and new insights into the metabolic syndrome: risk factors and emerging variables in the development of type 2 diabetes and cerebrocardiovascular disease. Medicina (Kaunas). 2023;59:561. https://doi.org/10.3390/medicina59030561.
115. Paublini H, López González AA, Busquets-Cortés C, Tomas-Gil P, Riutord-Sbert P, Ramírez-Manent JI. Relationship between atherogenic dyslipidaemia and lipid triad and scales that assess insulin resistance. Nutrients. 2023;15:2105. https://doi.org/10.3390/nu15092105.
116. Fahed G, Aoun L, Bou Zerdan M, Allam S, Bou Zerdan M, Bouferraa Y, et al. Metabolic syndrome: updates on pathophysiology and management in 2021. Int J Mol Sci. 2022;23:786. https://doi.org/10.3390/ijms23020786.
117. Muniyappa R, Sowers JR. Role of insulin resistance in endothelial dysfunction. Rev Endocr Metab Disord. 2013;14:5–12. https://doi.org/10.1007/s11154-012-9229-1.
118. Yan Y, Wang L, Zhong N, Wen D, Liu L. Multifaced roles of adipokines in endothelial cell function. Front Endocrinol (Lausanne). 2024;15:1490143. https://doi.org/10.3389/fendo.2024.1490143.
119. Laghlam D, Jozwiak M, Nguyen LS. Renin-angiotensin-aldosterone system and immunomodulation: a state-of-the-art review. Cells. 2021;10:1767. https://doi.org/10.3390/cells10071767.
120. Petramala L, Gigante A, Sarlo F, Servello A, Circosta F, Marino L, et al. Relevance of obesity-related organ damage and metabolic syndrome classification in cardiovascular and renal risk stratification in patients with essential hypertension. Front Cardiovasc Med. 2024;11:1369090. https://doi.org/10.3389/fcvm.2024.1369090.
121. Patel S, Rauf A, Khan H, Abu-Izneid T. Renin-angiotensin-aldosterone (RAAS): the ubiquitous system for homeostasis and pathologies. Biomed Pharmacother. 2017;94:317–25. https://doi.org/10.1016/j.biopha.2017.07.091.
122. Ma K, Gao W, Xu H, Liang W, Ma G. Role and mechanism of the renin-angiotensin-aldosterone system in the onset and development of cardiorenal syndrome. J Renin Angiotensin Aldosterone Syst. 2022;2022:3239057. https://doi.org/10.1155/2022/3239057.
123. Grassi G, Seravalle G, Mancia G. Sympathetic activation in cardiovascular disease: evidence, clinical impact and therapeutic implications. Eur J Clin Invest. 2015;45:1367–75. https://doi.org/10.1111/eci.12553.
124. Grassi G, Drager LF. Sympathetic overactivity, hypertension and cardiovascular disease: state of the art. Curr Med Res Opin. 2024;40(suppl. 1):5–13. https://doi.org/10.1080/03007995.2024.2305248.
125. Seravalle G, Grassi G. Sympathetic nervous system and hypertension: new evidences. Auton Neurosci. 2022;238:102954. https://doi.org/10.1016/j.autneu.2022.102954.
126. Ewen S, Ukena C, Linz D, Schmieder RE, Böhm M, Mahfoud F. The sympathetic nervous system in chronic kidney disease. Curr Hypertens Rep. 2013;15:370–6. https://doi.org/10.1007/s11906-013-0365-0.
127. van der Bel R, Verbree J, Gurney-Champion OJ, van Osch MJP, Stroes ESG, Nederveen AJ, et al. Sympathetic activation by lower body negative pressure decreases kidney perfusion without inducing hypoxia in healthy humans. Clin Auton Res. 2020;30:149–56. https://doi.org/10.1007/s10286-018-0570-7.
128. Bavishi C, Bangalore S, Messerli FH. Renin angiotensin aldosterone system inhibitors in hypertension: is there evidence for benefit independent of blood pressure reduction? Prog Cardiovasc Dis. 2016;59:253–61. https://doi.org/10.1016/j.pcad.2016.10.002.
129. Krzemińska J, Wronka M, Młynarska E, Franczyk B, Rysz J. Arterial hypertension—oxidative stress and inflammation. Antioxidants (Basel). 2022;11:172. https://doi.org/10.3390/antiox11010172.
130. Massy ZA, Drueke TB. Combination of cardiovascular, kidney, and metabolic diseases in a syndrome named cardiovascular-kidney-metabolic, with new risk prediction equations. Kidney Int Rep. 2024;9:2608–18. https://doi.org/10.1016/j.ekir.2024.05.033.

131. Pacurari M, Kafoury R, Tchounwou PB, Ndebele K. The renin-angiotensin-aldosterone system in vascular inflammation and remodeling. Int J Inflam. 2014;2014:689360. https://doi.org/10.1155/2014/689360.
132. Ames MK, Atkins CE, Pitt B. The renin-angiotensin-aldosterone system and its suppression. J Vet Intern Med. 2019;33:363–82. https://doi.org/10.1111/jvim.15454.
133. Oh GC, Cho HJ. Blood pressure and heart failure. Clin Hypertens. 2020;26:1. https://doi.org/10.1186/s40885-019-0132-x.
134. Vendeville N, Lepage MA, Festa MC, Mavrakanas TA. Clinical outcomes of renin-angiotensin-aldosterone blockade in patients with advanced chronic kidney disease: a systematic review and meta-analysis. Can J Cardiol. 2024;40:1718–28. https://doi.org/10.1016/j.cjca.2024.02.027.
135. Yanai K, Ishibashi K, Morishita Y. Systematic review and meta-analysis of renin-angiotensin-aldosterone system blocker effects on the development of cardiovascular disease in patients with chronic kidney disease. Front Pharmacol. 2021;12:662544. https://doi.org/10.3389/fphar.2021.662544.
136. Pecoits-Filho R, Fliser D, Tu C, Zee J, Bieber B, Wong MMY, et al. Prescription of renin-angiotensin-aldosterone system inhibitors (RAASi) and its determinants in patients with advanced CKD under nephrologist care. J Clin Hypertens (Greenwich). 2019;21:991–1001. https://doi.org/10.1111/jch.13563.
137. Bhandari S, Mehta S, Khwaja A, Cleland JGF, Ives N, Brettell E, et al. Renin-angiotensin system inhibition in advanced chronic kidney disease. N Engl J Med. 2022;387:2021–32. https://doi.org/10.1056/NEJMoa2210639.
138. Siragy HM, Carey RM. Role of the intrarenal renin-angiotensin-aldosterone system in chronic kidney disease. Am J Nephrol. 2010;31:541–50. https://doi.org/10.1159/000313363.
139. Batko K, Sączek A, Banaszkiewicz M, Małyszko J, Koc-Żórawska E, Żórawski M, et al. Comprehensive assessment of cardiovascular-kidney-metabolic (CKM) syndrome: novel tools for assessment of cardiovascular risk and kidney outcomes in long-term kidney transplant patients. Kardiol Pol. 2024;82:760–70. https://doi.org/10.33963/v.phj.101062.
140. Nordheim E, Jenssen TG. Chronic kidney disease in patients with diabetes mellitus. Endocr Connect. 2021;10:R151–9. https://doi.org/10.1530/EC-21-0097.
141. Zhao L, Zou Y, Liu F. Transforming growth factor-Beta1 in diabetic kidney disease. Front Cell Dev Biol. 2020;8:187. https://doi.org/10.3389/fcell.2020.00187.
142. Daiber A, Xia N, Steven S, Oelze M, Hanf A, Kröller-Schön S, et al. New therapeutic implications of endothelial nitric oxide synthase (eNOS) function/dysfunction in cardiovascular disease. Int J Mol Sci. 2019;20:187. https://doi.org/10.3390/ijms20010187.
143. Tran N, Garcia T, Aniqa M, Ali S, Ally A, Nauli SM. Endothelial nitric oxide synthase (eNOS) and the cardiovascular system: in physiology and in disease states. Am J Biomed Sci Res. 2022;15:153–77.
144. Schreibing F, Anslinger TM, Kramann R. Fibrosis in pathology of heart and kidney: from deep RNA-sequencing to novel molecular targets. Circ Res. 2023;132:1013–33. https://doi.org/10.1161/CIRCRESAHA.122.321761.
145. Ong CH, Tham CL, Harith HH, Firdaus N, Israf DA. TGF-β-induced fibrosis: a review on the underlying mechanism and potential therapeutic strategies. Eur J Pharmacol. 2021;911:174510. https://doi.org/10.1016/j.ejphar.2021.174510.
146. Mulsow JJ, Watson RW, Fitzpatrick JM, O'Connell PR. Transforming growth factor-beta promotes pro-fibrotic behavior by serosal fibroblasts via PKC and ERK1/2 mitogen activated protein kinase cell signaling. Ann Surg. 2005;242:880–7; ; discussion 887–9. https://doi.org/10.1097/01.sla.0000189606.58343.cd.
147. Meng XM, Nikolic-Paterson DJ, Lan HY. TGF-β: the master regulator of fibrosis. Nat Rev Nephrol. 2016;12:325–38. https://doi.org/10.1038/nrneph.2016.48.
148. Mazzarino M, Cetin E, Bartosova M, Marinovic I, Ipseiz N, Hughes TR, et al. Therapeutic targeting of chronic kidney disease-associated DAMPs differentially contributing to vascular pathology. Front Immunol. 2023;14:1240679. https://doi.org/10.3389/fimmu.2023.1240679.

149. Park CH, Yoo TH. TGF-β inhibitors for therapeutic management of kidney fibrosis. Pharmaceuticals. 2022;15:1485. https://doi.org/10.3390/ph15121485.
150. Chiuariu T, Şalaru D, Ureche C, Vasiliu L, Lupu A, Lupu VV, et al. Cardiac and renal fibrosis, the silent killer in the cardiovascular continuum: an up-to-date. J Cardiovasc Dev Dis. 2024;11:62. https://doi.org/10.3390/jcdd11020062.
151. Ha H, Lee HB. Reactive oxygen species and matrix remodeling in diabetic kidney. J Am Soc Nephrol. 2003;14(Suppl. 3):S246–9. https://doi.org/10.1097/01.asn.0000077411.98742.54.
152. Prasad GV. Metabolic syndrome and chronic kidney disease: current status and future directions. World J Nephrol. 2014;3:210–9. https://doi.org/10.5527/wjn.v3.i4.210.
153. Ren L, Cui H, Wang Y, Ju F, Cai Y, Gang X, Wang G. The role of lipotoxicity in kidney disease: from molecular mechanisms to therapeutic prospects. Biomed Pharmacother. 2023;161:114465. https://doi.org/10.1016/j.biopha.2023.114465.
154. Ge M, Fontanesi F, Merscher S, Fornoni A. The vicious cycle of renal lipotoxicity and mitochondrial dysfunction. Front Physiol. 2020;11:732. https://doi.org/10.3389/fphys.2020.00732.
155. Wende AR, Abel ED. Lipotoxicity in the heart. Biochim Biophys Acta. 2010;1801:311–9. https://doi.org/10.1016/j.bbalip.2009.09.023.
156. Li N, Li Y, Cui L, Shu R, Song H, Wang J, et al. Association between different stages of cardiovascular-kidney-metabolic syndrome and the risk of all-cause mortality. Atherosclerosis. 2024;397:118585. https://doi.org/10.1016/j.atherosclerosis.2024.118585.

Chapter 6
Inflammation and Oxidative Stress in Cardiovascular-Kidney-Metabolic Syndrome

Emilia Valasciuc, Evelina Maria Gosav, and Daniela Maria Tanase

Introduction

Cardiovascular kidney metabolic syndrome (CKM) is an emerging clinical and public health concern defined by interconnected cardiovascular disease and chronic kidney disease (CKD), along with a set of metabolic disorders including obesity, hypertension, and type 2 diabetes. Rather than representing a cluster of conditions, CKM syndrome encompasses a set of pathological processes that synergistically accelerate vascular damage and kidney failure [1, 2].

The epidemiology of CKM syndrome reveals an increase in disease burden with a growing prevalence of CKM-modifiable risk factors, such as poor diet, psychosocial stress, physical inactivity, and tobacco use, which precede the disease. The rising prevalence of CKM-related conditions in both developed and less developed countries poses a significant burden on the healthcare sector, with cardiovascular complications and CKD being the leading causes of mortality, particularly among undiagnosed or late-stage patients [3, 4].

Importantly, CKM syndrome is not solely a consequence of lifestyle and environmental factors. There are also genetic and epigenetic influences that contribute to behavioral and biological mechanisms underlying disease progression. However, at the core of CKM pathophysiology reside two interrelated processes—chronic inflammation and oxidative stress—which initiate and perpetuate endothelial dysfunction, insulin resistance, and target-organ damage, especially in the cardiovascular and renal systems [5].

E. Valasciuc (✉) · E. M. Gosav · D. M. Tanase
Grigore T. Popa University of Medicine and Pharmacy, Iasi, Romania

Saint Spiridon Emergency Hospital, Iasi, Romania

M. Floria, D. M. Tanase (eds.), *Cardiovascular-Kidney-Metabolic Syndrome*, https://doi.org/10.1007/978-3-032-11445-7_6

Chronic inflammation mediated by proinflammatory cytokines, such as tumor necrosis factor-alpha (TNF-α) and interleukin-6 (IL-6), and oxidative stress, primarily driven by reactive oxygen species (ROS), contribute significantly to cellular injury, fibrosis, and metabolic dysregulation. A deeper understanding of these mechanisms' involvement is critical to advancing therapeutic strategies. While antioxidant and anti-inflammatory interventions are explored, current approaches remain limited by inconsistent clinical outcomes. Therefore, a comprehensive evaluation of these processes represents a promising direction for improving prognosis and quality of life in CKM patients [6]. This chapter aims to examine current knowledge of the molecular mechanisms underlying chronic inflammation and oxidative stress, including the use of antioxidants, statins, angiotensin-converting enzyme (ACE) inhibitors, sodium-glucose cotransporter 2 (SGLT2) inhibitors, and glucagon-like peptide-1 (GLP1) receptor agonists, while addressing their clinical limitations as effective interventions for slowing CKM progression.

Chronic Inflammation as a Driver of Disease Progression

Chronic inflammation is defined as a prolonged and dysregulated immune response that results in progressive tissue damage and organ dysfunction. Compared to acute inflammation, which is a short-term protective response to infection, injury, or other stimuli, chronic inflammation persists over time, explaining its contribution to the pathogenesis of several chronic diseases. The sustained inflammatory milieu is marked by the continuous activation of immune cells, overproduction of proinflammatory cytokines, and excessive ROS generation, which further promote cellular injury and ongoing tissue damage [7].

In the context of CKM syndrome, chronic inflammation is now recognized as a central initiating factor where persistent inflammatory cytokines—mainly TNF- α, IL-6, and C-reactive protein (CRP)—are overproduced and apparently critical in the pathogenesis of atherosclerosis and insulin resistance. They are consistently elevated in individuals with CKM syndrome and strongly correlated with metabolic disturbances, such as obesity and type 2 diabetes, as well as cardiovascular and renal complications [8]. Importantly, chronic inflammation in CKM syndrome does not occur in isolation, as it is perpetuated by oxidative stress, genetic predisposition, and lifestyle related factors, including poor diet, physical inactivity, and even psychosocial stress. All of these elements interact in a feedback loop sustaining and amplifying the inflammatory state, disease progression, and target-organ damage [9].

Vascular Damage and Endothelial Dysfunction

A major consequence of chronic inflammation in CKM is the injury of the vascular endothelium, which plays a pivotal role in regulating vascular tone, blood flow, leukocyte infiltration, and hemostasis. Under normal physiological conditions, endothelial cells release nitric oxide (NO), a potent vasodilator that also possesses anti-inflammatory and antithrombotic properties. The aforementioned chronic inflammation impairs NO synthesis and bioavailability, while simultaneously increasing the expression of vasoconstrictor molecules such as endothelin-1, promoting early endothelial dysfunction; both are preliminary processes leading to the development of atherosclerosis and hypertension [10].

Proinflammatory cytokines, mainly TNF-α and IL-6, further exacerbate endothelial dysfunction by inducing the expression of adhesion molecules such as vascular cell adhesion molecule-1 (VCAM-1) and intracellular adhesion molecule-1 (ICAM-1), which assist in the adhesion and transmigration of circulating monocytes on the subendothelial space. Further, monocytes differentiate into macrophages and engulf particles of oxidized low-density lipoproteins (LDL), and then they transform into foam cells, an early and critical event in the development of atherosclerosis. This process initiates the formation of fatty streaks that transition into atherosclerotic plaques, ultimately compromising vascular integrity and reducing arterial compliance. As these plaques develop, they cause arterial stiffening and narrowing [11]. In addition, elevated cytokine levels increase the activity of matrix metalloproteinases (MMPs), which degrade the structural collagen components of the extracellular matrix (ECM). Degradation of the fibrous cap overlying atherosclerotic plaques increases plaque instability, promoting rupture of the plaque and the thinning of the arterial wall, which increases the risk of thrombosis and acute cardiovascular events such as myocardial infarction and stroke [11].

Simultaneously, chronic inflammation also has a deleterious impact on renal function. Persistent inflammatory signaling impairs renal hemodynamics, contributing to reduced glomerular filtration, functional decline, and progression of chronic kidney disease (CKD). In patients who already exhibit metabolic dysregulation and hypertension, chronic inflammation serves as a unifying and accelerating factor for end-stage renal disease [12].

Insulin Resistance

In CKM, insulin resistance is a core feature of metabolic dysfunction. It refers to the diminished ability of peripheral tissues, particularly muscle and adipose tissue, to respond effectively to insulin, leading to impaired glucose uptake and elevated blood glucose levels. Inflammation is intimately linked to the development of insulin resistance, as TNF-α disrupts insulin signaling pathways, particularly through PI3K-Akt [13, 14]. One key mechanism involves the serine phosphorylation of the insulin receptor substrate (IRS-1), a critical protein in insulin molecular signaling. Phosphorylation of specific serine residues inhibits the downstream transmission of insulin signals, effectively impairing glucose uptake into cells [13, 14]. This process contributes directly to the hyperglycemic state that promotes the systemic metabolic imbalance described in CKM [15].

In addition to TNF-α, IL-6 also contributes to insulin resistance by activating the Janus kinase/signal transducer and activator of transcription (JAK/STAT) pathway. Upon binding to its receptor, IL-6 promotes the phosphorylation of STAT3 via JAK1, leading to the transcription of genes associated with inflammation and insulin resistance. IL-6 also promotes serine phosphorylation of IRS family proteins, further diminishing their ability to exert their signaling function. Moreover, the enhancement in hepatic synthesis of acute-phase proteins such as CRP by IL-6 amplifies systemic inflammation and reduces insulin sensitivity [14]. This interplay between inflammatory signaling and metabolic dysfunction illustrates the bidirectional relationship between chronic inflammation and impaired glucose regulation involved in CKM syndrome.

The contribution of insulin resistance extends further to broader metabolic disturbances, including dyslipidemia, hypertension, and obesity. Elevated triglyceride levels and reduced high-density lipoprotein (HDL) cholesterol exacerbate endothelial dysfunction and atherosclerosis progression. Over time, the metabolic imbalances, in addition to hypertension, promote kidney fibrosis and CKD [16].

Synergistic Action of Inflammation
In the kidneys, persistent low-grade inflammation triggers a cascade of pathological events, including fibrosis, glomerulosclerosis, and a gradual decline in renal function. Fibroblasts, activated by TNF-α or IL-6, overproduce extracellular matrix components, disrupting normal tissue architecture, impairing the kidney's ability to filter blood and regulate fluid and electrolyte balance [17].

This inflammatory-mediated disruption from the normal glomerular structure leads to glomerulosclerosis, a key pathological hallmark of CKD, which clinically translates to impaired filtration efficiency and a reduction in glomerular filtration rate (GFR). The combined effects of inflammation alongside hypertension and oxidative stress in CKM patients creates a self-reinforcing cycle that accelerates the progression of CKD [18, 19].

Cardiac dysfunction is similarly influenced by inflammation. The activation of MMPs degrades structural proteins in the myocardium, leading to myocardial fibrosis. Fibrotic remodeling compromises the main cardiac functions, such as contraction and relaxation, creating the premises of heart failure development. In addition, the atherosclerosis sustained by the inflammatory milieu increases the risk of coronary artery disease and myocardial infarction, two common etiologies of heart failure [17].

Another well-established cause of target-organ damage in CKM syndrome is hypertension. Chronic high blood pressure promotes endothelial dysfunction, increased oxidative stress, and facilitates immune cell infiltration into cardiac and renal tissues, explaining the vicious cycle in which inflammation and hemodynamic stress synergistically deteriorate organ structure and function. Additionally, increased vascular permeability allows immune cell infiltration, perpetuating the inflammatory state [1].

A new concept regarding inflammation is called *inflammageing*, which consists of a state marked by chronically elevated levels of inflammatory markers, identified as risk factors for cardiovascular diseases and a higher risk of CKD, type 2 diabetes (Fig. 6.1) [20].

Factors that contribute to this new concept include genetic predisposition, altered intestinal microbiota, activation of the NLRP3 inflammasome, and oxidative stress.

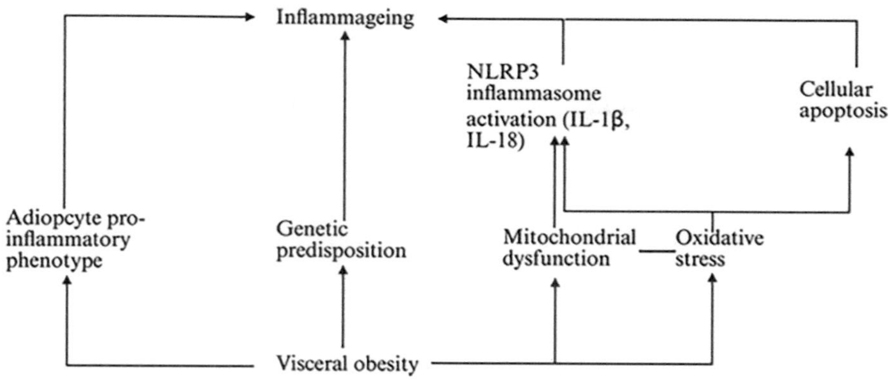

Fig. 6.1 Inflammageing concept

This age-related dysregulation of the immune system toward a proinflammatory state is a major contributor to the development and progression of:

- Cardiovascular diseases: Hypertension and atherosclerosis through activation of renin-angiotensin-aldosterone system (RAAS) leading to vasoconstriction, fluid retention and arterial stiffness.
- CKD: Through microvascular and fibrotic remodeling.
- Metabolic syndrome: By promoting insulin resistance and adipose tissue inflammation [20].

Obesity, particularly visceral fat and perivascular/perirenal adipose tissue act as an active endocrine organ that produces proinflammatory cytokines and adipokines. The dysfunctional adipocytes produce IL-6, TNF, and chemokines, as well as leptin and adiponectin—known hormones that modulate inflammation and insulin resistance in CKM syndrome. Furthermore, obesity induces the activation of the sympathetic nervous system and RAAS, impairing endothelial function and driving the progression of hypertension, glomerular injury, and systemic metabolic dysfunction [19, 21].

Ultimately, the interplay of insulin resistance, chronic inflammation, and oxidative stress contributes significantly to the poor clinical outcomes observed in CKM syndrome. These overlapping mechanisms underscore the importance of targeting inflammatory and metabolic pathways to mitigate organ damage and improve patient prognosis [22].

Oxidative Stress and Its Impact in CKM Syndrome

Oxidative stress is defined as a pathological state in which generation of ROS exceeds the normal capacity of antioxidant defense mechanisms to neutralize them. Typically, ROS are byproducts of normal cellular metabolism generated during oxidative phosphorylation within the mitochondrial electron transport chain. While ROS serves essential roles in cell signaling, immunity, and cellular homeostasis, excessive accumulation leads to oxidative damage at a macromolecular level involving lipids, proteins, and nucleic acids. Multiple risk factors already mentioned in CKM syndrome, such as chronic inflammation, dyslipidemia, obesity, and hypertension also promote increased ROS production [23, 24]. The self-reinforcing relationship that exists between oxidative stress, inflammation, and metabolic syndrome, creates a vicious cycle that accelerates disease progression across vascular, renal, and cardiac systems via endothelial dysfunction, renal fibrosis, and insulin resistance [25].

Mechanisms of Oxidative Stress in CKM Syndrome

ROS exert their pathogenic effects by damaging essential cellular components via lipid peroxidation, protein oxidation, and genotoxic effects. One of the primary targets of ROS is membrane lipids, especially polyunsaturated fatty acids, whose oxidation is implicated in the initiation and progression of atherosclerosis. The altered membrane integrity and increased permeability promoted by chronic inflammation allows oxidized lipids to deposit within the vascular intima, triggering immune cell recruitment and foam cells formation that further develop in atherosclerotic plaques [26]. Aberrant lipid peroxidation disrupts normal endothelial cell functions and enhances cardiovascular disease development and progression among patients with CKM.

Protein oxidation adversely impacts their enzyme activity, receptor function, and cellular architecture. In the context of CKM syndrome, oxidative stress affects several proteins involved in endothelial cell function, such as endothelial nitric oxide synthase (eNOS), which reduces the production of nitric oxide (NO), a key regulator of vascular tone. Reduced bioavailability of NO leads to vasoconstriction, increased vascular resistance, and hypertension—hallmark features of CKM [27, 28]. Additionally, oxidative stress activates the aforementioned MMPs, which degrade the ECM and destabilize atherosclerotic plaques, fueling acute vascular events such as myocardial infarction and stroke. Concurrent fibrosis and reduced cardiac contractility mark the onset of heart failure and arrhythmias [27, 28].

Genotoxic effects secondary to oxidative stress lead to cellular senescence and apoptosis. In CKM syndrome, oxidative DNA alterations impair the regenerative capacity of vascular, renal, and cardiac tissues, accelerating renal fibrosis and cardiac remodeling, which contributes to cumulative functional decline [12].

In hyperglycemic states, excess glucose is metabolized in the mitochondria, leading to an overproduction of superoxide. This is believed to be a primary initiating event in the development of diabetic complications involving both the cardiovascular and renal systems. The overproduction of ROS initiates and sustains multiple damaging pathways. Through polyol pathways, glucose is converted to sorbitol by aldose reductase, consuming NADPH also required for production of glutathione, a key antioxidant. Some excess glucose is diverted into the hexosamine pathway, where it leads to post-translational protein alterations promoting inflammation and fibrosis. The activation of protein kinase C (PKC) isoforms promotes vasoconstriction, increased vascular permeability, extracellular matrix deposition, and proinflammatory cytokine expression. Chronic high glucose levels also cause nonenzymatic glycation of proteins and lipids to form advanced glycation end-products (AGEs), which alter the structure of the extracellular matrix, leading to increased stiffness of blood vessels and myocardial tissue [29]. The consequence of these processes leads to diabetic cardiomyopathy characterized by myocardial fibrosis, hypertrophy, impaired contractility, and diabetic kidney disease, consisting of glomeruli basement membrane thickening, mesangial expansion, and tubulointerstitial fibrosis.

As for the pathogenesis of CKM syndrome, oxidative stress functions as both a driver and amplifier, as its interactions with inflammation foster a pathological cycle characterized by:

- Endothelial dysfunction;
- Increased insulin resistance;
- CKD progression;
- Cardiac remodeling and fibrosis.

Renal Dysfunction

Renal dysfunction occurring in CKM syndrome is closely associated with decreased NO production and increased ROS levels, which reduce renal perfusion and lead to ischemic injury. The kidneys are highly metabolically active and vascularized organs, rendering them vulnerable to oxidative damage [30]. In CKM syndrome, the interplay among inflammation, hyperglycemia, and hypertension, all of which enhance ROS production and directly damage endothelial, tubular, and mesangial cells. Under the influence of angiotensin II and aldosterone, the two major hormones that play significant roles in regulating blood pressure and fluid balance, ROS levels rise. When stimulated by these two hormones, the subunits of NADPH oxidase (NOX), especially from the vascular smooth muscle cells from the cortex and medulla, move into the mitochondrial membrane and amplify ROS production. Among NOX isoforms, NOX 4 is the most abundant in the kidney, predominantly in tubular epithelial cells and mesangial cells [31].

Under normal physiological conditions, NO plays a key role in maintaining renal blood flow, as it acts as a potent vasodilator in the afferent arterioles. Furthermore, it relaxes vascular smooth muscle cells, thereby promoting increased renal perfusion, facilitating natriuresis and regulating glomerular filtration, thus counteracting tubuloglomerular feedback. However, under increased ROS levels, NO bioavailability depletes, impairing vasodilatory effects, reducing renal blood flow, and promoting glomerular hypertension, which over time translates into glomerular injury and fibrosis. Local inflammation triggers fibroblast activation and the accumulation of ECM proteins, which additionally impair glomerular filtration. ROS also affects the balance of vasoactive substances by upregulation of cyclooxygenase (COX) enzymes. While normally COX modulates prostanoid production, when NO levels decline, COX activity increases in favor of vasoconstrictors, in particular the synthesis of thromboxane A_2 (TxA2) [32, 33]. Besides the imbalance in vasoactive substances, ROS exert direct effects on the structural and functional integrity of renal cells. One key process is epithelial-to-mesenchymal transition (EMT), during which tubular epithelial cells lose their tight junctions and apical-basal polarity and acquire mesenchymal characteristics, including enhanced motility and the ability to produce ECM, leading to renal fibrosis. ROS mediate EMT through activation of MAPK (ERK1/ERK2) and TGF-β1-/Smad-signaling pathways, which also promote mesangial cell apoptosis and cellular hypertrophy. Cumulative apoptosis, impaired repair, and excess ECM production lead to structural remodeling of nephrons and loss of function over time [34].

Through the oxidative activation of transcription factors such as nuclear factor-kappa B (NF-κB) and activator protein-1 (AP-1), ROS initiate proinflammatory transcriptional signals that upregulate genes responsible for phospholipase A2, monocyte chemoattractant protein-1 (MCP-1), and cyclooxygenase-2 (COX-2) [32]. The expression of these genes results in the recruitment of immune cells in the kidney interstitium, persistent inflammation, and further simulation of renal interstitial fibrosis, leading to progressive nephron loss and worsening renal function [32].

Overall, the pathophysiology of both cardiovascular and renal disease in CKM syndrome is related to oxidative stress. From disrupting renal blood flow and vasoactive balance, to inducing fibrosis and inflammatory gene expression, oxidative stress plays a central role in the progression of both kidney and cardiovascular diseases (Fig. 6.2) [32, 35].

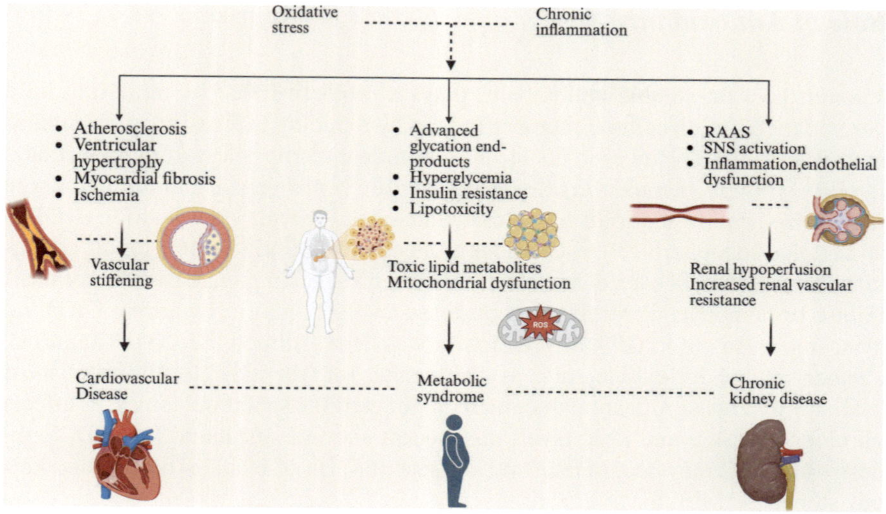

Fig. 6.2 The role of inflammation and oxidative stress in the pathophysiology of CKM syndrome

Therapeutic Strategies for Modulating Inflammation and Oxidative Stress

Given its systemic impact, addressing oxidative stress alongside inflammation may offer a viable strategy to slow CKM progression and improve patient outcomes. Future therapeutic approaches that target redox balance and protect vascular and renal functionality hold promise for better management for CKM syndrome. Several interventions have been explored to mitigate the detrimental effects of oxidative stress in cardiovascular and renal disease. Antioxidants such as vitamins E and C have demonstrated beneficial effects by enhancing endothelial function and delaying the progression of atherosclerosis. In addition, ACE inhibitors have shown efficacy in reducing oxidative stress and preserving renal function in CKM. But despite promising findings, there is still a need for robust clinical trials to confirm the long-term efficacy and safety of antioxidant therapies in the management of CKM syndrome [31, 36]. Key areas for further investigation include optimal dosage and treatment durations, as well as combined therapies with existing pharmacological interventions.

Additionally, novel therapeutic approaches such as gene therapy, targeted drug delivery, and nanomedicine may provide innovative alternatives for improving the prognosis of patients with CKM syndrome.

Role of Antioxidants

Vitamin E, a fat-soluble antioxidant, plays a protective role by inhibiting lipid peroxidation within cellular membranes and by reducing expression of proinflammatory cytokines. However, its strong antioxidant properties are demonstrated in vitro, while its therapeutic roles in humans are controversial and limited. Large randomized controlled trials like Heart Outcomes Prevention Evaluation (HOPE) and Alpha-Tocopherol, Beta-Carotene Cancer Prevention (ATBC) found no significant reduction in cardiovascular events, even suggesting increased risk of heart failure or hemorrhagic stroke at high doses (>400 IU/day). Regarding CKD, no clear improvement in GFR or proteinuria was demonstrated [37, 38]. Vitamin C, a water-soluble antioxidant, acts as a scavenger for free radicals. However, most trials showed no significant reduction in major cardiovascular outcomes, as effects on blood pressure and lipid levels are modest and not sustained. In CKD, high-dose vitamin C may accumulate and increase the risk of oxalate toxicity and kidney stones [39, 40].

Therefore, although antioxidants remain a potentially useful therapeutic tool, additional studies are necessary to optimize potential treatment regimens, to define patient-specific responses, and establish appropriate design protocols for CKM patients [41].

Anti-Inflammatory Therapies

Since chronic low-grade inflammation is a central pathological feature in the development and progression of CKM syndrome, targeting inflammatory pathways emerged as a critical strategy. Several pharmacological agents, including statins, ACE inhibitors, and biologic therapy targeting specific cytokines such as IL-6 and TNF-α, have shown therapeutic potential.

Statins, although primarily recognized for lipid-lowering properties, also exert anti-inflammatory and other pleiotropic properties. The key anti-inflammatory actions of statins reduce CRP, decrease production of TNF- α and IL-6, suppress NF-κB activation, and enhance NO bioavailability by reducing oxidative stress and preventing leukocyte adhesion to the endothelium. In this context, statins help by reducing vascular inflammation, improving renal hemodynamics, and slowing CKD progression, particularly in patients with proteinuria and diabetes, as well as by modulating dysregulated immune responses in obesity and insulin resistance [1, 42, 43].

Additionally, statins possess renoprotective effects and decrease the progression of kidney disease in CKM patients. For example, statins are known to decrease proteinuria, a marker of kidney dysfunction, and often improve renal function by mitigating oxidative stress and inflammation [42]. The Justification for the Use of Statins in Prevention: an Intervention Trial Evaluating Rosuvastatin

(JUPITER) reported that rosuvastatin significantly reduced the incidence of major cardiovascular events in individuals with elevated high-sensitivity C-reactive protein (hs-CRP). These findings were reinforced by the Study of Heart and Renal Protection (SHARP), which also demonstrated that simvastatin plus ezetimibe reduced major atherosclerotic events in patients with CKD [44, 45]. In conclusion, statins serve as effective anti-inflammatory agents in addition to their consecrated lipid-lowering role, improving endothelial function and slowing atherosclerotic progression [1].

ACE inhibitors are central to pharmacological management of CKM syndrome, particularly due to their antihypertensive, antioxidant, and anti-inflammatory effects. By reducing angiotensin II levels, ACE inhibitors facilitate vasodilatation, thereby improving vascular compliance, reduce left ventricular hypertrophy, and prevent myocardial remodeling, lowering the risk of myocardial infarction and heart failure hospitalization [1, 46]. Beyond their hemodynamic effects, ACE inhibitors also exhibit anti-inflammatory properties as they attenuate the expression of pro-inflammatory cytokines, and they enhance endothelial function by increasing NO bioavailability [12].

Clinical trials, including the Heart Outcomes Prevention Evaluation (HOPE) study, have demonstrated that ACE inhibitors such as enalapril and lisinopril reduce cardiovascular morbidity and mortality while slowing renal disease progression in high-risk CKM patients [38]. These findings support the use of ACE inhibitors as first-line therapy in patients with CKD, particularly those presenting with hypertension in the context of CKM syndrome.

SGLT2 inhibitor benefits extend beyond glycemic control as shown in landmark trials such as EMPA-KIDNEY, DAPA-HF, DAPA-CKD, and CREDENCE [47–49]. Nowadays, they are considered foundational therapy in patients with CKD, heart failure, and type 2 diabetes. Their ability to reduce heart failure hospitalization, CKD progression, and lower cardiovascular mortality effects arises from several pleiotropic mechanisms, such as:

- Reduced oxidative stress: Reduce mitochondrial dysfunction and oxidative stress, enhance autophagy.
- Anti-inflammatory effects: Suppress NLRP3 inflammasome, a key driver of IL-1β and IL-18 production, reduce systemic inflammatory markers such as CRP and TNF- α.
- Renal hemodynamics: Restore tubuloglomerular feedback, reduce intraglomerular pressure and proteinuria.
- Metabolic reprogramming: Promote ketogenesis and lipolysis, shift myocardial and renal substrate energy [12].

Glucagon-like peptide-1 receptor agonists (GLP-1RAs), originally also developed for glycemic control, now hold a prominent role in cardiometabolic therapy. A few trials such as LEADER, SUSTAIN-6, and REWIND demonstrated that GLP-1RAs reduced major adverse cardiovascular events (MACE) in patients at high risk for atherosclerotic cardiovascular disease [50]. Although their renal effects are not as pronounced as SGLT2 inhibitors, they reduce albuminuria and slow GFR decline. The benefits are mainly attributed to:

- Anti-inflammatory action: Reduce levels of pro-inflammatory cytokines (IL-6, TNF- α), decrease macrophage activation, and inhibit NF-κB signaling.
- Endothelial protection: Reduce nitric oxide production.
- Weight and appetite control: Sustained weight loss improves insulin sensitivity and systemic inflammation [50].

Combining SGLT2 inhibitors and GLP-1 RAs offers synergistic effects, addressing multiple aspects involved in CKM syndrome, such as hyperglycemic state, obesity, inflammation, and endothelial dysfunction [24, 51].

Emerging Therapies

Beyond conventional treatment, emerging anti-inflammatory strategies might be explored for their potential in managing CKM, including biologic agents targeting specific inflammatory cytokines such as IL-6 and IL- 1β.

Tocilizumab, a monoclonal antibody and antagonist blocking the activity of the IL-6 receptor and modulating systemic inflammation, was demonstrated in earlier research to prevent hyperlipidemia and improve insulin sensitivity in a rat model of induced insulin resistance [52]. Therefore, tocilizumab may be further proposed to be studied for prevention of both vascular and metabolic complications of CKM syndrome. By inhibiting one of the central cytokines in inflammatory cascades, these agents could interrupt atherogenesis and improve endothelial function [53]. Their proven efficacy in other inflammatory conditions such as rheumatoid arthritis lends further support to their potential applicability in CKM. A CANTOS trial with Canakinumab and IL- 1β blocker sustained the inflammation hypothesis of atherosclerosis [54]. However, immunosuppressive effects raised concerns about increased susceptibility to infections, emphasizing the need for further clinical studies to delineate the appropriate patient subgroup, treatment durations, and long-term safety profiles [54].

Other novel therapeutic approaches have included phytochemicals such as curcumin and resveratrol, which showed potential in preclinical studies using models of chronic kidney disease. However, their antioxidant and anti-inflammatory effects must be validated in clinical trials to evaluate their therapeutic value and safety (Table 6.1) [55].

In conclusion, the therapeutic landscape in CKM syndrome is continuously evolving. Conventional agents such as ACE inhibitors, SGLT2 inhibitors, GLP-1Ras, and statins have demonstrated considerable benefit, while newer strategies offer additional promise [68]. Nonetheless, more clinical trials are necessary to establish long-term efficacy, ensure safety, and define optimal therapeutics.

Table 6.1 Potential antioxidant and anti-inflammatory therapies in CKM syndrome

Therapy	Mechanism	References
Statins	Reduced IL-1 β levels Lower hsCRP levels	Ridker et al. [45] Koushki et al. [56]
ACE inhibitors	Decrease levels of IL-6, TNF- α, CRP	Awad et al. [57]
Dapagliflozin	Increases SOD activity Decreases NADPH activity and ROS formation	Hsieh et al. [58] Tsai et al. [59]
Empagliflozin	Increases heme oxygenase-1, Nrf-2 Decreases mitochondrial ROS in cardiac cells	Li et al. [60] Wang et al. [61] Uthman et al. [62]
GLP-1RAs	Increases SOD activity Decreases renal Nox, atrial and ventricular Nox2	Zhang et al. [63] Abdel-Latif et al. [64] Baylan et al. [65]
Colchicine	Inhibits inflammasome activation Reduces IL-18, IL-1 β	Tardif et al. [66]
Canakinumab	Reduces IL-1 β and hsCRP levels	Ridker et al. [54]
Ziltivekimab	Reduces IL-6 and hsCRP levels	Ridker et al. [67]

Learning Objectives

- Identify the roles of inflammation and oxidative stress in the pathophysiology of CKM syndrome.
- Recognize the molecular and cellular mechanisms linking chronic inflammation and oxidative stress to cardiovascular, renal, and metabolic dysfunction.
- Evaluate the impact of lifestyle factors and associated conditions on inflammatory and oxidative response.
- Discuss current and emerging therapeutic strategies targeting inflammation and oxidative stress in the management of CKM syndrome.
- Apply knowledge to clinical decision-making, including risk stratification and personalized treatment plans.

Key Reading

- *Chronic inflammation and oxidative stress* are central, interlinked mechanisms driving the development and progression of CKM syndrome.
- *Adipose tissue dysfunction*, particularly in visceral obesity, releases proinflammatory cytokines and adipokines, promoting systemic inflammation and oxidative imbalance.
- *Mitochondrial dysfunction and overproduction of ROS* impair nitric oxide bioavailability, contributing to endothelial dysfunction.

- *Oxidative stress* exacerbates glomerular hypertension, proteinuria, tubulointerstitial fibrosis, and decline in renal function.
- *Cardiac involvement* includes ROS-mediated myocardial remodeling, accelerated atherogenesis, and impaired ventricular function, contributing to heart failure.
- *Chronic inflammation and oxidative stress* form a feedback loop that accelerates endothelial injury, fibrosis, and CKM progression.
- *Insulin resistance*, a hallmark of metabolic syndrome and type 2 diabetes mellitus, establishes a self-reinforcing cycle of inflammation through altered glucose and lipid metabolism.
- *Endogenous antioxidant defense mechanisms*, such as glutathione and superoxide dismutase are diminished in CKM syndrome.
- *Therapeutic strategies* aimed at mitigating inflammation and oxidative stress through lifestyle modification, pharmacological agents, and emerging molecules represent a critical step for the prevention and management of CKM syndrome.

References

1. Ndumele CE, Neeland IJ, Tuttle KR, Chow SL, Mathew RO, Khan SS, et al. A synopsis of the evidence for the science and clinical management of Cardiovascular-Kidney-Metabolic (CKM) Syndrome: a scientific statement from the American Heart Association. Circulation [Internet]. 2023 [cited 2025 May 28];148(20):1636–64. Available from: https://www.ahajournals.org/doi/10.1161/CIR.0000000000001186. https://doi.org/10.1161/CIR.0000000000001186.
2. Medina E. CKM Syndrome: finally recognizing the connection between the heart, kidney & metabolic syndrome. metabolic syndrome [Internet]. Available from: https://www.kireportscommunity.org/post/ckm-syndrome-finally-recognizing-the-connection-between-the-heart-kidney-metabolic-syndrome
3. Braunwald E. Diabetes, heart failure, and renal dysfunction: the vicious circles. Prog Cardiovasc Dis [Internet]. 2019 Jul [cited 2025 May 28];62(4):298–302. Available from: https://linkinghub.elsevier.com/retrieve/pii/S0033062019301008. https://doi.org/10.1016/j.pcad.2019.07.003.
4. Braunwald E. From cardiorenal to cardiovascular–kidney–metabolic syndromes. Eur Heart J [Internet]. 2025 [cited 2025 May 28];46(8):682–4. Available from: https://academic.oup.com/eurheartj/article/46/8/682/7928657. https://doi.org/10.1093/eurheartj/ehae775
5. Sebastian SA, Padda I, Johal G. Cardiovascular-Kidney-Metabolic (CKM) syndrome: a state-of-the-art review. Curr Prob Cardiol [Internet]. 2024 [cited 2025 May 28];49(2):102344. Available from: https://linkinghub.elsevier.com/retrieve/pii/S0146280623007612. https://doi.org/10.1016/j.cpcardiol.2023.102344.
6. Kittelson KS, Junior AG, Fillmore N, da Silva Gomes R. Cardiovascular-kidney-metabolic syndrome – An integrative review. Prog Cardiovasc Dis [Internet]. 2024; Available from: https://www.sciencedirect.com/science/article/abs/pii/S0033062024001488?via%3Dihub. https://doi.org/10.1016/j.pcad.2024.10.012.

7. Charlton A, Garzarella J, Jandeleit-Dahm KAM, Jha JC. Oxidative stress and inflammation in renal and cardiovascular complications of diabetes. Biology [Internet]. 2020 [cited 2025 May 28];10(1):18. Available from: https://www.mdpi.com/2079-7737/10/1/18. https://doi.org/10.3390/biology10010018.
8. Mas-Fontao S, Civantos E, Boukichou-Abdelkader N, Soto-Catalan M, Romeo-Calas M, Marco A, et al. Oxidative stress and inflammation on metabolic abnormalities and renal involvement in prediabetic subjects across Europe. Nefrologia [Internet]. Available from: https://www.sciencedirect.com/science/article/pii/S0211699524000973?via%3Dihub. https://doi.org/10.1016/j.nefro.2024.10.003.
9. Cao Y, Wang W, Xie S, Xu Y, Lin Z. Joint association of the inflammatory marker and cardiovascular-kidney-metabolic syndrome stages with all-cause and cardiovascular disease mortality: a national prospective study. BMC Public Health [Internet]. 2025 [cited 2025 May 28];25(1):10. Available from: https://bmcpublichealth.biomedcentral.com/articles/10.1186/s12889-024-21131-2. https://doi.org/10.1186/s12889-024-21131-2.
10. Jamwal S, Sharma S. Vascular endothelium dysfunction: a conservative target in metabolic disorders. Inflamm Res [Internet]. 2018 [cited 2025 May 28];67(5):391–405. Available from: http://link.springer.com/10.1007/s00011-018-1129-8. https://doi.org/10.1007/s00011-018-1129-8.
11. Libby P. The changing landscape of atherosclerosis. Nature [Internet]. 2021 Apr 22 [cited 2025 May 28];592(7855):524–33. Available from: https://www.nature.com/articles/s41586-021-03392-8. https://doi.org/10.1038/s41586-021-03392-8.
12. Alicic RZ, Neumiller JJ, Tuttle KR. Combination therapy: an upcoming paradigm to improve kidney and cardiovascular outcomes in chronic kidney disease. Nephrol Dial Transplant [Internet]. 2025 [cited 2025 May 28];40(Supplement_1):i3–17. Available from: https://academic.oup.com/ndt/article/40/Supplement_1/i3/8002193. https://doi.org/10.1093/ndt/gfae212.
13. Wu H, Ballantyne CM. Metabolic inflammation and insulin resistance in obesity. Circ Res [Internet]. 2020 [cited 2025 May 29];126(11):1549–64. Available from: https://www.ahajournals.org/doi/10.1161/CIRCRESAHA.119.315896.
14. Shoelson SE, Lee J, Goldfine AB. Inflammation and insulin resistance. J Clin Investig [Internet]. 2006 [cited 2025 May 29];116(7):1793–801. Available from: http://www.jci.org/cgi/doi/10.1172/JCI29069. https://doi.org/10.1172/JCI29069.
15. Li W, Shen C, Kong W, Zhou X, Fan H, Zhang Y, et al. Association between the triglyceride glucose-body mass index and future cardiovascular disease risk in a population with Cardiovascular-Kidney-Metabolic syndrome stage 0–3: a nationwide prospective cohort study. Cardiovasc Diabetol [Internet]. 2024 [cited 2025 May 29];23(1):292. Available from: https://cardiab.biomedcentral.com/articles/10.1186/s12933-024-02352-6. https://doi.org/10.1186/s12933-024-02352-6.
16. Spoto B, Pisano A, Zoccali C. Insulin resistance in chronic kidney disease: a systematic review. Am J Physiol Renal Physiol [Internet]. 2016 [cited 2025 May 28];311(6):F1087–108. Available from: https://journals.physiology.org/doi/full/10.1152/ajprenal.00340.2016. https://www.physiology.org/doi/10.1152/ajprenal.00340.2016.
17. Marassi M, Fadini GP. The cardio-renal-metabolic connection: a review of the evidence. Cardiovasc Diabetol [Internet]. 2023; Available from: https://cardiab.biomedcentral.com/articles/10.1186/s12933-023-01937-x. https://doi.org/10.1186/s12933-023-01937-x
18. Baaten CCFMJ, Vondenhoff S, Noels H. Endothelial cell dysfunction and increased cardiovascular risk in patients with chronic kidney disease. Circ Res [Internet]. 2023 [cited 2025 May 29];132(8):970–92. Available from: https://www.ahajournals.org/doi/10.1161/CIRCRESAHA.123.321752. https://doi.org/10.1161/CIRCRESAHA.123.321752.
19. Kanbay M, Guldan M, Ozbek L, Copur S, Covic AS, Covic A. Exploring the nexus: the place of kidney diseases within the cardiovascular-kidney-metabolic syndrome spectrum. Eur J Int Med [Internet]. 2024 [cited 2025 May 28];127:1–14. Available from: https://linkinghub.elsevier.com/retrieve/pii/S0953620524003091. https://doi.org/10.1016/j.ejim.2024.07.014.

20. Ferrucci L, Fabbri E. Inflammageing: chronic inflammation in ageing, cardiovascular disease, and frailty. Nat Rev Cardiol [Internet]. 2018;15:505–22. Available from: https://www.nature.com/articles/s41569-018-0064-2. https://doi.org/10.1038/s41569-018-0064-2.
21. Koenen M, Hill MA, Cohen P, Sowers JR. Obesity, adipose tissue and vascular dysfunction. Circ Res [Internet]. 2021;128:951–68. Available from: https://www.ahajournals.org/doi/10.1161/CIRCRESAHA.121.318093. https://doi.org/10.1161/CIRCRESAHA.121.31809.
22. Massy ZA, Drueke TB. Combination of cardiovascular, kidney, and metabolic diseases in a syndrome named cardiovascular-kidney-metabolic, with new risk prediction equations. Kidney Int Rep [Internet]. 2024. Available from: https://www.kireports.org/article/S2468-0249(24)01757-1/fulltext. https://doi.org/10.1016/j.ekir.2024.05.033.
23. Cachofeiro V, Goicochea M, De Vinuesa SG, Oubiña P, Lahera V, Luño J. Oxidative stress and inflammation, a link between chronic kidney disease and cardiovascular disease. Kidney Int [Internet]. 2008 [cited 2025 May 28];74:S4–9. Available from: https://linkinghub.elsevier.com/retrieve/pii/S0085253815532328 https://doi.org/10.1038/ki.2008.516.
24. Valaitienė J, Laučytė-Cibulskienė A. Oxidative stress and its biomarkers in cardiovascular diseases. Artery Res [Internet]. 2024 [cited 2025 May 28];30(1):18. Available from: https://link.springer.com/10.1007/s44200-024-00062-8. https://doi.org/10.1007/s44200-024-00062-8.
25. Hill MA, Yang Y, Zhang L, Sun Z, Jia G, Parrish AR, et al. Insulin resistance, cardiovascular stiffening and cardiovascular disease. Metabolism [Internet]. 2021 [cited 2025 May 29];119:154766. Available from: https://linkinghub.elsevier.com/retrieve/pii/S0026049521000664. https://doi.org/10.1016/j.metabol.2021.154766.
26. Panth N, Paudel KR, Parajuli K. Reactive oxygen species: a key Hallmark of cardiovascular disease. Adv Med [Internet]. 2016 [cited 2025 May 28];2016:1–12. Available from: https://onlinelibrary.wiley.com/doi/10.1155/2016/9152732. https://doi.org/10.1155/2016/9152732.
27. García-Sánchez A, Miranda-Díaz AG, Cardona-Muñoz EG. The role of oxidative stress in physiopathology and pharmacological treatment with pro- and antioxidant properties in chronic diseases. Oxid Med Cell Long [Internet]. 2020 [cited 2025 May 28];2020:1–16. Available from: https://www.hindawi.com/journals/omcl/2020/2082145/. https://doi.org/10.1155/2020/2082145.
28. Akhigbe R, Ajayi A. The impact of reactive oxygen species in the development of cardiometabolic disorders: a review. Lipids Health Dis [Internet]. 2021 [cited 2025 May 28];20(1):23. Available from: https://lipidworld.biomedcentral.com/articles/10.1186/s12944-021-01435-7. https://doi.org/10.1186/s12944-021-01435-7.
29. Chen X, Xie N, Feng L, Huang Y, Wu Y, Zhu H, et al. Oxidative stress in diabetes mellitus and its complications: from pathophysiology to therapeutic strategies. Chinese Med J [Internet]. 2025 [cited 2025 May 28];138(1):15–27. Available from: https://journals.lww.com/10.1097/CM9.0000000000003230. https://doi.org/10.1097/CM9.0000000000003230.
30. Tirichen H, Yaigoub H, Xu W, Wu C, Li R, Li Y. Mitochondrial reactive oxygen species and their contribution in chronic kidney disease progression through oxidative stress. Front Physiol [Internet]. 2021 [cited 2025 May 28];12:627837. Available from: https://www.frontiersin.org/articles/10.3389/fphys.2021.627837/full. https://doi.org/10.3389/fphys.2021.627837
31. Verma S, Singh P, Khurana S, Ganguly NK, Kukreti R, Saso L, et al. Implications of oxidative stress in chronic kidney disease: a review on current concepts and therapies. Kidney Res Clin Pract [Internet]. 2021 [cited 2025 May 29];40(2):183–93. Available from: http://krcp-ksn.org/journal/view.php?doi=10.23876/j.krcp.20.163. https://doi.org/10.23876/j.krcp.20.163.
32. Kishi S, Nagasu H, Kidokoro K, Kashihara N. Oxidative stress and the role of redox signalling in chronic kidney disease. Nat Rev Nephrol [Internet]. 2024 [cited 2025 May 29];20(2):101–19. Available from: https://www.nature.com/articles/s41581-023-00775-0. https://doi.org/10.1038/s41581-023-00775-0.

33. Podkowińska A, Formanowicz D. Chronic kidney disease as oxidative stress- and inflammatory-mediated cardiovascular disease. Antioxidants [Internet]. 2020 [cited 2025 May 28];9(8):752. Available from: https://www.mdpi.com/2076-3921/9/8/752. https://doi.org/10.3390/antiox9080752.
34. Harlacher E, Wollenhaupt J. Impact of uremic toxins on endothelial dysfunction in chronic kidney disease: a systematic review. Int J Mol Sci [Internet]. 2022;23(531). Available from: https://www.mdpi.com/1422-0067/23/1/531. https://doi.org/10.3390/ijms23010531.
35. Rubattu S, Mennuni S, Testa M, Mennuni M, Pierelli G, Pagliaro B, et al. Pathogenesis of chronic cardiorenal syndrome: is there a role for oxidative stress? IJMS [Internet]. 2013 [cited 2025 May 29];14(11):23011–32. Available from: https://www.mdpi.com/1422-0067/14/11/23011. https://doi.org/10.3390/ijms141123011.
36. Młynarska E, Hajdys J, Czarnik W, Fularski P, Leszto K, Majchrowicz G, et al. The role of antioxidants in the therapy of cardiovascular diseases—a literature review. Nutrients [Internet]. 2024 [cited 2025 May 29];16(16):2587. Available from: https://www.mdpi.com/2072-6643/16/16/2587. https://doi.org/10.3390/nu16162587.
37. Yusuf S, Dagenais G, Pogue J, Bosch J, Sleight P. Vitamin E supplementation and cardiovascular events in high-risk patients. N Engl J Med [Internet]. 2000;342(3):154–60. Available from: https://www.nejm.org/doi/10.1056/NEJM200001203420302?url_ver=Z39.88-2003&rfr_id=ori:rid:crossref.org&rfr_dat=cr_pub%20%200www.ncbi.nlm.nih.gov. https://doi.org/10.1056/NEJM200001203420302.
38. Sleight P. The HOPE Study (Heart Outcomes Prevention Evaluation). J Renin Angiotensin Aldosterone Syst [Internet]. 2000 [cited 2025 May 29];1(1):18–20. Available from: https://journals.sagepub.com/doi/10.3317/jraas.2000.002. https://doi.org/10.3317/jraas.2000.002.
39. Sarandol E, Erdinc S, Senol E, Ersoy A, Surmen-Gur E. Effects of vitamin C supplementation on oxidative stress and serum paraoxonase/arylesterase activities in patients on long-term hemodialysis. Nefrología (English Edition) [Internet]. 2023 May [cited 2025 May 29];43(3):351–9. Available from: https://linkinghub.elsevier.com/retrieve/pii/S201325142200150X. https://doi.org/10.1016/j.nefroe.2022.11.024.
40. Karahan S, Afsar B, Kanbay M. Ascorbic acid: a promising agent in chronic kidney disease? Clin Kidney J [Internet]. 2018 [cited 2025 May 29];11(4):530–1. Available from: https://academic.oup.com/ckj/article/11/4/530/5045638. https://doi.org/10.1093/ckj/sfy044.
41. Park SK, Oh CM, Kim E, Jung JY. Dietary intake of antioxidant vitamins and its relation to the progression of chronic kidney disease in adults with preserved renal function. J Renal Nutr [Internet]. 2024 [cited 2025 May 29];34(5):438–46. Available from: https://linkinghub.elsevier.com/retrieve/pii/S1051227624000530. https://doi.org/10.1053/j.jrn.2024.03.005.
42. Esmeijer K, Dekkers OM, De Fijter JW, Dekker FW, Hoogeveen EK. Effect of different types of statins on kidney function decline and proteinuria: a network meta-analysis. Sci Rep [Internet]. 2019 [cited 2025 May 29];9(1):16632. Available from: https://www.nature.com/articles/s41598-019-53064-x. https://doi.org/10.1038/s41598-019-53064-x.
43. Oesterle A, Laufs U, Liao JK. Pleiotropic effects of statins on the cardiovascular system. Circ Res [Internet]. 2017 [cited 2025 May 29];120(1):229–43. Available from: https://www.ahajournals.org/doi/10.1161/CIRCRESAHA.116.308537. https://doi.org/10.1161/CIRCRESAHA.116.308537
44. Sharp Collaborative Group. Study of Heart and Renal Protection (SHARP): randomized trial to assess the effects of lowering low-density lipoprotein cholesterol among 9,438 patients with chronic kidney disease. Am Heart J [Internet]. 2010 Nov [cited 2025 May 29];160(5):785–794.e10. Available from: https://linkinghub.elsevier.com/retrieve/pii/S0002870310007593. https://doi.org/10.1016/j.ahj.2010.08.012.
45. Ridker PM. The JUPITER Trial: results, controversies, and implications for prevention. Circ Cardiovasc Qual Outcomes [Internet]. 2009 [cited 2025 May 29];2(3):279–85. Available from: https://www.ahajournals.org/doi/10.1161/CIRCOUTCOMES.109.868299.

46. Ndumele CE, Rangaswami J, Neeland IJ, Tuttle KR, Khan SS, Coresh J, et al. Cardiovascular-kidney-metabolic health: a presidential advisory from the American Heart Association. Available from: https://www.ahajournals.org/doi/10.1161/CIR.0000000000001184. https://doi.org/10.1161/CIR.0000000000001184.
47. Heerspink HJL, Stefánsson BV, Correa-Rotter R, Chertow GM, Greene T, Hou FF, et al. Dapagliflozin in Patients with chronic kidney disease. N Engl J Med [Internet]. 2020 [cited 2025 May 29];383(15):1436–46. Available from: http://www.nejm.org/doi/10.1056/NEJMoa2024816.
48. Perkovic V, Jardine MJ, Neal B, Bompoint S, Heerspink HJL, Charytan DM, et al. Canagliflozin and renal outcomes in type 2 diabetes and nephropathy. N Engl J Med [Internet]. 2019 [cited 2025 May 29];380(24):2295–306. Available from: http://www.nejm.org/doi/10.1056/NEJMoa1811744.
49. The EMPA-KIDNEY Collaborative Group. Empagliflozin in patients with chronic kidney disease. N Engl J Med [Internet]. 2023 [cited 2025 May 29];388(2):117–27. Available from: http://www.nejm.org/doi/10.1056/NEJMoa2204233.
50. Badve SV, Bilal A, Lee MMY, Sattar N, Gerstein HC, Ruff CT, et al. Effects of GLP-1 receptor agonists on kidney and cardiovascular disease outcomes: a meta-analysis of randomised controlled trials. Lancet Diab Endocrinol [Internet]. 2025 [cited 2025 May 29];13(1):15–28. Available from: https://linkinghub.elsevier.com/retrieve/pii/S2213858724002717. https://doi.org/10.1016/S2213-8587(24)00271-7.
51. Gaddy A, Elrggal M, Madariaga H, Lerma E, Colbert GB. Diabetic kidney disease. Dis Month [Internet]. 2025;71(4). Available from: https://www.sciencedirect.com/science/article/abs/pii/S0011502924001743?via%3Dihub. https://doi.org/10.1016/j.disamonth.2024.101848.
52. Abdelrahman AM, Al Suleimani YM, Ashique M, Manoj P, Ali BH. Effect of infliximab and tocilizumab on fructose-induced hyperinsulinemia and hypertension in rats. Biomed Pharmacother [Internet]. 2018 [cited 2025 May 29];105:182–6. Available from: https://linkinghub.elsevier.com/retrieve/pii/S0753332218319024. https://doi.org/10.1016/j.biopha.2018.05.118.
53. Gao C, Gao S, Zhao R, Shen P, Zhu Y, Duan C, et al. Association between systemic immune-inflammation index and cardiovascular-kidney-metabolic syndrome. Sci Rep [Internet]. 2024;14(1):19151. Available from: https://www.nature.com/articles/s41598-024-69819-0. https://doi.org/10.1038/s41598-024-69819-0.
54. Ridker PM, Everett BM, Thuren T, MacFadyen JG, Chang WH, Ballantyne C, et al. Antiinflammatory therapy with Canakinumab for atherosclerotic disease. N Engl J Med [Internet]. 2017 [cited 2025 May 29];377(12):1119–31. Available from: http://www.nejm.org/doi/10.1056/NEJMoa1707914.
55. Francini FP, Spinella P, Calò LA. Potential role of phytochemicals in metabolic syndrome prevention and therapy. DMSO [Internet]. 2019;12:1987–2002. Available from: https://www.dovepress.com/potential-role-of-phytochemicals-in-metabolic-syndrome-prevention-and%2D%2Dpeer-reviewed-article-DMSO. https://doi.org/10.2147/DMSO.S214550.
56. Koushki K, Shahbaz SK, Mashayekhi K, Sadeghi M, Zayeri ZD, Taba MY, et al. Anti-inflammatory Action of statins in cardiovascular disease: the role of inflammasome and toll-like receptor pathways. Clinic Rev Allerg Immunol [Internet]. 2021 [cited 2025 Jun 2];60(2):175–99. Available from: https://link.springer.com/10.1007/s12016-020-08791-9. https://doi.org/10.1007/s12016-020-08791-9.
57. Awad K, Zaki MM, Mohammed M, Banach M. Effect of the renin angiotensin system inhibitors on inflammatory markers: a systematic review and meta-analysis of 32 randomized controlled trials. Mayo Clin Proc [Internet]. 2022;97(10):1808–23. Available from: https://www.mayoclinicproceedings.org/article/S0025-6196(22)00439-6/abstract. https://10.1016/j.mayocp.2022.06.036

58. Hsieh PL, Chu PM, Cheng HC, Huang YT, Chou WC, Tsai KL, et al. Dapagliflozin Mitigates Doxorubicin-caused myocardium damage by regulating AKT-mediated oxidative stress, cardiac remodeling, and inflammation. IJMS [Internet]. 2022 [cited 2025 Jun 2];23(17):10146. Available from: https://www.mdpi.com/1422-0067/23/17/10146. https://doi.org/10.3390/ijms231710146.
59. Tsai KL, Hsieh PL, Chou WC, Cheng HC, Huang YT, Chan SH. Dapagliflozin attenuates hypoxia/reoxygenation-caused cardiac dysfunction and oxidative damage through modulation of AMPK. Cell Biosci [Internet]. 2021 [cited 2025 Jun 2];11(1):44. Available from: https://cellandbioscience.biomedcentral.com/articles/10.1186/s13578-021-00547-y. https://doi.org/10.1186/s13578-021-00547-y.
60. Li X, Flynn ER, Do Carmo JM, Wang Z, Da Silva AA, Mouton AJ, et al. Direct cardiac actions of Sodium-Glucose Cotransporter 2 inhibition improve mitochondrial function and attenuate oxidative stress in pressure overload-induced heart failure. Front Cardiovasc Med [Internet]. 2022 [cited 2025 Jun 2];9:859253. Available from: https://www.frontiersin.org/articles/10.3389/fcvm.2022.859253/full. https://doi.org/10.3389/fcvm.2022.859253.
61. Wang J, Huang X, Liu H, Chen Y, Li P, Liu L, et al. Empagliflozin Ameliorates diabetic cardiomyopathy via attenuating oxidative stress and improving mitochondrial function. Jiang DS, editor. Oxidative medicine and cellular longevity [Internet]. 2022 [cited 2025 Jun 2];2022:1–16. Available from: https://www.hindawi.com/journals/omcl/2022/1122494/. https://doi.org/10.1155/2022/1122494.
62. Uthman L, Li X, Baartscheer A, Schumacher CA, Baumgart P, Hermanides J, et al. Empagliflozin reduces oxidative stress through inhibition of the novel inflammation/NHE/[Na+]c/ROS-pathway in human endothelial cells. Biomed Pharmacother [Internet]. 2022 [cited 2025 Jun 2];146:112515. Available from: https://linkinghub.elsevier.com/retrieve/pii/S0753332221013020. https://doi.org/10.1016/j.biopha.2021.112515.
63. Zhang L, Li C, Zhu Q, Li N, Zhou H. Liraglutide, a glucagon-like peptide-1 analog, inhibits high glucose-induced oxidative stress and apoptosis in neonatal rat cardiomyocytes. Exp Ther Med [Internet]. 2019 [cited 2025 Jun 2]; Available from: http://www.spandidos-publications.com/10.3892/etm.2019.7388 https://doi.org/10.3892/etm.2019.7388.
64. Abdel-latif RG, Ahmed AF, Heeba GH. Low-dose lixisenatide protects against early-onset nephropathy induced in diabetic rats. Life Sci [Internet]. 2020 [cited 2025 Jun 2];263:118592. Available from: https://linkinghub.elsevier.com/retrieve/pii/S002432052031345X. https://doi.org/10.1016/j.lfs.2020.118592.
65. Baylan U, Korn A, Emmens RW, Schalkwijk CG, Niessen HWM, Krijnen PAJ, et al. Liraglutide treatment attenuates inflammation markers in the cardiac, cerebral and renal microvasculature in streptozotocin-induced diabetic rats. Eur J Clin Investig [Internet]. 2022 [cited 2025 Jun 2];52(9):e13807. Available from: https://onlinelibrary.wiley.com/doi/10.1111/eci.13807. https://doi.org/10.1111/eci.13807.
66. Tardif JC, Kouz S, Waters DD, Bertrand OF, Diaz R, Maggioni AP, et al. Efficacy and safety of low-dose Colchicine after myocardial infarction. N Engl J Med [Internet]. 2019 [cited 2025 Jun 2];381(26):2497–505. Available from: http://www.nejm.org/doi/10.1056/NEJMoa1912388
67. Ridker PM, Devalaraja M, Baeres FMM, Engelmann MDM, Hovingh GK, Ivkovic M, et al. IL-6 inhibition with ziltivekimab in patients at high atherosclerotic risk (RESCUE): a double-blind, randomised, placebo-controlled, phase 2 trial. Lancet [Internet]. 2021 May [cited 2025 Jun 2];397(10289):2060–9. Available from: https://linkinghub.elsevier.com/retrieve/pii/S0140673621005201. https://doi.org/10.1016/S0140-6736(21)00520-1.
68. Maack C, Lehrke M, Backs J, Heinzel FR, Hulot JS, Marx N, et al. Heart failure and diabetes: metabolic alterations and therapeutic interventions: a state-of-the-art review from the Translational Research Committee of the Heart Failure Association–European Society of Cardiology. Eur Heart J. 2018;39(48):4243–54. Available from: https://academic.oup.com/eurheartj/article/39/48/4243/5123540. https://doi.org/10.1093/eurheartj/ehy596.

Chapter 7
The Role of Gut Microbiota in Cardiovascular-Kidney-Metabolic Syndrome

Catalina Mihai, Mihaela Dranga, Otilia Nedelciuc, and Cristina Cijevschi Prelipcean

Introduction

Hippocrates, the father of medicine, stated that "all diseases begin in the gut." Indeed, modern research tends to confirm this statement, with the intestinal microbiota (IM) being involved in the pathogenesis of multiple diseases. The IM comprises all microorganisms (bacteria, viruses, protozoa, and fungi) in the digestive tract, while the intestinal microbiome refers to their genetic material [1]. The IM has multiple functions, including digestive, metabolic, and immunological, that contribute to maintaining health. Understanding the complexity of the interaction between microbiota disorders and various diseases creates the premises for new therapies that target intestinal dysbiosis [2].

About 100 trillion bacteria compose a healthy adult's gut microbiome, ten times more numerous than human cells. To describe the human microbiome, the National Institutes of Health spent $170 million on the Human Microbiome Project in 2007 [3]. According to the researchers, there are significant differences in the microbiome profile across people as well as within persons between various body parts. The gut is known to be colonized by more than 50 bacterial phyla, the most prevalent being *Bacteroidetes*, *Firmicutes*, and *Actinobacteria*.

According to the results of the Human Microbiome Project, every person has a different microbiome, with the gut microbiome exhibiting the highest variety and the slightest temporal fluctuations [3].

C. Mihai · M. Dranga (✉) · O. Nedelciuc · C. C. Prelipcean
Grigore T. Popa University of Medicine and Pharmacy Iași, Iași, Romania

Institute of Gastroenterology and Hepatology, St. Spiridon Emergency Hospital, Iași, Romania
e-mail: mihaela.dranga@umfiasi.ro

M. Floria, D. M. Tanase (eds.), *Cardiovascular-Kidney-Metabolic Syndrome*, https://doi.org/10.1007/978-3-032-11445-7_7

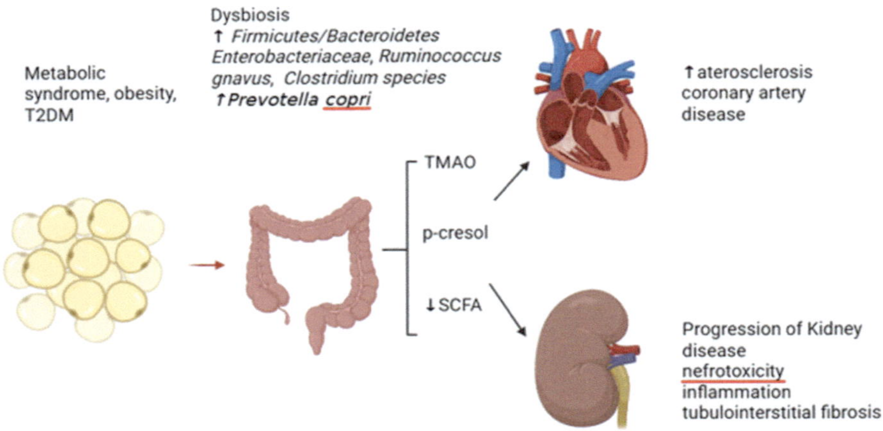

Fig. 7.1 Schematic representation of the association of dysbiotic gut microbiome, gut-derived uremic toxins, and the clinical manifestations of these uremic toxins

This complex ecosystem of microorganisms is instrumental in many physiological functions, including metabolism, immune response, and inflammation, which are vital to the development of CKM.

The intestinal microbiota alteration is one of the main etiopathology factors correlated with the occurrence of obesity, type 2 diabetes mellitus, and metabolic syndrome (MS), a fact proven both in epidemiological studies and in germ-free laboratory animal studies. It is a bidirectional nature of this etiopathology relationship, including complex connections, some of which are incompletely elucidated.

Cardio-metabolic diseases are often associated with gut dysbiosis, which is defined as the decrease of helpful bacteria and the enrichment of potentially harmful species (Fig. 7.1) [4].

Gut Microbiota and Cardiovascular Disease

Intestinal microbiota produces a range of compounds likely to impact cardiovascular health. Short-chain fatty acids (SCFAs), including butyrate and propionate, are released during dietary fiber fermentation. These acids have anti-inflammatory effects and contribute to maintaining the endothelial function. The gut bacteria transform dietary choline and carnitine into trimethylamine-N-oxide, which has been connected to increased cholesterol buildup and atherosclerosis [5].

The gut microbiota modulates the immune system, affecting systemic inflammation. Dysbiosis can trigger an exaggerated immune response, contributing to chronic inflammation, a key driver of atherosclerosis and other cardiovascular diseases. A healthy gut microbiota preserves the integrity of the intestinal barrier, preventing toxic substances from entering the bloodstream. Dysbiosis may weaken this barrier, leading to a more permeable intestine and heightened systemic inflammation, both connected to cardiovascular disease [6].

Clinical Evidence
Recent research has pointed to a link between specific microbial patterns and metabolites from the gut microbiota and the onset and progression of CVD [6, 7].

The advent of high-throughput sequencing technologies and advanced metabolomic techniques has allowed researchers to explore these associations at the taxonomic and functional levels. This process has revealed complex interactions between host physiology and microbial activity that had previously been overlooked [8, 9].

Recent breakthroughs in the field have shown changes in gut microbiota composition among individuals with cardiovascular conditions. Patients with atherosclerosis, coronary artery disease, or heart failure often suffer from microbial dysbiosis, characterized by low microbial diversity and an altered ratio of beneficial and potentially harmful bacterial taxa [10].

A frequent alteration consists of the modified *Firmicutes*-to-*Bacteroidetes* ratio.

The previously established connection between a higher *Firmicutes/Bacteroidetes* ratio and obesity, as well as MS, is under reevaluation, in light of emerging data suggesting that this imbalance may also lead to vascular dysfunction and atherogenesis [11].

Biomarkers
Trimethylamine-N-oxide—a molecule produced through gut microbial metabolism—constitutes another significant discovery in the field. Trimethylamine-N-oxide is formed using a two-step process: First, specific intestinal microorganisms turn dietary components such as choline, phosphatidylcholine, and L-carnitine (found in eggs, red meat, or some dairy products) into trimethylamine [12].

Trimethylamine is subsequently absorbed in the bloodstream and converted into trimethylamine-N-oxide in the liver by enzymes known as flavin-containing monooxygenases, particularly FMO3. Increased plasma levels of trimethylamine-N-oxide have been connected to a markedly increased risk of severe cardiovascular events (e.g., myocardial infarction, stroke, heart failure, or cardiovascular-related mortality) [13, 14].

A host of longitudinal and cross-sectional clinical studies have established TMAO levels as an independent predictor of future cardiovascular events, even in the case of traditional risk factors such as hypertension, dyslipidemia, smoking, and diabetes [15].

In addition to TMAO, various other compounds produced by microbes have emerged as potential indicators of cardiovascular risk. SCFAs, including propionate, acetate, or butyrate, are considered protective agents. These compounds are made through the fermentation of dietary fibers by gut commensal bacteria like *Faecalibacterium prausnitzii* or species of *Roseburia*. SCFAs are instrumental in regulating inflammatory responses, enhancing gut barrier integrity, and modulating blood pressure through interactions with G-protein-coupled receptors. Lower levels of SCFA-producing bacteria or reduced SCFA concentrations in plasma or feces have been associated with arterial stiffness, endothelial dysfunction, or chronic low-grade inflammation—all characteristic of cardiovascular disease [16].

Other metabolites, such as phenylacetylglutamine (PAGln), indoxyl sulfate, and p-cresyl sulfate, have equally stirred interest. PAGln has been correlated with heightened platelet hyperreactivity and an increased risk of thrombosis. These compounds result from amino acid metabolism by means of intestinal bacteria and are then processed in the liver or kidneys. Their presence in circulation correlates with adverse cardiovascular outcomes and may lead to increased severity of heart failure and chronic kidney disease, two often coexisting conditions [17].

An increased number of bacterial genera and species have been constantly associated with cardiovascular health or disease in microbial taxonomy. A significant presence of *Enterobacteriaceae*, *Ruminococcus gnavus*, and particularly *Clostridium species*, many of which can produce trimethylamine (TMA), has been noticed in patients with cardiovascular disease. Conversely, beneficial bacteria such as *Akkermansia muciniphila*, known for preserving mucosal integrity and regulating inflammation, are often diminished in individuals with cardiovascular disease. These findings indicate that both microbial composition and function significantly impact cardiovascular risk [18, 19].

Clinical trials and observational studies increasingly incorporate microbiome characterization into cardiovascular research methodologies [20, 21].

There are pilot programs that have categorized participants based on TMAO levels or gut microbial profiles in an attempt to assess varied responses to dietary modifications or pharmacological treatments [22].

Patients with high baseline TMAO levels may benefit more from dietary interventions that reduce the intake of choline and L-carnitine, such as plant-based diets. In contrast, others might need probiotic or prebiotic therapies to restore microbial balance. Furthermore, recent studies are investigating the potential of TMAO levels as a marker to assess the effectiveness of statin therapy or other cardiovascular medications, offering a new perspective for personalized medicine [23].

Despite the promising nature of these findings, several challenges remain valid. The gut microbiota is a dynamic and complex ecosystem that is influenced by a variety of factors, including age, geographical location, medication (antibiotics and proton pump inhibitors), diet, and health conditions. These factors can trigger significant interindividual variability, leading to a more difficult establishment of universal reference ranges or diagnostic thresholds for microbial biomarkers [24].

In addition, most recent studies are observational and cannot authoritatively demonstrate a causal relationship between changes in microbiota and disease outcomes [25].

Nevertheless, the clinical implications are considerable. Biomarkers derived from gut microbiota, such as TMAO and SCFAs, pose exciting possibilities for early diagnosis, risk stratification, or therapeutic monitoring. Ongoing research, particularly large-scale, longitudinal studies on diverse populations, is fundamental for validating these biomarkers and incorporating them into practical therapeutic strategies [26].

The gut microbiota and its metabolic byproducts are increasingly recognized as critical contributors to cardiovascular disease. Their potential as biomarkers used in early detection and risk assessment constitutes a significant advancement over traditional clinical parameters. With present-day increased understanding of these complex host–microbe interactions, microbiota-based therapies and diagnostics may become integral components of personalized cardiovascular care [27].

Gut Microbiota and Kidney Disease

Slow intestinal transit time, reduced protein absorption, decreased dietary fiber consumption, iron therapy, and frequent antibiotic usage are the main causes of gut microbiota dysbiosis in kidney disease patients [28].

There is preliminary evidence that renal disease patients have altered microbiomes. The authors of a study that employed DNA amplification report an overabundance of aerobic bacteria, including *Enterobacteriaceae* and *Enterococci* species. Anaerobic bacterial changes were also noted, with a marked decrease in *Bifidobacteria* and an increase in *Clostridium perfringens* [29]. According to Vaziri et al., there was a significant difference in the abundance of 190 microbial operational taxonomic units (OTUs) between individuals with end stage renal disease and those who appeared to be in good health [30]. It seems that bacterial families with urease, uricase, p-cresol, and indole-forming enzymes are more prevalent in end stage renal disease patients, while bacteria with short-chain fatty acid-forming enzymes are less prevalent. These alterations in the metabolism of gut microbes lead to inflammation and uremic toxicity [31].

Chronic kidney disease patients have lower levels of *Lactobacillus*, *Bactemides*, and *Bifidobacterium*. Additionally, research on this patient showed that the amount of *Parabacteroides, Enterococcus, Enterobacteriaceae,* and *Klebsiella* had increased while the proportion of *Prevotella, Ruminococcaceae, Roseburia,* and *Faecalibacterium* had decreased [32]. Systemic inflammation has been linked to higher percentages of *Bacterioidaceae* and *Clostridiaceae* [33]. On the other hand, individuals with CKD had lower levels of bacteria linked to anti-inflammatory effects and maintaining the integrity of the intestinal barrier, such as *Lactobacillaceae, Prevotellaceae,* and *Bifidobacteriacea* [34]. In a different study, the authors demonstrated that individuals with chronic kidney disease (CKD) had higher levels of pathogenic bacterial species, such as *Ruminococcus gnavus, Intestinibacter,* and *Erysipelatoclostridium*, than healthy subjects. Additionally, they observed a decrease in bacteria that produce SCFAs, including *Eubacterium, Coprococcus,* and *Bifidobacterium* [35]. In this regard, it has been demonstrated that patients with late stages of CKD have gradually fewer SCFA-producing bacteria [36]. Additionally, the scientists demonstrated that whereas *Ruminococcus gnavus* had an unfavorable relationship with the eGFR value, *Bifidobacterium* was positively connected with enhanced kidney function as measured by eGFR [35].

Along with inflammatory bowel disease and colon cancer, MS has also been associated with the proliferation of the gram-positive anaerobic bacterium *Ruminococcus gnavus* [37]. Furthermore, recent research has demonstrated that oral administration of *Ruminococcus gnavus* may exacerbate renal pathological alterations [38]. The bacterium's functions include producing uremic toxins, encouraging inflammatory processes, and decreasing the expression of proteins in the intestinal tight junction [38]. Therefore, in the context of CKD, these findings lend credence to the idea that dysbiosis, via the gut-kidney axis, contributes to the onset and advancement of kidney damage.

Protein-Bound Uremic Toxins in CKM Syndrome

Currently, the serum of CKD patients contains about 100 different uremic toxins. One of these, known as protein-bound uremic toxins (PBUT), is distinguished by its strong affinity for proteins. TMAO, p-cresol sulfate, and indoxyl sulfate (IS) are examples of PBUTs that are primarily produced by exogenous ingestion, gut dysbiosis, and endogenous metabolites. Dysbiosis of the gut microbiota, enzymatic alterations, and ineffective renal excretion cause PBUT to build up as kidney disease worsens, resulting in harm to multiple organs, including the kidney and heart [39].

CKD patients have alterations in the gut's "healthy" microbiome. Additionally, intestinal permeability is elevated in these people. Large quantities of PBUTs, including IS, PCS, and TMAO, are produced by the gut microbiota and are linked to kidney injury.

Because of increased intestinal permeability, PBUT can enter the circulation. According to certain research, changes in microbiota can impact how well the gut barrier works. This permits the translocation of potentially harmful bacteria into the systemic circulation along with their antigens, including endotoxins [40]. As toxins build up in the blood, they cause oxidative stress, chronic inflammation, metabolic abnormalities, and alterations in the composition of microorganisms. As a result of this vicious cycle, CKD and associated consequences develop and worsen [41].

Several genes encoding PBUT, antibiotic resistance, and virulence factors in functional groups were found to positively correlate with disease severity by the authors of a study that used deep metagenomic sequencing on various stages of kidney disease compared to healthy individuals. This suggests that PBUT plays a role in the development and progression of kidney disease [42].

After building up, the accumulated PBUTs suppress the expression of genes linked to tight junction proteins, including claudins and the occludens-1 zonula. This approach resulted in increased permeability and intestinal barrier damage [43]. The mRNA expression of tissue metalloprotease inhibitor-1 (TIMP-1) and transformer-β growth factor (TGF-β1) is markedly elevated by IS and PCS. This would ultimately result in renal tubular cell damage by raising the amount of reactive oxygen species (ROS) and the activity of triphosphopyridine nucleotide

(NADPH), which oxidizes based on time [44]. IS and PCS raise TGF-β1 levels and encourage chronic renal hyperfusion and fibrosis by stimulating the kidneys' renin-angiotensin system [45]. The gut's altered microbiota produces antigens that set off a series of inflammatory reactions that lead to tubulointerstitial fibrosis and glomerulosclerosis [46].

Studies have shown that TMAO can result in kidney damage and proinflammatory reactions. A greater reaction to the dietary precursor of TMAO is linked to a higher ratio of *Firmicutes* to *Bacteroidetes*, which is also present in CKD [47].

By changing the quantity of bacteria that produce TMAO, Yin et al. showed that dysbiosis can change TMAO levels [48]. Dysbiosis, increased intestinal permeability, and the impact of toxic metabolites in the intestine can also result in kidney disease [49].

Research has indicated that TMAO levels are elevated in CKD patients. It is linked to a higher chance of passing away. When TMAO and choline are fed to animal models, tubulointerstitial fibrosis and collagen deposition occur, and Smad3 phosphorylation rises noticeably as a result. A higher risk of significant cardiovascular adverse events is linked to elevated TMAO, which is a result of CKD [50].

Gut Microbial Metabolites SCFAs and Chronic Kidney Disease

Type 2 diabetes mellitus, obesity, hypertension, and disorders associated with MS are some of the primary causes of CKD.

Changes in intestinal flora cause systemic immunological imbalances in CKD patients, which worsen kidney disease over time and have an impact on other organs like the heart [51].

The number of bacteria in CKD patients' guts that produce SCFA has significantly decreased. The amount of flora decreases in tandem with the advancement of renal failure [52].

As chronic kidney disease worsens, a proinflammatory state develops. This is caused by intracellular nuclear activation factor-κB (NF-κB), which stimulates renal tissue cells to release proinflammatory cytokines and chemomymes. In CKD, this mechanism leads to fibrosis and inflammation [53].

By suppressing NF-kB activity, SCFAs reduce the expression of proinflammatory cytokines and chemokines such as IL-1β, IL-6, TNF-α, and COX-2, hence having an anti-inflammatory impact. Furthermore, SCFAs slowed the evolution of renal fibrosis by reducing the expression of the chemotactic protein monocyte-1 (MCP-1), a possible fibrosis inducer, that was produced by TNF-α [54].

Studies have demonstrated that SCFAs can lower immune cell motility, proliferation, and recruitment while also modifying their functions by directly or indirectly entering cells [55].

Reducing oxidative stress by controlling the activities of cellular oxidoreductase and P300-mediated nuclear factor is another crucial function [56].

Gut Microbiota, Obesity, Diabetes Mellitus, and Metabolic Syndrome

Microbiota Composition in Obesity and Metabolic Syndrome

It is not known whether IM composition induces obesity or whether specific diets modify IM composition and favor obesity. Obesity is associated with a particular profile of IM, with reduced diversity, microbial gene richness and composition, increased *Firmicutes-Bacteroidetes* ratio, decreased *Bacteroides*, and increased *Lactobacillus and Clostridium* [57, 58]. The increased *Firmicutes/Bacteroidetes* ratio can be considered a marker of individuals with obesity and MS. However, as long as this increased ratio is not found in all metabolic patients, this is controversial, demonstrating that other factors are involved in pathogenesis [57].

There are bacteria that, by increasing intestinal permeability and proinflammatory mechanisms, promote obesity (*Clostridium XIVb*, *Dorea* spp., *Enterobacter cloacae*, *Collinsella aerofaciens*). In contrast, others have a protective role (*Akkermansia muciniphila*, *Lactobacillus rhamnosus*, *Bifidobacterium longum*) [58]. Excess *Bacteroides thetaiotaomicron* is associated with obesity, T2DM, and MS [59]. *Prevotella copri* improves carbohydrate and lipid metabolism in patients consuming high-fiber diets but not those with high-fat diets [60]. Thus, *Prevotella copri* increases in diabetic patients' microbiota; it is thought to stimulate the production of branched-chain fatty acids and insulin resistance [61].

In general, butyrate-producing bacteria and those associated with fewer luminal lipopolysaccharides reduce visceral fat and increase intestinal barrier function (families *Rikenellaceae* and *Christensenellaceae*; genera *Bifidobacterium*, *Oscillospira*, *Akkermansia*; species *Alistipes finegoldii*, *Alistipes senegalensis*, and *Faecali prausnitzii*). In contrast, lipopolysaccharide-rich and hydrogen-producing bacteria are found in higher concentrations in obese patients (families *Prevotellaceae*, *Coriobacteriaceae*, *Erysipelotrichaceae*, *Alcaligenaceae*; genera *Roseburia*, *Fusobacterium*, *Escherichia-Shigella*, *Pseudomonas*, *Campylobacter*; species *Eubacterium dolichum*, *Staphylococcus aureus*) [62].

In turn, metabolic status influences the composition of the microbiota, perpetuating and amplifying obesity and metabolic dysfunction. Weight loss achieved through diet, medication, or bariatric surgery positively influences IM composition and comorbidities related to obesity and MS [63].

Recent research demonstrates a microbial signature in adipose tissue (especially the white one), most likely originating from bacterial translocation from the gut. Bacterial translocation refers to the movement of bacteria or their products from the gut to other body parts, which can occur in conditions of increased gut permeability, such as obesity. Obese patients with T2DM have a higher bacterial load and reduced diversity in adipose tissue [64].

Microbiota, Diet, and Energy Intake

Diet greatly influences the composition of IM. A high-fiber diet stimulates SCFAs-producing bacteria. In contrast, a Western diet rich in carbohydrates and saturated fats disrupts the IM balance, increasing the risk of obesity, T2DM, and MS. SCFAs provide 10% of the body's energy needs and provide 70% of the tryptophan produced in the colon [59]. At the same time, SCFAs (especially butyrate) have a lot of beneficial actions in host metabolism: they are the primary energy source for colonocytes, maintain the integrity of the intestinal barrier, reduce inflammation, inhibit hunger, stimulate AMP-activated protein kinase, and induce acid oxidation. However, their interaction with adipose tissue is complex, as, at the same time, butyrate and propionate can stimulate adipocyte differentiation and hyperplasia [65]. Excess SCFAs stimulate intestinal lipoprotein lipase, inducing triglyceride uptake and favoring the increase in fat deposits [66]. Some bacteria (*E. cloacae* and *C. aerofaciens*) favor the pro-lipogenesis effects of SCFAs. In contrast, others (*A. muciniphila*, *L. rhamnosus*, *Lactobacillus gasseri*, *B. longum*, and *Bifidobacterium animalis*) have anti-obesity effects [57].

The microbiota of obese individuals has an increased capacity to extract energy from food, increasing fat storage. Some bacterial species have an increased capacity to extract energy; for example, gram-positive bacteria, such as *Firmicutes*, boost the metabolism of unabsorbed carbohydrates and generate SCFAs with a role in glycolysis and lipogenesis, in contrast to gram-negative bacteria such as *Bacteroidetes* [59].

Metabolic Interactions

The components of undigested carbohydrates, lipids, and proteins reach the colon and serve as substrates for IM enzymes.

IM composition influences fat distribution, increasing visceral fat and promoting MS. IM influences lipid metabolism through multiple mechanisms; reduced fasting-induced adipocyte factor expression causes lipogenesis in peripheral tissues.

IM also influences the hormonal secretion of insulin and glucagon, affecting blood glucose levels. Particular bacterial species: *Akkermansia muciniphila*, *Bifidobacterium longum*, *Clostridium leptum* group, *Faecalibacterium prausnitzii*, and *Faecalibacterium* have a beneficial effect on glucose metabolism, while *Dorea*, *Shigella*, *Escherichia,* and *Ruminococci* promote insulin resistance and T2DM [67]. Although there are no diabetic gut microbial signatures, reduced microbial diversity is reported in most studies investigating the link between T2DM and IM [68].

Butyrate increases insulin sensitivity in peripheral tissues. Reduced butyrate production has been shown in patients with T2DM and prediabetes. Butyrate and propionate stimulate intestinal gluconeogenesis, regulate hepatic gluconeogenesis, and protect against obesity and T2DM [69].

Interestingly, the response or side effects to antidiabetic therapy are influenced by the composition of the IM. For example, an increased concentration of *Prevotella copri* reduces the ability of metformin to lower glycated hemoglobin, and *Streptococcus parasanguinis* increases the risk of side effects [70].

Dietary proteins influence IM by modulating amino acid metabolism and transport and regulating the immune system through interactions with toll-like receptors. Protein fermentation in the gut can produce harmful metabolites such as indoles, phenols, polyamines, hydrogen sulfide, amines, carnitine, and ammonia [71]. In turn, protein metabolites synthesized by IM influence host metabolic functions.

Phenylamine, tyrosine, and tryptophan synthesis, as well as glutamine/glutamate transport system and production of aromatic amino acids and branched-chain amino acids, are increased in obese patients compared to the general population [72]. Decreased glycine-producing bacterial species increase the risk of T2DM, while indole-propionic acid increases insulin secretion and sensitivity; N-acyl amides, mimicking endocannabinoids, influence carbohydrate metabolism.

Microbiota and Inflammation

Dysbiosis increases the permeability of the intestinal mucosa, allowing bacterial lipopolysaccharides to cross the intestinal wall and reach the bloodstream, triggering systemic inflammation with the production of cytokines (IL-6, TNF-beta). T helper lymphocytes and other cells involved in immunity influence metabolic health. Bacterial lipopolysaccharides interact with Toll-like receptor 4 on macrophages and activate nuclear factor-kappa B (NF-κB), which causes the release of cytokines (IL-6, TNF, IL-1β [73]. This "metabolic inflammation" leads to increased insulin resistance, a key factor in developing MS. A vicious cycle is created, with the inflammatory status amplifying the leaky gut and bacterial permeation.

In addition, lipopolysaccharides affect adipokines and inhibit peroxisome proliferator-activated receptor (PPAR) gamma, promoting lipogenesis and lipid storage. Interestingly, bacterial lipopolysaccharides can have different influences on the host immune system (immune tolerance or immune activation), depending on the bacterial species (pathogenic or commensal) from which they originate and on the microbial diversity [57].

Gut-Brain Axis

The brain-gut axis influences appetite and energy balance. Particular bacterial species produce neurotransmitters that modulate hunger and satiety (e.g., ClpB, a substance produced by *Escherichia coli,* determines the regulation of hunger [59]. *Enterococcus species* produce certain SCFAs that, crossing the blood-brain barrier, reduce appetite by stimulating the production of anorexigenic hormones like glucagon-like peptide 1 (GLP-1), peptide YY (PYY), and leptin through G protein-coupled receptors [74]. These hormones inhibit hunger, slow intestinal transit, and stimulate insulin secretion.

Other Mechanisms

The role of *bile acids* as promoters or protectors of lipogenesis is influenced by the composition of the IM. Bile acids act as ligands for the Farnesoid X receptor and inhibit gluconeogenesis, stimulating insulin secretion and hepatic glycogen production [75]. Beneficial bacteria (*L. rhamnosus*, *L. gasseri*, *B. longum*, *B. animalis*, *A. muciniphila*) increase insulin sensitivity and lipogenesis, while *E. cloacae* and *C. aerofaciens* induce lipogenesis [76].

Endocannabinoids play an essential role in carbohydrate and lipid metabolism. Their action on CB1 receptors, located mainly in the hypothalamus, determines hyperphagic behavior and increased lipogenesis. In contrast, their action on CB2 receptors in peripheral tissues and immune cells increases lipogenesis and has an anti-inflammatory effect. Beneficial bacteria (*A. muciniphila*, *L. rhamnosus*, *L. gasseri*, *B. longum*, and *E. coli Nissle* 1917) stimulate the action on receptors CB2, while *E. cloacae* and *C. aerofaciens* stimulate CB1 receptors, favoring obesity [59].

Other molecules involved in the pathogenesis of lipogenesis, obesity, insulin resistance, and MS are influenced by the composition of the IM: oxylipins, succinate, and fasting-induced adipose factor (angiopoietin-like protein 4) [59].

Therapeutic Interventions

Mediterranean Diet

The Mediterranean diet (MD) promotes the consumption of lean proteins and is typified by a high intake of fruits, vegetables, legumes, nuts, whole grains, and dairy products, as well as by the extensive use of extra virgin olive oil [77]. Recent studies showed that it can have an essential role in the prevention and treatment of obesity, diabetes, chronic renal disease, cardiovascular disorders, and CKD syndrome [78]. The risk of major chronic diseases (T2DM, CKD, and CVD) was examined in a meta-analysis of 70 trials. The results consistently showed a substantial negative link between higher adherence to the MD and the risk of these chronic diseases [79].

Vegetable-based diets were significantly associated with higher levels of fecal SCFAs, *Prevotella*, and specific fiber-degrading *Firmicutes*, according to an analysis of the gut microbiota and metabolome of 153 people with varying dietary regimens, stratified by diet type and MD adherence. On the other hand, those who adhered to the MD less frequently had greater amounts of TMAO in their urine [80]. An 8-week isocaloric MD dietary intervention research ($n = 82$) revealed improvements in cardiovascular metabolic indicators, a decrease in PBUT metabolites, and a rise in the abundance of key dietary fiber metabolites, among other microbial characteristics in the gut [80].

Probiotics, Prebiotics, Fecal Microbiota Transplantation

Probiotics are live microorganisms that inhibit the proliferation of harmful bacteria by attaching to their binding sites and competing for nutrients [81].

Probiotics, which usually contain live bacterial strains like *Bifidobacteria*, *Lactobacilli*, and *Streptococci*, are an inexpensive, minimally invasive treatment with few adverse effects. By producing bacteriocins, these probiotics can have antimicrobial effects [82], improve intestinal barrier function to decrease the absorption of enterogenic uremic toxins in patients with chronic kidney disease, slow down the growth of harmful bacteria, increase waste-molecule catabolism, reduce inflammation by blocking receptors, and engage in immune responses [83].

Randomized studies have shown that probiotics can lead to weight loss and improve MS parameters [84]. Bacterial species considered beneficial for preventing and treating obesity are *A. muciniphila* and *D. welbionis*, *Lactobacillus spp*, and *Bifidobacterium spp*, while *E. cloacae*, *C. aerofaciens*, *Dorea formicigenerans*, *Dorea longicatena*, and the *Collinsella genus* promote the occurrence of obesity through various pathogenic mechanisms [3].

Prebiotics are mostly indigestible carbohydrates such as inulin, oligofructose, oligogalactose, oligosoybean sugar, and oligo xylose are examples of nearly or that are part of prebiotics [85]. These carbohydrates encourage the growth of beneficial bacteria like *Bifidobacterium* and *Lactobacillus* in the gastrointestinal tract while suppressing other bacterial species.

Fecal microbiota transplantation (FMT) entails transferring stool from a healthy donor to a patient with dysbiosis. Engineered probiotics consist of genetically modified strains designed to deliver specific therapeutic molecules or modulate host–microbe interactions in a targeted manner. Although these strategies remain largely experimental about cardiovascular disease, preliminary data point to their potential as viable options in the future, especially for patients with severe or treatment-resistant conditions. FMT has shown efficacy in managing diabetes [86], obesity, MS [87], and CKD [88].

However, there is insufficient evidence to support using FMT as a therapeutic method in obesity, T2DM, or MS. Its combination as an adjuvant to other therapies (e.g., Incretins) could modulate IM in the long term [58].

Advanced therapeutic approaches are currently under investigation. Obese and T2DM patients have altered virus-bacterial correlation at the level of IM; Bacteriophages could modify metabolite levels and have potential therapeutic effects in T2DM and MS [89]. The so-called psychobiotics can influence eating behavior. Using IM-related molecules as biomarkers and therapeutic targets (SCFAs, fasting-induced adipose factors, AMP-activated protein kinase, bile acids, farnesoid X receptor (FXR) pathways) seems promising [60]. Although the studies are encouraging, the same therapeutic intervention may lead to different outcomes depending on genetic factors, the particular configuration of the IM, diet, therapies, metabolic profile, etc.

There are currently no firm recommendations regarding the composition, dose, duration, or mode of administration of therapies based on microbiota modulation in obesity, diabetes, and MS. There are multiple ongoing studies regarding pre, probiotics, postbiotics, and fecal transplant in CKM syndrome.

Future Directions

Multiple barriers exist to understanding and modulating the relationship between IM, obesity, and MS. Animal studies cannot be fully extrapolated to humans. Various factors influence IM. Obesity and MS are diseases with complex etiopathogenesis in which IM is only one interconnected player among other pathogenic mechanisms. Understanding the molecular mechanisms by which IM and its metabolic products interact with the host organism is crucial for preventing and treating obesity and MS. The multiomics approach (metagenomics, metabolomics, and proteomics) will open new directions for understanding the complex interaction mechanisms between microbiota, the immune system, and metabolism. Biomarkers derived from microbiota could lead to the early detection of metabolic diseases. Personalized nutrition, genetic engineering, and manipulation of IM will lead to optimal metabolic health and reduce the complications associated with obesity and CKM syndrome.

Conclusion

The gut microbiota is instrumental for CKM syndrome, by means of a variety of mechanisms, such as the synthesis of metabolites, modulation of the immune system, and preservation of gut barrier integrity. Gaining insight into the intricate interactions between gut microbiota and CKM syndrome fosters new research directions for prevention and treatment. Ongoing research is vital in accounting for the complexities of this relationship and in designing targeted therapies aimed at enhancing cardiovascular, metabolic, and renal health.

Learning Objectives

- Evaluation of the complex role of microbiota in the cardio-kidney-metabolic syndrome
- Explanation of pathophysiological mechanisms linking intestinal dysbiosis and cardio-kidney-metabolic syndrome
- Understanding microbiota-derived biomarkers in cardio-kidney-metabolic syndrome
- Evaluation of new therapeutic interventions on the microbiota in cardio-kidney-metabolic syndrome

Key Reading

- *CKM syndrome* defines a group of interrelated health conditions that include CVD, CKD, and metabolic disorders, such as obesity and diabetes.
- *Gut microbiota* represents a complex ecosystem of microorganisms that is instrumental in many physiological functions, including metabolism, immune response, and inflammation, factors vital to the development of obesity, T2DM, CVD, and CKD.
- *Obesity and adipose tissue dysfunction* are key contributors to CKM syndrome, facilitating inflammation, oxidative stress, and insulin resistance, impacting cardiovascular and renal systems.

- *Type 2 diabetes mellitus* is associated with chronic hyperglycaemia and insulin resistance, contributing to vascular and glomerular injury.
- *CKD* is often related to dysbiosis, which correlates with elevated levels of uremic toxins, subsequently accelerating CKD progression and can negatively impact cardiovascular health.
- *CVD and dysbiosis*—disturbed gut microbiota correlate with intestinal inflammation and reduced gut barrier integrity, which causes higher circulating levels of bacterial structural components and microbial metabolites, such as trimethylamine-N-oxide and short-chain fatty acids, that may promote the onset of CVD.

References

1. D'Argenio V, Salvatore F. The role of the gut microbiome in the healthy adult status. Clin Chim Acta. 2015;451:97–102. https://doi.org/10.1016/j.cca.2015.01.003.
2. Ene-Iordache B, Perico N, Bikbov B, Carminati S, Remuzzi A, Perna A, et al. Chronic kidney disease and cardiovascular risk in six regions of the world (ISN-KDDC): a cross-sectional study. Lancet Global Health. 2016;4:e307–19. https://doi.org/10.1016/S2214-109X(16)00071-1.
3. Turnbaugh PJ, Ley RE, Hamady M, Fraser-Liggett CM, Knight R, Gordon JI. The human microbiome project. Nature. 2007;449:804–10. https://doi.org/10.1038/nature06244.
4. Li Q, Gao B, Siqin B, He Q, et al. Gut microbiota: a novel regulator of cardiovascular disease and key factor in the therapeutic effects of flavonoids. Front Pharmacol. 2021;12:651926. https://doi.org/10.3389/fphar.2021.651926.
5. Novakovic M, Rout A, Kingsley T, et al. Role of gut microbiota in cardiovascular diseases. World J Cardiol. 2020;12(4):110–22. https://doi.org/10.4330/wjc.v12.i4.110.
6. Tang WH, Kitai T, Hazen SL. Gut microbiota in cardiovascular health and disease. Circ Res. 2017;120(7):1183–96. https://doi.org/10.1161/CIRCRESAHA.117.309715.
7. Rahman MM, Islam F, Or-Rashid MH, et al. The gut microbiota (microbiome) in cardiovascular disease and its therapeutic regulation. Front Cell Infect Microbiol. 2022;12:903570. https://doi.org/10.3389/fcimb.2022.903570.
8. Di Bella JM, Bao Y, Gloor GB, Burton JP, Reid G. High throughput sequencing methods and analysis for microbiome research. J Microbiol Methods. 2013;95(3):401–14. https://doi.org/10.1016/j.mimet.2013.08.011.
9. Interino N, Vitagliano R, D'Amico, et al. Microbiota–gut–brain axis: mass-spectrometry-based metabolomics in the study of microbiome mediators—stress relationship. Biomolecules. 2025;15(2):243. https://doi.org/10.3390/biom15020243.
10. Kazemian N, Mahmoudi M, Halperin F, Wu JC, Pakpour S. Gut microbiota and cardiovascular disease: opportunities and challenges. Microbiome. 2020;8(1):36. https://doi.org/10.1186/s40168-020-00821-0.
11. Magne F, Gotteland M, Gauthier L, et al. The Firmicutes/Bacteroidetes ratio: a relevant marker of gut dysbiosis in obese patients? Nutrients. 2020;12(5):1474. https://doi.org/10.3390/nu12051474.
12. Wang Z, Klipfell E, Bennett BJ, et al. Gut flora metabolism of phosphatidylcholine promotes cardiovascular disease. Nature. 2011;472(7341):57. https://doi.org/10.1038/nature09922.

13. Canyelles M, Borràs C, Rotllan N, Tondo M, Escolà-Gil JC, Blanco-Vaca F. Gut microbiota-derived TMAO: a causal factor promoting atherosclerotic cardiovascular disease? Int J Mol Sci. 2023;24(3):1940. https://doi.org/10.3390/ijms24031940.
14. Roncal C, Martínez-Aguilar E, Orbe J, et al. Trimethylamine-N-Oxide (TMAO) predicts cardiovascular mortality in peripheral artery disease. Sci Rep. 2019;9:15580. https://doi.org/10.1038/s41598-019-52082-z.
15. Tang WHW, Li XS, Wu Y, et al. Plasma trimethylamine N-oxide (TMAO) levels predict future risk of coronary artery disease in apparently healthy individuals in the EPIC-Norfolk prospective population study. Am Heart J. 2021;236:80–6. https://doi.org/10.1016/j.ahj.2021.01.020.
16. Hu T, Wu Q, Yao Q, Jiang K, Yu J, Tang Q. Short-chain fatty acid metabolism and multiple effects on cardiovascular diseases. Ageing Res Rev. 2022;81:101706. https://doi.org/10.1016/j.arr.2022.101706.
17. Zhu W, Gregory JC, Org E, et al. Gut microbial metabolite TMAO enhances platelet hyperreactivity and thrombosis risk. Cell. 2016;165(1):111–24. https://doi.org/10.1016/j.cell.2016.02.011.
18. Witkowski M, Weeks TL, Hazen SL. Gut microbiota and cardiovascular disease. Circ Res. 2020;127(4):553–70. https://doi.org/10.1161/CIRCRESAHA.120.316242.
19. Azzouz D, Omarbekova A, Heguy A, et al. Lupus nephritis is linked to disease-activity associated expansions and immunity to a gut commensal. Ann Rheum Dis. 2019;78:947–56. https://doi.org/10.1136/annrheumdis-2018-214856.
20. Dean YE, Shebl MA, Doma M, et al. Intestinal microbiome as a diagnostic marker of coronary artery disease: a systematic review and meta-analysis. Ann Med Surg (Lond). 2024;86(10):6105–20. https://doi.org/10.1097/MS9.0000000000002516.
21. Li C, Stražar M, Mohamed AMT, et al. Gut microbiome and metabolome profiling in Framingham heart study reveals cholesterol-metabolizing bacteria. Cell. 2024;187(8):1834–52. https://doi.org/10.1016/j.cell.2024.03.014.
22. Jing L, Zhang H, Xiang Q, et al. Targeting Trimethylamine N-oxide: a new therapeutic strategy for alleviating atherosclerosis. Front Cardiovasc Med. 2022;9:864600. https://doi.org/10.3389/fcvm.2022.864600.
23. Jaworska K, Kopacz W, Koper M, Ufnal M. Microbiome-Derived Trimethylamine N-Oxide (TMAO) as a multifaceted biomarker in cardiovascular disease: challenges and opportunities. Int J Mol Sci. 2024;25(23):12511. https://doi.org/10.3390/ijms252312511.
24. Favari C, Rinaldi de Alvarenga JF, Sánchez-Martínez L, et al. Factors driving the inter-individual variability in the metabolism and bioavailability of (poly)phenolic metabolites: a systematic review of human studies. Redox Biol. 2024;71:103095. https://doi.org/10.1016/j.redox.2024.103095.
25. Xie S, Meng Q, Wang L. The effect of gut microbiome and plasma metabolome on systemic sclerosis: a bidirectional two-sample Mendelian randomization study. Front Microbiol. 2024;15:1427195. https://doi.org/10.3389/fmicb.2024.1427195.
26. Petrosino JF. The microbiome in precision medicine: the way forward. Genome Med. 2018;10(1):12. https://doi.org/10.1186/s13073-018-0525-6.
27. Nesci A, Carnuccio C, Ruggieri V, et al. Gut microbiota and cardiovascular disease: evidence on the metabolic and inflammatory background of a complex relationship. Int J Mol Sci. 2023;24(10):9087. https://doi.org/10.3390/ijms24109087.
28. Ramezani A, Massy ZA, Meijers B, Evenepoel P, Vanholder R, Raj DS. Role of the gut microbiome in Uremia: a potential therapeutic target. Am J Kidney Dis. 2016;67(3):483–98. https://doi.org/10.1053/j.ajkd.2015.09.027.
29. Hida M, Aiba Y, Sawamura S, Suzuki N, Satoh T, Koga Y. Inhibition of the accumulation of uremic toxins in the blood and their precursors in the feces after oral administration of Lebenin, a lactic acid bacteria preparation, to uremic patients undergoing hemodialysis. Nephron. 1996;74(2):349–55. https://doi.org/10.1159/000189334.

30. Vaziri ND, Wong J, Pahl M, et al. Chronic kidney disease alters intestinal microbial flora. Kidney Int. 2013;83(2):308–15. https://doi.org/10.1038/ki.2012.345.
31. Wong J, Piceno YM, Desantis TZ, Pahl M, Andersen GL, Vaziri ND. Expansion of urease- and uricase-containing, indole- and p-cresol-forming and contraction of short-chain fatty acid-producing intestinal microbiota in ESRD. Am J Nephrol. 2014;39(3):230–7. https://doi.org/10.1159/000360010.
32. Iatcu CO, Steen A, Covasa M. Gut microbiota and complications of Type-2 diabetes. Nutrients. 2021;14(1):166. https://doi.org/10.3390/nu14010166.
33. Vaziri ND, Yuan J, Nazertehrani S, Ni Z, Liu S. Chronic kidney disease causes disruption of gastric and small intestinal epithelial tight junction. Am J Nephrol. 2013;38:99–103. https://doi.org/10.1159/000353764.
34. Kanbay M, Onal EM, Afsar B, et al. The crosstalk of gut microbiota and chronic kidney disease: role of inflammation, proteinuria, hypertension, and diabetes mellitus. Int Urol Nephrol. 2018;50:1453–66. https://doi.org/10.1007/s11255-018-1873-2.
35. Dissayabutra T, Chuaypen N, Somnark P, et al. Characterization of gut dysbiosis and intestinal barrier dysfunction in patients with metabolic dysfunction-associated steatotic liver disease and chronic kidney disease: a comparative study. 2025;15:15481. https://doi.org/10.1038/s41598-025-00237-6.
36. He M, Wei W, Zhang Y, et al. Gut microbial metabolites SCFAs and chronic kidney disease. J Transl Med. 2024;22(1):172. https://doi.org/10.1186/s12967-024-04974-6.
37. Crost EH, Coletto E, Bell A, Juge N. Ruminococcus gnavus: friend or foe for human health. FEMS Microbiol Rev. 2023;47(2):fuad014. https://doi.org/10.1093/femsre/fuad014.
38. Jourde-Chiche N, Burtey S. Accumulation of protein-bound uremic toxins: the kidney remains the leading culprit in the gut-liver-kidney axis. Kidney Int. 2020;97:1102–4. https://doi.org/10.1016/j.kint.2020.02.026.
39. Zaky A, Glastras SJ, Wong MYW, Pollock CA, Saad S. The role of the gut microbiome in diabetes and obesity-related kidney disease. Int J Mol Sci. 2021;22:17. https://doi.org/10.3390/ijms22179641.
40. Glorieux G, Gryp T, Perna A. Gut-derived metabolites and their role in immune dysfunction in chronic kidney disease. Toxins. 2020;12(4):245. https://doi.org/10.3390/toxins12040245.
41. Tang S, Wu G, Liu Y, Xue B, Zhang S, Zhang W, et al. Guild-level signature of gut microbiome for diabetic kidney disease. MBio. 2024;15(7):e0073524. https://doi.org/10.1128/mbio.00735-24.
42. Huang Y, Zhou J, Wang S, Xiong J, Chen Y, Liu Y, et al. Indoxyl sulfate induces intestinal barrier injury through IRF1-DRP1 axis-mediated mitophagy impairment. Theranostics. 2020;10:7384–400. https://doi.org/10.7150/thno.45455.
43. Watanabe H, Miyamoto Y, Honda D, Tanaka H, Wu Q, Endo M, et al. p-Cresyl sulfate causes renal tubular cell damage by inducing oxidative stress by activation of NADPH oxidase. Kidney Int. 2013;83:582–92. https://doi.org/10.1038/ki.2012.448.
44. Jing YJ, Ni JW, Ding FH, Fang YH, Wang XQ, Wang HB, et al. p-Cresyl sulfate is associated with carotid arteriosclerosis in hemodialysis patients and promotes atherogenesis in apoE−/− mice. Kidney Int. 2016;89:439–49. https://doi.org/10.1038/ki.2015.287.
45. Rayego-Mateos S, Rodrigues-Diez RR, Fernandez-Fernandez B, Mora-Fernández C, Marchant V, Donate-Correa J, et al. Targeting inflammation to treat diabetic kidney disease: the road to 2030. Kidney Int. 2023;103:282–96. https://doi.org/10.1016/j.kint.2022.10.030.
46. Subramaniam S, Fletcher C. Trimethylamine N-oxide: breathe new life. Br J Pharmacol. 2018;175:1344–53. https://doi.org/10.1111/bph.13959.
47. Miller MJ. Risk factors for cardiovascular disease: a cautionary tale of diet-microbiome interactions. J Am Coll Nutr. 2013;32:75–8. https://doi.org/10.1080/07315724.2013.799982.
48. Yin J, Liao SX, He Y, Wang S, Xia GH, Liu FT, et al. Dysbiosis of gut microbiota with reduced trimethylamine-N-oxide level in patients with large-artery atherosclerotic stroke or transient ischemic attack. J Am Heart Assoc. 2015;4(11):e002699. https://doi.org/10.1161/JAHA.115.002699.

49. Tang WH, Wang Z, Kennedy DJ, et al. Gut microbiota-dependent trimethylamine N-oxide (TMAO) pathway contributes to both development of renal insufficiency and mortality risk in chronic kidney disease. Circ Res. 2015;116(3):448–55. https://doi.org/10.1161/CIRCRESAHA.116.305360.
50. Tang WH, Wang Z, Levison BS, et al. Intestinal microbial metabolism of phosphatidylcholine and cardiovascular risk. N Engl J Med. 2013;368(17):1575–84. https://doi.org/10.1056/NEJMoa1109400.
51. Cooper TE, Khalid R, Chan S, et al. Synbiotics, prebiotics and probiotics for people with chronic kidney disease. Cochrane Database Syst Rev. 2023;10(10):013631. https://doi.org/10.1002/14651858.CD013631.pub2.
52. Khan S, Jena G. Sodium butyrate, a HDAC inhibitor ameliorates eNOS, iNOS and TGF-β1-induced fibrogenesis, apoptosis and DNA damage in the kidney of juvenile diabetic rats. Food Chem Toxicol. 2014;73:127–39. https://doi.org/10.1016/j.fct.2014.08.010.
53. Ratliff BB, Abdulmahdi W, Pawar R, Wolin MS. Oxidant mechanisms in renal injury and disease. Antioxid Redox Signal. 2016;25(3):119–46. https://doi.org/10.1089/ars.2016.6665.
54. Gong J, Noel S, Pluznick JL, Hamad ARA, Rabb H. Gut microbiota-kidney cross-talk in acute kidney injury. Semin Nephrol. 2019;39(1):107–16. https://doi.org/10.1016/j.semnephrol.2018.10.009.
55. Yao Y, Cai X, Fei W, et al. The role of short-chain fatty acids in immunity, inflammation and metabolism. Crit Rev Food Sci Nutr. 2022;62(1):1–12. https://doi.org/10.1080/10408398.2020.1854675.
56. Lanza M, Campolo M, Casili G, et al. Sodium butyrate exerts neuroprotective effects in spinal cord injury. Mol Neurobiol. 2019;56(6):3937–47. https://doi.org/10.1007/s12035-018-1347-7.
57. Grigor'eva IN. Gallstone disease, obesity and the firmicutes/bacteroidetes ratio as a possible biomarker of gut dysbiosis. J Pers Med. 2020;11(1):13. https://doi.org/10.3390/jpm11010013.
58. Iqbal M, Yu Q, Tang J, Xiang J. Unraveling the gut microbiota's role in obesity: key metabolites, microbial species, and therapeutic insights. J Bacteriol. 2025;22;207(5):e0047924. https://doi.org/10.1128/jb.00479-24.
59. Li H, Wang XK, Tang M, et al. Bacteroides thetaiotaomicron ameliorates mouse hepatic steatosis through regulating gut microbial composition, gut-liver folate and unsaturated fatty acids metabolism. Gut Microbes. 2024;16(1):2304159. https://doi.org/10.1080/19490976.2024.2304159.
60. Pillai SS, Gagnon GA, Foster C, Ashraf AP. Exploring the gut microbiota: key insights into its role in obesity, metabolic syndrome, and type 2 diabetes. J Clin Endocrinol Metab. 2024;109(11):2709–19. https://doi.org/10.1210/clinem/dgae499.
61. Pedersen HK, Gudmundsdottir V, Nielsen HB, et al. Human gut microbes impact host serum metabolome and insulin sensitivity. Nature. 2016;535(7612):376–81. https://doi.org/10.1038/nature18646.
62. Van Hul M, Cani PD. The gut microbiota in obesity and weight management: microbes as friends or foe? Nat Rev Endocrinol. 2023;19(5):258–71. https://doi.org/10.1038/s41574-022-00794-0.
63. Gentile JKA, Oliveira KD, Pereira JG, et al. The intestinal microbiome in patients undergoing bariatric surgery: a systematic review. Arq Bras Cir Dig. 2022;35:e1707. https://doi.org/10.1590/0102-672020220002e1707.
64. Anhê FF, Jensen BAH, Varin TV, Servant F, Van Blerk S, Richard D, Marceau S, Surette M, Biertho L, Lelouvier B, Schertzer JD, Tchernof A, Marette A. Type 2 diabetes influences bacterial tissue compartmentalisation in human obesity. Nat Metab. 2020;2:233–42. https://doi.org/10.1038/s42255-020-0178-9.
65. Yu H, Li R, Huang H, Yao R, Shen S. Short-chain fatty acids enhance the lipid accumulation of 3T3-L1 cells by modulating the expression of enzymes of fatty acid metabolism. Lipids. 2018;53:77–84. https://doi.org/10.1002/lipd.12005.

66. Upadhyaya S, Banerjee G. Type 2 diabetes and gut microbiome: at the intersection of known and unknown. Gut Microbes. 2015;6(2):85–92. https://doi.org/10.1080/19490976.2015.1024918.
67. Palmnäs-Bédard MSA, Costabile G, Vetrani C, Åberg S, Hjalmarsson Y, Dicksved J, et al. The human gut microbiota and glucose metabolism: a scoping review of key bacteria and the potential role of SCFAs. Am J Clin Nutr. 2022;116(4):862–74. https://doi.org/10.1093/ajcn/nqac217.
68. Bednarska NG, Håberg AK. Understanding patterns of the gut microbiome may contribute to the early detection and prevention of type 2 diabetes mellitus: a systematic review. Microorganisms. 2025;13(1):134. https://doi.org/10.3390/microorganisms13010134.
69. Dabke K, Hendrick G, Devkota S. The gut microbiome and metabolic syndrome. J Clin Invest. 2019;129(10):4050–7. https://doi.org/10.1172/JCI129194.
70. Elbere I, Silamikelis I, Dindune II, et al. Baseline gut microbiome composition predicts metformin therapy short-term efficacy in newly diagnosed type 2 diabetes patients. PLoS One. 2020;15(10):e0241338. https://doi.org/10.1371/journal.pone.0241338.
71. Windey K, de Preter V, Verbeke K. Relevance of protein fermentation to gut health. Mol Nutr Food Res. 2012;56(1):184–96. https://doi.org/10.1002/mnfr.201100542.
72. Oduro-Donkor D, Turner MC, Farnaud S, Renshaw D, Kyrou I, Hanson P, et al. Modification of fecal microbiota as a mediator of effective weight loss and metabolic benefits following bariatric surgery. Expert Rev Endocrinol Metab. 2020;15(5):363–73. https://doi.org/10.1080/17446651.2020.1801412.
73. Zhang K, Zhang R, Zhang Y, Zhang M, Su H, Zhao F, et al. Regulation of LPS-Induced inflammatory responses in bovine mammary epithelial cells via TLR4-mediated NF-κB and MAPK signaling pathways by lactoferrin. Life (Basel). 2025;15:69. https://doi.org/10.3390/life15010069.
74. Abenavoli L, Scarpellini E, Colica C, Boccuto L, Salehi B, Sharifi-Rad J, et al. Gut microbiota and obesity: a role for probiotics. Nutrients. 2019;11(11):2690. https://doi.org/10.3390/nu11112690.
75. Crudele L, Gadaleta RM, Cariello M, Moschetta A. Gut microbiota in the pathogenesis and therapeutic approaches of diabetes. EBioMedicine. 2023;97:104821. https://doi.org/10.1016/j.ebiom.2023.104821.
76. Zeng Z, Chen M, Liu Y, Zhou Y, Liu H, Wang S, Ji Y. Role of Akkermansia muciniphila in insulin resistance. J Gastroenterol Hepatol. 2025;40:19–32. https://doi.org/10.1111/jgh.16747.
77. Serra-Majem L, Tomaino L, Dernini S, Berry EM, Lairon D, Ngo de la Cruz J, et al. Updating the mediterranean diet pyramid towards sustainability: focus on environmental concerns. Int J Environ Res Public Health. 2020;17(23):8758. https://doi.org/10.3390/ijerph17238758.
78. Dinu M, Pagliai G, Casini A, Sofi F. Mediterranean diet and multiple health outcomes: an umbrella review of meta-analyses of observational studies and randomised trials. Eur J Clin Nutr. 2018;72:30–43. https://doi.org/10.1038/ejcn.2017.58.
79. Galbete C, Schwingshackl L, Schwedhelm C, Boeing H, Schulze MB. Evaluating Mediterranean diet and risk of chronic disease in cohort studies: an umbrella review of meta-analyses. Eur J Epidemiol. 2018;33:909–31. https://doi.org/10.1007/s10654-018-0427-3.
80. De Filippis F, Pellegrini N, Vannini L, Jeffery IB, La Storia A, Laghi L, et al. High-level adherence to a Mediterranean diet beneficially impacts the gut microbiota and associated metabolome. Gut. 2016;65:1812–21. https://doi.org/10.1136/gutjnl-2015-309957.
81. Goderska K, Agudo Pena S, Alarcon T. Helicobacter pylori treatment: antibiotics or probiotics. Appl Microbiol Biotechnol. 2018;102(1):1–7. https://doi.org/10.1007/s00253-017-8535-7.
82. Cotter PD, Hill C, Ross RP. Bacteriocins: developing innate immunity for food. Nat Rev Microbiol. 2005;3(10):777–88. https://doi.org/10.1038/nrmicro1273.

83. Resta-Lenert S, Barrett KE. Probiotics and commensals reverse TNF-alpha- and IFN-gamma-induced dysfunction in human intestinal epithelial cells. Gastroenterology. 2006;130(3):731–46. https://doi.org/10.1053/j.gastro.2005.
84. Raygan F, Rezavandi Z, Bahmani F, et al. The effects of probiotic supplementation on metabolic status in type 2 diabetic patients with coronary heart disease. Diabetol Metab Syndr. 2018;10:51. https://doi.org/10.1186/s13098-018-0353-2.
85. Sarao LK, Arora M. Probiotics, prebiotics, and microencapsulation: a review. Crit Rev Food Sci Nutr. 2017;57(2):344–71. https://doi.org/10.1080/10408398.2014.887055.
86. Li YJ, Chen X, Kwan TK, Loh YW, Singer J, Liu Y, et al. Dietary Fiber protects against diabetic nephropathy through short-chain fatty acid-mediated activation of G protein-coupled receptors GPR43 and GPR109A. J Am Soc Nephrol. 2020;31:1267–81. https://doi.org/10.1681/ASN.2019101029.
87. Yu EW, Gao L, Stastka P, Cheney MC, Mahabamunuge J, Torres Soto M, et al. Fecal microbiota transplantation for the improvement of metabolism in obesity: the FMT-TRIM double-blind placebo-controlled pilot trial. PLoS Med. 2020;17:e1003051. https://doi.org/10.1371/journal.pmed.1003051.
88. Bian J, Liebert A, Bicknell B, Chen XM, Huang C, Pollock CA. Faecal microbiota transplantation and chronic kidney disease. Nutrients. 2022;14(12):2528. https://doi.org/10.3390/nu14122528.
89. Wu J, Yang K, Fan H, Wei M, Xiong Q. Targeting the gut microbiota and its metabolites for type 2 diabetes mellitus. Front Endocrinol (Lausanne). 2023;14:1114424. https://doi.org/10.3389/fendo.2023.1114424.

Chapter 8
The Role of Insulin Resistance and Metabolic Dysregulation in Cardiovascular-Kidney-Metabolic Syndrome

Laura Mihalache and Lidia Iuliana Graur

Introduction

Metabolic syndrome is a cluster of metabolic risk factors characterized by abdominal obesity, dyslipidemia, hypertension, and dysglycemia. Cardiovascular-kidney-metabolic (CKM) syndrome is defined as a constellation of health impairments attributable to the complex connections between obesity, diabetes, chronic kidney disease, and cardiovascular disease, including heart failure, atrial fibrillation, coronary artery disease, stroke, and peripheral arterial disease [1]. It is a systemic alteration that can lead to organ failure and an increased rate of cardiovascular events.

The clinical implications of this pathological entity include increased risk of premature mortality, excessive morbidity, and multiorgan failure, as well as associated healthcare costs. It is widely recognized that metabolic alterations play a key role in the pathophysiology of this syndrome, with complex cardiovascular and renal connections and bidirectional interactions. Dysfunctional excess adipose tissue (particularly perivisceral and ectopically stored adipose tissue) causes chronic low-grade inflammation, insulin resistance with all its metabolic consequences, and an increased cardiovascular risk. Renal function impairment is now recognized as a central mediator of the relationship between metabolic risk factors and cardiovascular disease. As a result, the recent proposal to use the concept of CKM syndrome tries to replace the previous approach of considering cardio-renal syndrome and cardiometabolic disease as separate entities, especially since they are interconnected by common mechanisms and mutually influence each other [1].

L. Mihalache (✉) · L. I. Graur
Grigore T. Popa University of Medicine and Pharmacy, Iasi, Romania

Saint Spiridon Emergency Hospital, Iasi, Romania
e-mail: laura.mihalache@umfiasi.ro

M. Floria, D. M. Tanase (eds.), *Cardiovascular-Kidney-Metabolic Syndrome*,
https://doi.org/10.1007/978-3-032-11445-7_8

Cardiovascular-kidney-metabolic syndrome is essentially a progressive pathological condition entailing the alteration of the health status due to the pathological connections between obesity, diabetes, cardiovascular, and kidney disease, partially overlapping with the components of the classic metabolic syndrome. The onset is early in life, and the principal element seems to be represented by the excessive accumulation of dysfunctional adipose tissue (adiposopathy) characterized by inflammation, insulin resistance, and oxidative stress. Frequently, there is progression toward the development of metabolic risk factors (hypertension, dyslipidemia, and type 2 diabetes mellitus—elements traditionally united under the name of metabolic syndrome) and chronic kidney disease. Over time, these comorbidities will progress and will cause the appearance of subclinical lesions of atherosclerotic disease and subclinical abnormalities of myocardial structure and function, concurrently with the progressive decline of kidney function, so that ultimately we witness the appearance of clinical cardiovascular disease, with or without renal failure [1].

The constellation of factors brought together under the name of metabolic syndrome (abdominal obesity, dysglycemia, dyslipidemia, and hypertension) are an integral part of the CKM syndrome and have numerous pathophysiological consequences (endothelial dysfunction, atherogenesis, thrombosis, myocardial ischemia and fibrosis, cardiac remodeling) that will contribute to the development of all subtypes of cardiovascular disease (including coronary artery disease, cerebrovascular disease, peripheral arterial disease, cardiac arrhythmias, and heart failure) [1]. In this context, insulin resistance is one of the physiopathogenic mechanisms with a central role in the occurrence and progression of metabolic alterations that underlie the definition of CKM syndrome.

Insulin Resistance: Definition and Clinical Implications

Insulin is an anabolic hormone with major roles in regulating cellular energy metabolism and in modulating the pathways for cellular growth and development, particularly in certain tissues such as adipose tissue, skeletal muscle tissue, liver, or brain. The reduction in the response of target tissues to the action of insulin is known as insulin resistance, a complex physiopathological condition in which there is a reduction in insulin sensitivity, an alteration in the ability of insulin to inhibit glucose production, and to stimulate peripheral glucose uptake [2].

The existence of insulin resistance as a pathogenic mechanism was first suggested in 1936 by Himsworth, who showed that in people with obesity and diabetes, glucose uptake is reduced after insulin administration [3]. However, the first evidence of insulin resistance belongs to Yalow and Berson, two researchers who showed in 1960 that insulinemia is increased in patients with type 2 diabetes [4].

Insulin resistance is a multifaceted medical condition characterized by the inability of insulin, which is effective in normal individuals, to elicit its typical biological effects, particularly in adipose tissue, muscle tissue, and the liver. Consequently, in the context of insulin resistance, there is a compensatory elevation in insulin secretion, resulting in relative hyperinsulinemia, and the progression of metabolic changes may finally culminate in the onset of type 2 diabetes. Insulin resistance, among several pathogenic processes and pathways, is the pivotal factor that underpins the emergence of most chronic pathologies, together referred to as CKM syndrome. This condition is defined by a failure of insulin's physiological effects on target tissues, influenced by causes including oxidative stress, chronic subclinical inflammation, lipid metabolic impairment, microbiome alterations, and epigenetic modifications. Insulin resistance is critical in the onset of various chronic diseases, including type 2 diabetes, cardiovascular and cerebrovascular diseases, chronic kidney disease, metabolic liver disease, certain neoplastic disorders, and conditions associated with cognitive impairments, which are significant contributors to global morbidity and mortality. Chronic disorders resulting from metabolic changes associated with insulin resistance would adversely affect individuals, leading to physical and psychological modifications, as well as burdening the healthcare system with increasing medical and economic costs [5]. Furthermore, individuals with metabolic disorders are susceptible populations during epidemic circumstances, as evidenced by the current COVID-19 pandemic [6].

Insulin exerts its effects at the cellular level via a particular receptor situated on cell membranes. The insulin receptor belongs to a family of structurally related receptor tyrosine kinases that interact with a common set of intracellular proteins, including the IRS (insulin receptor substrate) family. Two main post-receptor signaling pathways have been identified: the phosphatidylinositol 3-kinase/protein kinase B (PI3K/Akt) pathway (which is the traditional insulin signaling pathway) and the Ras/mitogen-activated protein kinase (RAS/MAPK) pathway. The PI3K enzyme has two subunits, a catalytic subunit (p110) and a regulatory subunit (p85) [7]. The activation of the PI3K/Akt pathway plays a crucial role in cell growth and proliferation, but also in the normal metabolism of glucose and fatty acids, while the activation of the RAS/MAPK signaling pathway contributes to the regulation of various pathophysiological processes involved in cell growth, proliferation, differentiation and apoptosis, without being involved in the regulation of intermediary metabolisms [8–10].

The physiological effects of insulin are multiple, as it is a hormone significantly involved in the regulation of energy metabolism, influencing and regulating intermediary metabolic processes, resulting in an anabolic effect.

The etiology and pathogenesis of insulin resistance are complex aspects of human pathology. Factors that could be involved in the etiology of insulin resistance may be represented by genetic predisposition, aging, environmental factors, and lifestyle risk factors (food intake and meal composition, sedentary lifestyle, smoking, inadequate sleep, certain pollutants), though obesity remains one of the major contributing factors to the development of insulin resistance [11]. Abnormalities in the insulin signaling pathway result in the manifestation of insulin resistance within the body. The main mechanisms of insulin resistance are represented by abnormalities of binding to the specific receptor or abnormalities of the receptor, abnormalities of the internal environment that favor insulin resistance, metabolic alterations in muscle or liver tissue, intracellular factors, etc. [11]. It is important to note that these pathways can interact with each other and cause a state of systemic insulin resistance that underlies the occurrence of metabolic disorders and CKM syndrome.

The alteration of insulin signaling can be explained by two main contexts: On the one hand, it can be secondary to the inactivation of the protein that represents the insulin receptor substrate (IRS), including the down-regulation of the number of receptors or their binding affinity; on the other hand, it may be secondary to the impairment of post-receptor signaling pathways or their intracellular signaling efficacy. The cellular mechanisms responsible for the reduction of insulin action may be located at the level of hormone binding to the receptor or at a more distal stage called "postreceptor". In subjects with obesity without diabetes, it seems that the predominant impairment is at the receptor level, with a decrease in the number of receptors on the membrane surface (negative regulation due to hyperinsulinemia). Physiologically, the two insulin signaling pathways at the cellular level are represented by:

- The mitogen-activated protein kinase pathway, which is a proatherogenic pathway
- The phosphatidylinositol-3-kinase-activated pathway, which is a protective pathway through nitric oxide synthesis

In the presence of insulin resistance, there is an imbalance between these two pathways, in the sense that there is a blockage in the phosphatidylinositol-3-kinase pathway, so that hyperinsulinemia, which is a corollary of insulin resistance, ultimately leads to the stimulation of the other pathway, which is not blocked, namely, the mitogen-activated protein kinase pathway; this pathway is involved in the growth effect of endothelin, cell adhesion molecules, and in the growth and migration of vascular smooth muscle cells. As a result, in the presence of insulin resistance, the PI3K/Akt signaling pathway is altered, with the preservation of the functionality of the MAPK signaling pathway, which is involved in the occurrence and progression of atherosclerotic lesions [12, 13].

Metabolic Syndrome and Cardiovascular Kidney Metabolic Syndrome: The Role of Insulin Resistance

Obesity and Adiposopathy: Key Role in Insulin Resistance

Obesity is a chronic disease characterized by complex etiopathogenesis and progressive evolution, serving as the primary risk factor for the development of insulin resistance and various metabolic, cardiovascular, renal, and hepatic diseases, often constituting the principal condition for the appearance of CKM syndrome [14]. In the presence of an energy imbalance, excess energy is stored in the form of adipose tissue, from where it can be quickly used as an energy substrate when conditions require it. The storage of this excess energy in adipocytes is associated with ischemia and local hypoxia, cellular apoptosis, fibrosis, and a reduction in capillary density in the extracellular matrix, with the subsequent accumulation of monocytes and macrophages. This results in increased secretion of proinflammatory cytokines and changes in adipokines secretion, including reduced synthesis and release of adiponectin, the main insulin-sensitizing hormone. Inflammation and secretory dysfunction of adipose tissue will subsequently exacerbate the insulin resistance found in individuals with obesity [15].

Currently, adipose tissue is no longer considered an inert energy store, but is a metabolically active tissue, with several types described, depending on location and metabolic profile. Thus, white adipose tissue can be located subcutaneously or viscerally and can vary in terms of its distribution, morphology, and function. Excess lipids are stored at the level of adipocytes, increasing their size and number in direct relation to the excess energy quantity. The size of adipocytes suggests their function, larger adipocytes (thus fuller with lipid deposits) being more insulin-resistant, hyperlipolytic, and resistant to the anti-lipolytic action of insulin [16]. When there is dysfunction and inability of the subcutaneous adipose tissue to expand proportionally to the energy excess due to alteration of adipogenesis or restrictive hyperplasia, ectopic lipid storage is observed in the liver, skeletal muscle tissue, and myocardial tissue, with both structural and functional alterations of tissues and organs [17].

The central accumulation of excess adipose tissue, particularly at the abdominal, perivisceral level, is most strongly associated with insulin resistance, risk of type 2 diabetes, and cardiovascular, kidney, and hepatic disease. The liver and muscle tissue are the main sites of ectopic accumulation of excess lipids when the storage capacity of adipose tissue is exceeded. Ectopic lipid accumulation is generally associated with the onset and progression of both insulin resistance and subclinical inflammation, thus contributing to an increased risk of CKM syndrome. Increased visceral adipose tissue mass is closely correlated with ectopic lipid deposition in metabolically active organs and contributes to the pathophysiology of CKM syndrome through its dysfunction, expressed by pathological secretion of adipocytokines, subclinical inflammation, and increased release of free fatty acids (FFA) into the circulation [17]. Additionally, the accumulation of ectopic adipose tissue at the epicardial and perivascular level is an essential factor in the development and progression of coronary disease, the dysfunction of this type of tissue being associated with increased local levels of proinflammatory adipokines [18]. Similarly, the accumulation of ectopic adipose tissue at the peri- and intrarenal level will contribute to the development and worsening of hypertension [19]. At the same time, in the presence of dysfunctional adipose tissue, mitochondrial dysfunction is also observed, with an increase in the production of reactive oxygen species and lipid peroxidation [20].

In addition to the increased risk of metabolic disorders, cardiovascular and renal pathologies, there has been demonstrated a strong and direct relationship between obesity and metabolic liver disease, a higher rate of sleep apnea syndrome, and even the risk of certain types of cancer [1]. The development of metabolic dysfunction-associated steatotic liver disease (MASLD) will further amplify the phenomena of insulin resistance and systemic inflammation. The release of pro-oxidative and proinflammatory mediators into the systemic circulation will exacerbate the pathophysiological processes involved in atherogenesis and myocardial injury, glomerulosclerosis, tubulointerstitial inflammation, and renal fibrosis [21, 22].

In conclusion, the accumulation of excessive adipose tissue is frequently associated with dysfunctional, inflammatory adipose tissue, the deposition of ectopic adipose tissue, and systemic hemodynamic stress and endothelial dysfunction. At the adipose tissue level, insulin resistance will promote the stimulation of lipolysis and the release of FFA. The accumulation of FFA at the hepatocyte level will cause hepatic insulin resistance, steatosis, increased gluconeogenesis, and hepatic glucose production, thus contributing to the increase in basal plasma glucose. The accumulation of FFA in the skeletal muscle also contributes to the increase in local insulin resistance, with the deviation of metabolism toward the use and oxidation of FFA, to the detriment of the use of glucose as an energy substrate, thus contributing to the decrease in glucose tolerance. In the initial stages, hyperinsulinemia secondary to the increase in insulin secretion by pancreatic β cells is observed. However, in the presence of glucotoxicity and lipotoxicity, there is a progressive decline in the insulin secretory capacity of β cells, with all the implicit consequences [15].

Insulin Resistance and Hyperglycemia

The biological effects of insulin on glucose metabolism are crucial: insulin decreases hepatic glucose production (inhibiting both gluconeogenesis and hepatic glycogenolysis) and stimulates glucose uptake and utilization, especially in muscle, but also in adipose and hepatic tissue (increasing intracellular glucose consumption by activating glycolysis and hepatic and muscle glycogenesis). The primary role of insulin is to facilitate glucose transport across cell membranes, following its coupling with its specific receptor at this level.

Insulin resistance and decreased insulin secretion are essential elements involved in the pathogenesis of type 2 diabetes mellitus, in varying proportions. Numerous epidemiological studies show that insulin resistance is usually detected before changes in the insulin secretory response can be identified. In the initial stages, increased insulin secretion is sufficient to maintain glycemic values within the normal range [23]. In the presence of predisposing environmental and genetic factors and the persistence of insulin resistance, a vicious circle is created that will ultimately lead to beta-cell failure, possibly due to the mechanisms of gluco- and lipotoxicity along with other factors that favor the development of type 2 diabetes [24]. As a result, insulin resistance can be identified before glucose tolerance deteriorates, and prophylactic intervention aimed at reducing insulin resistance may be effective at this time.

Given that insulin is a hormone with a central role in the regulation of glucose metabolism, insulin resistance is closely correlated with all stages of dysglycemia, from prediabetes to diabetes, with or without its specific complications. The alteration of compensatory insulin hypersecretion in response to increased insulin resistance is one of the pathophysiological factors associated with reduced glucose tolerance and will contribute to the development of diabetes mellitus.

At the hepatic level, insulin resistance causes increased endogenous glucose production due to inadequate suppression of hepatic gluconeogenesis, concurrently with reduced glycogen synthesis, which will ultimately result in basal hyperglycemia [24]. At the muscle level, insulin resistance is accompanied by decreased glucose utilization through proximal defects in insulin signaling, contributing to increased blood glucose levels [24].

Hyperglycemia can contribute to the establishment of a vicious circle, as it has been demonstrated that hyperglycemia exerts an unfavorable role on the insulin secretory function of the beta cell and the utilization of glucose in skeletal muscle under the action of insulin. Thus, glucotoxicity accentuates insulin secretion deficits (decreases GLUT-2 expression in the beta cell or increases the glycogen content of these cells) and decreases insulin sensitivity (reduces GLUT-4 expression or limits the activity of key enzymes in glucose metabolism) [25].

Insulin Resistance and Dyslipidemia

Insulin is deeply involved in the regulation of lipid metabolism and plays a central role in establishing the anti-atherogenic lipid profile. The biological effects of insulin on lipid metabolism are multiple: It stimulates intravascular lipolysis, inhibits lipolysis in adipose tissue (by inhibiting lipase), increases lipogenesis in adipose tissue, and decreases hepatic production of very-low-density lipoprotein (VLDL). Insulin accelerates hepatic synthesis of fatty acids, reduces their oxidative degradation (directing them towards triglyceride synthesis), and stimulates cholesterol synthesis by activating 3-Hydroxy-3-MethylGlutaryl-Coenzyme A (HMGCoA)-reductase. When these effects are intact, the consequence is a decrease in serum glucose, triglycerides, and FFA, as well as an increase in lipoprotein lipase activity in adipose tissue.

Lipid alterations particular to insulin resistance are specific to atherogenic dyslipidemia and are represented by hypertriglyceridemia, increased concentration of VLDL, reduced concentration of high-density lipoprotein (HDL), and the formation of small dense LDL cholesterol particles (sdLDL). The alteration of the lipid profile in insulin resistance includes increased plasma levels of FFA. It is well known that VLDL particles are synthesized in the liver through an insulin-regulated process that promotes the degradation of apoprotein B (apoB) via the PI3K pathway. In the presence of insulin resistance, the alteration of this process will lead to increased production of triglyceride-rich VLDL [26], concurrently with the reduction in the clearance of these lipoproteins [27], which further contributes to an increase in the circulating levels of these particles.

The formation of sdLDL cholesterol particles is a secondary process to the alteration of the function of the cholesteryl ester transfer protein (CETP) and hepatic lipase. CETP promotes the transfer of triglycerides from VLDL to LDL and HDL, thus causing an increase in the triglyceride content of these lipoproteins. These triglyceride-rich lipoproteins will become a substrate for hepatic lipase, which will convert LDL particles to sdLDL and increase the catabolism of HDL with a decrease in the concentration of apoprotein A (apoA) [28, 29].

The lipid profile specific to insulin resistance is highly atherogenic, with sdLDL having greater ease of penetration of the vascular wall, an increased half-life, being much more easily oxidized, and having a lower affinity for LDL receptors [30]. At the same time, hypertriglyceridemia boosts the hyperactivation of the renin-angiotensin-aldosterone System (RAAS), which will promote mechanisms associated with an increased risk of developing diabetic cardiomyopathy [31].

Lipoprotein lipase is also present in muscle tissue. Its experimental overexpression leads to a marked increase in muscle triglycerides, a defect in the ability of IRS 1 to activate PI-3-kinase, and a decrease in insulin-mediated glucose transport, thus leading to the institution of insulin resistance [32]. Under normal conditions, insulin decreases the activity of lipoprotein lipase at the muscle level, an action which, together with its stimulation at the adipose tissue level, will maintain lipids at the fat mass level. In obese and insulin-resistant individuals, increased activity of muscle lipoprotein lipase has been observed with excessive accumulation of lipids in myocytes and decreased muscle glucose uptake, through the transmembrane transport inhibition [33]. It has been proven that insulin resistance at the muscle level is manifested by reduced glucose uptake and is a consequence of both altered glucose transport and phosphorylation of glucose molecules, reduced glucose oxidation, and glycogen synthesis. At the same time, altered lipid metabolism contributes to the pathogenesis of insulin resistance at the muscle level, with mitochondrial defects in oxidative phosphorylation being reported in skeletal muscle [33].

In adipose tissue, lipoprotein lipase hydrolyzes triglycerides from chylomicrons and VLDL, providing FFA for the synthesis of storage triglycerides. Under physiological conditions, insulin increases lipoprotein lipase activity in adipose tissue, an effect that is altered under conditions of insulin resistance. In patients with type 2 diabetes mellitus, a reduction in lipoprotein lipase activity has been observed in adipose tissue, which slows down the clearance of VLDL particles and chylomicrons. Consequently, patients with type 2 diabetes have a higher amount of triglycerides and FFA in plasma compared to healthy subjects, at the same plasma insulin concentration, suggesting that adipose tissue is also affected by insulin resistance. The consequence of the increase in FFA is their preferential consumption over glucose, and the unused glucose will contribute to the worsening of hyperglycemia. In addition, the increased turnover of FFA will lead to an increase in their quantity at the hepatic level, a phenomenon followed by their excessive hepatic oxidation and the increase in substrates used in gluconeogenesis, a mechanism that further contributes to the exacerbation of hyperglycemia [23]. As the concentration of FFAs increases, triglycerides are mobilized from adipose tissue, leading to their accumulation in insulin-dependent tissues, particularly in the liver and skeletal muscle, which results in increased insulin resistance and its consequences. The unfavorable role of increased FFA in the pathophysiology of type 2 diabetes has been known for many years and is explained by the interference of substrates with insulin action, either in the liver or in skeletal muscle. The demonstration of an unfavorable effect of FFA on insulin secretion is more recent. Animal studies have shown that an increase in fatty acid levels increases the triglyceride content of β cells, decreases GLUT-2 expression, and reduces the insulin secretory response to glucose. Conversely, a decrease in the concentration of fatty acids allows the reversibility of all these anomalies. These results can be extrapolated to humans, because a chronic increase in circulating FFA has been reported to accompany the decrease in insulin secretory capacity, while their decrease allows the improvement of β-cell function. By analogy with glucotoxicity, this interference has been called lipotoxicity.

The increase in circulating FFA specific to the alteration of lipid metabolism in insulin resistance will be accompanied by their storage in non-adipose tissues, such as the liver and kidneys. This ectopic deposition will contribute to the development of chronic kidney disease and the appearance of liver damage in a metabolic context, pathological conditions that will mutually worsen as the disease progresses to advanced forms, with the exacerbation of dyslipidemia, thus constituting a vicious circle with complex bidirectional relationships [34].

Insulin Resistance and Hypertension

Hypertension is a component of the metabolic syndrome often encountered in clinical practice, and patients with hypertension are frequently hyperinsulinemic and have impaired glucose tolerance. Epidemiological studies show that the incidence of hypertension is very high among people with type 2 diabetes, including hypertension resistant to treatment and/or associated with cardiovascular disease. A meta-analysis conducted on 10,230 people with hypertension showed that insulin resistance and insulinemia are independent risk factors for the development of hypertension [35]. In the Framingham Heart Study, type 2 diabetes was associated with a two to four times greater risk of developing hypertension, peripheral arterial disease, and myocardial infarction [36].

The mechanisms by which insulin resistance is involved in the development of hypertension are numerous, with obesity contributing both to the development and worsening of insulin resistance. Insulin resistance and diabetes promote arterial stiffness, thus contributing to the development of hypertension. Relatively recent data further suggest that hyperinsulinemia associated with insulin resistance is an independent risk factor for vascular stiffness [37]. We can conclude that insulin resistance has a two-pronged effect: it contributes to both hyperinsulinemia and hyperglycemia, which synergistically influence vascular stiffness. This dual impact plays a key role in the early pathophysiological stages of hypertension and cardiovascular injury in CKM syndrome.

The activation of the renin-angiotensin-aldosterone system (RAAS) both at the systemic and local levels in the presence of insulin resistance and the subsequent hyperglycemia is another mechanism that contributes to the development of hypertension. Studies conducted in vitro and in vivo have shown that insulin resistance and hyperglycemia induce systemic RAAS activation with increased vascular resistance and blood pressure. The RAAS activation observed in insulin resistance and type 2 diabetes is accompanied by increased levels of angiotensin II and aldosterone, with altered insulin signaling, reduced activation of endothelial nitric oxide synthase (eNOS), and reduced nitric oxide (NO)-mediated vasodilation [38]. Furthermore, hyperinsulinemia associated with insulin resistance stimulates the MAPK pathway with the production of the vasoconstrictor substance endothelin 1 (ET-1), which contributes to increased vascular insulin resistance, excessive vascular stiffness, and hypertension [38].

The activation of the sympathetic nervous system is another contributing mechanism to the development of hypertension associated with insulin resistance, having been documented both in animal models and in human subjects with hypertension [39]. The increase in sympathetic tone induces the stimulation of β-adrenergic receptors that promote insulin resistance, and the increase in blood pressure in response to hyperinsulinemia can also be mediated by changing the baroreflex sensitivity.

Insulin resistance is also associated with mitochondrial dysfunction and increased production of reactive oxygen species, creating an imbalance between vasoconstrictor and vasodilator endothelium-derived factors, leading to an increased vascular tone. Excessive amounts of reactive oxygen species will cause reduced NO production and increased NO destruction, which will cause decreased NO bioavailability, thus contributing to worsening arterial stiffness and hypertension [40].

Systemic inflammation is a key contributor to the development of hypertension in the context of insulin resistance. Proinflammatory cytokines can cause and worsen insulin resistance, simultaneously with the reduction of insulin-mediated NO production, ultimately leading to increased blood pressure values. In the presence of insulin resistance, perivascular adipose tissue becomes active and secretes reactive oxygen species and proinflammatory adipokines, contributing to vascular insulin resistance and impaired relaxation [41].

In insulin resistance, altered glycemic homeostasis is also driven by increased renal glucose reabsorption via SGLT2 in the proximal tubule, a mechanism responsible for reclaiming approximately 90% of filtered glucose. In people with insulin resistance and type 2 diabetes, an increase in the threshold of glucose reabsorption is observed due to the upregulation of SGLT2 (sodium/glucose cotransporter 2) with increased absorption of glucose and sodium at the proximal tubular level, thus contributing to the occurrence of hypertension and associated cardiovascular diseases [42]. Recent large, randomized, placebo-controlled trials have demonstrated that treatment with SGLT2 inhibitors significantly reduces blood pressure and the risk of cardiovascular events and prevents the progression of kidney disease in people with diabetes.

All these vascular changes that occur due to insulin resistance are frequently linked to alterations in the heart. The heart, the muscular pump of the human body, requires a large amount of ATP, the energy currency at the cellular level. Myocardial metabolism is largely influenced by the availability of energy substrates, which will depend on the actions of insulin at the level of peripheral tissues. In this context, the heart is one of the organs that requires good insulin signaling to correctly manipulate the energy substrates necessary for the contractile function and the action of ion pumps, so that insulin resistance can also have adverse consequences at the level of cardiac metabolism. Insulin resistance can exacerbate the mechanisms of atherosclerosis, myocardial fibrosis, and ventricular hypertrophy, with the subsequent occurrence of diastolic dysfunction and eventual occurrence and progression of heart failure phenomena. In particular, insulin resistance is responsible for the development of diabetic-specific cardiomyopathy through pathophysiological mechanisms that include altered insulin signaling at the myocardial cell level, cardiac mitochondrial dysfunction, endoplasmic reticulum stress, altered autophagy, altered myocardial calcium handling, alterations in cardiac microcirculation, inappropriate neurohormonal activation, and maladaptive immune responses [43–45]. Regardless of the phenotype, both hyperglycemia and hyperinsulinemia in the context of insulin resistance, as well as lipotoxicity and endothelial dysfunction, may play a crucial role in the development of abnormalities specific to diabetic cardiomyopathy. The accumulation of advanced glycation end products (AGEs), maladaptive calcium homeostasis, and the activation of the local RAAS, together with insulin resistance-induced myocardial energy inefficiency, are mechanisms that will promote alterations in myocardial contractility, myocardial stiffness, and fibrosis, aspects that will additionally contribute to the cardiac dysfunction specific to diabetic cardiomyopathy [46–49]. In conclusion, insulin resistance is directly related to hypertrophy, fibrosis, and diastolic and systolic dysfunction, exacerbating the risk of coronary heart disease and heart failure. Thus, we are currently talking about a proper insulin–heart axis, with numerous influences of insulin on the modulation of cardiac functions being described, from metabolic regulation to the development of cardiac hypertrophy. The binding of insulin to its specific receptor will activate certain signaling pathways that will modulate glucose and fatty acid metabolism at the cardiomyocyte level, having a central role in maintaining cardiac energy homeostasis. Under conditions of insulin resistance, important cardiac metabolic disorders occur, including autonomic dysfunction, abnormalities of intracellular signaling, and the activation of the RAAS. All these mechanisms that appear and worsen under conditions of insulin resistance will contribute to the emergence and progression of specific cardiomyopathy.

Impact of Insulin Resistance on Cardiovascular and Kidney Axis

The Global Impact of Insulin Resistance and Type 2 Diabetes on the Cardiovascular System

The first study to assess the relationship between insulin resistance and cardiovascular disease was the Insulin Resistance Atherosclerosis Study (IRAS), a multiethnic cohort study. The resulting data showed that insulin resistance is an independent predictor of increased risk of cardiovascular disease in people without diabetes, a relationship maintained even after adjusting for the presence of other risk factors (high cholesterol, smoking, hypertension, weight status assessed based on the body mass index (BMI) value) [50].

Insulin resistance and type 2 diabetes are strongly associated with the development of atherosclerotic lesions, the clinical manifestations of which are coronary artery disease, peripheral arterial disease, and stroke. As previously mentioned, hyperglycemia is closely related to endothelial dysfunction, vascular abnormalities, and chronic low-grade inflammation, phenomena that underlie the formation and progression of atherosclerotic plaque [51]. At the same time, insulin resistance is closely related to atherogenic dyslipidemia, characterized by increased levels of sdLDL cholesterol particles and low levels of HDL cholesterol [52]. In the presence of hyperglycemia, glycation of LDL particles occurs, which will increase their atherogenic potential. Glycated LDL particles are recognized by receptors expressed on macrophages, with the intracellular accumulation of cholesterol and the increased formation of atherosclerotic plaque [53]. Atherosclerotic lesions have an increased incidence and are diffuse and serial; stenoses are more severe and usually distal, affecting all vascular territories, making the therapeutic approach difficult. In the presence of insulin resistance and hyperglycemia, arterial hypertension commonly coexists, driven by a predominance of vasoconstrictive over vasodilatory endothelial signals, as well as by increased arterial stiffness. These mechanisms play a pivotal role in the early development of hypertension and cardiovascular disease [54]. There is therefore a wealth of data showing the direct relationship between obesity, insulin resistance, and atherosclerotic cardiovascular disease, a relationship explained by numerous pathogenic mechanisms involving the classical risk factors represented by hypertension, dyslipidemia, and diabetes. However, epidemiological data and clinical trials strongly support a causal link between obesity and heart failure, mediated by a range of mechanisms—metabolic, hemodynamic, inflammatory, cellular, and mechanical—that contribute to the progression of cardiac dysfunction [55]. Moreover, obesity is associated with an increased risk of atrial fibrillation [56] and thromboembolic disease [57], pathologies that contribute to the increase in the risk of morbidity and mortality for these people.

The Global Impact of Insulin Resistance and Type 2 Diabetes on Kidney Function

The kidneys are a major target of the mechanisms involved in the development of chronic complications specific to diabetes, and diabetic kidney disease (DKD) is a major cause of morbidity and mortality. In recent years, the scientific community has moved away from the concept of "diabetic nephropathy" to increasingly use the term "diabetic kidney disease." This paradigm shift is justified by the scientific accumulations regarding the abnormalities that may be associated with the presence of insulin resistance and chronic hyperglycemia. Thus, diabetic nephropathy was defined by increased urinary albumin excretion, being traditionally recognized as a condition characterized by the progressive decline of kidney function, which can be classified into five evolutionary stages [58]. The term "diabetic kidney disease" is a broader term that includes all possible renal abnormalities that occur in the presence of diabetes mellitus [59]. In conclusion, diabetic kidney disease represents the renal manifestation of gluco- and lipotoxicity-induced damage. One of the earliest changes is represented by glomerular hyperfiltration, subsequent to the alteration of tubulo-glomerular feedback and glomerular hemodynamic abnormalities that occur in the diabetic environment [60]. Persistent hyperfiltration causes progressive and irreversible damage to the nephron with a decline in eGFR, possibly even progression to end-stage renal disease. Renal tissue damage will have as clinical manifestation the emergence of urinary protein excretion, associated with functional and structural cellular alterations favored by metabolic imbalances [61]. Thus, multiple mechanisms underlying the occurrence of diabetic kidney disease are currently being discussed (structural and cellular lesions in tubular cells, podocytes, mesangial cells, local activation of the RAAS), to which other cardiovascular risk factors that promote renal injury (high blood pressure, obesity, hyperuricemia, inflammation) may possibly be associated. Furthermore, compared to the traditional approach, it is known that there is the possibility of a nonalbuminuric phenotype of diabetic kidney disease, with mechanisms at the macrovascular and tubulointerstitial levels as contributing factors [62].

Alteration of Cardiovascular and Kidney Function and the Risk of Developing Type 2 Diabetes Mellitus

Traditionally, type 2 diabetes is considered a major cardiovascular and renal risk factor. However, the relationship is not unidirectional, and there is currently an accumulation of data and results that support the fact that cardiovascular dysfunction and renal disease can cause metabolic alterations and increase the risk of developing type 2 diabetes mellitus.

Insulin resistance plays an important role in the complex relationship between hypertension, type 2 diabetes, and cardiovascular and chronic kidney disease. For several years, there have been data showing that insulin resistance can occur in both conventional tissues (represented by liver, muscle, and adipose tissue), as well as in renal and cardiovascular tissue. The activation of the RAAS with increased angiotensin II levels is a characteristic of the cardiometabolic syndrome and contributes to the alteration of the insulin signaling pathway and the formation of reactive oxygen species, with the induction of endothelial dysfunction [63].

The mechanisms underlying the negative impact of cardiovascular and renal dysfunction on the risk of developing type 2 diabetes are not fully elucidated, although numerous hypotheses have been proposed. For example, endothelial dysfunction is increasingly cited as the common ground for glycemic and cardiovascular homeostasis dysregulation [64]. This hypothesis is supported by the close, bidirectional relationship between insulin resistance (the central mechanism in the physiopathology of type 2 diabetes) and endothelial dysfunction (one of the crucial steps that initiate specific events in the pathogenesis of cardiovascular diseases) [65]. Additionally, heart failure can be considered a state of insulin resistance due, among other things, to specific neurohormonal activation: Hyperactivation of the sympathetic nervous system in heart failure will cause alteration of glycemic homeostasis via stimulation of alpha-adrenergic receptors, with hypoperfusion in skeletal muscle and decreased tissue glucose uptake at this level [66, 67]. At the same time, the chronic activation of the sympathetic nervous system stimulates lipolysis, increasing the level of FFA that will be stored ectopically, promoting hepatic gluconeogenesis and altering the insulin secretion from pancreatic ß-cells [68]. The activation of the RAAS in heart failure is another mechanism proposed to be involved in the development of type 2 diabetes. Angiotensin II induces vasoconstriction in the muscles and reduced peripheral glucose uptake, mechanisms associated with reduced insulin sensitivity [69]. Additionally, angiotensin II can induce β-cell dysfunction through a mechanism dependent on endoplasmic reticulum alteration, with the alteration of insulin secretion and the promotion of β-cell apoptosis [70]. Furthermore, heart failure is a proinflammatory condition, and proinflammatory cytokines play an important role in the development of insulin resistance and subsequently type 2 diabetes. Patients with heart failure exhibit varying degrees of physical activity limitation, which may contribute to disturbances in glucose metabolism. Reduced skeletal muscle perfusion and generalized muscle atrophy are frequently associated with an ensuing reduction in peripheral glucose utilization (muscle being one of the organs that consumes the most glucose as an energy substrate) and decreased insulin sensitivity [67].

This mechanism of insulin resistance at the muscle level is also present in patients with chronic kidney disease, caused by the alteration of postreceptor insulin signaling pathways in the context of oxidative stress and chronic inflammation [71, 72]. In the context of chronic kidney disease, other mechanisms also contribute to the exacerbation of insulin resistance. Thus, metabolic acidosis, a common complication of chronic kidney disease, impairs the biological response to insulin [73], as well as the accumulation of uremic toxins with the progression of the disease [74].

Vitamin D deficiency, which is common in patients with chronic kidney disease, is another factor that may contribute to impaired glucose metabolism. A randomized trial of non-diabetic patients with chronic kidney disease showed that the incidence of insulin resistance was higher in patients with vitamin D deficiency compared to those with normal vitamin D levels, and vitamin D supplementation significantly improved insulin resistance, suggesting a direct role for vitamin D in regulating glycemic homeostasis in patients with chronic kidney disease [75].

Therapeutic Strategies to Improve Insulin Sensitivity

Nutritional Interventions

Lifestyle optimization, and in particular nutritional interventions, are a central element in the therapeutic approach to metabolic syndrome in general, and insulin resistance in particular. Specific dietary modifications—such as reducing caloric intake, improving food quality, or adjusting macronutrient distribution within the daily energy intake—have been shown to improve various components of metabolic syndrome and positively influence individual metabolic parameters.

Numerous studies have attempted to demonstrate the effectiveness of different types of diets in improving metabolic parameters, using varying degrees of macronutrient restrictions or various dietary patterns, without being able to precisely establish the most effective dietary pattern for the management of insulin resistance syndrome. However, current scientific evidence is in favor of the Mediterranean diet and the DASH (Dietary Approaches to Stop Hypertension) diet as effective nutritional interventions in the prevention and treatment of metabolic syndrome [76]. The nutritional quality and nutrient distribution within these dietary patterns correspond to the recommendations of a dietary plan associated with metabolic health, being easy to put into practice without assuming unnecessary dietary restrictions, difficult to follow in the long term.

The Mediterranean diet is a highly studied dietary pattern, for which there is extensive data in the specialized literature confirming the health benefits, the effects of primary and secondary prevention in both type 2 diabetes and cardiovascular diseases, and the components of the insulin resistance syndrome [77]. Numerous scientific evidence show that the Mediterranean diet not only has positive effects on health but also presents benefits in terms of sustainability and culture, being recognized by UNESCO as part of the Intangible Cultural Heritage of Humanity [78]. A review of the nutritional strategies used in the management of insulin resistance syndrome showed that adopting the Mediterranean diet can prevent excess adiposity and adiposopathy (expressed by a dysfunctional adipose tissue inflammatory response), can reduce the risk of developing metabolic syndrome, improve its individual components (such as reducing abdominal circumference, blood pressure, triglyceride levels and increasing HDL cholesterol), reduce the incidence of type 2 diabetes and cardiovascular disease (including coronary heart disease and stroke), reduce mortality, and is associated with a reduction in the incidence of cancer and neurodegenerative diseases. Moreover, adopting a Mediterranean diet also has favorable effects in terms of body composition, with a reduction in total and segmental adipose tissue being demonstrated, with favorable consequences on the metabolic profile [76]. The higher the Mediterranean diet adherence scores, the more pronounced the beneficial effects, and the improvement or even reversal of the components of the insulin resistance syndrome is more important. Accumulated scientific data show that the Mediterranean diet reduces the incidence of the metabolic syndrome and its components, improves insulin sensitivity, reduces systemic inflammation, and significantly reduces cardiovascular risk [78]. Considering all these health benefits, associated with the ease and feasibility of implementing its specific elements that differentiate it from other types of dietary patterns, the Mediterranean diet is currently considered the first-line nutritional strategy and can be implemented from the first stages in the prevention and management of insulin resistance syndrome.

The Dietary Approaches to Stop Hypertension (DASH) diet has been a promising nutritional strategy for the treatment of hypertension since 1977, and subsequent studies have confirmed its effectiveness. Over time, evidence has accumulated supporting the DASH diet's favorable impact on weight, including modest reductions in BMI and waist circumference, improvements in cardiometabolic parameters, and a lower risk of cardiovascular disease [76].

In nutritional interventions targeting insulin resistance, carbohydrate-restricted diets have been proposed as a potential treatment. However, evidence from the literature suggests that when caloric intake is restricted for weight control, the amount or source of carbohydrates does not appear to be a decisive factor in improving insulin sensitivity. Instead, in this context, food quality becomes more relevant—particularly dietary fiber, glycemic index, and lipid composition—which may play a significant role in enhancing insulin sensitivity [79].

Various types of intermittent fasting diets have also demonstrated their potential in reducing weight as assessed by BMI, reducing abdominal circumference, with additional benefits represented by improved glycemic control and reduced inflammation. The beneficial effects reported at the liver level, although of low significance, seem to be due to the reduction of enzymatic activity and liver stiffness [80, 81]. Fasting mimicking diet (FMD) is a form of periodic intermittent fasting, in which caloric intake is restricted for 5 days each month, and has been shown to have beneficial effects on the components of metabolic syndrome by reducing BMI and abdominal circumference, preserving lean mass, and improving the metabolic profile [82]. An even greater effect has been reported in individuals with higher BMI values and in individuals with a higher number of metabolic syndrome components, but the reported limitations are quite large, which does not allow generalization of the data, and further studies are needed to confirm these effects.

Plant-based diets are increasingly gaining attention at the population level and are now widely recognized as part of healthy dietary patterns. In this respect, the Planetary Health Diet introduced by the EAT-Lancet Commission is such a dietary model designed to protect global health in the face of the challenges posed by the issue of sustainability, promoting the consumption of plant-based foods while reducing the consumption of animal-based foods. This type of diet offers substantial health benefits—reduces abdominal circumference and improves metabolic status, reduces the risk of type 2 diabetes and improves glycemic control in people already diagnosed, and produces a favorable lipid profile with a reduction in LDL cholesterol, critical elements in the prevention of atherosclerosis and cardiovascular diseases [83].

Physical Activity

The close link between regular physical activity, longevity, and health was mentioned over 2000 years ago by Hippocrates and has been epidemiologically proven by numerous studies that have shown that a sedentary lifestyle is correlated with an increased prevalence of cardiovascular diseases.

During physical activity, metabolic and mitochondrial adaptations occur, facilitating insulin-dependent glucose uptake by skeletal muscle, reducing hyperinsulinemia. Myokines secreted at the muscle level after short periods of physical exercise exert endocrine functions and appear to increase GLP-1 (glucagon-like peptide-1) secretion, lipolysis and glucose uptake by adipocytes, with a net promotion of insulin sensitivity [84]. Irisin is one of these myokines that facilitates glucose uptake in skeletal muscle, improves glucose and lipid metabolism in the liver, acting as an insulin-sensitizing molecule [85].

High-intensity interval training (HIIT) has the ability to induce the secretion of VEGF (vascular endothelial growth factor), increase NO production, and stimulate anti-oxidative enzymes, with a favorable effect on insulin sensitivity [86].

Regular physical activity plays a key beneficial role in patients with metabolic syndrome. Cardiorespiratory fitness is a critical factor that reduces cardiovascular risk in a dose-dependent manner, regardless of the patient's weight status [87]. The duration of physical activity is another important element, with 60 min per week of vigorous physical activity significantly reducing the rate of metabolic syndrome [88].

Recent data from the literature suggest that resistance training increases insulin sensitivity and glucose tolerance in different population groups, regardless of age or the presence of hypertension or diabetes. A growing body of evidence suggests that aerobic exercise and resistance training provide benefits through different mechanisms [89].

Pharmacotherapy

From a pharmacological point of view, the available therapeutic arsenal with direct action on reducing insulin resistance and increasing insulin sensitivity is limited, and currently, no drug with a specific role in reducing insulin resistance is approved. The therapeutic classes that have demonstrated this effect of reducing insulin resistance are represented by biguanides and thiazolidinediones, although some authors consider that the only class that has a truly direct effect of increasing insulin sensitivity is the thiazolidinediones class, since all other molecules have an indirect effect [90]. Advances in therapeutic possibilities for insulin resistance syndrome have not been notable recently, but a lot of evidence has accumulated confirming that effective treatment of obesity will also have favorable effects in terms of improving insulin resistance. Thus, drugs that initially proved their efficacy and safety in the therapeutic regimens of patients with type 2 diabetes mellitus as antidiabetic agents are currently being successfully used as a treatment for obesity, with the potential to indirectly improve insulin sensitivity, through favorable effects on weight but also by reducing gluco- and lipotoxicity [91]. Moreover, protective effects at a cardiovascular and renal level have been demonstrated for the new antidiabetic therapeutic classes, which have led to the recommendation of their use and inclusion in therapeutic guidelines from the early stages of the disease's evolution, immediately after diagnosis.

Thiazolidinediones are drugs that increase insulin sensitivity in muscle, liver and adipose tissue, while promoting the redistribution of adiposity to peripheral adipocytes. The effect of thiazolidinediones on insulin sensitivity is mediated by the activation of PPARγ, a nuclear receptor that regulates the transcription of multiple genes involved in carbohydrate and lipid metabolism, energy balance, and lipid oxidation. This activation promotes adipocyte differentiation, enhances lipogenesis with redistribution of adipose tissue, and lowers circulating levels of FFAs and pro-inflammatory cytokines, ultimately contributing to a reduction in cardiovascular risk [16]. Furthermore, the use of thiazolidinediones contributes to the delay of β-cell dysfunction, exerting protective effects against oxidative stress and contributing to the preservation of the composition and structure of pancreatic islets [92, 93].

The efficacy of thiazolidinediones in reducing insulin resistance has been demonstrated in several randomized clinical trials, along with the reduction of hepatic and visceral adiposity [94, 95], a delay in the formation of atherosclerotic plaques and the amelioration of other cardiovascular risk factors [96], but also the resolution of specific NASH (nonalcoholic steatohepatitis) lesions and the improvement of peripheral insulin sensitivity [97]. However, the practical use of thiazolidinediones in therapeutic regimens is currently increasingly reduced due to adverse effects such as weight gain, water retention, or even the worsening of heart failure phenomena in certain situations [98].

Metformin belongs to the class of biguanides and is the most commonly prescribed drug used in the therapeutic algorithm of people with type 2 diabetes, which has proven its effectiveness and safety in the long term. Its mechanism of action involves increasing insulin sensitivity, especially at the hepatic level, leading to a reduction in endogenous hepatic glucose production [16]. Additionally, metformin also acts on adipocytes and muscle cells, causing fatty acid reesterification and inhibiting lipolysis, which will increase insulin sensitivity indirectly by reducing lipotoxicity [99]. Numerous studies conducted on experimental models and human subjects have shown that the mechanism of action for metformin includes an interference with insulin signaling pathways, the activation of the AMPK signaling pathway and an increased production and expression of specific GLUT4 transporters, but also increases glycogen synthesis, suggesting that metformin improves insulin sensitivity through multiple mechanisms, potentially delaying or even preventing the onset of type 2 diabetes while improving cardiovascular status [100, 101].

GLP-1 receptor agonists (GLP-1 RAs) increase glucose-dependent insulin secretion, contributing to improved glycemic control. Additionally, they inhibit glucagon release, reducing hepatic glucose production and contributing to reduced basal plasma glucose. GLP-1 RAs also act at the level of lipid metabolism, resulting in improved lipid profiles by reducing plasma triglycerides and LDL cholesterol levels [102, 103]. The combined effects of improved glycemic and lipid control will lead to more efficient mobilization and use of the body's energy stores, reducing the accumulation of excess fat. GLP-1 RAs also cause an increase in thermogenesis, which will lead to an increase in the body's energy expenditure with the modulation of the energy balance [104]. In addition to their effects on energy and intermediary metabolism, GLP-1 receptor agonists improve adipose tissue function by reducing inflammation, thereby decreasing insulin resistance and metabolic dysfunction in adipose tissue [105]. At the same time, it promotes the redistribution of adiposity from the abdominal, perivisceral level to the subcutaneous deposits, thus further reducing the risk of type 2 diabetes and cardiovascular or kidney diseases [106].

Glucose-dependant insulinotropic polypeptide receptor agonists (GIP RAs) contribute to weight control by modulating both lipid and glycemic metabolism, causing increased insulin secretion and reduced glucagon secretion, while promoting lipogenesis in certain tissues and inhibiting lipid storage in others [107]. The beneficial effects are therefore multifaceted: They include direct improvements in glycemic control and lipid profiles, as well as enhanced metabolic flexibility, allowing more efficient switching between glucose and lipid utilization as energy sources. The use of the dual GLP-1 and GIP Rc agonist allows for a greater impact by synergistically modulating multiple metabolic pathways [108].

Sodium-glucose cotransporter 2 (SGLT2) inhibitors are molecules initially introduced in the management guidelines for people with type 2 diabetes, being effective in lowering plasma glucose by inhibiting glucose reabsorption at the level of the proximal tubule, and therefore causing an increase in glucosuria. Numerous preclinical and clinical studies have shown that SGLT2i can reduce hyperinsulinemia and/or decrease insulin resistance, with significant improvements in skeletal muscle and myocardial microperfusion, improvement of arterial stiffness, and improvement of endothelial function, signs of improved vascular insulin sensitivity [91].

Evidence from the literature suggests several mechanisms through which SGLT2 inhibitors may improve insulin sensitivity. These include the reduction of glucotoxicity and lipotoxicity, weight loss accompanied by decreased adipocytokine levels, attenuation of inflammation via lower proinflammatory cytokine expression, improvement of β-cell function through modulation of apoptosis-related pathways, and the amelioration of oxidative stress [16]. Additionally, SGLT2 inhibitors promote a shift in energy substrate utilization in the heart, liver, and kidneys toward ketone bodies and short-chain fatty acids instead of glucose. This metabolic adaptation, along with improved glomerular hemodynamics, contributes to both cardiac and renal protection in individuals with or without type 2 diabetes [109].

Possible *therapeutic targets for the future* are certain molecular receptors and cellular sites that can be used in the development of new molecules for the treatment of insulin resistance in general and type 2 diabetes in particular. Thus, among the current research mentioned in the literature on the possibility of improving insulin sensitivity, we can mention: blocking the enzyme 11b-hydroxysteroid dehydrogenase (the enzyme involved in the activation of cortisone), increasing the circulating level of adiponectin (a protein secreted by adipose tissue positively correlated with insulin sensitivity), blocking fetuin-A (a protein synthesized by the liver necessary for FFA transport, involved in insulin resistance), modulating the plasma level of visfatin (it is assumed that it would improve insulin sensitivity), modulating Metrnl (an adipokine secreted predominantly by subcutaneous white adipose tissue, involved in the regulation of energy and lipid metabolism, cardiovascular function, inflammation, and insulin sensitivity), reducing the level of PEDF (pigment epithelium-derived factor) (a glycoprotein secreted by adipose tissue that promotes insulin resistance and inflammation), increasing the level of vaspin (a glycoprotein produced by adipose tissue that modulates insulin action), modulating the level of GPER (G protein-coupled estrogen receptor) (a protein that interacts with and is stimulated by estradiol, involved in the control of blood pressure, lipid and carbohydrate metabolism, inflammation), or even gene therapy (the modification of the genes involved, in order to treat or even cure the disease) [11, 110] . Another direction of research is to find effective solutions to suppress lipid synthesis in the liver or to stimulate lipid oxidation in the muscle mass with the aim of reducing intramyocellular lipid accumulation and possibly improving insulin sensitivity [24]. Of course, research is at its early stages, and the vast majority of published data comes from experimental studies on animal models, but the future sounds promising, and the path to personalized medicine is open, the aim being to find an effective and safe therapeutic regimen for each individual.

Metabolic Surgery

Metabolic surgery is associated with greater average weight loss compared to non-surgical obesity treatment modalities, regardless of the procedure performed [111], although a direct comparison with new generations of anti-obesity drugs has not yet been made. The benefits of metabolic surgery extend beyond weight loss, and the results are the consequence of numerous mechanisms and interrelationships between various organs and systems, peripheral and central, secondary to the modification of the gastrointestinal tract, more than the simple gastric restriction or nutrient malabsorption. Numerous studies published in the literature have demonstrated the metabolic effects of surgical interventions, which is also the reason why the term metabolic surgery replaced the name bariatric surgery. The resulting data confirm that surgical treatment is associated with a lower incidence of certain types of cancer (ovarian, breast, and endometrial), with reduced cardiovascular risk and mortality, reduced prevalence of depression and anxiety, improved glycemic control with reduced need for medication, prevention or even remission of type 2 diabetes, reduced blood pressure values, improvement of dyslipidemia, and improved kidney function [112–116].

Conclusions

Insulin resistance is a pathological condition that plays a central role in the development of various metabolic disorders, including type 2 diabetes, dyslipidemia, hypertension, and even certain neoplastic diseases. It is determined by abnormalities in the insulin signaling cascade, including insulin receptor abnormalities and metabolic disorders. Insulin resistance is one of the mechanisms that contribute to the emergence of clinical conditions united under the name of CKM syndrome. Excessive/dysfunctional adipose tissue accumulation is most often the initial element in the development of pathogenic mechanisms that underlie the development of chronic pathologies and the potentiation of cardiovascular-kidney-metabolic interactions. In this context, early intervention is essential, even from the initial stages of the development of CKM syndrome. The implementation of effective therapeutic strategies for optimizing lifestyle and preventing or even treating obesity is vital, with the aim of reducing cardiovascular and renal risk, using strategies that have demonstrated their cardio- and reno-protective effect. At the same time, it is necessary to implement therapeutic strategies for people with cardiovascular and/or renal diseases in a multidisciplinary context, using therapies that have demonstrated their long-term effectiveness and safety and that address multiple pathogenic links.

Learning Objectives

- Understand the mechanisms underlying the occurrence of insulin resistance
- Identify and describe the main risk factors of insulin resistance
- Explain the complex pathophysiological mechanisms linking insulin resistance to cardiovascular, metabolic, and renal pathology
- Understand and apply current therapeutic methods to improve insulin resistance and reduce cardio-reno-metabolic risk

Key Reading

- *Insulin resistance* can be defined as the state in which insulin levels, effective in normal subjects, do not produce their known biological effects, especially at the level of adipose tissue, muscle tissue, and liver.
- *Insulin resistance* is one of the central mechanisms involved in the emergence of the constellation of chronic diseases united under the name of cardiovascular-kidney-metabolic syndrome.
- *Excessive/dysfunctional adipose tissue accumulation*, including ectopic deposits, is most often the initial element in the development of pathogenic mechanisms that underlie the development of chronic pathologies and the potentiation of cardiovascular-kidney-metabolic interactions.
- *The early implementation of therapeutic strategies* for obesity management is an essential step in the treatment of cardiovascular-kidney-metabolic syndrome.

References

1. Ndumele CE, Rangaswami J, Chow SL, Neeland IJ, Tuttle KR, Khan SS, Coresh J, Mathew RO, Baker-Smith CM, Carnethon MR, et al. Cardiovascular-kidney-metabolic health: a presidential advisory from the American Heart Association. Circulation. 2023;148:1606–35. https://doi.org/10.1161/CIR.0000000000001184.
2. Bugianesi E, McCullough AJ, Marchesini G. Insulin resistance: a metabolic pathway to chronic liver disease. Hepatol Baltim Md. 2005;42:987–1000. https://doi.org/10.1002/hep.20920.
3. Himsworth HP. Diabetes mellitus: its differentiation into insulin-sensitive and insulin-insensitive types. Int J Epidemiol. 1936;2013(42):1594–8. https://doi.org/10.1093/ije/dyt203.
4. Yalow RS, Berson SA. Immunoassay of endogenous plasma insulin in man. 1960. Obes Res. 1996;4:583–600. https://doi.org/10.1002/j.1550-8528.1996.tb00274.x.
5. Saklayen MG. The global epidemic of the metabolic syndrome. Curr Hypertens Rep. 2018;20:12. https://doi.org/10.1007/s11906-018-0812-z.
6. Steenblock C, Schwarz PEH, Ludwig B, Linkermann A, Zimmet P, Kulebyakin K, Tkachuk VA, Markov AG, Lehnert H, de Angelis MH, et al. COVID-19 and metabolic disease: mechanisms and clinical management. Lancet Diabetes Endocrinol. 2021;9:786–98. https://doi.org/10.1016/S2213-8587(21)00244-8.
7. Fan Y, Yan Z, Li T, Li A, Fan X, Qi Z, Zhang J. Primordial drivers of diabetes heart disease: comprehensive insights into insulin resistance. Diabetes Metab J. 2024;48:19–36. https://doi.org/10.4093/dmj.2023.0110.
8. Saltiel AR. Insulin signaling in health and disease. J Clin Invest. 2021;131:e142241, 142241. https://doi.org/10.1172/JCI142241.
9. Petersen MC, Shulman GI. Mechanisms of insulin action and insulin resistance. Physiol Rev. 2018;98:2133–223. https://doi.org/10.1152/physrev.00063.2017.
10. Plotnikov A, Zehorai E, Procaccia S, Seger R. The MAPK cascades: signaling components, nuclear roles and mechanisms of nuclear translocation. Biochim Biophys Acta. 2011;1813:1619–33. https://doi.org/10.1016/j.bbamcr.2010.12.012.

11. Mir MM, Jeelani M, Alharthi MH, Rizvi SF, Sohail SK, Wani JI, Sabah ZU, BinAfif WF, Nandi P, Alshahrani AM, et al. Unraveling the mystery of insulin resistance: from principle mechanistic insights and consequences to therapeutic interventions. Int J Mol Sci. 2025;26:2770. https://doi.org/10.3390/ijms26062770.
12. Harmancey R, Haight DL, Watts KA, Taegtmeyer H. Chronic hyperinsulinemia causes selective insulin resistance and down-regulates Uncoupling Protein 3 (UCP3) through the activation of Sterol Regulatory Element-Binding Protein (SREBP)-1 transcription factor in the mouse heart. J Biol Chem. 2015;290:30947–61. https://doi.org/10.1074/jbc.M115.673988.
13. Wang CCL, Gurevich I, Draznin B. Insulin affects vascular smooth muscle cell phenotype and migration via distinct signaling pathways. Diabetes. 2003;52:2562–9. https://doi.org/10.2337/diabetes.52.10.2562.
14. Cases A, Broseta JJ, Marqués M, Cigarrán S, Julián JC, Alcázar R, Ortiz A. Cardiovascular-kidney-metabolic syndrome definition and its role in the prevention, risk staging, and treatment. An opportunity for the nephrology. Nefrologia. 2024;44:771–83. https://doi.org/10.1016/j.nefroe.2024.11.011.
15. Rubino F, Cummings DE, Eckel RH, Cohen RV, Wilding JPH, Brown WA, Stanford FC, Batterham RL, Farooqi IS, Farpour-Lambert NJ, et al. Definition and diagnostic criteria of clinical obesity. Lancet Diabetes Endocrinol. 2025;13:221–62. https://doi.org/10.1016/S2213-8587(24)00316-4.
16. Kosmas CE, Bousvarou MD, Kostara CE, Papakonstantinou EJ, Salamou E, Guzman E. Insulin resistance and cardiovascular disease. J Int Med Res. 2023;51:3000605231164548. https://doi.org/10.1177/03000605231164548.
17. Stefan N. Causes, consequences, and treatment of metabolically unhealthy fat distribution. Lancet Diabetes Endocrinol. 2020;8:616–27. https://doi.org/10.1016/S2213-8587(20)30110-8.
18. Iacobellis G. Epicardial fat links obesity to cardiovascular diseases. Prog Cardiovasc Dis. 2023;78:27–33. https://doi.org/10.1016/j.pcad.2023.04.006.
19. Parvanova A, Reseghetti E, Abbate M, Ruggenenti P. Mechanisms and treatment of obesity-related hypertension-part 1: mechanisms. Clin Kidney J. 2024;17:sfad282. https://doi.org/10.1093/ckj/sfad282.
20. Masenga SK, Kabwe LS, Chakulya M, Kirabo A. Mechanisms of oxidative stress in metabolic syndrome. Int J Mol Sci. 2023;24:7898. https://doi.org/10.3390/ijms24097898.
21. Neeland IJ, Ross R, Després J-P, Matsuzawa Y, Yamashita S, Shai I, Seidell J, Magni P, Santos RD, Arsenault B, et al. Visceral and ectopic fat, atherosclerosis, and cardiometabolic disease: a position statement. Lancet Diabetes Endocrinol. 2019;7:715–25. https://doi.org/10.1016/S2213-8587(19)30084-1.
22. Kreiner FF, Schytz PA, Heerspink HJL, von Scholten BJ, Idorn T. Obesity-related kidney disease: current understanding and future perspectives. Biomedicine. 2023;11:2498. https://doi.org/10.3390/biomedicines11092498.
23. Reaven GM, Banting Lecture. Role of insulin resistance in human disease. Diabetes. 1988;1988(37):1595–607. https://doi.org/10.2337/diab.37.12.1595.
24. Lee S-H, Park S-Y, Choi CS. Insulin resistance: from mechanisms to therapeutic strategies. Diabetes Metab J. 2022;46:15–37. https://doi.org/10.4093/dmj.2021.0280.
25. Bloomgarden ZT. Insulin resistance concepts. Diabetes Care. 2007;30:1320–6. https://doi.org/10.2337/dc07-zb05.
26. Taghibiglou C, Carpentier A, Van Iderstine SC, Chen B, Rudy D, Aiton A, Lewis GF, Adeli K. Mechanisms of hepatic very low density lipoprotein overproduction in insulin resistance. Evidence for enhanced lipoprotein assembly, reduced intracellular ApoB degradation, and increased microsomal triglyceride transfer protein in a Fructose-Fed Hamster Model. J Biol Chem. 2000;275:8416–25. https://doi.org/10.1074/jbc.275.12.8416.

27. Gaggini M, Gorini F, Vassalle C. Lipids in atherosclerosis: pathophysiology and the role of calculated lipid indices in assessing cardiovascular risk in patients with hyperlipidemia. Int J Mol Sci. 2022;24:75. https://doi.org/10.3390/ijms24010075.
28. Ormazabal V, Nair S, Elfeky O, Aguayo C, Salomon C, Zuñiga FA. Association between insulin resistance and the development of cardiovascular disease. Cardiovasc Diabetol. 2018;17:122. https://doi.org/10.1186/s12933-018-0762-4.
29. Goldberg IJ. Clinical review 124: diabetic dyslipidemia: causes and consequences. J Clin Endocrinol Metab. 2001;86:965–71. https://doi.org/10.1210/jcem.86.3.7304.
30. Ikezaki H, Lim E, Cupples LA, Liu C-T, Asztalos BF, Schaefer EJ. Small dense low-density lipoprotein cholesterol is the most atherogenic lipoprotein parameter in the prospective Framingham Offspring study. J Am Heart Assoc. 2021;10:e019140. https://doi.org/10.1161/JAHA.120.019140.
31. Zhou M-S, Schulman IH, Zeng Q. Link between the renin-angiotensin system and insulin resistance: implications for cardiovascular disease. Vasc Med Lond Engl. 2012;17:330–41. https://doi.org/10.1177/1358863X12450094.
32. Ferreira LD, Pulawa LK, Jensen DR, Eckel RH. Overexpressing human lipoprotein lipase in mouse skeletal muscle is associated with insulin resistance. Diabetes. 2001;50:1064–8. https://doi.org/10.2337/diabetes.50.5.1064.
33. Abdul-Ghani MA, DeFronzo RA. Pathogenesis of insulin resistance in skeletal muscle. J Biomed Biotechnol. 2010;2010:476279. https://doi.org/10.1155/2010/476279.
34. Rong J, Zhang Z, Peng X, Li P, Zhao T, Zhong Y. Mechanisms of hepatic and renal injury in lipid metabolism disorders in metabolic syndrome. Int J Biol Sci. 2024;20:4783–98. https://doi.org/10.7150/ijbs.100394.
35. Wang F, Han L, Hu D. Fasting insulin, insulin resistance and risk of hypertension in the general population: a meta-analysis. Clin Chim Acta Int J Clin Chem. 2017;464:57–63. https://doi.org/10.1016/j.cca.2016.11.009.
36. Fox CS. Cardiovascular disease risk factors, type 2 diabetes mellitus, and the Framingham heart study. Trends Cardiovasc Med. 2010;20:90–5. https://doi.org/10.1016/j.tcm.2010.08.001.
37. Koenen M, Hill MA, Cohen P, Sowers JR. Obesity, adipose tissue and vascular dysfunction. Circ Res. 2021;128:951–68. https://doi.org/10.1161/CIRCRESAHA.121.318093.
38. Sowers JR. Diabetes mellitus and vascular disease. Hypertens Dallas Tex. 1979;2013(61):943–7. https://doi.org/10.1161/HYPERTENSIONAHA.111.00612.
39. Jia G, Sowers JR. Hypertension in diabetes: an update of basic mechanisms and clinical disease. Hypertens Dallas Tex. 1979;2021(78):1197–205. https://doi.org/10.1161/HYPERTENSIONAHA.121.17981.
40. Montezano AC, Touyz RM. Reactive oxygen species, vascular Noxs, and hypertension: focus on translational and clinical research. Antioxid Redox Signal. 2014;20:164–82. https://doi.org/10.1089/ars.2013.5302.
41. Jia G, Aroor AR, Sowers JR. The role of mineralocorticoid receptor signaling in the cross-talk between adipose tissue and the vascular wall. Cardiovasc Res. 2017;113:1055–63. https://doi.org/10.1093/cvr/cvx097.
42. Aroor AR, Das NA, Carpenter AJ, Habibi J, Jia G, Ramirez-Perez FI, Martinez-Lemus L, Manrique-Acevedo CM, Hayden MR, Duta C, et al. Glycemic control by the SGLT2 inhibitor empagliflozin decreases aortic stiffness, renal resistivity index and kidney injury. Cardiovasc Diabetol. 2018;17:108. https://doi.org/10.1186/s12933-018-0750-8.
43. Zhao X, An X, Yang C, Sun W, Ji H, Lian F. The crucial role and mechanism of insulin resistance in metabolic disease. Front Endocrinol. 2023;14:1149239. https://doi.org/10.3389/fendo.2023.1149239.
44. Jia G, Whaley-Connell A, Sowers JR. Diabetic cardiomyopathy: a hyperglycaemia- and insulin-resistance-induced heart disease. Diabetologia. 2018;61:21–8. https://doi.org/10.1007/s00125-017-4390-4.

45. Jia G, DeMarco VG, Sowers JR. Insulin resistance and hyperinsulinaemia in diabetic cardiomyopathy. Nat Rev Endocrinol. 2016;12:144–53. https://doi.org/10.1038/nrendo.2015.216.
46. Lombardi C, Spigoni V, Gorga E, Dei Cas A. Novel insight into the dangerous connection between diabetes and heart failure. Herz. 2016;41:201–7. https://doi.org/10.1007/s00059-016-4415-7.
47. Dunlay SM, Givertz MM, Aguilar D, Allen LA, Chan M, Desai AS, Deswal A, Dickson VV, Kosiborod MN, Lekavich CL, et al. Type 2 diabetes mellitus and heart failure: a scientific statement from the American Heart Association and the Heart Failure Society of America: this statement does not represent an update of the 2017 ACC/AHA/HFSA heart failure guideline update. Circulation. 2019;140:e294–324. https://doi.org/10.1161/CIR.0000000000000691.
48. Lebeche D, Davidoff AJ, Hajjar RJ. Interplay between impaired calcium regulation and insulin signaling abnormalities in diabetic cardiomyopathy. Nat Clin Pract Cardiovasc Med. 2008;5:715–24. https://doi.org/10.1038/ncpcardio1347.
49. Basta G, Schmidt AM, De Caterina R. Advanced glycation end products and vascular inflammation: implications for accelerated atherosclerosis in diabetes. Cardiovasc Res. 2004;63:582–92. https://doi.org/10.1016/j.cardiores.2004.05.001.
50. Howard G, O'Leary DH, Zaccaro D, Haffner S, Rewers M, Hamman R, Selby JV, Saad MF, Savage P, Bergman R. Insulin sensitivity and atherosclerosis. The Insulin Resistance Atherosclerosis Study (IRAS) Investigators. Circulation. 1996;93:1809–17. https://doi.org/10.1161/01.cir.93.10.1809.
51. Sena CM, Pereira AM, Seiça R. Endothelial dysfunction - a major mediator of diabetic vascular disease. Biochim Biophys Acta. 2013;1832:2216–31. https://doi.org/10.1016/j.bbadis.2013.08.006.
52. Musunuru K. Atherogenic Dyslipidemia: cardiovascular risk and dietary intervention. Lipids. 2010;45:907–14. https://doi.org/10.1007/s11745-010-3408-1.
53. Aronson D, Rayfield EJ. How Hyperglycemia promotes atherosclerosis: molecular mechanisms. Cardiovasc Diabetol. 2002;1:1. https://doi.org/10.1186/1475-2840-1-1.
54. Jia G, Bai H, Mather B, Hill MA, Jia G, Sowers JR. Diabetic vasculopathy: molecular mechanisms and clinical insights. Int J Mol Sci. 2024;25:804. https://doi.org/10.3390/ijms25020804.
55. Borlaug BA, Jensen MD, Kitzman DW, Lam CSP, Obokata M, Rider OJ. Obesity and heart failure with preserved ejection fraction: new insights and pathophysiological targets. Cardiovasc Res. 2023;118:3434–50. https://doi.org/10.1093/cvr/cvac120.
56. Pontiroli AE, Centofanti L, Le Roux CW, Magnani S, Tagliabue E, Folli F. Effect of prolonged and substantial weight loss on incident atrial fibrillation: a systematic review and meta-analysis. Nutrients. 2023;15:940. https://doi.org/10.3390/nu15040940.
57. Larsson SC, Bäck M, Rees JMB, Mason AM, Burgess S. Body mass index and body composition in relation to 14 cardiovascular conditions in UK biobank: a Mendelian randomization study. Eur Heart J. 2020;41:221–6. https://doi.org/10.1093/eurheartj/ehz388.
58. Fineberg D, Jandeleit-Dahm KAM, Cooper ME. Diabetic nephropathy: diagnosis and treatment. Nat Rev Endocrinol. 2013;9:713–23. https://doi.org/10.1038/nrendo.2013.184.
59. Usman MS, Khan MS, Butler J. The interplay between diabetes, cardiovascular disease, and kidney disease. In: Chronic kidney disease and type 2 diabetes. Arlington: ADA Clinical Compendia Series; American Diabetes Association; 2021.
60. Premaratne E, Verma S, Ekinci EI, Theverkalam G, Jerums G, MacIsaac RJ. The impact of hyperfiltration on the diabetic kidney. Diabetes Metab. 2015;41:5–17. https://doi.org/10.1016/j.diabet.2014.10.003.
61. Jefferson JA, Shankland SJ, Pichler RH. Proteinuria in diabetic kidney disease: a mechanistic viewpoint. Kidney Int. 2008;74:22–36. https://doi.org/10.1038/ki.2008.128.

62. Pugliese G, Penno G, Natali A, Barutta F, Di Paolo S, Reboldi G, Gesualdo L, De Nicola L. Italian Diabetes Society and the Italian Society of Nephrology Diabetic Kidney Disease: new clinical and therapeutic issues. Joint position statement of the Italian diabetes society and the Italian Society of Nephrology on "The Natural History of Diabetic Kidney Disease and Treatment of Hyperglycemia in Patients with Type 2 Diabetes and Impaired Renal Function.". J Nephrol. 2020;33:9–35. https://doi.org/10.1007/s40620-019-00650-x.
63. Cooper SA, Whaley-Connell A, Habibi J, Wei Y, Lastra G, Manrique C, Stas S, Sowers JR. Renin-Angiotensin-Aldosterone system and oxidative stress in cardiovascular insulin resistance. Am J Physiol Heart Circ Physiol. 2007;293:H2009–23. https://doi.org/10.1152/ajpheart.00522.2007.
64. Kim J, Montagnani M, Koh KK, Quon MJ. Reciprocal relationships between insulin resistance and endothelial dysfunction: molecular and pathophysiological mechanisms. Circulation. 2006;113:1888–904. https://doi.org/10.1161/CIRCULATIONAHA.105.563213.
65. Cersosimo E, DeFronzo RA. Insulin resistance and endothelial dysfunction: the road map to cardiovascular diseases. Diabetes Metab Res Rev. 2006;22:423–36. https://doi.org/10.1002/dmrr.634.
66. Swan JW, Walton C, Godsland IF, Clark AL, Coats AJ, Oliver MF. Insulin resistance in chronic heart failure. Eur Heart J. 1994;15:1528–32. https://doi.org/10.1093/oxfordjournals.eurheartj.a060425.
67. Palazzuoli A, Iacoviello M. Diabetes leading to heart failure and heart failure leading to diabetes: epidemiological and clinical evidence. Heart Fail Rev. 2023;28:585–96. https://doi.org/10.1007/s10741-022-10238-6.
68. Kostis JB, Sanders M. The Association of Heart Failure with insulin resistance and the development of type 2 diabetes. Am J Hypertens. 2005;18:731–7. https://doi.org/10.1016/j.amjhyper.2004.11.038.
69. Jandeleit-Dahm KAM, Tikellis C, Reid CM, Johnston CI, Cooper ME. Why blockade of the renin-angiotensin system reduces the incidence of new-onset diabetes. J Hypertens. 2005;23:463–73. https://doi.org/10.1097/01.hjh.0000160198.05416.72.
70. Chan SMH, Lau Y-S, Miller AA, Ku JM, Potocnik S, Ye J-M, Woodman OL, Herbert TP. Angiotensin II causes β-cell dysfunction through an ER stress-induced proinflammatory response. Endocrinology. 2017;158:3162–73. https://doi.org/10.1210/en.2016-1879.
71. Thomas SS, Zhang L, Mitch WE. Molecular mechanisms of insulin resistance in chronic kidney disease. Kidney Int. 2015;88:1233–9. https://doi.org/10.1038/ki.2015.305.
72. Spoto B, Pisano A, Zoccali C. Insulin resistance in chronic kidney disease: a systematic review. Am J Physiol Renal Physiol. 2016;311:F1087–108. https://doi.org/10.1152/ajprenal.00340.2016.
73. Bellasi A, Di Micco L, Santoro D, Marzocco S, De Simone E, Cozzolino M, Di Lullo L, Guastaferro P, Di Iorio B. UBI study investigators correction of metabolic acidosis improves insulin resistance in chronic kidney disease. BMC Nephrol. 2016;17:158. https://doi.org/10.1186/s12882-016-0372-x.
74. Zhang S, Tang S, Liu Y, Xue B, Xie Q, Zhao L, Yuan H. Protein-bound uremic toxins as therapeutic targets for cardiovascular, kidney, and metabolic disorders. Front Endocrinol. 2025;16:1500336. https://doi.org/10.3389/fendo.2025.1500336.
75. Lu Y, Wang Y, Sun Y, Li Y, Wang J, Zhao Y, Yang F, Gao X, Xu J, Tong Z. Effects of active vitamin D on insulin resistance and islet β-cell function in non-diabetic chronic kidney disease patients: a randomized controlled study. Int Urol Nephrol. 2022;54:1725–32. https://doi.org/10.1007/s11255-021-02968-7.
76. Castro-Barquero S, Ruiz-León AM, Sierra-Pérez M, Estruch R, Casas R. Dietary strategies for metabolic syndrome: a comprehensive review. Nutrients. 2020;12:2983. https://doi.org/10.3390/nu12102983.
77. Fahed G, Aoun L, Bou Zerdan M, Allam S, Bou Zerdan M, Bouferraa Y, Assi HI. Metabolic syndrome: updates on pathophysiology and management in. Int J Mol Sci. 2021;2022(23):786. https://doi.org/10.3390/ijms23020786.

78. Scaglione S, Di Chiara T, Daidone M, Tuttolomondo A. Effects of the Mediterranean diet on the components of metabolic syndrome concerning the cardiometabolic risk. Nutrients. 2025;17:358. https://doi.org/10.3390/nu17020358.
79. Muscogiuri G, Barrea L, Caprio M, Ceriani F, Chavez AO, El Ghoch M, Frias-Toral E, Mehta RJ, Mendez V, Paschou SA, et al. Nutritional guidelines for the management of insulin resistancE. Crit Rev Food Sci Nutr. 2022;62:6947–60. https://doi.org/10.1080/10408398.2021.1908223.
80. Heath RJ, Welbourne J, Martin D. What are the effects of time-restricted eating upon metabolic health outcomes in individuals with metabolic syndrome: a scoping review. Physiol Rep. 2025;13:e70338. https://doi.org/10.14814/phy2.70338.
81. Jurek JM, Zablocka-Sowinska K, Clavero Mestres H, Reyes Gutiérrez L, Camaron J, Auguet T. The impact of dietary interventions on metabolic outcomes in Metabolic Dysfunction-Associated Steatotic Liver Disease (MASLD) and comorbid conditions, including obesity and type 2 diabetes. Nutrients. 2025;17:1257. https://doi.org/10.3390/nu17071257.
82. Popa AD, Gherasim A, Mihalache L, Arhire LI, Graur M, Niță O. Fasting mimicking diet for metabolic syndrome: a narrative review of human studies. Meta. 2025;15:150. https://doi.org/10.3390/metabo15030150.
83. Muszalska A, Wiecanowska J, Michałowska J, Pastusiak-Zgolińska KM, Polok I, Łompieś K, Bogdański P. The role of the planetary diet in managing metabolic syndrome and cardiovascular disease: a narrative review. Nutrients. 2025;17:862. https://doi.org/10.3390/nu17050862.
84. Ruegsegger GN, Booth FW. Health benefits of exercise. Cold Spring Harb Perspect Med. 2018;8:a029694. https://doi.org/10.1101/cshperspect.a029694.
85. Arhire LI, Mihalache L, Covasa M. Irisin: a hope in understanding and managing obesity and metabolic syndrome. Front Endocrinol. 2019;10:524. https://doi.org/10.3389/fendo.2019.00524.
86. Ben-Zeev T, Okun E. High-intensity functional training: molecular mechanisms and benefits. NeuroMolecular Med. 2021;23:335–8. https://doi.org/10.1007/s12017-020-08638-8.
87. Katzmarzyk PT, Church TS, Blair SN. Cardiorespiratory fitness attenuates the effects of the metabolic syndrome on all-cause and cardiovascular disease mortality in men. Arch Intern Med. 2004;164:1092–7. https://doi.org/10.1001/archinte.164.10.1092.
88. Laaksonen DE, Lakka H-M, Salonen JT, Niskanen LK, Rauramaa R, Lakka TA. Low levels of leisure-time physical activity and cardiorespiratory fitness predict development of the metabolic syndrome. Diabetes Care. 2002;25:1612–8. https://doi.org/10.2337/diacare.25.9.1612.
89. Roberts CK, Hevener AL, Barnard RJ. Metabolic syndrome and insulin resistance: underlying causes and modification by exercise training. Compr Physiol. 2013;3:1–58. https://doi.org/10.1002/cphy.c110062.
90. Abdul-Ghani M, Maffei P, DeFronzo RA. Managing insulin resistance: the forgotten pathophysiological component of type 2 diabetes. Lancet Diabetes Endocrinol. 2024;12:674–80. https://doi.org/10.1016/S2213-8587(24)00127-X.
91. Horton WB, Love KM, Gregory JM, Liu Z, Barrett EJ. Metabolic and vascular insulin resistance: partners in the pathogenesis of cardiovascular disease in diabetes. Am J Physiol Heart Circ Physiol. 2025;328:H1218–36. https://doi.org/10.1152/ajpheart.00826.2024.
92. Del Prato S, Marchetti P. Targeting insulin resistance and beta-cell dysfunction: the role of Thiazolidinediones. Diabetes Technol Ther. 2004;6:719–31. https://doi.org/10.1089/dia.2004.6.719.
93. Campbell IW, Mariz S. Beta-cell preservation with Thiazolidinediones. Diabetes Res Clin Pract. 2007;76:163–76. https://doi.org/10.1016/j.diabres.2006.08.015.
94. Scheen AJ. DREAM study: prevention of type 2 diabetes with ramipril and/or rosiglitazone in persons with dysglycaemia but no cardiovascular desease. Rev Med Liege. 2006;61:728–32.
95. Punthakee Z, Alméras N, Després J-P, Dagenais GR, Anand SS, Hunt DL, Sharma AM, Jung H, Yusuf S, Gerstein HC. Impact of rosiglitazone on body composition, hepatic fat, fatty acids, adipokines and glucose in persons with impaired fasting glucose or impaired glucose

tolerance: a sub-study of the DREAM trial. Diabet Med J Br Diabet Assoc. 2014;31:1086–92. https://doi.org/10.1111/dme.12512.
96. Betteridge DJ. CHICAGO, PERISCOPE and PROactive: CV risk modification in diabetes with Pioglitazone. Fundam Clin Pharmacol. 2009;23:675–9. https://doi.org/10.1111/j.1472-8206.2009.00741.x.
97. Cusi K, Orsak B, Bril F, Lomonaco R, Hecht J, Ortiz-Lopez C, Tio F, Hardies J, Darland C, Musi N, et al. Long-term Pioglitazone treatment for patients with nonalcoholic steatohepatitis and prediabetes or type 2 diabetes Mellitus: a randomized trial. Ann Intern Med. 2016;165:305–15. https://doi.org/10.7326/M15-1774.
98. Colca JR, Tanis SP, Kletzien RF, Finck BN. Insulin sensitizers in 2023: lessons learned and new avenues for investigation. Expert Opin Investig Drugs. 2023;32:803–11. https://doi.org/10.1080/13543784.2023.2263369.
99. Li M, Chi X, Wang Y, Setrerrahmane S, Xie W, Xu H. Trends in insulin resistance: insights into mechanisms and therapeutic strategy. Signal Transduct Target Ther. 2022;7:216. https://doi.org/10.1038/s41392-022-01073-0.
100. Herman R, Kravos NA, Jensterle M, Janež A, Dolžan V. Metformin and insulin resistance: a review of the underlying mechanisms behind changes in GLUT4-mediated glucose transport. Int J Mol Sci. 2022;23:1264. https://doi.org/10.3390/ijms23031264.
101. Giannarelli R, Aragona M, Coppelli A, Del Prato S. Reducing insulin resistance with metformin: the evidence today. Diabetes Metab. 2003;29:6S28–35. https://doi.org/10.1016/s1262-3636(03)72785-2.
102. Lecis D, Prandi FR, Barone L, Belli M, Sergi D, Longo S, Muscoli S, Romeo F, Federici M, Lerakis S, et al. Beyond the cardiovascular effects of Glucagon-like Peptide-1 receptor agonists: body slimming and plaque stabilization. Are new statins born? Biomolecules. 2023;13:1695. https://doi.org/10.3390/biom13121695.
103. Piccirillo F, Mastroberardino S, Nusca A, Frau L, Guarino L, Napoli N, Ussia GP, Grigioni F. Novel antidiabetic agents and their effects on lipid profile: a single shot for several cardiovascular targets. Int J Mol Sci. 2023;24:10164. https://doi.org/10.3390/ijms241210164.
104. Beiroa D, Imbernon M, Gallego R, Senra A, Herranz D, Villarroya F, Serrano M, Fernø J, Salvador J, Escalada J, et al. GLP-1 Agonism stimulates Brown adipose tissue thermogenesis and Browning through hypothalamic AMPK. Diabetes. 2014;63:3346–58. https://doi.org/10.2337/db14-0302.
105. Alharbi SH. Anti-inflammatory role of Glucagon-like Peptide 1 receptor agonists and its clinical implications. Ther Adv Endocrinol Metab. 2024;15:20420188231222367. https://doi.org/10.1177/20420188231222367.
106. Zhao L, Zhu C, Lu M, Chen C, Nie X, Abudukerimu B, Zhang K, Ning Z, Chen Y, Cheng J, et al. The key role of a Glucagon-like Peptide-1 receptor agonist in body fat redistribution. J Endocrinol. 2019;240:271–86. https://doi.org/10.1530/JOE-18-0374.
107. Moiz A, Filion KB, Tsoukas MA, Yu OH, Peters TM, Eisenberg MJ. Mechanisms of GLP-1 receptor agonist-induced weight loss: a review of central and peripheral pathways in appetite and energy regulation. Am J Med. 2025;S0002-9343(25):00059–2. https://doi.org/10.1016/j.amjmed.2025.01.021.
108. De Fano M, Malara M, Vermigli C, Murdolo G. Adipose tissue: a novel target of the incretin Axis? A paradigm shift in obesity-linked insulin resistance. Int J Mol Sci. 2024;25:8650. https://doi.org/10.3390/ijms25168650.
109. Marton A, Kaneko T, Kovalik J-P, Yasui A, Nishiyama A, Kitada K, Titze J. Organ protection by SGLT2 inhibitors: role of metabolic energy and water conservation. Nat Rev Nephrol. 2021;17:65–77. https://doi.org/10.1038/s41581-020-00350-x.
110. Wolosowicz M, Prokopiuk S, Kaminski TW. Recent advances in the treatment of insulin resistance targeting molecular and metabolic pathways: fighting a losing battle? Med Kaunas Lith. 2022;58:472. https://doi.org/10.3390/medicina58040472.

111. Sjöström L. Review of the key results from the Swedish Obese Subjects (SOS) trial - a prospective controlled intervention study of bariatric surgery. J Intern Med. 2013;273:219–34. https://doi.org/10.1111/joim.12012.
112. Liao J, Yin Y, Zhong J, Chen Y, Chen Y, Wen Y, Cai Z. Bariatric surgery and health outcomes: an umbrella analysis. Front Endocrinol. 2022;13:1016613. https://doi.org/10.3389/fendo.2022.1016613.
113. Caiazzo R, Marciniak C, Rémond A, Baud G, Pattou F. Future of bariatric surgery beyond simple weight loss: metabolic surgery. J Visc Surg. 2023;160:S55–62. https://doi.org/10.1016/j.jviscsurg.2023.01.005.
114. Singh P, Subramanian A, Adderley N, Gokhale K, Singhal R, Bellary S, Nirantharakumar K, Tahrani AA. Impact of bariatric surgery on cardiovascular outcomes and mortality: a population-based cohort study. Br J Surg. 2020;107:432–42. https://doi.org/10.1002/bjs.11433.
115. Chandrakumar H, Khatun N, Gupta T, Graham-Hill S, Zhyvotovska A, McFarlane SI. The effects of bariatric surgery on cardiovascular outcomes and cardiovascular mortality: a systematic review and meta-analysis. Cureus. 2023;15:e34723. https://doi.org/10.7759/cureus.34723.
116. Ardiles LG. Obesity and renal disease: benefits of bariatric surgery. Front Med. 2023;10:1134644. https://doi.org/10.3389/fmed.2023.1134644.

Chapter 9
Diagnosis and Biomarkers of CKM Syndrome

Minela Aida Maranduca, Tudor Cristian Cozma, Dragomir Nicolae Serban, and Ionela Lacramioara Serban

Introduction

As the name suggests, cardiovascular-kidney-metabolic syndrome involves a multi-organ interplay between several physiopathological factors and pathways mainly targeting—but not limited to—the cardiovascular and renal systems. Owing to extensive systemic damage and propensity for disability, CKM has definitely turned into a major public health issue, leading to increased medical care costs on a global scale. Defined by the American Heart Association in late October 2023, the central mechanism underlying the initiation of CKM is a release into the systemic circulation of proinflammatory and prooxidative factors, derived from an excessive amount of dysfunctional adipose tissue with an often peri-visceral distribution. The main targets of these mediators are the heart, kidneys, and arteries, thus initiating and amplifying the atherosclerotic process at these levels. This inflammatory activity is also the consequence of a decrease in glucose tolerance by reducing the insulin sensitivity of the tissues. By virtue of these changes, the hepatocytes undergo a sustained metabolic hit, which translates into the onset of non-alcoholic steatohepatitis (NASH). Through a positive feedback mechanism, NASH exacerbates the inflammatory and pro-oxidant phenomena, closing a self-sustained destructive cycle characterized by systemic inflammation and insulin resistance [1].

Obesity essentially revolves around deposition of excess triglycerides in the so-called ectopic sites—liver, skeletal muscle, cardiac muscle—aside from the typical volume increase of adipose cells. Ectopic adipose tissue can cause additional organ

---

M. A. Maranduca (✉)
Grigore T. Popa University of Medicine and Pharmacy, Iasi, Romania

Department of Physiology, Faculty of Medicine, Iasi, Romania
e-mail: minela.maranduca@umfiasi.ro

T. C. Cozma · D. N. Serban · I. L. Serban
Grigore T. Popa University of Medicine and Pharmacy, Iasi, Romania

M. Floria, D. M. Tanase (eds.), *Cardiovascular-Kidney-Metabolic Syndrome*,
https://doi.org/10.1007/978-3-032-11445-7_9

damage through local release of proinflammatory and prooxidative mediators. For example, perirenal fat can lead to the development of hypertension, while epicardial and pericardial fat deposition can constitute the substrate for coronary atherosclerotic phenomena. Obesity disturbs the body's metabolic balance by increasing insulin resistance and initiating the process of atherosclerosis. This ultimately led to cardiovascular, cerebrovascular, and nonalcoholic liver diseases. Obesity, which is known to be an independent risk factor for cardiovascular disease (CVD), has a major impact on the cardiovascular system, leading to important structural and functional changes such as cellular remodeling, inflammation, neurohormonal, altogether reunited into an array of disruptive hemodynamic changes. The risk of developing atherosclerosis is 49% higher in obese than in nonobese individuals due to the release of proinflammatory adipokines and oxygen free radicals from visceral adipose tissue, causing endothelial dysfunction and activation of lymphocytes and macrophages [2, 3].

The developmental framework for CKM syndrome relies on a four-stage concept, characterized by a progressively increasing number of systems entangled in determining the surge in cardiovascular burden. While the first stage of disease involves solely the adipose tissue, the consequences of obesity are limited to the adipocyte and an impaired fatty acid metabolism, the latter stages gradually engage more metabolic disruptions, and, critically, the development and progression of chronic kidney disease. The commencement of chronic kidney disease is encountered in early phases of CKM syndrome as soon as stage 2, obesity, and hyperglycemia representing the key contributors to the onset and advancement of impaired renal function [4].

The association between abdominal obesity, altered basal blood glucose, dyslipidemia, and hypertension is recognized today as metabolic syndrome. This facilitates the evolution of cardiovascular disease, which promotes endothelial dysfunction, atherothrombosis, and fibrosis. Furthermore, the progression of occasional hyperglycemia to type 2 diabetes mellitus serves to amplify the pathophysiological mechanisms that contribute to vascular, cardiac, and renal injury [5].

Stemming from an important hemodynamic load—that is, endothelial shear stress—hyperglycemia promotes endothelial injury and atherosclerosis. Increased hemodynamic burden is similarly responsible for the development of glomerulosclerosis by means of hyperfiltration. The formation of glycation end products, the consequence of impaired intracellular glucose metabolism, favors inflammatory and fibrotic processes, ultimately leading to hyperglycemic-mediated vascular and renal dysfunction. These metabolic systemic disturbances are perpetuated due to the prolonged release fashion of end products of glycation, acting on proinflammatory and profibrotic genes and determining gain-of-function epigenetic switches [6].

The risk of developing cardiovascular disease is increased in the presence of chronic kidney disease, the latter being driven by and giving rise to a significant proinflammatory state. Increased systemic inflammation is simply proven by elevated inflammatory markers. Nevertheless, there is a vicious, intertwined network comprised of the kidneys and blood vessels. Reduced glomerular filtration rate worsens fluid retention, causing vascular congestion. Should the transmural pressure regulatory mechanisms be overwhelmed, a persistent increase in systemic blood pressure would surpass the vessel's physiological compliance range and activate the endothelial cell layer, eventually leading to pathological vascular wall adaptations. The resulting atherosclerotic process will take place on a systemic scale, renal vessel injury chiefly leading to overt hypertension and heart failure [6].

CKM Physiopathology

Renal artery denervation is a minimally invasive procedure that targets the sympathetic nervous system activity in the renal arteries, leading to a reduction in BP levels. The sympathetic nervous system plays a pivotal role in the regulation of BP through its effects on vascular tone, heart rate, and renal function. In hypertensive patients, increased sympathetic nervous system activity is often observed, contributing to elevated BP levels and cardiovascular complications. The kidneys are key targets of sympathetic innervation, with the renal nerves located in the adventitia of the renal arteries. A simplified scheme of the problematic exchanges occurring in CKM syndrome can be found in Fig. 9.1.

The Interplay Between Obesity and CVD

Obesity, defined by an increase in body mass index above 25 kg/m^2 and morbid over 30 kg/m^2, exerts direct and indirect effects on the cardiovascular system, with major implications for the structure and function of the heart and blood vessels. Obesity is not only an independent traditional risk factor but also the root cause for several other risk factors for cardiovascular disease: diabetes mellitus, hypertension, dyslipidemia, and chronic kidney disease.

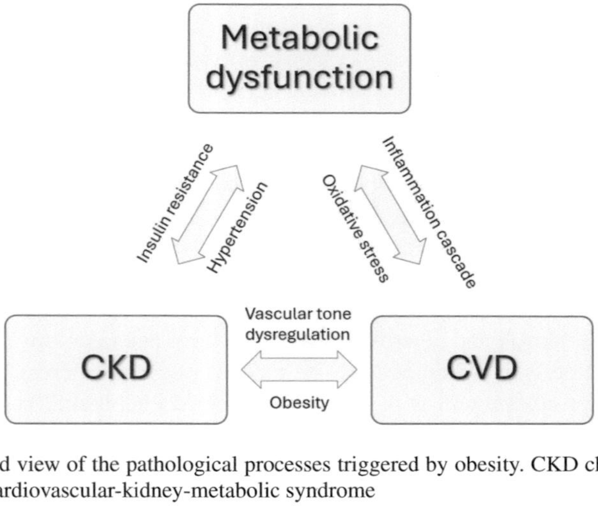

Fig. 9.1 A simplified view of the pathological processes triggered by obesity. CKD chronic kidney disease, CKM cardiovascular-kidney-metabolic syndrome

Adipose tissue is an important organ involved in immunity and inflammation through the secretion of adipokines. In individuals with obesity, the surplus of circulating fatty acids—the result of excessive food consumption but not the sole cause—and their accumulation in critical metabolic organs (such as the liver, pancreas, and skeletal muscle) lead to oxidative damage, inflammation, and metabolic dysfunction. The disturbed balance of fatty acids is an integrated part of the concept of "adipose tissue dysfunction." The more severe effects are represented by increased release of proinflammatory mediators, together promoting and perpetuating atherosclerosis. Aside from the dispersed secretion of cytokines, obese patients often present substantial epicardial fat deposits, which exacerbate the local damage, leading to coronary atherosclerosis, atrial fibrillation, and congestive heart failure [7].

The pathological alterations brought by obesity are commonly complemented by increased vascular stiffness, calcification, and altered intima-media ratio in the coronary arteries. Primary atheromatous plaque formation is the histological outcome of apolipoprotein B oxidation and endothelial dysfunction, which occurs as a consequence of the inflammation and oxidative stress induced and maintained by obesity. Thus, beyond the direct consequence of obesity, endothelial dysfunction commences through the indirect impact of obesity upon other traditional risk factors for cardiovascular disease, jointly contributing to development and progression of coronary atherosclerosis and ischemic heart disease [8].

Impaired cardiac hemodynamics, the consequence of changes on both structural and functional levels—are associated with obesity. Impaired left ventricular systolic function with diastolic function impairment are the immediate results of left ventricular hypertrophy, the dominant manner of cardiac remodeling in obesity. Accordingly, ventricular filling pressures and pulmonary arterial pressure increase. Prolonged diastolic heart failure and ventricular remodeling ultimately drive a gradual decrease in cardiac output and the ensue of global heart failure [9].

The pathophysiologic mechanism through which the obesity-hypertension dyad exerts its effects is the activation of the Renin-Angiotensin-Aldosterone system (RAAS). RAAS depicts a multifaceted influence on sodium retention, encompassing both indirect and direct mechanisms. The indirect pathway involves brain-mediated activation of the sympathetic nervous system, while the direct component is characterized by the augmentation of Angiotensin II and Aldosterone activities and proinflammatory cytokines production. Restoration of hydro-electrolytic balance following RAAS activation is achieved by a corresponding increase in arterial pressure in order to eliminate excess water and salt. The rise in systemic blood pressure is, on one hand, the inherent outcome of the spike in RAAS activity, while on the other hand, it is a requirement for return to homeostasis. This translates into a right-shift of the pressure-natriuresis curve [10, 11].

Atherosclerosis and atherosclerotic CVD have been demonstrated to be primarily associated with dyslipidemia. The process of atherosclerosis is initiated by the entry of apo-lipoprotein B past the disorganized endothelial barrier deep into the vascular wall. The oxidated fraction of proatherogenic LDL fraction is represented to a more significant extent since obesity constitutionally prompts an excess circulating quantity of LDL, with a subsequent reduction in the affinity of the LDL receptor, and lastly an increased half-life for LDL particles. Dyslipidemia is further driven by an increased release of fatty acids and triglycerides from the liver, resulting in excess adipose tissue formation. This in turn encloses a self-propelled vicious cycle by an increase in insulin resistance and proinflammatory cytokines synthesis [12, 13].

Obesity, Hyperglycemia, and Diabetes: An Impending Stepwise Complication?

Adipose tissue, a vital component in the regulation of glucose homeostasis, plays a pivotal role in lipid mobilization through its function as energy storage. Obesity has been demonstrated to induce insulin resistance, which largely manifests in the liver. The accumulation of adipose tissue in the liver serves as a reliable clue for insulin resistance, most likely determined by an inappropriate glucose response of the beta pancreatic cells [14, 15].

The distribution of adipose tissue has been identified as an independent risk factor in the development of insulin resistance. There is strong evidence for a higher risk of developing insulin resistance in patients where the quantity of visceral fat exceeds that of subcutaneous abdominal fat.

The reduced insulin sensitivity and impaired glucose tolerance that are observed in obesity are part of the aftermath of the proinflammatory and pro-oxidant status. Chronic hyperglycemia, a hallmark of type 2 diabetes mellitus, has been proven to increase the formation of glycation end products and the secretion of reactive oxygen species on a cellular level, stemming from the impaired glucose metabolism within the cell itself. A sequence of intracellular signals is initiated, leading to the synthesis of proinflammatory mediators, profibrotic factors, and various molecules that contribute to the recruitment of immune cells [16, 17]. One would consider aggressive glycemic control to be a reasonable strategy toward preventing the progression to diabetes mellitus and its deleterious effects. However, the implementation of strict measures to regulate hyperglycemia has demonstrated a limited impact on the progression of microvascular and macrovascular complications in diabetic patients. It is imperative to acknowledge that these metabolic alterations are perpetuated by a series of epigenetic changes that inevitably occur upon proinflammatory and profibrotic genes.

The development of type 2 diabetes mellitus is the unfortunate result of chronic insulin resistance, which, over time, leads to pancreatic beta-cell dysfunction. Hyperglycemia has been demonstrated to induce changes in renal hemodynamics, manifesting as glomerular hyperfiltration and hypertension [18]. These alterations initiate and exacerbate renal damage, which, in conjunction with obesity and systemic hypertension, contribute to endothelial dysfunction, atherosclerosis, and glomerulosclerosis.

Obesity and CKD: The Often-Overlooked CVD Culprit

Obesity bears an astounding impact upon renal function and structure. The increase in renal reabsorption of sodium, coupled with altered natriuresis, is driven by the activation of the Renin-Angiotensin-Aldosterone system and increased firing of the sympathetic nervous system. These lead to circulating volume expansion and the undesired building blocks of CKD: increased GFR, hyperfiltration, and, eventually, glomerular injury.

The mechanical compression of the kidney by visceral, perirenal, and renal sinus fat has been demonstrated to increase tubular sodium reabsorption and arterial pressure. Furthermore, obesity-driven uncontrolled activation of the immune system prompts an unregulated secretion of proinflammatory cytokines, their accumulation in the mesangial space having a detrimental effect upon the kidneys [19].

Obesity definitely induces a series of phenomena, including, but not limited to, increased blood pressure, release of inflammatory mediators, and various metabolic pathways impairment. These in turn gradually lead to the development of organ damage—again, including, but not limited to, the kidneys. A schematic view of the biomarkers touched over the course of this review, and the three main pillars on which the pathology and development of CKM are shown in Fig. 9.2.

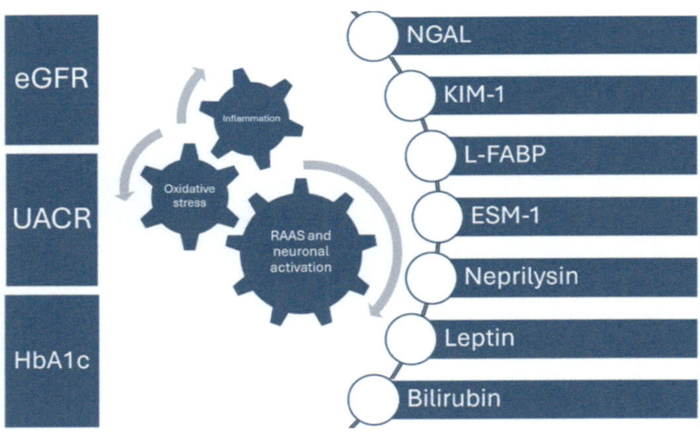

Fig. 9.2 Schematic depiction of the most important contents of this chapter. On the left side of the figure, the traditional diagnostic measures include eGFR, estimated glomerular filtration rate; UACR, urinary albumin-to-creatinine ratio; HbA1c, glycosylated hemoglobin. In the center of the image, the three interlocked gears denote three pivotal mechanisms for CKM syndrome, where RAAS is the Renin-Angiotensin-Aldosterone system. To the right, 7 of the most representative new diagnostic tools. NGAL neutrophil gelatinase-associated lipocalin, KIM-1 kidney-associated injury molecule 1, L-FABP liver-associated fatty acid-binding protein, ESM-1 endocan or endothelium-specific molecule 1

Biomarkers of Cardiovascular, Kidney, and Metabolic Syndrome

The incidence of CKM continues to rise, and so is the incidence of cardiovascular and chronic kidney disease, given this syndrome's multiorgan targeting mechanism. Given the negative impact on lifestyle and the following significant financial implications, guidelines for early diagnosis and prompt commencement of therapy for CKM are mandatory. The reduction in complication incidence rate would benefit not only the patient from a quality-of-life perspective but also reduce the load on the health system worldwide.

The utilization of biomarkers is paramount in the diagnosis, monitoring, and prognosis of CKM syndrome, with their application being instrumental in the initiation of treatment at the earliest notice. These quantifiable markers provide extremely useful information about the pathophysiological mechanisms of CKM syndrome and are of crucial value in highlighting the response to therapeutic interventions, as well as in personalizing therapy. Personalized medicine has been demonstrated to enhance quality of life by mitigating the inherent adverse effects of classical therapy through implementation of more effective management strategies. Newer updated biomarkers have been designed to provide information concerning the early, subtle changes that CKM causes, enabling the detection of the disease long before the traditional tests would depict significant changes.

Traditional Biomarkers

Serum creatinine—used for calculating the estimated glomerular filtration rate (eGFR—urea nitrogen, urinary albumin/creatinine ratio (uACR), and glycosylated hemoglobin are additional indicators of renal function, comprising the traditional markers employed in the diagnosis and prognosis of patients diagnosed and/or at risk of developing chronic kidney disease (CKD).

Estimated Glomerular Filtration Rate (eGFR)

Ideal blueprint in identification and description of the severity of CKM syndrome, eGFR (estimated glomerular filtration rate) evaluates glomerular function by calculating the fluid filtered by all glomerular capillaries over a given unit of time. In clinical practice, eGFR calculation relies on serum and urinary creatinine concentration. With respect to aging, eGFR is directly proportional to muscle mass and therefore decreases with increasing age. The normal range value of this index is 80–140 ml/min/1.73 m^2, irrespective of age and sex.

With respect to eGFR, renal function damage is classified into five mutually exclusive stages:

- eGFR equal, or higher than 90 ml\min\1.73 m^2 (other tests show inceptive renal damage)
- 60 to 89 ml/min/1.73 m^2 (development of the initial lesions)
- 45 to 59 ml/min/1.73 m^2 (discernible drop in renal function)
- 30 to 44 ml/min/1.73 m^2 (filtration rate continues to plummet)
- 15 to 29 ml/min/1.73 m^2 (renal function approaches insufficiency)
- Less than 15 ml/min/1.73 m^2 (renal failure)

Creatinine, however, the main byproduct of muscle protein metabolism, is not a reliable indicator of intrinsic renal pathology. The clearance of creatinine is subject to wide timewise variation, mainly due to autoregulation of the glomerular afferent arterioles. This, in turn, is altered by an array of underlying pathologies, the most evocative counting diabetes mellitus, hypertension, and heart failure.

Hypervolemia, irrespective of the GFR value, consistently and accurately predicts odds for mortality. This correlation is attributable to the occurrence of systemic inflammation and the subsequent triggering of cardiac remodeling. The primary objective of dialysis in patients with end-stage chronic kidney disease is to preserve residual renal function, thereby facilitating euvolemia and lessening the progression of cardiac remodeling. Systemic inflammation mediates the deleterious effects of hypervolemia through a surge in cytokine synthesis. The latter has been independently associated with malnutrition typically observed in end-stage CKD, but inversely with residual renal function [20].

Progression of CKD and mortality have been consistently associated with eGFR variability in both short and long-term. It is important to note that the hydration status greatly influences the short-term variability of eGFR. Unexpectedly, the inadvertent decrease in GFR occurring during rigorous blood pressure control does not increase the risk of CKD progression to end-stage but actually confers a protective effect on renal function in certain populations. The prompt initiation of aggressive diuretic therapy for restoring adequate volume loading in patients suffering from decompensated heart failure has demonstrated long-term benefits concerning preservation of renal function [21].

The introduction of additional markers of glomerular filtration, alongside creatinine, has the potential to enhance the predictive capacity of eGFR. A model based on creatinine, cystatin C, and the inverse of β2-microglobulin would result in a significantly more robust prediction for end-stage renal disease. Consequently, the eGFR would be calculated with greater accuracy in the context of sarcopenia, while the use of formulas that include cystatin C would cancel the requirement of adjusting for race [22].

Reduced renal function, as indicated by decreased eGFR, has been demonstrated to accelerate the metabolic imbalance associated with CKM syndrome and to increase the risk of developing cardiovascular complications. It is imperative to accurately monitor renal function in order to swiftly implement the necessary therapeutic interventions, thereby delaying the progression of renal impairment and preventing the installation of its severe adverse effects [23].

Urinary Albumin to Creatinine Ratio (uACR)

uACR has been identified as a highly specific biomarker of CKM syndrome, serving as an early indicator of renal impairment by quantifying the presence of albumin in the urine. Owing to the intricate intertwining of the pathophysiological mechanisms between metabolic, renal, and cardiovascular dysfunctions, increased uACR translates to higher odds for developing cardiovascular disease in CKM syndrome. Similar to eGFR, there is a significant daily individual variability in uACR of up to 40%, possible confounding factors including blood pressure, race, sex, muscle mass, diet, and water intake. Three measurements recorded within one-month intervals are recommended for accuracy.

Proteinuria represents a powerful predictor of end-stage CKD, irrespective of eGFR. A composite renal profile consisting of an eGFR ranging from 45 to 60 ml/min/1.73 m^2 and a recent increase in uACR value greater than 0.3 (dimensionless) is associated with higher mortality compared to a different profile consisting of an eGFR between 30 and 45 ml/min/1.73 m^2, albeit low albuminuria. Low proteinuria associated with reduced yet stable eGFR could signal the onset of cardiorenal syndrome, dehydration, or obstructive sleep apnea, rather than intrinsic renal pathology [20]. Albuminuria, even in small amounts (microalbuminuria), has been associated with an increased risk of major adverse cardiovascular events such as myocardial infarction and stroke, as well as with an increased mortality from cardiovascular causes. In individuals diagnosed with CKM syndrome stage 2 or higher, annual UACK is recommended, as its increase is associated with an elevated risk of developing subclinical heart failure. Even if the structural and functional changes could go unnoticed for years, tapering CVD progression becomes increasingly difficult with advanced stages of CKM.

Glycosylated Hemoglobin

Glucose binding to hemoglobin, a protein found exclusively in erythrocytes, results in the formation of glycosylated hemoglobin. Following non-enzymatic first-order kinetics, a persistent increase in blood glucose levels translates to an increase in the amount of glucose that binds to hemoglobin. As a surrogate indicator for the last three-month blood glucose history, glycosylated hemoglobin emerges as a fundamental biomarker for patients with CKM syndrome who present diabetes mellitus. Traditionally, glycosylated hemoglobin (HbA1c) is a valuable tool in the management of diabetes mellitus, with the potential to not only help the patient better control their blood glucose levels. Owing to the significant predictive value for lipidic profile, HbA1c also works as an indicator of the risk for cardiovascular and chronic kidney disease. The level of glycosylated hemoglobin parallels the concentration of triglycerides, cholesterol, and LDL-cholesterol and is inversely proportional to the concentration of HDL-cholesterol. Maintaining glycosylated hemoglobin levels around 7% has been shown to correlate with a reduced incidence of diabetic nephropathy.

Concerning acute cardiovascular events, levels of glycosylated hemoglobin correlate with an elevated risk of recurrence of atrial tachyarrhythmia and paroxysmal atrial fibrillation in patients diagnosed with diabetes mellitus. From a chronic perspective of disease evolution, glycosylated hemoglobin is independently and inversely linked to coronary artery reserve flow, with an increase in HbA1c signaling an unfavorable prognosis [24].

Novel Biomarkers

Neutrophil Gelatinase-Associated Lipocalin (NGAL)

NGAL is a protein expressed in a variety of tissues, initially found and described in the granules of activated neutrophils. The presence of NGAL is not confined to white blood cells, since it is expressed in the kidney and cardiomyocytes. Its novel use as an indicator for renal health status arises from its secretion by injured nephron epithelia. Under normal circumstances, NGAL is reabsorbed almost entirely in the proximal part of the nephron, and plasma concentration should be less than 20 ng/ml [25]. However, kidney injury, regardless of acute or chronic character, would lead to higher values of this biomarker both in plasma, through increased release from the directly damaged nephrons, and in urine, through a decreased reabsorbtion ability in the proximal convolute tubules of the disturbed nephrons. Alongside hypertension and eGFR, serum NGAL concentration has been identified as a risk factor for the development of renal injury [26]. The plasma concentration of this molecule is subject to variation due to its unpredictable release in systemic inflammation or in the presence of other comorbidities. Exceptionally, an elevated preoperative plasma NGAL has higher predictive value than troponin I with respect to the occurrence of renal injury in postoperative cardiac surgery patients. Moreover, in patients diagnosed with acute coronary syndrome, an increase in plasma NGAL concentration was consistently observed. These findings suggest that this biomarker might hold a significant predictive value for renal injury in CVD-challenged patients.

Kidney Injury Molecule-1 (KIM-1)

Similar to NGAL, KIM-1 is a transmembrane glycoprotein secreted by nephron proximal convoluted tubule cells and has been observed to increase in urinary concentration following postischemic and/or posthypoxic tubular injury. It has been established as a biomarker indicative of progression from chronic kidney disease to end-stage renal disease, pinpointing when initiation of renal replacement therapy becomes mandatory [27].

Liver Fatty Acid–Binding Protein (L-FABP)

In opposition to the first two molecules described in this section, human L-FABP is a constitutively renal tissue expressed 14 kDa molecular weight protein, which can be encountered both during normal conditions and under injury. Unlike NGAL and KIM-1, which flag the extent of damage undertaken by the nephron pool, L-FABP activity involves a reparatory role by binding the excess of soluble fatty acids. These fatty acids represent a concern for the normal renal function since their accumulation triggers aberrant mitochondrial activity, promoting progression of any initial lesion (most often tubular damage) and accelerating kidney interstitial fibrosis. Therefore, a persistent increase in L-FABP plasma level can indirectly point out an early destructive process targeting either the kidneys or the liver, without any constraint regarding the acute or chronic character of the underlying etiology [28].

Leptin

Discovered in 1994, leptin is encoded by the "obesity gene" and participates in the body's energy homeostasis. Synthesis of leptin, a protein hormone that belongs to the adipokine family, takes place in adipocytes within an amount that is directly proportional to the volume of subcutaneous white adipose tissue, whereas the visceral fraction of adiposity has less impact upon the quantity of leptin. Consequently, the concentration of leptin increases in obesity [8]. Following release into the bloodstream, leptin crosses the blood-brain barrier and exerts its effects primarily in the central nervous system (CNS) by binding to specific membrane receptors (LEPR-B). These receptors are predominantly expressed in the hypothalamus, with additional expression observed in other brain regions and extracranial organs, including the heart, liver, lungs, and small intestine. Receptors for leptin are categorized as type I cytokine receptors, their broad presence in apparently miscellaneous tissues underscoring the pleiotropic nature of its effects [8].

Leptin exhibits a circadian pattern of secretion, with the maximum recorded at night, and in higher concentrations in women than in men of equivalent body weight. This protein exerts autocrine, paracrine, and endocrine effects. Conventionally viewed as an anorexigenic hormone, leptin thus plays a crucial role in the regulation of body weight by reducing food intake. In addition, leptin acts upon muscular tissue through an increase in fatty acid oxidation.

Insulin is a strong regulator for the production of leptin, in such a way that prolonged hyperinsulinemia exerts positive feedback and increases leptin release into circulation. The mechanisms of action of leptin are interlinked with those of insulin, both acting on the same neuronal phenotype toward promoting satiety and inhibiting hunger. While leptin directly acts on neurogenesis and shapes neuronal excitability in various parts of the hypothalamus, the combined effects of leptin and insulin tightly regulate food intake and metabolic control. In spite of elevated levels of circulating leptin in obese patients, the anorexigenic effect of this hormone is impeded due to leptin resistance—much like insulin resistance—in these individuals. Leptin resistance is the main driver of obesity, with food intake happening in a less controlled manner. Consequently, fat deposition occurs in peripheral tissues such as the liver, myocardium, pancreas, and blood vessels, shaping the picture of metabolic syndrome. As previously described, the onset of metabolic syndrome draws severe pathophysiological issues, namely: endothelial dysfunction, stimulation of atherothrombotic mechanisms, myocardial injury with stimulation of fibrosis and cardiac remodeling [9].

The phenomenon of chronic inflammation, a condition prevalent among individuals with a BMI in the overweight and obese categories, is theorized as an effect of leptin-mediated activation of the immune system. Indeed, leptin has been demonstrated to increase the secretion of proinflammatory cytokines at the macrophage level (IL-6, IL-12, and TNF-alpha). These cytokines act through a positive feedback mechanism, which in turn increases the expression of leptin in adipose tissue, as well as the secreted leptin fraction. Therefore, this hormone can be perceived as an acute phase protein, initiating and increasing inflammation. The presence of a high number of adipocytes and macrophages in obesity is a key factor in the accelerated development of inflammation. This provides a comprehensive explanation for the chain reaction driven by obesity and chronic inflammation, whereby the production of proinflammatory cytokines and the increased levels of acute phase proteins are all orchestrated by the immune system in the context of adipose tissue dysfunction [8, 9].

There is solid evidence supporting that the development of diabetes mellitus and obesity is tightly linked to the presence of leptin resistance and hyperleptinemia. Furthermore, leptin plays a pivotal role in triggering major adverse cardiovascular events, since the severity of coronary artery disease and heart failure directly follows the trend of circulating leptin concentration.

Endocan

Discovered 20 years ago, Endothelial cell specific molecule-1 (ESM-1), also known as Endocan, is a low molecular weight proteoglycan currently considered a marker of endothelial dysfunction. Structurally, it is a soluble sulfated dermatan, with a short-acting period but high binding sensitivity. Endocan is secreted by endothelial cells under the stress of proinflammatory factors (TNF-alpha, IL-1). It is expressed at increased levels in adipocytes and in organs involved in regulating cell proliferation (liver, kidney, heart, neurons). Endocan plays a role in leukocyte migration and adhesion processes, as well as in vascular smooth muscle cell proliferation, all these acting as mechanisms that soar especially in the pathogenesis of endothelial dysfunction. ESM-1 is therefore a key element involved in the early stages of atherosclerosis [29].

Obesity is recognized as a risk factor for CKM syndrome and is associated with a low degree of chronic inflammation on behalf of the secretion of proinflammatory cytokines and adipokines by adipocytes. Evidence suggests that in cases of obesity, there is an increase in the adipocyte expression of endocan, which further plays a role in the inflammatory response associated with obesity. The latter ultimately stimulates atherogenesis and the development of atherosclerotic cardiovascular disease, aligning with the other proinflammatory molecules already described.

Metabolic syndrome, a hard component of the CKM triad, is an expression of endothelial dysfunction. Increased serum endocan concentration in the otherwise normal postprandial lipemia and nonalcoholic hepatic steatosis has been identified as an independent risk factor for atherosclerotic cardiovascular disease. Endocan has also been advanced as a prognostic factor for the decline in pancreatic beta-cell function in diabetic patients or those with impaired glucose tolerance, proven by the consistent association between the steep levels of glycosylated hemoglobin and increased serum endocan. Accordingly, endocan becomes an independent risk factor for subclinical atherosclerosis in prediabetic patients [30].

Neprilysin

Neprilysin is a zinc-dependent membrane-bound endopeptidase that plays a crucial role in determining the half-life time of certain vasoactive molecules, including vasoconstrictors (neurotensin, angiotensin I and II, and endothelin I) and vasodilators (adrenomedullin, substance P, bradykinin). Its presence has been detected in various tissues, among which the vascular endothelium and cardiomyocytes, and renal tubules are most representative for this review.

Adrenomedullin is key in preserving the functionality of the vascular endothelium in patients with overt heart failure, by limiting vessel fluid extravasation on both peripheral and pulmonary levels, thereby maintaining the barrier function of the inner layer of the vascular wall. Substance P has been demonstrated to exert a positive inotropic and chronotropic effect through an increase in cholinergic transmission. Lastly, bradykinin elicits a robust vasodilator effect by increasing the bioavailability of prostacyclin and nitric oxide [31]. Neprilysin is responsible for the natural degradation of both vasodilators and vasoconstrictors. A variation in the peptidase activity would not lead to an apparent change in the vascular tone, owing to the reciprocating effects of the mediators controlled through enzymatic degradation. The reality of an obese individual is, however, markedly different.

In obesity, a concurrent increase in neprilysin activity and decrease in endogenous natriuretic peptides are the outcome of an intricate interaction between leptin, the renin-angiotensin system (RAAS), and the renal sympathetic nervous system. The aforementioned factors lead to Aldosterone release, which, through a positive feedback mechanism, stimulate adipogenesis, adipocyte dysfunction, and adipose tissue inflammation [32].

Inhibition of neprilysin stimulates diuresis and natriuresis, reduces sympathetic activation, restores vascular tone regulation, and exerts anti-inflammatory, antifibrotic, and antihypertrophic effects on cardiomyocytes in vivo. Long-term suppression of neprilysin enzymatic activity is a therapeutic target in heart failure, clinical trials proving improved endothelial function and renovascular protection [32].

With a key role in the pathophysiological mechanisms that drive heart failure, neprilysin is a biomarker used in the prediction of hospitalization and death from cardiovascular causes. In obese individuals, there is a directly proportional increase in concentration of soluble neprilysin (shed extracellular domain) with body mass [31].

Uric Acid

Serum uric acid, an indirect biomarker of oxidative stress, is formed by the breakdown of purines. Albeit a standard byproduct of metabolism, an elevated level of serum uric acid has been demonstrated to be a contributing factor to the onset of gout. Recent studies provide substantial evidence supporting that serum uric acid levels play a significant role in the initiation and progression of cardiovascular and metabolic diseases. At present, serum uric acid is a relevant cardiometabolic risk factor.

Furthermore, hyperuricemia is a constant feature in patients suffering from chronic kidney disease, and there is solid proof backing the bidirectional character of the relationship between hyperuricemia and chronic kidney disease. There is uniform linear correlation between hyperuricemia and chronic kidney disease, the severity of hyperuricemia paralleling the advancement of CKD. According to recent research, hyperuricemia appears more often in patients with microalbuminuria; contrastingly, in patients with an eGFR below 40 ml/min, the prevalence of hyperuricemia decreases in the presence of macroalbuminuria. This surprising phenomenon may be explained by the fact that the most common cause of chronic kidney disease is diabetic nephropathy. In such instances, urinary uric acid excretion approaches normal levels, attributable to high daily diuresis, the consequence of osmotic diuresis [33].

Reduced eGFR in the presence of microalbuminuria has a significant impact on cardiovascular risk and mortality. Serum uric acid fuels renal impairment, thus instigating a vicious cycle that drives progression of CKD to end-stage renal disease—an undisputed risk factor for cardiovascular mortality [34]. Nevertheless, high plasma uric acid values stimulate inflammatory processes, endothelial dysfunction, renal interstitial tissue damage, activation of the RAAS, and accelerating alterations in renal hemodynamics. Toward the final phases of the disease, glomerulosclerosis and fibrosis ensue, which contribute to renal and systemic vascular damage.

Aldosterone

It is widely acknowledged that obesity exerts a deleterious effect on renal function, the association between obesity and hypertension representing a major mechanism. The latter results from the activation of components within the Renin-Angiotensin-Aldosterone system (RAAS) in response to obesity.

In obese individuals, there is an increase in aldosterone synthesis, as well as an enhanced sensibility of mineralocorticoid receptors through a process that is not directly influenced by aldosterone. The increase in plasma aldosterone concentration is the result of two main factors. First, excess formation of angiotensin II leads to increased renin secretion and activation of the sympathetic nervous system. Second, there is an increase in leptin concentration, which independently drives Aldosterone levels. Cortisol, adipocyte-derived cytokines, hyperglycemia, and oxidative stress separately stimulate the activation of mineralocorticoid receptors via aldosterone-independent pathways [35]. Research conducted on both animals and obese humans has returned a reduction in blood pressure of 50% upon administration of mineralocorticoid receptor inhibitors by decreasing renal sodium reabsorption and rescue of glomerular filtration rate. A further benefit is the decrease in urinary albumin excretion. Conversely, the administration of leptin receptor antagonists to mice led to enhanced endothelial function through a reduction in plasma aldosterone concentration and the desensitization of mineralocorticoid receptors [36].

Bilirubin

Bilirubin, a pigment resulting from the degradation of hemoglobin, is now considered a new biomarker for the early diagnosis of CKM syndrome. It is widely accepted that an elevation in plasma bilirubin concentration is instrumental in the diagnosis and prognosis of chronic liver conditions. Contemporary science recognizes bilirubin as an atypical hormone with significant antioxidant potency and functioning as a cardiometabolic signaling molecule [37]. It has been observed that metabolic dysfunction is associated with a decrease in serum bilirubin concentration below 6 μM, and this increases the risk of cardiovascular complications such as stroke. Furthermore, the decline in serum bilirubin concentration is a reliable indicator of obesity and progression to type 2 diabetes.

Shifting the perspective toward the cardiac tissue, here bilirubin decreases the formation of oxygen-free radicals and increases the bioavailability of nitric oxide. In adipose tissue, a slight increase in serum bilirubin concentration has been negatively associated with hypertriglyceridemia and abdominal obesity. Also, bilirubin, in conjunction with biliverdin A, concurrently limits hepatic steatosis [38].

In light of the beneficial antioxidative actions of bilirubin, one would assume that moderately increased levels should clinically translate into improved prognosis. Indeed, an important change in lipid metabolism has been observed in Gilbert's syndrome, which is known to be associated with mild hyperbilirubinemia. In this particular instance, there is a decline in proatherogenic markers evidenced by a decrease in LDL-C, triglycerides, and total cholesterol [36]. Mild elevations in serum bilirubin have been demonstrated to be associated with enhanced cellular sensitivity to glucose and insulin. This phenomenon may be attributed to bilirubin's property of impeding the signaling pathways associated with inflammation.

Lipocalin-Type Prostaglandin D Synthase (L-PGDS)

L-PGDS is a small extracellular protein member of the lipocalin family. It is characterized by its protective, anti-atherogenic role in the myocardial infarction-mediated hypoxic injury. The molecule is unique due to its dual character, in that it plays both the role of an enzyme involved in the synthesis of prostaglandin D2 (PG D2) and that of a protein transporter of lipophilic ligands [39].

Recent studies have demonstrated L-PGDS accumulation in atherosclerotic plaque of coronary arteries with severe stenosis. Furthermore, this protein may be involved in glucocorticoid-mediated protection during myocardial ischemia/reperfusion lesion, through a local biosynthesis of PG D2 from myocyte reserve of L-PGDS [40].

The presence of L-PGDS in myocardial cells, atrial endocardial cells, and atherosclerotic intimal smooth muscle cells alike suggests that it could yield diagnostic and/or prognostic value. Additionally, it could become a therapeutic target, the rescue of the cellular pool requiring enhancement of L-PGDS levels, especially in the injuries determined by coronary artery disease and myocardial infarction.

Conclusions

From a molecular standpoint, a wide array of pathogenic mechanisms lay at the foundation of CKM syndrome, the most representative including chronic inflammation, oxidative stress, and endothelial dysfunction. These damage-inflicting processes are fueled by an imbalanced vascular tone, a tendency toward insulin resistance, and dysregulated activation of RAAS axis, which in turn fosters adverse outcomes such as arterial stiffness and atherosclerosis. A hallmark chronic condition driven by CKM from the early stages of the syndrome is a profound dysregulation of the immune system, through an uncontrolled synthesis of proinflammatory cytokines. Furthermore, there is a trend toward higher plasma glycemia values, contributing to systemic inflammation, insulin resistance, and kidney damage. All previous pathological instances lay the foundation for endothelial dysfunction, which encloses an autocatalyzed vicious circle wrapped around cardiovascular disease.

Personalized therapeutic intervention should address not only the individual components of the CKM syndrome but also target the linking mechanisms that allow progression toward advanced stages of the disease. The discovery and confirmation of newer, more reliable biomarkers for accurately diagnosing CKM in the earliest phases is paramount, but researchers have to keep in mind that these "ideal" molecules will be found in close proximity to the underlying mechanisms of the disease. Traditional or otherwise unremarkable molecules may hold significant meaning—as is the case of bilirubin—while other markers involved in apparently harmless molecular networks may reveal their true identity only under the impaired conditions triggered by obesity—as depicted in the situation of neprilysin.

Learning Objectives

- Understanding the physiopathological network in the center of which the cardiovascular-kidney-metabolic syndrome is located
- Highlighting the critical role of endothelial dysfunction as a common mediator and effector for the disruptive actions in CKM syndrome both from a physiopathological and diagnostic standpoints
- Recognizing the limited diagnostic power of the traditional biomarkers within the intricate net of CKM syndrome
- Remarking part of the novel indicators are molecular indicators of injury of the organs involved in the pathological cascade
- Surfacing of common laboratory tests and their prognostic significance with respect to life-threatening complications of CKM syndrome

Key Reading

- *CKM syndrome* is a self-fueled vicious cycle relying upon early life occurrence of obesity, renal function impairment, and low-grade chronic inflammation, culminating in the development of endothelial dysfunction. Ensue of cardiovascular disease defines mild stages of CKM, subsequent multiple organ damage pushing the advance of the disease.
- *Traditional diagnostic markers* are the clinicians' tool for assessing the severity of each component disease within the syndrome. While the primary driving factor, obesity, is defined by anthropometric measures, the onset of the disease may be suggested by corroborating insulin resistance and functional decline of glomerular filtration capacity.
- *Novel biomarkers of CKM* rely upon the significant contribution of inflammatory and RAAS cascades activation. Centered on endothelial dysfunction, surrogate markers of oxidative stress have also proven useful.
- *The intricate picture* of CKM syndrome puts stress on healthcare professionals, since adequate management of the disease must encompass all individual suffering organs. Prompt identification using emerging diagnostic tests should be guided by the supposed degree of systemic damage, since many molecules serve as indicators for the extent of injury.

References

1. Ndumele CE, Neeland IJ, Tuttle KR, Chow SL, Mathew RO, Khan SS, Coresh J, Baker-Smith CM, Carnethon MR, Després J-P, et al. A synopsis of the evidence for the science and clinical management of cardiovascular-kidney-metabolic (CKM) syndrome: a scientific statement from the American Heart Association. Circulation. 2023;148:1636–64. https://doi.org/10.1161/CIR.0000000000001186.
2. Despres JP, Carpentier AC, Tchernof A, Neeland IJ, Poirier P. Management of obesity in cardiovascular practice: JACC focus seminar. J Am Coll Cardiol. 2021;78:513–31. https://doi.org/10.1016/j.jacc.2021.05.035.
3. Rangaswami J, Bhalla V, Blair JEA, Chang TI, Costa S, Lentine KL, Lerma EV, Mezue K, Molitch M, Mullens W, et al. Cardiorenal syndrome: classification, pathophysiology, diagnosis, and treatment strategies: a scientific statement from the American Heart Association. Circulation. 2019;139:e840–78. https://doi.org/10.1161/CIR.0000000000000664.
4. Claudel SE, Verma A. Cardiovascular-kidney-metabolic syndrome: a step toward multidisciplinary and inclusive care. Cell Metab. 2025;35(12):2104–6. https://doi.org/10.1016/j.cmet.2023.10.015.
5. Amdur RL, Feldman HI, Dominic EA, Anderson AH, Beddhu S, Rahman M, Wolf M, Reilly M, Ojo A, Townsend RR, et al. Use of measures of inflammation and kidney function for prediction of atherosclerotic vascular disease events and death in patients with CKD: findings from the CRIC study. Am J Kidney Dis. 2019;73:344–53. https://doi.org/10.1053/j.ajkd.2018.09.012.
6. Baccarelli AA, Ordovas J. Epigenetics of early cardiometabolic disease: mechanisms and precision medicine. Circ Res. 2023;132:1648–62. https://doi.org/10.1161/CIRCRESAHA.123.322135.
7. Rana MN, Neeland IJ. Adipose tissue inflammation and cardiovascular disease: an update. Curr Diab Rep. 2022;22:27–37. https://doi.org/10.1007/s11892-021-01446-9.
8. Vilariño-García T, Polonio-González ML, Pérez-Pérez A, Ribalta J, Arrieta F, Aguilar M, Obaya JC, Gimeno-Orna JA, Iglesias P, Navarro J, Durán S, et al. Role of Leptin in obesity, cardiovascular disease, and type 2 diabetes. Int J Mol Sci. 2024;25(4):2338. https://doi.org/10.3390/ijms25042338.
9. Landecho MF, Tuero C, Valenti V, Bilbao I. Relevance of Leptin and other Adipokines in obesity-associated cardiovascular risk. Nutrients. 2019;11:2664. https://doi.org/10.3390/nu11112664.
10. Hall JE, do Carmo JM, da Silva AA, Wang Z, Hall ME. Obesity-induced hypertension— interaction of neurohumoral and renal mechanisms. Circ Res. 2015;116:991–1006. https://doi.org/10.1161/CIRCRESAHA.116.305697.
11. Wickramasinghe M, Weaver JU. Practical guide to obesity. St Louis: Elsevier; 2018. p. 99–108. https://doi.org/10.1016/C2016-0-01351-7.
12. Klop B, Elte JW, Cabezas MC. Dyslipidemia in obesity: mechanisms and potential targets. Nutrients. 2013;5:1218–40. https://doi.org/10.3390/nu5041218.
13. Rosell M, Appleby P, Spencer E, Key T. Weight gain over 5 years in 21,966 meat-eating, fish-eating, vegetarian, and vegan men and women in EPIC-Oxford. Int J Obes. 2006;30:1389–96. https://doi.org/10.1038/sj.ijo.0803305.
14. D'Adamo E, Cali AMG, Weiss R, Santoro N, Pierpont B, Northrup V, Caprio S. Central role of fatty liver in the pathogenesis of insulin resistance in obese adolescents. Diabetes Care. 2010;33:1817–22. https://doi.org/10.2337/dc10-0284.
15. Mutruc V, Bologa C, Sorodoc V, Ceasovschih A, Morarasu BC, Sorodoc L, Catar OE, Lionte C. Cardiovascular-kidney-metabolic syndrome: a new paradigm in clinical medicine or going back to basics? J Clin Med. 2025;14, 8:2833. https://doi.org/10.3390/jccm14082833.
16. Sánchez-Margalet V, Martín-Romero C, Santos-Alvarez J, Goberna R, Najib S, Gonzalez-Yanes C. Role of leptin as an immunomodulator of blood mononuclear cells: mechanisms

of action. Clin Exp Immunol. 2003;133:11–9. https://doi.org/10.1046/j.1365-2249.2003.02190.x.
17. Fernández-Riejos P, Najib S, Santos-Alvarez J, Martín-Romero C, Pérez-Pérez A, González-Yanes C, Sánchez-Margalet V. Role of leptin in the activation of immune cells. Mediat Inflamm. 2010;2010:568343. https://doi.org/10.1155/2010/568343.
18. Bell BB, Rahmouni K. Leptin as a mediator of obesity-induced hypertension. Curr Obes Rep. 2016;5:397–404. https://doi.org/10.1007/s13679-016-0231-x.
19. Ali MM, Parveen S, Williams V, Dons R, Uwaifo GI. Cardiometabolic comorbidities and complications of obesity and chronic kidney disease (CKD). J Clin Transl Endocrinol. 2024;36:100341. https://doi.org/10.1016/j.jcte.2024.100341.
20. Zsom L, Zsom M, Salim SA, Fülöp T. Estimated glomerular filtration rate in chronic kidney disease: a critical review of estimate-based predictions of individual outcomes in kidney disease. Toxins (Basel). 2022;14(2):127. https://doi.org/10.3390/toxins14020127.
21. Alaini A, Malhotra D, Rondon-Berrios H, Argyropoulos CP, Khitan ZJ, Raj DSC, Rohrscheib M, Shapiro JI, Tzamaloukas AH. Establishing the presence or absence of chronic kidney disease: uses and limitations of formulas estimating the glomerular filtration rate. World J Methodol. 2017;7:73–92. https://doi.org/10.5662/wjm.v7.i3.73.
22. Pottel H, Björk J, Rule AD, Ebert N, Eriksen BO, Dubourg L, Vidal-Petiot E, Grubb A, Hansson M, Lamb EJ, et al. Cystatin C-based equation to estimate GFR without the inclusion of race and sex. N Engl J Med. 2023;388:333–43. https://doi.org/10.1056/NEJMoa2203769.
23. Quiroga B, Díez J. Estimation of glomerular filtration rate in cardiorenal patients: a step forward. Clin Kidney J. 2023;16(7):1049–55. https://doi.org/10.1093/ckj/sfad083.
24. Sherwani SI, Khan HA, Ekhzaimy A, Masood A, Sakharkar MK. Significance of HbA1c test in diagnosis and prognosis of diabetic patients. Biomark Insights. 2016;11:95–104. https://doi.org/10.4137/BMI.S38440.
25. Yang H, Chen Y, He J, Li Y, Feng Y. Advances in the diagnosis of early biomarkers for acute kidney injury: a literature review. BMC Nephrol. 2025;26(1):115. https://doi.org/10.1186/s12882-025-04040-3.
26. Albert C, Zapf A, Haase M, Röver C, Pickering JW, Albert A, Bellomo R, Breidthardt T, Camou F, Chen Z, et al. Neutrophil Gelatinase-Associated Lipocalin measured on clinical laboratory platforms for the prediction of acute kidney injury and the associated need for dialysis therapy: a systematic review and meta-analysis. Am J Kidney Dis. 2020;76(6):826–e411. https://doi.org/10.1053/j.ajkd.2020.05.015.
27. Xie Y, Wang Q, Wang C, Qi C, Ni Z, Mou S. High urinary excretion of kidney injury molecule-1 predicts adverse outcomes in acute kidney injury: a case control study. Crit Care. 2016;20(1):286. https://doi.org/10.1186/s13054-016-1455-6.
28. Voth M, Verboket R, Henrich D, Marzi I. L-FABP and NGAL are novel biomarkers for detection of abdominal injury and hemorrhagic shock. Injury. 2023;54(5):1246–56. https://doi.org/10.1016/j.injury.2023.01.001.
29. Klisic A, Patoulias D. The role of Endocan in cardiometabolic disorders. Meta. 2023;13(5):640. https://doi.org/10.3390/metabo13050640.
30. Khalaji A, Behnoush AH, Mohtasham Kia Y, Alehossein P, Bahiraie P. High circulating endocan in chronic kidney disease? A systematic review and meta-analysis. PLoS One. 2023;18(8):e0289710. https://doi.org/10.1371/journal.pone.0289710.
31. Núñez J, Núñez E, Revuelta-López E, Miñana G, Barallat J, Bodi V, Sanchis J, Aimo A, Emdin M, Lupón J, Husser O, Bayes-Genis A. The influence of sex and body mass index on the association between soluble neprilysin and risk of heart failure hospitalizations. Sci Rep. 2021;11(1):5940. https://doi.org/10.1038/s41598-021-85490-1.
32. Rajzer P, Biegus J. Sacubitril/valsartan in a wide spectrum of heart failure patients (from mechanisms of action to outcomes in specific populations). Heart Fail Rev. 2025;30(2):387–405. https://doi.org/10.1007/s10741-024-10471-1.
33. Gesteiro E, Megía A, Guadalupe-Grau A, Fernandez-Veledo S, Vendrell J, González-Gross M. Early identification of metabolic syndrome risk: a review of reviews and proposal for defin-

ing pre-metabolic syndrome status. Nutr Metab Cardiovasc Dis. 2021;31(9):2557–74. https://doi.org/10.1016/j.numecd.2021.05.022.
34. Srikanthan K, Feyh A, Visweshwar H, Shapiro JI, Sodhi K. Systematic review of metabolic syndrome biomarkers: a panel for early detection, management, and risk stratification in the West Virginian population. Int J Med Sci. 2016;13(1):25–38. https://doi.org/10.7150/ijms.13800.
35. Funder JW. Apparent mineralocorticoid excess. J Steroid Biochem Mol Biol. 2017;165:151–3. https://doi.org/10.1016/j.jsbmb.2016.03.010.
36. Hall JE, do Carmo JM, da Silva AA, Wang Z, Hall ME. Obesity, kidney dysfunction and hypertension: mechanistic links. Nat Rev Nephrol. 2019;15:367–85. https://doi.org/10.1038/s41581-019-0145-4.
37. Creeden JF, Gordon DM, Stec DE, Hinds TD Jr. Bilirubin as a metabolic hormone: the physiological relevance of low levels. Am J Physiol Endocrinol Metab. 2021;320(2):E191–207. https://doi.org/10.1152/ajpendo.00405.2020.
38. Wallner M, Marculescu R, Doberer D, Wolzt M, Wagner O, Vitek L, Bulmer AC, Wagner KH. Protection from age-related increase in lipid biomarkers and inflammation contributes to cardiovascular protection in Gilbert's syndrome. Clin Sci (Lond). 2013;125:257–64. https://doi.org/10.1042/CS20120661.
39. Yang HH, Wang X, Li S, Liu Y, Akbar R, Fan GC. Lipocalin family proteins and their diverse roles in cardiovascular disease. Pharmacol Ther. 2023;244:108385. https://doi.org/10.1016/j.pharmthera.2023.108385.
40. Urade Y. Biochemical and structural characteristics, gene regulation, physiological, pathological and clinical features of Lipocalin-type Prostaglandin D2 synthase as a multifunctional Lipocalin. Front Physiol. 2021;12:718002. https://doi.org/10.3389/fphys.2021.718002.

Chapter 10
Stages of Disease Progression in Cardiovascular-Kidney-Metabolic Syndrome

Maria Mihaela Godun, Diana Elena Floria, and Mariana Floria

Introduction

Cardiovascular-kidney-metabolic (CKM) syndrome represents a progressive condition that most frequently begins early in life. It is caused by a combination of biological, social, and environmental influences, which contribute to the accumulation of excessive and dysfunctional adipose tissue. The dysfunctional adiposity is correlated with chronic inflammation, oxidative stress, and insulin resistance—the key mechanisms that disrupt normal metabolic regulation. This excess/dysfunctional adiposity frequently leads to the development of metabolic risk factors such as high blood pressure, hypertriglyceridemia, type 2 diabetes, metabolic syndrome, and chronic kidney disease (CKD) [1].

As a systemic disorder, it involves complex interactions among metabolic syndrome (MetS), chronic kidney disease (CKD), and cardiovascular disease (CVD), resulting in multiorgan dysfunction and a high risk of adverse cardiovascular complications, such as atherosclerotic cardiovascular disease (ATCVD) and heart failure (HF) [2].

Eventually, the interconnection of these risk factors can lead to subclinical coronary atherosclerosis, detectable through imaging markers such as coronary artery calcium (CAC). Additionally, subclinical pathologies across various CKM pathways may be present before clinical symptoms arise, suggesting that early detection can be crucial. Clinical outcomes can be significantly improved by the identification and modification of these risk factors.

M. M. Godun (✉) · D. E. Floria · M. Floria
Grigore T. Popa University of Medicine and Pharmacy, Iasi, Romania

Saint Spiridon Emergency Hospital, Iasi, Romania
e-mail: godun.maria-mihaela@d.umfiasi.ro

M. Floria, D. M. Tanase (eds.), *Cardiovascular-Kidney-Metabolic Syndrome*,
https://doi.org/10.1007/978-3-032-11445-7_10

The pathophysiology of CKM syndrome involves complex interactions of hemodynamic and neurohormonal mechanisms, including sympathetic overactivity, renin-angiotensin-aldosterone system (RAAS) activation, oxidative stress, and chemical mediators like nitric oxide and endothelins [3, 4]. In diabetes, hyperglycemia triggers mitochondrial superoxide production, leading to oxidative stress and tissue damage through pathways such as advanced glycation end-products (AGEs), protein kinase C activation, and endothelial dysfunction [4–6]. AGEs contribute to organ damage by increasing tissue stiffness and leading to diabetic complications such as atherosclerosis, diabetic cardiomyopathy, and diabetic kidney disease. RAAS activation exacerbates organ dysfunction through vasoconstriction and fibrosis [7]. Excessive adipose tissue and carbohydrate intake activate the mTOR/S6K1 pathway, further promoting insulin resistance and organ damage. This mechanism highlights the interconnected processes leading to CKM syndrome, which are useful for early prevention [8].

The key components of CKM syndrome are:

1. Metabolic risk factors
    - Obesity
    - Diabetes
    - Metabolic syndrome (abdominal obesity, high blood pressure, impaired fasting glucose, high triglyceride levels, low HDL cholesterol)
2. Chronic kidney disease (CKD)
    - Decline in kidney function
    - Albuminuria as a predictor of cardiovascular risk
3. Cardiovascular disease (CVD)
    - Subclinical CVD (coronary artery calcification, elevated cardiac biomarkers)
    - Clinical CVD (heart failure, coronary artery disease, stroke, peripheral artery disease, atrial fibrillation)
4. Interconnected pathophysiology
    - Systemic inflammation
    - Oxidative stress
    - Insulin resistance
5. Multiorgan dysfunction
    - The outcomes of the CKM syndrome affect all organs, including liver (nonalcoholic fatty liver disease), pancreas (impaired insulin secretion), blood vessels (atherosclerosis), brain (cognitive impairment), and lungs (sleep apnea)
6. Social determinants of health (SDOH)
    - The social problems that might lead to metabolic risk factors and CKM syndrome (food insecurity, housing instability, limited health care access)

Stages of Cardiovascular-Kidney-Metabolic Syndrome

The stages of CKM syndrome, as described by the American Heart Association (AHA), are categorized into five distinct levels, from 0 to 4 (Fig. 10.1). These stages reflect the different degrees of progression and severity of the pathologies included in the syndrome, requiring proper management and intervention to address the specific challenges associated with each stage.

Key pathophysiological mechanisms across stages:

- Chronic inflammation
- Oxidative stress
- RAAS activation
- Advanced glycation end-products
- Endoplasmic reticulum stress [4]

Stage 0: No Risk Factors

In the earliest stage, stage 0, there are no CKM risk factors. This is the moment to start the prevention by modifying the lifestyle. AHA created the "Life's Essential 8" (eat better, be more active, stop smoking, get healthy sleep, manage weight, control cholesterol, manage blood sugar, manage blood pressure) (Fig. 10.2). These are the main measures to be taken to maintain cardiovascular health [9, 10].

Individuals in this stage have:

- Normal body mass index (BMI) and waist circumference
- Normal glycemia, lipid profile, and blood pressure
- There is no evidence of CKD or subclinical/clinical CVD

This stage is typically seen in youth and young adults as CKM risk factors tend to develop with aging. At this stage, there is no evidence of metabolic dysfunction

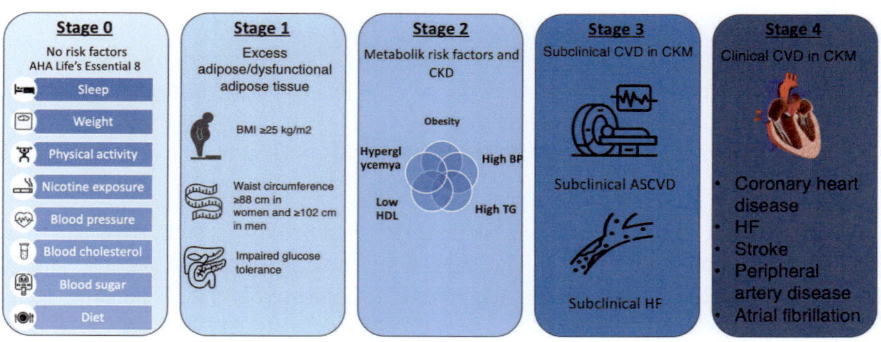

Fig 10.1 The stages of cardiovascular-kidney-metabolic (CKM) syndrome

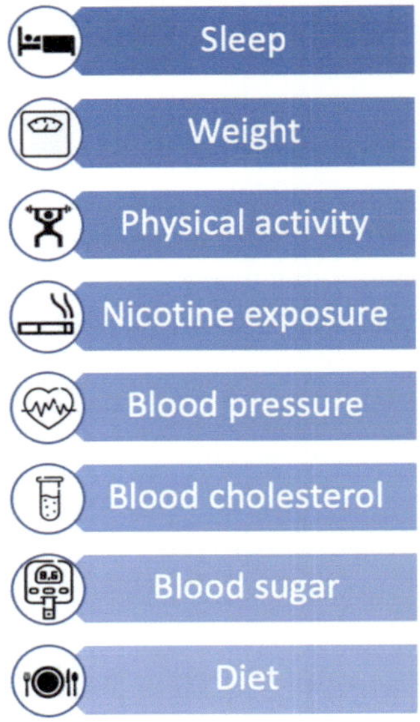

Fig. 10.2 Life's Essential 8. The eight components of cardiovascular health: healthy sleep, healthy weight, physical activity, avoidance of nicotine, healthy blood pressure, levels of blood lipids, blood glucose, and a healthy diet

or organ damage. The focus is on maintaining cardiovascular health and preventing the onset of risk factors.

Intervention: Primordial prevention through healthy eating, maintaining a normal BMI, physical activity, quitting tobacco, and proper sleep. Screening every 3–5 years for blood pressure, triglyceride, HDL cholesterol, and blood sugar is recommended [11].

Stage 1: Excess or Dysfunctional Adipose Tissue

This stage involves individuals with excess body fat or an unhealthy distribution of fat, such as abdominal obesity, impaired glucose tolerance, or prediabetes. Risk factors include:

- Overweight/obesity (BMI ≥25 kg/m^2; ≥23 kg/ m^2 for Asian population)
- Abdominal obesity (waist circumference ≥88 cm for women and ≥102 cm for men; ≥80/90 cm for Asian population).
- Fasting blood glucose levels of 100–124 mg/dl or HbA1c between 5.7% and 6.4% [12].

Interventions: Healthy eating and regular physical activity, weight loss, and treat glucose intolerance if needed. The screening indicated in this stage is every 2–3 years to assess blood pressure, triglycerides, cholesterol, and blood sugar.

Stage 2: Metabolic Risk Factors and Chronic Kidney Disease

This stage includes the population with metabolic risk factors (type 2 diabetes mellitus (DM), high blood pressure, high triglycerides (≥135 mg/dl), metabolic syndrome (MetS), or kidney disease (low estimated filtration rate or albuminuria persisting for ≥3 months).

Metabolic risk factors such as hypertension and diabetes lead to CKD, while CKD exacerbates hypertension and metabolic dysfunction. These associated conditions increase systemic inflammation, endothelial dysfunction, and oxidative stress, leading over time to subclinical CVD.

Stage 2 signifies a turning point in CKM syndrome progression, as metabolic risk factors and CKD substantially raise the risk of cardiovascular complications. Important factors to consider include [13]:

- Lifestyle modification: Addressing the metabolic syndrome components through dietary changes, physical activity, and weight loss.
- Pharmacological management: Using medication to control blood pressure, levels of cholesterol and triglycerides, and glucose levels. The medication includes antihyperglycemic, lipid-lowering, and antiplatelets. To lower cardiovascular risk, treatment with SGLT2 inhibitor or GLP-1 receptor agonist is advised in patients with high predicted risk or certain comorbidities. If the targets are not achieved by these modifications, the alternative of bariatric surgery should be taken into account.
- Kidney protection: Implementing therapies to slow CKD progression and reduce cardiovascular risk, such as angiotensin-converting enzyme (ACE) inhibitors/angiotensin II receptor blockers (ARBs), SGLT2 inhibitors, and nonsteroidal mineralocorticoid antagonists [14].

Interventions:

- Hypertension control: Reaching the target blood pressure (<130/80 mmHg)
- Diabetes management: A value of HbA1c lower than 7% is recommended
- CKD monitoring: regular assessments of eGFR and urine albumin-creatine ratio (UACR) to track kidney function and guide interventions

Stage 3: Subclinical Cardiovascular Disease in Cardiovascular-Kidney-Metabolic Syndrome

This phase is characterized by early cardiovascular disease without symptoms, such as subclinical heart failure (elevated cardiac biomarkers or imaging abnormalities), or subclinical atherosclerosis (coronary artery calcification (CAC)), in individuals with metabolic risk factors, kidney disease, or those at high predicted risk for CVD.

Essential aspects in the management of this stage are:

- Early detection: Using imaging and biomarkers to identify subclinical disease.
- Risk stratification: There are new prediction algorithms that have to be applied to quantify absolute risk and guide therapy.
- Preventive therapies: Introducing lifestyle and pharmacological interventions to delay the progression of the disease [15].

Intervention:

- In case of subclinical atherosclerosis:
  - If CAC is >0: Statin use is recommended for intermediate risk.
  - If CAC is >100: Aspirin use is recommended if there is low bleeding risk.
- In case of subclinical heart failure:
  - Patients with ejection fraction <40%: angiotensin-converting enzyme inhibitors (ACEIs)/angiotensin II receptor blockers (ARBs) and beta-blockers.
  - Patients with diabetes: SGLT2 inhibitors to reduce HF risk.

Subclinical cardiovascular disease indicates organ damage in the early stage, marked by disorders in vascular integrity, myocardial function, and cardiac conduction. These changes significantly increase the risk of progression to clinical CVD and kidney failure.

Stage 4: Clinical Cardiovascular Disease in Cardiovascular-Kidney-Metabolic Syndrome

This stage targets individuals with symptomatic CVD in the presence of excess body fat, metabolic risk factors, or kidney disease. It is further divided into:

- *Stage 4a*: Clinical CVD without kidney failure
- *Stage 4b*: Clinical CVD with kidney failure

Stage 4 reflects a progressed stage of disease, where cardiovascular, kidney, and metabolic conditions occur together, leading to significant cardiovascular and kidney dysfunction. Clinical CVD includes: heart failure, coronary heart disease, peripheral artery disease, atrial fibrillation, and stroke. Kidney failure exacerbates cardiovascular complications, leading to a high-risk condition marked by elevated morbidity and mortality [16]. The two-way interaction between CKD and CVD intensifies disease severity, as CKD contributes to cardiovascular damage while CVD further impairs kidney function [17].

Unlike the other stages, stage 4 management focuses on secondary prevention and optimizing care for patients with multiorgan disease through:

- Comprehensive risk reduction: Approaching all CKM risk factors to prevent further deterioration
- Guideline-directed medical therapy (GDMT): Implementing evidence-based treatments for CVD and CKD
- Multidisciplinary care: Integrating care among various specialties to effectively manage multiple coexisting conditions

Cardiovascular-Kidney-Metabolic Syndrome and Heart Failure Staging

The stages of HF and CKM syndrome are closely interrelated, reflecting the progression of disease across cardiovascular, kidney, and metabolic health. The ACC/AHA HF stages range from stage A (at risk for HF) to stage D (advanced HF with severe symptoms). Both staging systems underscore the critical importance of early detection and intervention to prevent disease progression. This alignment between HF and CKM stages (Table 10.1) demonstrates the importance of the integrated, preventive strategies that address cardio-reno-metabolic health to reduce the burden and progression of HF [18].

Nowadays there are well-known management strategies in different pathologies

1. *Heart Failure*

HF is the last step in the cardiovascular continuum. The treatment is complex depending on the disease etiology in association with the recommendation to follow the specific guideline-directed medical therapy (β-blokers, angiotensin receptor/neprilysin inhibitors or ARNIs, mineralocorticoid receptor agonists, and SGLT2 inhibitors) [19]. The first definition of heart failure supports the standardization of cardiac pathologies from a diagnostic point of view and, obviously, a unitary therapy based primarily on prevention. Therefore, physicians can intervene in each step of CKM with prevention measures and equally with pharmacologic or interventional or surgical therapies.

Appropriate medical therapy for HF is recommended in patients with atrial fibrillation and HF with impaired left ventricular ejection fraction to reduce symptoms and/or HF hospitalization and prevent atrial fibrillation recurrence. Sodium-glucose

Table 10.1 Correlation between heart failure (HF) and cardiovascular-kidney-metabolic (CKM) syndrome staging

	No risk factors	At risk of HF	Pre-HF	HF	Advanced HF
HF stage	0	A	B	C	D
CKM stage	0	1–2	3	4	4
Characteristics	Healthy	≥1 risk factors for HF	Subclinical disease	Clinical HF	Advanced HF

cotransporter-2 inhibitors are recommended for patients with HF and atrial fibrillation regardless of left ventricular global systolic function to reduce the risk of HF hospitalization and cardiovascular death.

Key therapeutic classes, including SGLT2 inhibitors, GLP-1 receptor agosnists, mineralocorticoid receptor antagonists (MRAs), and angiotensin-aldosteron system inhibitors (RAASi) have demonstrated significant benefits in reducing HF risk and improving cardiovascular and kidney outcomes. Combined with antihypertensive agents, beta-blokers, and statins, these therapies form the foundation of HF management in CKM syndrome.

- *RAASi*: Reduce blood pressure, prevent cardiac remodeling, regulate fluid balance and vascular remodeling, and improve kidney function.
- *SGLT2 inhibitors*: Reduce glucose reabsorbtion in the kidneys, leading to improved glycemic control and diuresis, and reduce cardiac preload and afterload. Many studies have shown that SGLT2 inhibitors reduce the risk of incident HF and HF hospitalizations [20].
- *GLP1 receptor agonists*: Improve glycemic control, promote weight loss, and reduce inflammation and oxidative stress. Many cardiovascular benefits were documented, including reduced major adverse cardiovascular events [21].
- *MRAs*: The mechanism of this therapy is blocking the aldosterone receptors, reducing sodium retention, fibrosis, and inflammation. Finerenone, a nonsteroidal MRA, offers a more targeted approach, reducing inflammation and fibrosis while minimizing hyperkalemia risk. By reducing albuminuria and maintaining kidney function, it plays a crucial role in slowing CKD progression and preventing HF [22].

2. *Atherosclerotic Cardiovascular Disease*

In atherosclerotic cardiovascular disease (ASCVD), the physician can intervene for secondary prevention with Aspirin or P2Y12 inhibitors. High-intensity statin therapy should be initiated, with additional LDL-lowering agents such as ezetimibe or PCSK9 inhibitors for patients at high-risk ASCVD or for those unable to achive target LDL levels with statin therapy alone [23]. Drugs such as Bempedoic acid or inclisiran can be used for patients with statin intolerance [24]. Depending on additional cardiovascular risk in secondary prevention, the cut-off for LDL-c is variable; in high and very high cardiovascular risk, high doses of statin are necessary. The elevated triglyceridemia or other atherosclerotic factors linked to dyslipidemia (as lipoprotein (a) and apolipo proteins A or B) must be diagnosed and treated appropriately. A great attention must be accorded to the low HDL cholesterol (or greater).

Lifestyle modification represents the first step in the management of ASCVD and consists of a healthy diet, weight management, smoking cessation, stress management, healthy sleep, and regular physical activity.

Key components of treatment [12, 25]:

- Lipid-lowering therapy: High-intensity statins, ezetimibe or PCSK9 inhibitors, bempedoic acid or inclisiran

- Antiplatelet therapy: Aspirin or P2Y12 inhibitors
- Blood pressure management: ACE inhibitors or ARBs (target blood pressure <130/80 mmHg)
- Antihyperglycemic agents: SGLT2 inhibitors or GLP-1 receptor agonists

Regular follow-up is important to assess lipid profiles, blood pressure, and glycemic control. Coronary artery calcium scoring can be used to screen for subclinical ASCVD in intermediate-risk patients to guide decisions on therapy intensification.

3. *Diabetes and Chronic Kidney Disease*

Proven interventions for preventing CKD in people with diabetes include blood glucose management (A1C < 7%) and blood pressure control. Intensive glucose control close to normoglycemia has been shown to delay the onset of albuminuria and progression in both diabetes and CKD.

ACE inhibitors and ARBs represent the key treatments for individuals with CKD and albuminuria, as well as for the treatment of hypertension in people with diabetes (with or without CKD). In the situation of established CKF (eGFR <60 mL/min/1.73 m^2 and urine albumin-to-creatinine ratio (UACR) ≥300 mg/g creatinine), ACE inhibitors or ARBs were proven to reduce the risk of progression to end-stage kidney disease and cardiovascular disease.

Patients with diabetes mellitus and chronic kidney disease have a very high cardiovascular risk. Nowadays, there are new classes of drugs that can be administered to prevent decline in kidney function. Treatment with SGLT2 inhibitors is recommended for all patients with CKD, regardless of diabetes status, to preserve kidney function and reduce cardiovascular mortality. SGLT2 inhibitors slow CKD progression and reduce the risk of heart failure, independent of their effects on blood glucose levels [26].

The GLP-1 receptor agonists should be considered for patients with diabetes and CKD who are unable to use SGLT2 inhibitors due to advanced kidney disease [27]. GLP-1 receptor agonists are recommended for reducing cardiovascular risk when it is a primary concern, as they reduce the risk of CV events, minimize the risk of hypoglycemia, and help slow the progression of CKD [28].

Treatment with Finerenone for patients with kidney disease and proteinuria to lower the risk of adverse cardiovascular and renal outcomes is recommended [29].

Interventions that lower albuminuria:

- Optimize glucose management (HbA1c < 7%)
- Optimize blood pressure management (<130/80 mmHg)
- Treatment with ACE inhibitors or ARBs
- Stop smoking
- Lose weight
- Decrease salt intake and/or protein intake
- Treatment with SGLT2 inhibitors, MRAs, or GLP-1 receptor agonists [30]

4. *Atrial Fibrillation*

The most frequently encountered arrythmia in clinical practice in patients with cardiovascular comorbidities is atrial fibrillation. The 2024 European Society of Cardiology guidelines for the management of atrial fibrillation were conceived according to the CARE-AF pathway.

The guideline document recommends treatment using the AF-CARE pathway, which is comprised of:

[C] Comorbidity and risk factor management
[A] Avoiding stroke and thromboembolism
[R] Reducing symptoms by rate and rhythm control
[E] Evaluating and reassessing as patients' disease and comorbidities progress

The identification and appropriate treatment of all patient comorbidities are mandatory to prevent integrated risk factor atrial fibrillation occurrence. The primary management is based, therefore, on lifestyle changes, including: encouraging physical activity, promoting weight loss, smoking cessation, treating obstructive sleep apnea, arterial hypertension, diabetes mellitus, and chronic obstructive pulmonary disease. A patient-centered and integrated approach to atrial fibrillation management means working with a model of care that respects the patient's experience.

Joint decision-making regarding the best option for atrial fibrillation management should be made between the patient and the provider, supported by a multidisciplinary team. Education for patients, family members, caregivers, and health care professionals is recommended.

Hypertension, HF, T2DM, obesity, obstructive sleep apnea, physical inactivity, and high alcohol intake should be evaluated and managed to avoid recurrences and progression of this arrhythmia, improve success of all treatments, and prevent adverse outcomes.

Metformin or SGLT2 inhibitors should be considered for individuals needing pharmacological management of diabetes mellitus to prevent the most frequent arrhythmia in clinical practice.

Weight loss is recommended as part of comprehensive risk factor management in overweight and obese individuals with AF to reduce symptoms and arrhythmia burden, with a target of $\geq$10% reduction in body weight. Management of obstructive sleep apnea may be considered as part of a comprehensive management of risk factors in individuals with atrial fibrillation to reduce recurrence and progression. When screening for obstructive sleep apnea in individuals with atrial fibrillation, using only symptom-based questionnaires is not recommended. A tailored exercise program is recommended for individuals with paroxysmal or persistent atrial fibrillation to improve cardiorespiratory fitness and reduce AF recurrence. Maintaining an active lifestyle is recommended to prevent atrial fibrillation, with the equivalent of 150–300 min per week of moderate-intensity or 75–150 min per week of vigorous-intensity aerobic physical activity.

Reducing alcohol consumption to ≤3 standard drinks (≤30 grams of alcohol) per week is recommended as part of comprehensive risk factor management to reduce AF recurrence.

Assessment of the risk of thromboembolism may be done with locally validated risk tools or the CHA2DS2-VA score and assessment of other risk factors.

Oral anticoagulants are recommended for all eligible patients: If CHA2DS2-VA = 1, anticoagulation should be considered; if CHA2DS2-VA ≥2, anticoagulation is recommended.

Direct oral anticoagulants as apixaban, dabigatran, edoxaban, and rivaroxaban are preferred over vitamin K antagonists, except in patients with mechanical heart valves and mitral stenosis.

Adding antiplatelet treatment to oral anticoagulation is not recommended in atrial fibrillation patients for the goal of preventing ischemic stroke or thromboembolism. Anticoagulants and antiplatelet agents should not be combined, unless the patient has an acute vascular event or needs interim treatment for procedures. Anticoagulation should be pursued according to the patient's individual risk of thromboembolism, irrespective of whether they are in atrial fibrillation or sinus rhythm. Oral anticoagulation is recommended in all patients with atrial fibrillation and hypertrophic cardiomyopathy or cardiac amyloidosis, regardless of CHA2DS2-VA score. A reduced dose of DOAC therapy is not recommended, unless patients meet DOAC-specific criteria, to prevent underdosing and avoidable thromboembolic events. All patients should be kept on an oral anticoagulant for ≥2 months after an atrial fibrillation ablation procedure, irrespective of estimated thromboembolic risk.

For a formal risk-score-based assessment of bleeding risk, the HAS-BLED score should be considered to help address modifiable bleeding risk factors and to identify patients at high risk of bleeding (HAS-BLED score ≥3) for early and more frequent clinical review and follow-up.

Beta-blockers (in any left ventricular ejection fraction), digoxin (any left ventricular ejection fraction), or diltiazem/verapamil (for left ventricular ejection fraction >40%) may be used as initial therapy, as an adjunct to rhythm control therapies, or as a sole treatment strategy to control heart rate and symptoms.

Rhythm control should be considered in all suitable atrial fibrillation patients, including a cardioversion, antiarrhythmic drugs, and catheter or surgical ablation to reduce symptoms and morbidity. The primary indication for rhythm control is reduction in atrial fibrillation-related symptoms and improvement in the quality of life. Implementation of a rhythm control strategy should be considered within 12 months of diagnosis in selected patients with atrial fibrillation at risk of thromboembolic events to reduce the risk of cardiovascular death or hospitalization. Electrical cardioversion as a diagnostic tool should be considered in patients with persistent atrial fibrillation where there is uncertainty about the value of sinus rhythm restoration on symptoms, or to assess improvement in left ventricular function. Catheter ablation should be considered as a second-line option if antiarrhythmic drugs fail to control atrial fibrillation in persistent atrial fibrillation, or as a first-line option in patients with paroxysmal atrial fibrillation. Repeat atrial fibrillation catheter ablation should be considered in patients with atrial fibrillation recurrence after initial catheter ablation, provided the patient's symptoms were improved after the initial pulmonary vein isolation or after failed initial pulmonary vein isolation, to reduce symptoms, recurrence, and progression of atrial fibrillation.

Endoscopic or hybrid ablation should be considered if catheter ablation fails, or as an alternative to catheter ablation in persistent AF despite antiarrhythmic drugs.

Continuation of oral anticoagulation is recommended in patients with atrial fibrillation at elevated thromboembolic risk after concomitant, endoscopic, or hybrid atrial fibrillation ablation, independent of rhythm outcome or left atrial appendage exclusion, to prevent ischemic stroke and thromboembolism.

Atrial fibrillation ablation during cardiac surgery should be performed in centers with experienced teams, especially for patients undergoing mitral valve surgery. Surgical closure of the left atrial appendage should be considered as an adjunct to oral anticoagulation in patients with atrial fibrillation undergoing endoscopic or hybrid ablation to prevent ischemic stroke and thromboembolism.

Patients should be periodically reassessed with attention to new modifiable risk factors that could slow or reverse the progression of atrial fibrillation, increase quality of life, and prevent adverse outcomes.

Anticoagulation for stroke prophylaxis, with dose adjustments for direct oral anticoagulants in patients with advanced CKD. Patients with hemodialysis are a special category. In hemodialysis patients with atrial fibrillation and mechanical valve replacement, the treatment with antivitamin K is the only treatment allowed with oral anticoagulants. In those without mechanical valve replacement (but with atrial fibrillation) the physician must assess the dialysis risk score which is the sum of the following parameters: prior transient ischemic stroke or stroke (plus 3 points), diabetes mellitus (plus 1 point), age >75 years (plus 1 point) and gastrointestinal bleeding <1 year (minus 1 point). Depending on this score value: (1) In patients with dialysis risk score <2, left atrial appendage closure may be considered as an alternative to oral anticoagulation; (2) in patients with dialysis risk score ≥2, Apixaban 2.5 mgx2/day or rivaroxaban 10 mg/day or left atrial appendage closure is recommended.

5. *Obesity and Metabolic Syndrome*

In patients with obesity and metabolic syndrome, structured weight loss intervention is recommended to improve metabolic risk factors and functional status under nutrition counseling. Ligestyle change is mandatory. Lifestyle modification supported by multidisciplinary care teams, including pharmacotherapy or bariatric surgery, is recommended for severe obesity [31].

A key component in the management of obesity in CKM syndrome is the use of GLP-1 receptor agonists, such as liraglutide, semaglutide, and tirzepatide. These medications promote substantial weight loss, while also providing additional benefits for cardiovascular and kidney health. Semaglutide has demonstrated a 20% reduction in major adverse cardiovascular events in individuals with obesity and atherosclerotic cardiovascular disease, as well as decreasing the risk of renal complications in those with type 2 diabetes. Tirzepatide offers additional benefits by reducing sleep apnea severity and improving overall metabolic health. GLP-1 receptor agonists represent a significant advancement in the treatment of obesity and its associated complications in CKM syndrome. The mechanism of action includes:

- Stimulating insulin secretion
- Suppressing glucagon release
- Regulating appetite
- Delaying gastric emptying
- Providing cardiorenal benefits [32]

SGLT2 inhibitors play a significant role in the treatment of obesity by promoting weight loss and improving adipose tissue function. SGLT2 inhibitor treatment has been shown to reduce total body weight, with an average weight loss of approximately 2 kg, having the highest effect over the first weeks of treatment [33]. The mechanism of weight loss is driven by the decrease in serum glucose, leading to changes in the insulin/glucagon ratio. This promotes lipolysis and lipid oxidation, while the associated reduction in insulin levels further enhances fat breakdown. With chronic use, SGLT2inhibitors may stimulate endogenous production from amino acids, favoring lipolysis. SGLT2 inhibitors reduce visceral and subcutaneous adipose tissue without negatively affecting bone mineral density or markers of bone turnover [34].

Prevention

The prevention of CKM syndrome focuses on addressing risk factors and implementing lifestyle interventions. The purpose of primordial prevention is to prevent the development of risk factors, while primary prevention targets the optimization of existing risk factors [35].

American Heart Association developed in 2023 the PREVENT risk prediction equations, useful tools for estimating 10- to 30-year absolute risk of total CVD, including both heart failure and ASCVD. These sex-specific models include traditional risk factors such as smoking, cholesterol, and blood pressure, along with eGFR as a main predictor. Optional measurements to enhance the risk prediction are: urine albumin-to-creatine ratio, hemoglobin A1c, and social determinants of health. By incorporating up-to-date data and adjusting for competing risks such as non-CVD mortality, PREVENT offers a comprehensive, individualized approach for cardiovascular risk assessment and prevention, guiding personalized treatment strategies for diverse populations and healthcare settings [36].

The screening for CKM syndrome should start in young patients from the age of 3 with annual assessments for overweight/obesity, blood pressure, and mental health. Blood tests, including lipids and glucose tolerance tests, are recommended for children with obesity or additional risk factors [37].

On the other hand, adult screening is performed through regular measurement of BMI, waist circumference, and metabolic syndrome components (triglycerides,

HDL cholesterol, glycemia, blood pressure). The screening frequency depends on CKM stages. Screening every 3–5 years for adults in stage 0 CKM, every 2–3 years in stage 1 CKM, and annual assessments are recommended in stage 2 CKM or higher [38].

Screening for CKD and utilizing kidney-protective treatments, including SGLT2 inhibitors, GLP-1 receptor agonists, and nonsteroidal mineralocorticoid receptor agonists, is essential for preventing CKM syndrome progression [22].

Early intervention to regress CKM stages and address SDOH can further reduce the risk of CKM syndrome and its related complications. A systematic screening for factors like housing instability, mental health, and food insecurity needs to be implemented, and also to connect the patients to programs that address social needs [39].

Learning Objectives

1. Understand the progression of CKM syndrome:
   - Become familiar with the stages of cardiovascular-kidney-metabolic (CKM) syndrome, ranging from stage 0 (no risk factors) to stage 4 (established cardiovascular disease with or without kidney failure).
   - Recognize the interconnected pathophysiological mechanisms, including chronic inflammation, oxidative stress, RAAS activation, and insulin resistance.
2. Identify risk factors and enable early detection:
   - Identify key metabolic risk factors such as obesity, diabetes, hypertension, and chronic kidney disease (CKD).
   - Understand the importance of early detection through imaging markers (e.g., coronary artery calcium) and biomarkers to identify subclinical disease.
3. Explore preventive strategies:
   - Learn about lifestyle interventions, including the "Life's Essential 8" framework (healthy eating, physical activity, weight management, etc.) for primordial prevention.
   - Understand screening recommendations for blood pressure, cholesterol, and blood sugar across different stages of CKM syndrome.
4. Examine evidence-based management approaches:
   - Review pharmacologic therapies such as SGLT2 inhibitors, GLP-1 receptor agonists for the management of CKD and cardiovascular disease.
   - Explore multidisciplinary care strategies for advanced stages of CKM syndrome.

5. Apply risk prediction tools:
    - Evaluate how to use the American Heart Association's PREVENT equations for estimating long-term cardiovascular risk.
    - Learn how to incorporate traditional and optional measurements for personalized risk assessment.

Key Reading

- *Definition and Overview of CKM Syndrome*
    - CKM syndrome represents a progressive condition caused by biological, social, and environmental factors, leading to excess and dysfunctional adipose tissue.
    - It involves complex interactions among metabolic syndrome (MetS), cardiovascular disease (CVD), and chronic kidney disease (CKD), ultimately leading to multiorgan dysfunction.
- *Pathophysiology*
    - Fundamental pathological processes include chronic inflammation, oxidative stress, insulin resistance, and neurohormonal mechanisms.
    - Other underlying mechanisms involve advanced glycation end-products (AGEs), endoplasmic reticulum stress, and mTOR/S6K1 pathway activation.
- *Stages of CKM Syndrome*
    - Stage 0: No risk factors; focus on primordial prevention via "Life's Essential 8" (defined by the American Heart Association).
    - Stage 1: Excess or dysfunctional adiposity; target weight reduction and early glucose control.
    - Stage 2: Presence of metabolic risk factors and/or CKD; implement lifestyle and pharmacologic therapies.
    - Stage 3: Subclinical CVD; proactive screening and early intervention.
    - Stage 4: Clinical CVD with or without kidney failure; requires secondary prevention and integrated, multidisciplinary care.
- *Management Strategies*
    - Lifestyle interventions: Diet, physical activity, smoking cessation, sleep, etc.
    - Pharmacologic treatments: Include SGLT2 inhibitors, GLP-1 receptor agonists, statins, MRAs, ACEIs/ARBs, and antiplatelet agents based on disease stage and comorbidities.
    - Multidisciplinary care is crucial for advanced stages.

- *Prevention and Screening*
  - Early screening starts in childhood for at-risk individuals.
  - AHA's "Life's Essential 8" promotes cardiovascular health from a young age.
  - Address social determinants of health (SDOH) like food insecurity and housing instability.
  - Screening recommendation: Annual assessments for children and adults based on CKM stages.
- *Multiorgan Impact and Comorbidities*
  - CKM syndrome affects multiple organs, including the liver, pancreas, blood vessels, brain, and lungs.
  - Comorbidities like diabetes, obesity, atrial fibrillation, and CKM require integrated management.
- *Emerging Therapies*
  - SGLT2 inhibitors and GLP-1 receptor agonists for cardiorenal benefits and weight loss.
  - High-intensity statins, PCSK9 inhibitors, and bempedoic acid are used for lipid lowering in ASCVD management.
  - Finerenone, a nonsteroidal MRA, reduces fibrosis and inflammation in CKD.
- *Risk Prediction*
  - The AHA's PREVENT equation estimates 10- to 30-year CVD risk.
  - Useful in tailoring long-term prevention strategies across diverse populations.

References

1. Ndumele CE, Rangaswami J, Chow SL, et al. On behalf of the American Heart Association. Cardiovascular-kidney-metabolic health: a presidential advisory from the American Heart Association. Circulation. 2023;148:1606–35. https://doi.org/10.1161/CIR.0000000000001184.
2. Braunwald E. From cardiorenal to cardiovascular–kidney–metabolic syndromes. Eur Heart J. 2024;00:1–3. https://doi.org/10.1093/eurheartj/ehae775.
3. Marassi M, Fadini GP. The cardio-renal-metabolic connection: a review of the evidence. Cardiovasc Diabetol. 2023;22(1):195. https://doi.org/10.1186/s12933-023-01937-x.
4. Kadowaki T, Maegawa H, Watada H, et al. Interconnection between cardiovascular, renal and metabolic disorders: a narrative review with a focus on Japan. Diabetes Obes Metab. 2022;24(12):2283–96. https://doi.org/10.1111/dom.14829.

5. Forbes JM, Cooper ME. Mechanisms of diabetic complications. Physiol Rev. 2013;93(1):137–88. https://doi.org/10.1152/physrev.00045.2011.
6. Giacco F, Brownlee M. Oxidative stress and diabetic complications. Circ Res. 2010;107(9):1058–70. https://doi.org/10.1161/CIRCRESAHA.110.223545.
7. Lim HS, MacFadyen RJ, Lip GY. Diabetes mellitus, the renin-angiotensin-aldosterone system, and the heart. Arch Intern Med. 2004;164(16):1737–48. https://doi.org/10.1001/archinte.164.16.1737.
8. Whaley-Connell A, Sowers JR. Oxidative stress in the cardiorenal metabolic syndrome. Curr Hypertens Rep. 2012;14(4):360–5. https://doi.org/10.1007/s11906-012-0279-2.
9. Pulakat L, DeMarco VG, Ardhanari S, et al. Adaptive mechanisms to compensate for overnutrition-induced cardiovascular abnormalities. Am J Physiol Regul Integr Comp Physiol. 2011;301(4):R885–95.
10. Lloyd-Jones DM, Allen NB, Anderson CAM, Black T, Brewer LC, Foraker RE, Grandner MA, Lavretsky H, Perak AM, Sharma G, Rosamond W, American Heart Association. Life's essential 8: updating and enhancing the American Heart Association's construct of cardiovascular health: a presidential advisory from the American Heart Association. Circulation. 2022;146(5):e18–43. https://doi.org/10.1161/CIR.0000000000001078. Epub 2022 Jun 29. PMID: 35766027; PMCID: PMC10503546
11. Sebastian SA, Padda I, Johal G. Cardiovascular-Kidney-Metabolic (CKM) syndrome: a state-of-the-art review. Curr Probl Cardiol. Published online December 14, 2023. 2023; https://doi.org/10.1016/j.cpcardiol.2023.102344.
12. Grundy SM, Cleeman JI, Daniels SR, Donato KA, Eckel RH, Franklin BA, Gordon DJ, Krauss RM, Savage PJ, Smith SC Jr, et al. Diagnosis and management of the metabolic syndrome: an American Heart Association/National Heart, Lung, and Blood Institute scientific statement [published corrections appear in Circulation. 2005;112:e297 and Circulation. 2005;112:e298]. Circulation. 2005;112(17):2735–52. https://doi.org/10.1161/CIRCULATIONAHA.105.169404.
13. ElSayed NA, Aleppo G, Aroda VR, Bannuru RR, Brown FM, Bruemmer D, Collins BS, Das SR, Hilliard ME, Isaacs D, et al. 10: cardiovascular disease and risk management: standards of care in diabetes–2023. Diabetes Care. 2023;46:S158–90. https://doi.org/10.2337/dc23S010.
14. Webster AC, Nagler EV, Morton RL, Masson P. Chronic kidney disease. Lancet. 2017;389:1238–52. https://doi.org/10.1016/S0140-6736(16)32064-5.
15. Rinella ME, Neuschwander-Tetri BA, Siddiqui MS, Abdelmalek MF, Caldwell S, Barb D, Kleiner DE, Loomba R. AASLD practice guidance on the clinical assessment and management of nonalcoholic fatty liver disease. Hepatology. 2023;77:1797–835. https://doi.org/10.1097/HEP.0000000000000323.
16. US Renal Data System. 2022 USRDS annual data report: epidemiology of kidney disease in the United States. Accessed 1 June 2023. https://adr.usrds.org/2022.
17. Rangaswami J, Bhalla V, Blair JEA, Chang TI, Costa S, Lentine KL, Lerma EV, Mezue K, Molitch M, Mullens W, on behalf of the American Heart Association Council on the Kidney in Cardiovascular Disease and Council on Clinical Cardiology, et al. Cardiorenal syndrome: classification, pathophysiology, diagnosis, and treatment strategies: a scientific statement from the American Heart Association. Circulation. 2019;139:e840–78. https://doi.org/10.1161/CIR.0000000000000664.
18. Khan SS, Breathett K, Braun LT, Chow SL, Gupta DK, Lekavich C, Lloyd-Jones DM, Ndumele CE, Rodriguez CJ, Allen LA, on behalf of the American Heart Association Prevention Science Committee of the Council on Epidemiology and Prevention; Council on Cardiovascular and Stroke Nursing; Council on Basic Cardiovascular Sciences; Council on Clinical Cardiology; Council on Hypertension; and Council on Quality of Care and Outcomes Research. Risk-based primary prevention of heart failure: a scientific statement from the American Heart Association. Circulation. 2025;152:e1006–26. https://doi.org/10.1161/CIR.0000000000001307.

19. Ledwidge M, Gallagher J, Conlon C, Tallon E, O'Connell E, Dawkins I, Watson C, O'Hanlon R, Bermingham M, Patle A, et al. Natriuretic peptidebased screening and collaborative care for heart failure: the STOP-HF randomized trial. JAMA. 2013;310:66–74. https://doi.org/10.1001/jama.2013.7588.
20. Giugliano D, Longo M, Signoriello S, Maiorino MI, Solerte B, Chiodini P, Esposito K. The effect of DPP-4 inhibitors, GLP-1 receptor agonists and SGLT-2 inhibitors on cardiorenal outcomes: a network meta-analysis of 23 CVOTs. Cardiovasc Diabetol. 2022;21:42. https://doi.org/10.1186/s12933-022-01474-z.
21. Marso SP, Bain SC, Consoli A, Eliaschewitz FG, Jódar E, Leiter LA, Lingvay I, Rosenstock J, Seufert J, Warren ML, et al. SUSTAIN-6 Investigators. Semaglutide and cardiovascular outcomes in patients with type 2 diabetes. N Engl J Med. 2016;375:1834–44. https://doi.org/10.1056/NEJMoa1607141.
22. Naaman SC, Bakris GL. Diabetic nephropathy: update on pillars of therapy slowing progression. Diabetes Care. 2023;46:1574–86. https://doi.org/10.2337/dci23-0030.
23. Arnett DK, Blumenthal RS, Albert MA, Buroker AB, Goldberger ZD, Hahn EJ, Himmelfarb CD, Khera A, Lloyd-Jones D, McEvoy JW, et al. 2019 ACC/AHA guideline on the primary prevention of cardiovascular disease: a report of the American College of Cardiology/American Heart Association Task Force on Clinical Practice Guidelines [published corrections appear in Circulation. 2019;140:e649–e650, Circulation. 2020;141:e60, and Circulation. 2020;141:e774]. Circulation. 2019;140:e596–646. https://doi.org/10.1161/CIR.0000000000000678.
24. Visseren FLJ, Mach F, Smulders YM, Carballo D, Koskinas KC, Back M, Benetos A, Biffi A, Boavida JM, Capodanno D, et al. 2021 ESC guidelines on cardiovascular disease prevention in clinical practice. Eur Heart J. 2021;42:3227–337. https://doi.org/10.1093/eurheartj/ehab484.
25. Giovannucci E, Harlan DM, Archer MC, Bergenstal RM, Gapstur SM, Habel LA, Pollak M, Regensteiner JG, Yee D. Diabetes and cancer: a consensus report. Diabetes Care. 2010;33:1674–85. https://doi.org/10.2337/dc10-0666.
26. Emdin CA, Rahimi K, Neal B, Callender T, Perkovic V, Patel A. Blood pressure lowering in type 2 diabetes: a systematic review and meta-analysis. JAMA. 2015;313(6):603–15. https://doi.org/10.1001/jama.2015.276.
27. McGuire DK, Shih WJ, Cosentino F, et al. Association of SGLT2 inhibitors with cardiovascular and kidney outcomes in patients with type 2 diabetes: a metaanalysis. JAMA Cardiol. 2021;6:148–58.
28. Tuttle KR, Lakshmanan MC, Rayner B, Busch RS, Zimmermann AG, Woodward DB, Botros FT. Dulaglutide versus insulin glargine in patients with type 2 diabetes and moderate-to-severe chronic kidney disease (AWARD-7): a multicentre, open label, randomised trial. Lancet Diabetes Endocrinol. 2018;6:605–17. https://doi.org/10.1016/s2213-8587(18)30104-9.
29. Perkovic V, Tuttle KR, Rossing P, et al. FLOW Trial Committees and Investigators. Effects of semaglutide on chronic kidney disease in patients with type 2 diabetes. N Engl J Med. 2024;391:109–21.
30. Agarwal R, Filippatos G, Pitt B, Anker SD, Rossing P, Joseph A, Kolkhof P, Nowack C, Gebel M, Ruilope LM, et al. Cardiovascular and kidney outcomes with finerenone in patients with type 2 diabetes and chronic kidney disease: the FIDELITY pooled analysis. Eur Heart J. 2022;43:474–84. https://doi.org/10.1093/eurheartj/ehab777.
31. American Diabetes Association Professional Practice Committee. 11. Chronic kidney disease and risk management: standards of care in diabetes—2025. Diabetes Care. 2025;48(Supplement_1):S239–51. https://doi.org/10.2337/dc25-S011.
32. McDowell K, Petrie MC, Raihan NA, Logue J. Effects of intentional weight loss in patients with obesity and heart failure: a systematic review. Obes Rev. 2018;19:1189–204. https://doi.org/10.1111/obr.12707.
33. Drucker DJ. Discovery of GLP-1-based drugs for the treatment of obesity. N Engl J Med. 2025;392(6):612–5. https://doi.org/10.1056/NEJMcibr2409089. Epub 2024 Sep 19. PMID: 39297560

34. D'Marco L, Morillo V, Gorriz JL, Suarez MK, Nava M, Ortega Á, Parra H, Villasmil N, Rojas-Quintero J, Bermúdez V. SGLT2i and GLP-1RA in cardiometabolic and renal diseases: from Glycemic control to adipose tissue inflammation and senescence. J Diabetes Res. 2021;2021:9032378. https://doi.org/10.1155/2021/9032378.
35. Bolinder J, Ljunggren Ö, Johansson L, et al. Dapagliflozin maintains glycaemic control while reducing weight and body fat mass over 2 years in patients with type 2 diabetes mellitus inadequately controlled on metformin. Diabetes Obes Metab. 2014;16:159–69.
36. Lloyd-Jones DM, Hong Y, Labarthe D, Mozaffarian D, Appel LJ, Van Horn L, Greenlund K, Daniels S, Nichol G, Tomaselli GF, et al. American Heart Association Strategic Planning Task Force and Statistics Committee. Defining and setting national goals for cardiovascular health promotion and disease reduction: the American Heart Association's strategic impact goal through 2020 and beyond. Circulation. 2010;121:586–613. https://doi.org/10.1161/CIRCULATIONAHA.109.192703.
37. Khan SS, Coresh J, Pencina MJ, Ndumele CE, Rangaswami J, Chow SL, Palaniappan LP, Sperling LS, Virani SS, Ho JE, Neeland IJ, Tuttle KR, Rajgopal Singh R, MSV E, Lloyd-Jones DM, on behalf of the American Heart Association. Novel prediction equations for absolute risk assessment of total cardiovascular disease incorporating cardiovascular kidney-metabolic health: a scientific statement from the American Heart Association. Circulation. 2023;148:1982–2004. https://doi.org/10.1161/CIR.0000000000001191.
38. Hampl SE, Hassink SG, Skinner AC, Armstrong SC, Barlow SE, Bolling CF, Avila Edwards KC, Eneli I, Hamre R, Joseph MM, et al. Clinical practice guideline for the evaluation and treatment of children and adolescents with obesity. Pediatrics. 2023;151 https://doi.org/10.1542/peds.2022-060640.
39. Shelton RC, Adsul P, Oh A. Recommendations for addressing structural racism in implementation science: a call to the field. Ethn Dis. 2021;31:357–64. https://doi.org/10.18865/ed.31.S1.357.

Chapter 11
Obesity as a Central Factor in Cardiovascular–Kidney–Metabolic Syndrome

Evelina Maria Gosav, Emilia Valasciuc, and Daniela Maria Tanase

Introduction

World Health Organization (WHO) reported that, over 390 million children and adolescents aged 5–19 years were overweight, while 160 million were reported obese a obesity. In adults, over 890 million (16%) of the world's population have obesity. The prevalence of overweight individuals varies by region and continent, ranging from 31% in Southeast Asia and Africa to 67% in North America. The worldwide prevalence of obesity doubled between 1990 and 2022. In 2024, the NCD Risk Factor Collaboration (NCD-RisC) and the World Obesity Federation's analysis updates show that up to 3 billion people live with overweight or obesity. Additionally, the Global Burden of Disease (GBD) Obesity Collaborators found an increase in the burden of elevated BMI, with high BMI accounting for 4.0 million deaths in 2015, more than two-thirds of which were caused by cardiovascular diseases (CVD), even after accounting for smoking and ill health [1, 2]. Metabolically healthy obesity (MHO) has a higher risk of CVD and, implicitly, chronic kidney disease (CKD) [3].

The WHO defines overweight as a body mass index (BMI) $\geq$25 kg/m^2 and obesity as a BMI $\geq$30 kg/m^2 (Table 11.1).

Obesity is a multifactorial disease that results from an imbalance between energy intake and energy expenditure. Other contributing factors include obesogenic environments, genetic and psychosocial influences, monogenic diseases or genetic syndromes, medications, coexisting conditions, and iatrogenic procedures. A deficient

E. M. Gosav (✉) · E. Valasciuc · D. M. Tanase
Grigore T. Popa University of Medicine and Pharmacy, Iasi, Romania

Saint Spiridon Emergency Hospital, Iasi, Romania
e-mail: evelina.maria.gosav@umfiasi.ro

M. Floria, D. M. Tanase (eds.), *Cardiovascular-Kidney-Metabolic Syndrome*,
https://doi.org/10.1007/978-3-032-11445-7_11

Table 11.1 WHO classification of overweight and obesity in adults

BMI 20 to <25 kg/m^2: Normal weight
BMI 25 to <30 kg/m^2: Overweight
BMI ≥30 kg/m^2: Obesity
BMI 30 to <35 kg/m^2: Obesity class 1
BMI 35 to <40 kg/m^2: Obesity class 2
BMI ≥40 kg/m^2: Obesity class 3 (severe obesity)

health system, coupled with a lack of access to healthy sustainable foods and the absence of food regulations, promotes unhealthy behaviors that worsen the progression of obesity. Notably, the global costs of being overweight and obese are expected to double in the next few years, and the rising incidence in low- and middle-income countries represents a health burden that cannot be ignored. The WHO and the World Health Assembly Global Nutrition Targets recognize these challenges and aim to halt the rise of diabetes and obesity by endorsing a global plan that is essential for sustainable change [1, 2].

Notably, over the years, a wide range of research has demonstrated the impact of BMI on noncommunicable diseases (NCDs) such as CVD, diabetes, metabolic syndrome, neoplasia, chronic respiratory issues, arthritis, neurological conditions, and digestive disorders. Recent reviews and relevant literature suggest that BMI is a valuable survey and primary healthcare screening tool that can guide nutritional and exercise counseling. However, there are limitations in assessing excess fat and predicting the risk of chronic disease. BMI cut-off values should be reconsidered across populations, considering age, ethnicity, and different body builds.

The intricate mechanism through which obesity promotes the development and progression of diseases involves shared pathways, with the central issue being the presence of metabolic syndrome (MetS) [4]. MetS is a cluster of interrelated risk factors, and its prevalence has risen alarmingly over the last decade, from 27.6% to 32.3%, showing a higher prevalence but lower risk in females compared to males. MetS is characterized by abdominal obesity, insulin resistance, hypertension, and hypertriglyceridemia. It is also associated with a high risk of CVD, the development of type 2 diabetes mellitus (T2DM), and vascular and neurological complications. Patients with diabetes are particularly vulnerable to CVD and renal disease, while individuals with established CVD may develop kidney disease due to vascular impairment. Chronic and acute kidney diseases are common comorbidities among these patients. Obesity and MetS play central roles in this triad, promoting disease onset, progression, and the occurrence of adverse events. Thus, in recent years, attention has shifted toward cardiovascular–kidney–metabolic (CKM) syndrome, a health disorder defined by the interconnectedness of heart disease, kidney disease, diabetes, and obesity, which can lead to poor health outcomes [5].

Adipose Tissue Features

Adipose tissue is one of the largest endocrine organs in the body. Mesenchymal stem cells differentiate into white, brown, and beige adipocytes, known as an intermediary phenotype. Each one has molecular features and specific functions. White adipose tissue is responsible for energy and triglyceride storage, while brown adipose tissue specializes in thermogenesis and oxidation. Brown-to-white adipocyte transdifferentiation is characterized by the downregulation of peroxisome proliferator-activated receptor-γ coactivator 1-α (a protein essential for many vital cellular events). Visceral fat owns certain properties, for example, the epicardial adipose tissue (EAT), which originally derives from brown tissue, exhibits neonatal thermogenic functions. After its transformation into adulthood as a beige phenotype, its function diversifies to cardiac energy storage purposes. Under normal conditions, this tissue regulates oxidative stress and inflammation via cardioprotective lipogenesis, fatty acid metabolism, and release of adipokines [6].

Obesity and Cardiovascular Disease

Obesity promotes CVD appearance and CVD mortality independently of other cardiovascular risk factors. The recent European Obesity–CVD Society of Cardiology consensus statement focuses on raising awareness of obesity as a major risk factor. It also provides guidance for implementing evidence-based practices for obesity prevention and optimal management within the context of primary and secondary cardiovascular disease prevention [7]. Abdominal obesity, determined by waist circumference (WC), is a marker of CVD risk independent of BMI. "Normal-weight obesity" patients with excess fat but not obesity, and with associated cardiometabolic disease, in many cases they are misclassified via BMI. Thus, experts suggest that all patients are evaluated with WC and BMI acquisition. Ectopic fat depots and all adipose tissue are correlated; attention is required to individual variations in visceral adipose tissue (VAT) and the quantity of subcutaneous adiposity. Due to easier access to imaging techniques such as computed tomography (CT) and magnetic resonance imaging (MRI), the study of the human body and its composition has identified visceral fat and its impact on organs. VAT and/or retroperitoneal fat (i.e., centrally located body fat) are reliable indicators of health risk, even in normal BMI subjects, suggesting an underlying dysmetabolic state. Often, VAT is accompanied by higher liver fat accumulation, diagnosed as nonalcoholic fatty liver disease (NAFLD), recently entitled metabolic fatty liver disease (MAFLD) [8].

Ectopic fat depots are of interest, as they have distinct anatomic locations depending on the presence of comorbidities. Pericardial and epicardial adipose tissue are often identified in metabolic patients, even on transthoracic echocardiography or in a CT scan. Epicardial adipose tissue is the visceral fat between the outer wall of the myocardium and the visceral layer of the pericardium. It originates from embryonic brown adipose tissue, which promotes vascular pro-inflammatory cell release and is highly associated with arterial stiffness in subjects with CVD and T2MD. Cardiac fat is associated with traditional CVD risk factors, raised BMI, and the presence of atherogenic lipoproteins. Additionally, epicardial adipose tissue thickness is insulin resistant and is highly associated with blood pressure, dyslipidemia, and even sleep apnea independently of BMI [8, 9]. In the Multi-Ethnic Study of Atherosclerosis (MESA), pericardial fat was correlated with a higher prevalence of cardiometabolic risk factors, adiposity-associated inflammation, and poorer CVD prognosis and left-ventricular (LV) remodeling, independent of insulin resistance, and CT measures of hepatic fat [10].

Over the years, scientific research has investigated the role of obesity and MetS in CVD and the underlying pathways and mechanisms involved. Diseases such as chronic or acute coronary syndromes, arterial hypertension, and cardiac arrhythmias are often accompanied and determined by dysmetabolic changes due to obesity, which may lead to CKM (Fig. 11.1).

- *Chronic and Acute Coronary Artery Disease*

In coronary artery disease (CAD) and atherosclerosis, central obesity is a main contributor to disease onset and progression. Many studies demonstrated that BMI in overweight and obese patients is linked with a higher risk of incident CAD. There are conflicting results in the literature on the association between obesity and CAD and its independence from metabolic cardiovascular risk factors (hypertension, diabetes, dyslipidemia/other comorbidities) [11]. Others showed that obesity without MetS is not linked with incident myocardial infarction [12].

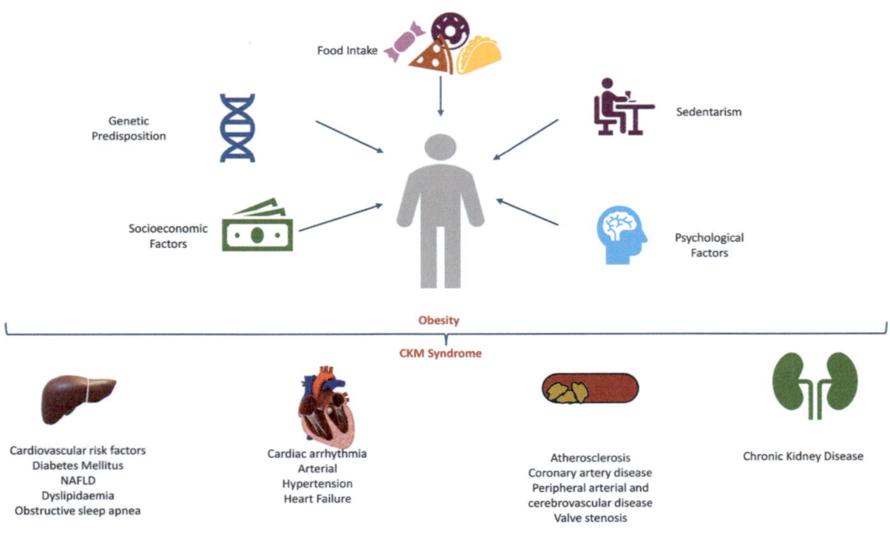

Fig. 11.1 Impact of obesity on cardiovascular and renal systems

Visceral obesity, including in the pericardial and epicardial spaces, participates in atherosclerotic and atherothrombotic processes through systemic and vascular inflammation, which promotes oxidative stress, low-density lipoprotein oxidation, and endothelial dysfunction. The continuous production of adipocytokines can modulate vessel biology via vasa vasorum and paracrine signaling, maintaining a prothrombotic state. Carotid intima-media thickness is a strong indicator of atherosclerosis in patients with obesity. Importantly, obesity impairs the structure and function of coronary microvasculature, as reflected in coronary flow reserve (CFR), hyperemic myocardial blood flow (MBF) impairment, and small-vessel remodeling, which is shown to be a precursor and long-term predictor of clinically relevant cardiovascular events [8, 13].

The presence of MetS is an additional risk factor for the development of CAD, major adverse cardiovascular events (MACE), and major cerebrovascular events (MCCE). Hosseini et al. [14] demonstrated in over 13,000 patients with acute coronary syndrome (ACS) after percutaneous coronary intervention (PCI) that MetS components (hypertension and impaired fasting glucose) were significantly associated with a higher incidence of *major adverse cardiac and cerebrovascular events* (MACCE).

- *Arterial Hypertension*

Research consistently noted the involvement of MetS and obesity in arterial hypertension, as well as their effects on arterial pressure fluctuations. There appears to be a positive correlation between age and the risk of hypertension in obese individuals, including children and adults, across both sexes. Obese women face a five-fold risk of incidence of hypertension, while a modest weight reduction can decrease blood pressure in these patients [15]. An evaluation encompassed by WC/waist-to-hip ratio (WHR) and blood pressure (BP) independent of BMI values is more reliable in predicting obesity-related cardiometabolic risk.

The putative mechanism between obesity and hypertension entails cumulative involvement between metabolic, neuroendocrine, and renal pathways. Adipose-derived cytokines (e.g., leptin) alteration, insulin resistance, structural renal debilitation, the stimulation of the renin–angiotensin–aldosterone system (RAAS), and the sympathetic nervous system (SNS) overactivation are the main contributors. When SNS overactivity occurs, the α-adrenergic and β-adrenergic receptors are directly and indirectly stimulated (through other systems like RAAS). Renal and muscle SNS activity is elevated in obese subjects; however, it is not uniformly distributed across all organs. Interestingly, chronic elevation of SNS in resting heart rate is believed to be mediated by reduced parasympathetic tone. Its overactivity appears to be influenced by factors such as visceral adiposity, sex, and ethnicity. Compared to lean patients, obese subjects have higher levels of plasma renin activity, angiotensin-converting enzyme, angiotensinogen, and aldosterone. The formation of angiotensin II through RAAS activation leads to systemic vasoconstriction and aldosterone production from the adrenal cortex, with subsequently raised kidney tubular sodium reabsorption, intravascular volume expansion, and arterial hypertension [16].

There is a bidirectional circuit between SNS and RAAS; one stimulates the other, with a secondary release of renin from the juxtaglomerular cells. This action lowers renal tubular blood flow and sodium delivery. Adipocytes themselves own intrinsic RAAS and can secrete mineralocorticoid-secreting factors that enhance aldosterone production from the adrenal gland. Mechanical renal compression due to water retention and the presence of perirenal fat leads to renal medulla compression and diminished renal tubular blood flow. Secondarily, lower sodium delivery triggers a feedback-mediated reduction in afferent arteriolar resistance, raised kidney blood flow, and renin release. These mechanisms increase blood pressure and elevate glomerular hydrostatic pressure, leading to progressive glomerular sclerosis and damaged renal function [16]. Weight loss and MetS risk factors management may prevent the onset of hypertension and renal impairment.

In addition, obesity and MetS are marked by leptin resistance, hyperleptinemia, insulin resistance, and hyperinsulinemia. As is known, leptin (adipose-derived cytokine) participates in energy homeostasis and can stimulate the central nervous system activity, and pressure effects on the cardiovascular system. Its full role in obesity-related hypertension is not elucidated; more research is needed. Insulin affects the sympathetic–excitatory system, with increased stimulation of SNS activity and paraventricular nucleus neurons. It promotes kidney sodium retention in the proximal convoluted tubule via sodium–hydrogen exchanger 3 (NHE3) activation. Additionally, insulin is a vasodilator; however, in obese patients, this response is affected due to endothelial dysfunction, which leads to an increased vasoconstrictor tone state [16, 17].

- *Cardiac Arrhythmias*

Growing evidence points out that patients with similar BMI have different CVD risk profiles. Obesity and MetS are independently associated with the risk of cardiac arrhythmias such as atrial fibrillation (AF). The ongoing Framingham Heart Study noted that obesity raises the risk of developing new-onset AF by 50%, and other CVDs that can contribute individually to the development of AF. The pathogenesis of AF-obesity is complex and multifactorial. It involves increased left-atrial, left-ventricular, and arterial pressure with secondary diastolic dysfunction and left-ventricular workload, myocyte hypertrophy, and chamber dilatation. Cardiac fibrosis is more often seen in hypertensive–obese patients. Studies show that EAT is independently and strongly associated with AF, owning a particular role in AF pathogenesis through paracrine signaling [6, 18].

AF is characterized by a pro-inflammatory pattern that involves the upregulation of cytokines, adipokines (including chemerin and resistin, which are linked to atrial remodeling), interleukins (except interleukin-1β), C-reactive protein (CRP), and tumor necrosis factor (TNF-α). These cytokines enhance collagen deposition, oxidative stress, and abnormal calcium modulation, promoting tissue damage, fibrosis, and impaired electrophysiology of the atria. Inflammation and oxidative stress, as noted, are significant contributors to AF. Interestingly, when a subject loses weight, the number of infiltrating macrophages and inflammatory factors decreases [19]. Medications with anti-inflammatory effects, such as statins, angiotensin-converting enzyme inhibitors, angiotensin II receptor blockers, and even antiarrhythmic drugs (e.g., amiodarone), can reduce the prevalence of AF. TNF-α activates myofibroblasts through the transforming growth factor (TGF)-β signaling pathway and increases the expression of matrix metalloproteinase-2 and matrix metalloproteinase-9 (MMP9), which promotes myocardial remodeling. Furthermore, TNF-α increases the intracellular Ca^{2+} concentration during diastole and lowers the Ca^{2+} content in the sarcoplasmic reticulum, leading to ectopic triggering activity and causing AF. Similar fibrotic and remodeling effects but via activating the pSTAT3/STAT3 signaling pathway are engaged by interleukin-6 (IL-6). Il-6 prolongs the expression of α-smooth muscle actin (α-SMA), type I collagen, and type III collagen by inhibiting Tregs function. Additionally, it directly damages the production of connexin (e.g., connexin 40 and connexin 43) in myocardial cells, thereby inducing atrial electrical remodeling and risk of AF [20].

Oxidative stress is seen as an early event in obesity and CVD. Interestingly, for every 10% increase in redox glutathione, the odds of developing AF increased by 30%. Oxidative stress promotes atrial fibrillation (AF) via reactive oxygen species (ROS) that enhance late sodium currents and early depolarization, and by affecting L-type calcium channels and the ryanodine receptor 2 (RyR2). ROS endorses atrial fibroblast proliferation and expression of pro-fibrotic factors like MMP9, p38, and c-Jun. Influenced by angiotensin II and dependent on reduced nicotinamide adenine dinucleotide phosphate (NADPH) oxidase and ROS production, oxidative stress is a major contributor to CVD development and progression [8, 18].

Atrial electrical remodeling is caused by increased outward potassium (K^+) current, leading to accelerated repolarization and hyperpolarization of atrial cells, and ultimately conduction abnormalities. Conduction delay and local conduction block by localized fibrosis of the atrium underlie the formation of reentrant arrhythmias [18]. In AF pathogenesis, adipose tissue, specifically EAT, contributes through neurohormonal changes mediated by numerous ganglionic plexi (GP). GP plays both vagal and sympathetic roles, which are essential for contractility. Hyperactivity of the GP and increased atrial sympathetic responses drive amplification of calcium transients and autonomic dysfunction, resulting in increased effective refractory period heterogeneity and arrhythmogenesis. Obesity maintains an imbalance in the autonomic nervous system, induced by hyperleptinemia, insulin resistance, and hypoxemia. Myocardial remodeling is driven by EAT sympathetic hyperactivity, combined with the release of pro-inflammatory cells, which subsequently activates the obesity-mediated RAAS. Moreover, angiotensin II enhances fibrosis by suppressing metalloproteinase-1 expression and inducing collagen type 1 synthesis in cardiac fibroblasts. Pro-fibrotic EAT cytokines/chemokines such as YKL-70 and cTGF are linked with total collagen content. EAT promotes an imbalance in Ca^{2+} hemostasis that influences electrical changes in the atrium, while fibroblasts also affect the electrical activity of cardiomyocytes via paracrine-bioactive substances. These intricate mechanisms are observed in autopsy studies that support the concept that "AF begets AF." Overall, central obesity and local obesity are major contributors to the development of cardiac arrhythmia, with higher risk when components of MetS are added (Fig. 11.1) [11, 18, 21].

Patients with prediabetes and diabetes have a 20% higher risk of developing atrial fibrillation (AF). For every 20 mg/dL increase in blood glucose, there is an 11% added risk. Obesity is a major contributor to diabetes, while diabetes-induced atrial fibrosis has increased the incidence of AF. In addition to the previously discussed mechanism, hyperglycemia introduces other complex mechanisms that lead to further structural and electrophysiological changes in the heart. Through the receptor for advanced glycation end products (AGE) pathway and oxidative stress, hyperglycemia facilitates the accumulation of AGEs, which transmit fibrotic signals.

All evidence shows that obesity and MetS are major participants in vascular and cellular changes via complex mechanisms and pathways, raising the risk of CVD and cardiac atrial and ventricular arrhythmia. A healthier lifestyle and loss of weight reduce this risk and slow disease progression. Each overweight or obese patient should be examined and searched for all metabolic risk factors to prevent disease onset (Fig. 11.2).

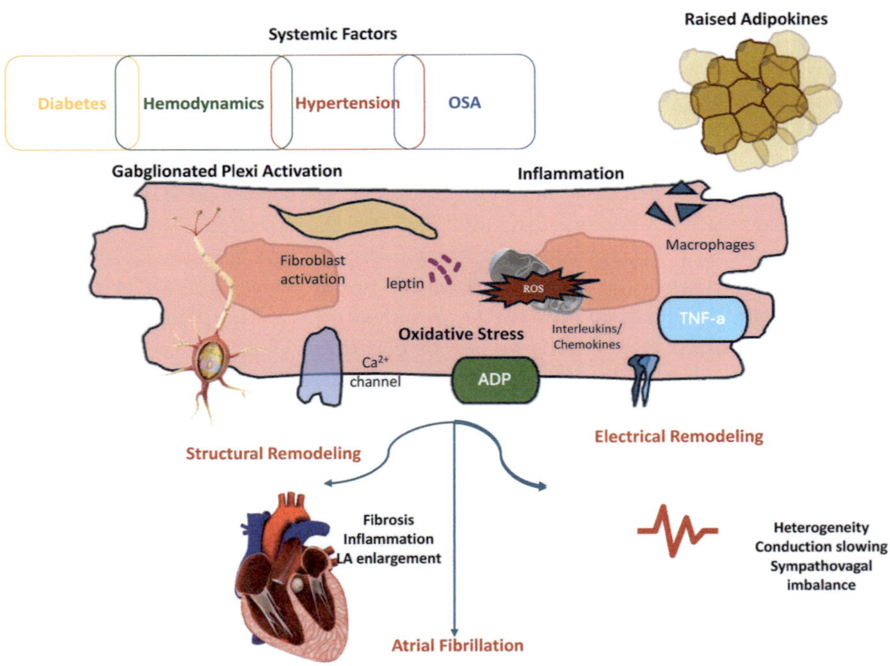

Fig. 11.2 Arrhythmogenic effects of obesity and left atrial (LA) epicardial adipose tissue (EAT) on myocardial structure and function

Obesity and Renal Disease

The first studies that investigated the relationship between kidney disease and obesity emerged almost a century ago [22]. Since then, substantial research has shown that being overweight, obese, or having metabolic syndrome (MetS) is a strong independent risk factor for chronic kidney disease (CKD) and end-stage renal disease (ESRD). The incidence of obesity-related kidney disease increases each year. Analysis using genetic methods reveals that for every 0.06 increase in waist-to-hip ratio, the risk for CKD rises by nearly 30%, and for every 5 kg/m^2 increase in BMI, the risk of CKD increases by 50%. BMI is associated with obesity-related kidney injury; however, it depends on body composition distribution. Individuals with excess visceral adipose tissue (VAT) are linked to higher insulin resistance and an increased risk of CKD compared to those with subcutaneous adipose tissue (SAT). Waist circumference and waist-to-hip ratio serve as better indicators of mortality and cardiometabolic risk than BMI [23].

There are numerous predisposing factors for obesity and hypertension, including low birth weight, preterm delivery, low nephron count, and intrauterine growth restriction. In cases of reduced nephron numbers, patients have a higher likelihood of developing hyperfiltering nephropathies. Additionally, individuals with unilateral nephrectomy and higher BMI are more susceptible to proteinuria and kidney dysfunction. Genetic determinants characterize obesity nephropathy; therefore, early evaluation through metabolomics tools may aid in preventing disease onset and progression [24].

The pathophysiology of CKD, obesity, and MetS is complex and characterized by lipotoxicity, insulin resistance, adipocytokine dysregulation, increased blood pressure, and enhanced glomerular blood pressure (Fig. 11.3). However, it is difficult to determine whether the effect of obesity on CKD is independent of these metabolic factors. Interestingly, MHO, a dynamic condition that changes over time, is generally associated with incident CKD, but these associations must be interpreted with care [3].

- *Inflammation and RAAS in Obesity-Related CKD*

Adipose cells are a significant source of inflammation, particularly visceral adipose tissue, which is a primary source of cytokine release. Individuals with obesity exhibit low-grade inflammatory responses, accompanied by macrophage infiltration that depends on fat localization and distribution. There are two types of macrophages involved: M1 with pro-inflammatory effects and M2 with anti-inflammatory effects. Macrophage infiltration is associated with the injury and apoptosis of adipocytes due to hypoxia—induced by obesity and vascular thinning. Obesity promotes the conversion of M2 to the M1 phenotype, which further enhances inflammatory cell expression and ROS production. Supplementary, miRNAs own key roles in macrophage polarization; however, more studies are needed to elucidate their full function [23].

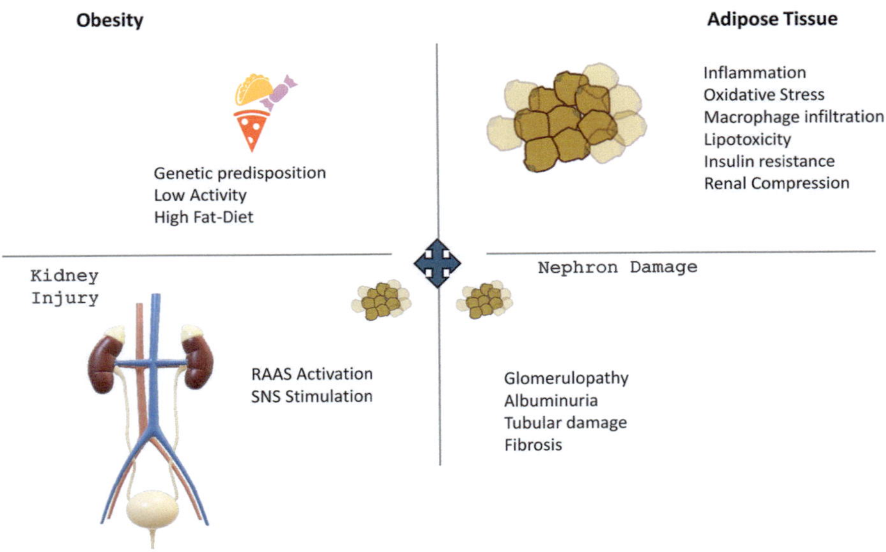

Fig. 11.3 Role of obesity in chronic kidney disease

Persistent inflammation is a known pattern of CKD. Leptin, adiponectin, monocyte chemoattractant protein-1, TNF-α, transforming growth factor, and ANG II play significant roles. The NF-κB pathway, activation of the mitogen-activated protein kinase cascade, and the JAK-STAT signaling pathway are also implicated in renal injury. MCP-I is associated with fat accumulation, driven by elevated levels of TNF-α. Interestingly, TNF-α deficiency protects the renal system from albuminuria in obesity [25]. Recently, the pathogenic effects of nucleotide-binding oligomerized structural domain-like receptor protein 3 (NLRP3) inflammasome have been demonstrated in obesity-associated nephropathy. NLRP3 activation operates through the caspase-1-IL-1β/IL-18 axis and may result from hyperfiltration induced by the RAAS system, activation of ER, and mitochondrial impairment. These cytokines promote podocyte damage, with inflammasome signaling contributing to the onset of obesity-associated nephropathy as early as the glomerular hyperfiltration stage [23].

As previously mentioned, obesity is associated with raised RASS activity. Obese individuals have higher levels of angiotensinogen, ACE, renin, and aldosterone, which alter natriuresis, with secondary increased renal tubular salt reabsorption, volume expansion, and hypertension. Aldosterone further enhances ANG II effects, resulting in renal vascular inflammation, fibrosis, podocyte impairment, and proliferation of thylakoid cells. Utilization of MR antagonists can delay CKD progression also in nondiabetic patients [26, 27].

- *Lipotoxicity and Insulin Resistance in Obesity-Related CKD*

Almost 30 years ago, Moorhead et al. [28] described the role of lipid toxicity in CKD pathogenesis. A normal kidney contains approximately 3% lipids. The adipose tissue accumulated around the kidneys determines local pressure and hemodynamic effects. On the other hand, the local visceral adipose tissue regulates kidney metabolism through secretory agents. Altered lipid metabolism and dyslipidemia (hypercholesterolemia and/or hypertriglyceridemia) influence the pathogenesis and progression of CKD. Elevated TG and reduced HDL levels seem to be independent of the onset of CKD. Nevertheless, there are conflicting results in the literature regarding serum lipids and the development of CKD, mainly attributed to differences in the ethnicities of the groups studied [24].

The perirenal fat via adipokine secretion exerts pro-inflammatory effects, stimulates RAAS, and increases the endocrine and paracrine roles in lipid and glucose homeostasis. Many recent studies suggest that perirenal fat thickness may predict CFR reduction and incidence of proteinuria in obese patients [29]. There are many aspects of how perirenal fat induces kidney injury that remain to be elucidated. Perirenal fat deposition determines raised interstitial hydrostatic pressure, renin release, sodium tubular reabsorption, and kidney disease progression. A recent meta-analysis and systematic review that included 2576 patients demonstrated the association of perirenal fat thickness and its relation with CKD and highlighted the importance of its diagnosis when treating CKD patients [30].

Insulin resistance is also a key to obesity, overnutrition, and MetS by activating SNS and RAAS, oxidative stress, and adipokines. The hypersecretion of adipocytokines generates a cellular imbalance. TNF-α inhibits insulin activity by inducing phosphorylation of insulin receptor substrate-1 (IRS-1). With time and CKD progression, adipocyte atrophy starts kipolysis and release of free fatty acids (FFA), which can accumulate as intrahepatic lipids and skeletal muscle intracellular (intramyocellular lipid) and promote insulin resistance. Studies performed on patients with early-stage CKD showed that the connection between insulin resistance and renal function is influenced by BMI. Homeostatic model assessment for insulin resistance (HOMA-IR), a viable tool in assessing insulin resistance in CKD patients, correlated with inflammatory markers, CKD progression, and albuminuria. The negative effects of insulin resistance are seen in mesangial cells, podocytes, and tubular epithelial cells. Involved in diabetes and MAFLD, insulin resistance, along with gut microbiota, is a key component and driver of CVD and kidney disease development [31, 32].

- *Leptin, Adiponectin, and Insulin Resistance in Obesity-Related CKD*

Leptin is an adipocyte-derived hormone produced primarily in white adipose tissue and mostly eliminated by the kidneys. Leptin enhances oxidative stress and endothelial dysfunction, and promotes platelet aggregation. Obese patients and those with CKD have higher leptin expression compared to individuals with normal weight. The amount of leptin in the blood is proportional to the fat content, with obese subjects being characterized by "leptin resistance." The central nervous system acts on the leptin receptor (LepR), stimulating its effects as an activator of Janus kinase 2 (JAK2). Leptin levels can also stimulate the cardiovascular sympathetic nerve activity and the renal sympathetic nerve activity. Interestingly, raised plasma leptin can determine activation of RAAS via increased renal sympathetic nerve activity and subsequently hemodynamic changes. As leptin levels continue to increase, due to elevated TGF-β expression in glomerular cells and activation of the JAK/STAT signaling pathway, the renal filtration rate declines, accompanied by the development of glomerulosclerosis and profibrotic effects on mesangial cells [24].

Adiponectin is an amino acid protein expressed in myocytes, hepatic parenchymal cells, and epithelial cells. It has three structural forms and acts like a polypotent hormone, with both anti-inflammatory (via promoting the conversion to the M2 phenotype) and pro-inflammatory effects, and antifibrotic and cardioprotective effects. Patients with MetS, obesity, T2DM, and hyperlipidemia have lower levels of adiponectin. This reduction in adiponectin can be attributed to the suppression of adiponectin transcription due to the obesity's persistent chronic inflammatory state. Its function is generated by interacting with adiponectin receptors such as adiponectin receptor 1 (AdipoR1), adiponectin receptor 2 (AdipoR2), and T-cadherin (T-cadherin). AdipoR1 and AdipoR2 are expressed in the liver and skeletal muscle and participate in the regulation of metabolic processes. Adiponectin is also expressed in the renal artery endothelium, capillary endothelium, and renal smooth muscle cells. Obesity is an independent risk factor for CKD; adiponectin levels are raised in patients with severe renal dysfunction estimated glomerular filtration rate (eGFR) <15 mL/min/1.73 m^2. Moreover, stages 3 and 4 of CKD were associated with increased adiponectin and increased risk of mortality. Leptin and adiponectin, together with TNF-α and IL-6, increase urinary albumin excretion and further damage the vascular endothelium and alter the renal hemodynamics [24, 33].

- *Hemodynamic Changes in Obesity-Related CKD*

GFR is determined by renal plasma flow (RPF), the hydraulic pressure gradient across the kidney membrane, and ultrafiltration coefficient, which normally ranges from 90 to 120 mL/min/1.73 m^2 [27]. A high majority of obese patients develop hypertension, the main precursor for other CVD and renal disease. Hypoxia and increased metabolic demand characterize early obesity. Thus, increased renal plasma flow and increased renal glomerular filtration rate stimulate the glomerular–tubular balance, causing increased sodium–water reabsorption by the proximal tubules, which subsequently raises blood pressure. Moreover, natriuretic peptides, which have higher concentrations in obese subjects, cause a decrease in plasma natriuretic peptide concentration, which weakens the inhibitory effect on the RAAS and increases sodium and water retention [34]. The main mechanism of hypertension developing in obesity is RAAS activation. In unhealthy metabolically obese subjects, the afferent tone is changed to an efferent arteriolar tone. Salt-sensitive hypertension was reported to relate to glomerular hyperfiltration, neurohumoral mechanisms, and metabolic changes determined by long-term overweight and obesity. Activation of RAAS, as seen, promotes fibrogenic factor production and matrix renal deposition. Obesity raises glomerular capillary blood pressure and expansion of the basement membrane, which determines deformation and detachment of the podocytes, and renal damage. Thus, studies across time showed the indubitable beneficial impact of weight loss on renal function and on CVD [34].

- *Histopathology in Obesity-Related CKD*

In obesity-related nephropathy, generally, histopathologic changes are represented by the hypodensity of podocytes, glomerulomegaly with mesangial proliferation, matrix buildup, and decreased density of more focally effaced, hypertrophied podocytes with milder foot process fusion, and finally glomerulomegaly, and focal segmental glomerulosclerosis (FSGS) [34]. A unique feature of obesity-related nephropathy is the slight disappearance of the foot processes. Compared with 75% in primary FSGS, the mean rate of foot process loss in obesity was 40% [35]. Along with other renal cellular changes in obesity, of importance is the development of focal lipid vacuoles in the mesangial cells and tubular epithelial cells' cytoplasms due to excessive lipid accumulation. All modifications are histopathologically relevant for disease diagnosis and proper treatment Table 11.2.

In experimental studies, glomerular cluster volume increases exponentially with body weight, which causes decreased density and number of podocytes, increased width of the peduncle, and mild and segmental loss of the peduncle. As podocytes are unable to proliferate, their detachment is stimulated by the glomerular volume expanding, mechanical strain due to tensile tension, and shear stress reaching a breaking point. These mechanisms play a crucial role in proteinuria and obesity-related nephropathy. Interestingly, compared with primary FSGS, obesity-FSGS is adaptative, the proliferation of podocyte stress zones enhances the expansion of segmental lesions with, finally, total glomerular fibrosis [36].

Table 11.2 Pathological/histopathological changes in obesity-related nephropathy

Kidney injury	Pathological renal damage
Glomerural injury	Low glomerular density Podocyte injury Glomerulosclerosis Mesangial expansion Glomerulomegaly Global or focal segmental Glomerulosclerosis
Kidney tubules injury	Proximal tubular epithelial Hypertrophy Tubular cell apoptosis Tubulointerstitial fibrosis Tubular atrophy

It is important to point out that, although typically found in obesity, these changes in glomerulomegaly with FSGS are not CKD-specific; thus, diseases related to obesity such as diabetic glomerulosclerosis or hypertensive nephrosclerosis should be excluded. These findings only suggest that kidney biopsy, although invasive, may be a significant tool in the correct treatment of patients with severe obesity and renal disease.

Obesity and Cardiovascular–Kidney–Metabolic Syndrome

Concerning, the pathologies interested, the American Heart Association (AHA) collectedly named in 2023 the correlation between obesity, T2DM, CVD, and CKD into cardiovascular–kidney–metabolic (CKM). The molecular intricate pathways are interconnected via a common mechanism involving persistent obesity-chronic inflammation, hyperglycemia, insulin resistance, the heightened activity of the RAAS, the generation of advanced glycation end-products, oxidative stress, lipotoxicity, ER stress, abnormalities in calcium handling, malfunctioning of mitochondria, and impaired energy production (Fig. 11.4) [37]. Taken separately, as seen, each disease is marked by obesity, depending on the grade of fat deposition and localization. The impairment in CKM, however, is more complex and is fundamentally characterized by changes that are dependent on each disease's severity.

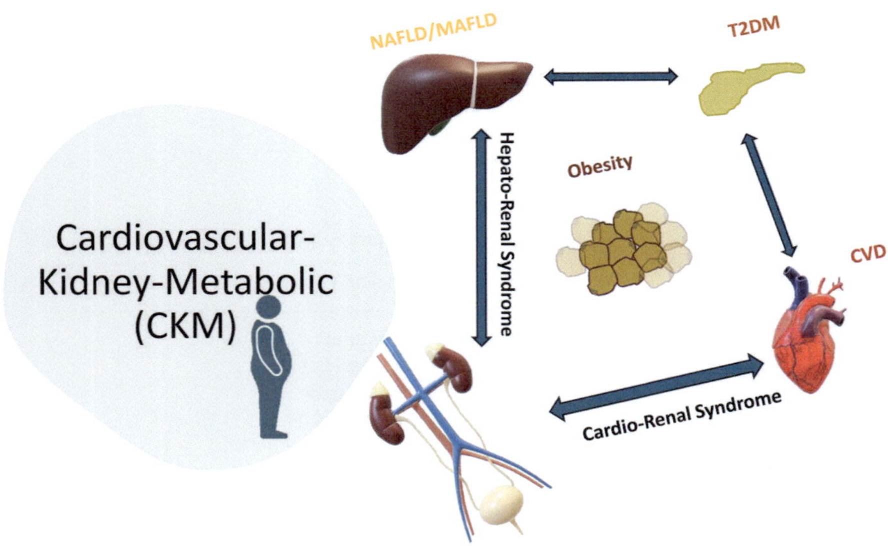

Fig. 11.4 The intricate relationship in CKM syndrome

Even if liver impairment and MAFLD are known metabolic diseases associated with CVD or CKD, CKM seems to omit the hepatic involvement. Therefore, recent field specialists recommend an expanded framework of the cardiovascular–renal–hepatic–metabolic (CRHM) syndrome to more comprehensively capture the broader interorgan dynamics [38]. Interestingly, the bidirectional pathophysiological mechanism involved in CKM is also influenced by the lymphatic vascular system. Fowler et al. [39] described the role of lymphatics in CKM obesity. Humans with morbid obesity often display altered but reversible weight loss, lymphatic function, and lymphedema. Their study highlights that improvement in the lymphatic vascular network could represent a novel therapeutic avenue in CKM, obesity, and/or their comorbidities.

The "butterfly effect," as some researchers state, in chronic cardiovascular and kidney disorders, describes a phenomenon in which acute injuries in one organ lead to dysfunction in the other. Although this chapter focuses on chronic disease, acute kidney injury, and acute heart disease are two major risks of CKM, which are aggravated in obese subjects [40].

Considering the wide spectrum of pathophysiological changes in CKM, various pharmacological and non-pharmacological approaches alongside weight loss, led by an interdisciplinary coordinated team, should help with primary and secondary care in these patients.

As the burden of obesity and CKM continues to increase, the interdisciplinary team may improve the patient's experience, optimize resources, and lead to efficiencies and cost savings. Implementation of innovative and integrated care delivery models and new CKM syndrome guidelines will be essential for disease management and may improve patients' quality of life [40].

Learning Objectives

- Obesity is a central contributor to metabolic syndrome and cardiovascular kidney metabolic syndrome.
- The multifactorial pathways of obesity involve pro-inflammatory cell release by adipokines, oxidative stress, immune system activation, insulin resistance, lipotoxicity, and enhanced RAAS activity.
- Patients with overweight and obesity, especially those with visceral adipose tissue surplus, are prone to develop earlier cardiovascular or renal disease and associated complications.
- Targeting obesity via weight loss is an imperative management strategy that has demonstrated beneficial effects in CKM syndrome.

Key Reading

- Cardiovascular–kidney–metabolic syndrome encompasses a gamut of pathophysiological changes driven by common pathways that ultimately lead to cardiac and renal impairment.
- Obesity with increased prevalence and incidence continues to raise global health issues, promoting the development of metabolic syndrome even in the younger population.
- A deficient health system, coupled with a lack of access to healthy sustainable foods and the absence of food regulations, promotes unhealthy behaviors that worsen the progression of obesity.
- Metabolic syndrome is characterized by abdominal obesity, insulin resistance, hypertension, and hypertriglyceridemia, which increases the risk of diabetes, renal dysfunction, and cardiovascular diseases.
- For a comprehensive evaluation of obesity risk, it is recommended to evaluate BMI, waist circumference (WC), and ectopic VAT.
- Management of obesity can alleviate CKM and its related complications.

References

1. Worldwide trends in underweight and obesity from 1990 to 2022: a pooled analysis of 3663 population-representative studies with 222 million children, adolescents, and adults. Lancet. 2024;403(10431):1027–50. Epub 20240229. https://doi.org/10.1016/s0140-6736(23)02750-2. PubMed PMID: 38432237; PubMed Central PMCID: PMC7615769.
2. Global burden and strength of evidence for 88 risk factors in 204 countries and 811 subnational locations, 1990–2021: a systematic analysis for the Global Burden of Disease Study 2021. Lancet. 2024;403(10440):2162–203. https://doi.org/10.1016/s0140-6736(24)00933-4. PubMed PMID: 38762324; PubMed Central PMCID: PMC11120204.
3. Cho YK, Lee J, Kim HS, Park J-Y, Lee WJ, Kim Y-J, et al. Impact of transition in metabolic health and obesity on the incident chronic kidney disease: a nationwide cohort study. J Clin Endocrinol Metab. 2020;105(3):e148–e57. https://doi.org/10.1210/clinem/dgaa033.
4. Wu Y, Li D, Vermund SH. Advantages and limitations of the body mass index (BMI) to assess adult obesity. Int J Environ Res Public Health. 2024;21(6) Epub 20240610. https://doi.org/10.3390/ijerph21060757. PubMed PMID: 38929003; PubMed Central PMCID: PMC11204233.
5. Di Pietro P, Izzo C, Carrizzo A. Editorial: the role of metabolic syndrome and disorders in cardiovascular disease. Front Endocrinol. 2023;14:1327394. https://doi.org/10.3389/fendo.2023.1327394.
6. Sha R, Baines O, Hayes A, Tompkins K, Kalla M, Holmes AP, et al. Impact of obesity on atrial fibrillation pathogenesis and treatment options. J Am Heart Assoc. 2024;13(1):e032277. https://doi.org/10.1161/JAHA.123.032277.
7. Koskinas KC, Van Craenenbroeck EM, Antoniades C, Blüher M, Gorter TM, Hanssen H, et al. Obesity and cardiovascular disease: an ESC clinical consensus statement. Eur Heart J. 2024;45(38):4063–98. https://doi.org/10.1093/eurheartj/ehae508.

8. Powell-Wiley TM, Poirier P, Burke LE, Després J-P, Gordon-Larsen P, Lavie CJ, et al. Obesity and cardiovascular disease: a scientific statement from the American Heart Association. Circulation. 2021;143(21):e984–1010. https://doi.org/10.1161/CIR.0000000000000973.
9. Al-Talabany S, Mordi I, Graeme Houston J, Colhoun HM, Weir-McCall JR, Matthew SZ, et al. Epicardial adipose tissue is related to arterial stiffness and inflammation in patients with cardiovascular disease and type 2 diabetes. BMC Cardiovasc Disord. 2018;18(1):31. Epub 20180213. https://doi.org/10.1186/s12872-018-0770-z. PubMed PMID: 29433433; PubMed Central PMCID: PMC5809843.
10. Shah RV, Anderson A, Ding J, Budoff M, Rider O, Petersen SE, et al. Pericardial, but not hepatic, fat by CT is associated with CV outcomes and structure: the multi-ethnic study of atherosclerosis. JACC Cardiovasc Imaging. 2017;10(9):1016–27. Epub 20170315. https://doi.org/10.1016/j.jcmg.2016.10.024. PubMed PMID: 28330662; PubMed Central PMCID: PMC5591038.
11. Ndumele CE, Matsushita K, Lazo M, Bello N, Blumenthal RS, Gerstenblith G, et al. Obesity and subtypes of incident cardiovascular disease. J Am Heart Assoc. 2016;5(8) Epub 20160728. https://doi.org/10.1161/jaha.116.003921. PubMed PMID: 27468925; PubMed Central PMCID: PMC5015307.
12. Mørkedal B, Vatten LJ, Romundstad PR, Laugsand LE, Janszky I. Risk of myocardial infarction and heart failure among metabolically healthy but obese individuals: HUNT (Nord-Trøndelag Health Study), Norway. J Am Coll Cardiol. 2014;63(11):1071–8. Epub 20131215. https://doi.org/10.1016/j.jacc.2013.11.035. PubMed PMID: 24345592.
13. Spezia M, Bonato A, De Fortunato G, Bossi A, Glauber M. The role of obesity and adipokines in coronary microvascular dysfunction: a systematic review and meta-analysis. Eur Heart J Cardiovasc Imaging. 2021;22(Supplement_1):jeaa356–83. https://doi.org/10.1093/ehjci/jeaa356.383.
14. Hosseini K, Khalaji A, Behnoush AH, Soleimani H, Mehrban S, Amirsardari Z, et al. The association between metabolic syndrome and major adverse cardiac and cerebrovascular events in patients with acute coronary syndrome undergoing percutaneous coronary intervention. Sci Rep. 2024;14(1):697. https://doi.org/10.1038/s41598-024-51157-w.
15. Faulkner JL, Belin de Chantemèle EJ. Sex differences in mechanisms of hypertension associated with obesity. Hypertension. 2018;71(1):15–21. Epub 20171113. https://doi.org/10.1161/hypertensionaha.117.09980. PubMed PMID: 29133358; PubMed Central PMCID: PMC5730468.
16. Shariq OA, McKenzie TJ. Obesity-related hypertension: a review of pathophysiology, management, and the role of metabolic surgery. Gland Surg. 2020;9(1):80–93. https://doi.org/10.21037/gs.2019.12.03. PubMed PMID: 32206601; PubMed Central PMCID: PMC7082272.
17. Quesada O, Claggett B, Rodriguez F, Cai J, Moncrieft AE, Garcia K, et al. Associations of insulin resistance with systolic and diastolic blood pressure: a study from the HCHS/SOL. Hypertension. 2021;78(3):716–25. https://doi.org/10.1161/HYPERTENSIONAHA.120.16905.
18. Shu H, Cheng J, Li N, Zhang Z, Nie J, Peng Y, et al. Obesity and atrial fibrillation: a narrative review from arrhythmogenic mechanisms to clinical significance. Cardiovasc Diabetol. 2023;22(1):192. Epub 20230729. https://doi.org/10.1186/s12933-023-01913-5. PubMed PMID: 37516824; PubMed Central PMCID: PMC10387211.
19. Weisberg SP, McCann D, Desai M, Rosenbaum M, Leibel RL, Ferrante AW Jr. Obesity is associated with macrophage accumulation in adipose tissue. J Clin Invest. 2003;112(12):1796–808. https://doi.org/10.1172/jci19246. PubMed PMID: 14679176; PubMed Central PMCID: PMC296995.
20. Lazzerini PE, Laghi-Pasini F, Acampa M, Srivastava U, Bertolozzi I, Giabbani B, et al. Systemic inflammation rapidly induces reversible atrial electrical remodeling: the role of Interleukin-6-mediated changes in Connexin expression. J Am Heart Assoc. 2019;8(16):e011006. Epub 20190819. https://doi.org/10.1161/jaha.118.011006. PubMed PMID: 31423933; PubMed Central PMCID: PMC6759884.

21. Lee SY, Lee SR, Choi EK, Kwon S, Yang S, Park J, et al. Association between change in metabolic syndrome status and risk of incident atrial fibrillation: a nationwide population-based study. J Am Heart Assoc. 2021;10(16):e020901. https://doi.org/10.1161/JAHA.121.020901.
22. Preble WE. Obesity: observations on one thousand cases. Boston Med Surg J. 1923;188(17):617–21. https://doi.org/10.1056/NEJM192304261881701.
23. Hao M, Lv Y, Liu S, Guo W. The new challenge of obesity - obesity-associated nephropathy. Diabetes Metab Syndr Obes. 2024;17:1957–71. Epub 20240506. https://doi.org/10.2147/dmso.S433649. PubMed PMID: 38737387; PubMed Central PMCID: PMC11086398.
24. Jiang Z, Wang Y, Zhao X, Cui H, Han M, Ren X, et al. Obesity and chronic kidney disease. Am J Physiol Endocrinol Metab. 2023;324(1):E24–41. https://doi.org/10.1152/ajpendo.00179.2022. PubMed PMID: 36383637.
25. Wang H, Li J, Gai Z, Kullak-Ublick Gerd A, Liu Z. TNF-α deficiency prevents renal inflammation and oxidative stress in obese mice. Kidney Blood Press Res. 2017;42(3):416–27. https://doi.org/10.1159/000478869.
26. Verma A, Vaidya A, Subudhi S, Waikar SS. Aldosterone in chronic kidney disease and renal outcomes. Eur Heart J. 2022;43(38):3781–91. https://doi.org/10.1093/eurheartj/ehac352.
27. Stevens PE, Ahmed SB, Carrero JJ, Foster B, Francis A, Hall RK, et al. KDIGO 2024 clinical practice guideline for the evaluation and management of chronic kidney disease. Kidney Int. 2024;105(4):S117–314. https://doi.org/10.1016/j.kint.2023.10.018.
28. Moorhead JF, El-Nahas M, Chan MK, Varghese Z. Lipid nephrotoxicity in chronic progressive glomerular and tubulo-interstitial disease. Lancet. 1982;320(8311):1309–11. https://doi.org/10.1016/S0140-6736(82)91513-6.
29. Foster MC, Hwang S-J, Porter SA, Massaro JM, Hoffmann U, Fox CS. Fatty kidney, hypertension, and chronic kidney disease. Hypertension. 2011;58(5):784–90. https://doi.org/10.1161/HYPERTENSIONAHA.111.175315.
30. Kang P, Sun B, Hao J, Wang C, Chen X. Perirenal fat and chronic kidney disease: a systematic review and meta-analysis. Kidney Blood Press Res. 2025;50(1):240–8. https://doi.org/10.1159/000543989.
31. Nakashima A, Kato K, Ohkido I, Yokoo T. Role and treatment of insulin resistance in patients with chronic kidney disease: a review. Nutrients. 2021;13(12):4349. PubMed PMID. https://doi.org/10.3390/nu13124349.
32. Zaky A, Glastras SJ, Wong MYW, Pollock CA, Saad S. The role of the gut microbiome in diabetes and obesity-related kidney disease. Int J Mol Sci. 2021;22(17):9641. PubMed PMID. https://doi.org/10.3390/ijms22179641.
33. Beberashvili I, Cohen-Cesla T, Khatib A, Hamad RA, Azar A, Stav K, et al. Comorbidity burden may explain adiponectin's paradox as a marker of increased mortality risk in hemodialysis patients. Sci Rep. 2021;11(1):9087. https://doi.org/10.1038/s41598-021-88558-0.
34. Jiang Z, Wang Y, Zhao X, Cui H, Han M, Ren X, et al. Obesity and chronic kidney disease. Am J Physiol Endocrinol Metab. 2023;324(1):E24–e41. Epub 20221116. https://doi.org/10.1152/ajpendo.00179.2022. PubMed PMID: 36383637.
35. Kambham N, Markowitz GS, Valeri AM, Lin J, D'Agati VD. Obesity-related glomerulopathy: an emerging epidemic. Kidney Int. 2001;59(4):1498–509. https://doi.org/10.1046/j.1523-1755.2001.0590041498.x.
36. De Vriese AS, Wetzels JF, Glassock RJ, Sethi S, Fervenza FC. Therapeutic trials in adult FSGS: lessons learned and the road forward. Nat Rev Nephrol. 2021;17(9):619–30. https://doi.org/10.1038/s41581-021-00427-1.
37. Sebastian SA, Padda I, Johal G. Cardiovascular-kidney-metabolic (CKM) syndrome: a state-of-the-art review. Curr Probl Cardiol. 2024;49(2):102344. Epub 20231214. https://doi.org/10.1016/j.cpcardiol.2023.102344. PubMed PMID: 38103820.

38. Theodorakis N, Nikolaou M. From cardiovascular-kidney-metabolic syndrome to cardiovascular-renal-hepatic-metabolic syndrome: proposing an expanded framework. Biomolecules. 2025;15(2) Epub 20250202. https://doi.org/10.3390/biom15020213. PubMed PMID: 40001516; PubMed Central PMCID: PMC11853431.
39. Fowler J, Song L, Tam K, Roth Flach R. Targeting lymphatic function in cardiovascular-kidney-metabolic syndrome: preclinical methods to analyze lymphatic function and therapeutic opportunities. Front Cardiovasc Med. 2024;11:1412857. https://doi.org/10.3389/fcvm.2024.1412857.
40. Bedo D, Beaudrey T, Florens N. Unraveling chronic cardiovascular and kidney disorder through the butterfly effect. Diagnostics. 2024;14(5):463. PubMed PMID. https://doi.org/10.3390/diagnostics14050463.

Chapter 12
The Role of the Kidney in Cardiovascular–Kidney–Metabolic Syndrome

Crischentian Brinza, Adrian Covic, and Alexandru Burlacu

Introduction

Cardiovascular–renal–metabolic (CKM) syndrome represents a complex interplay among the cardiovascular, renal, and metabolic systems, where dysfunction in one organ often exacerbates pathology in others [1]. The kidney plays a central role in maintaining homeostasis through its regulatory functions in fluid balance, electrolyte control, blood pressure regulation, and metabolic waste excretion. However, in the context of CKM syndrome, renal impairment contributes significantly to cardiovascular and metabolic complications, creating a vicious cycle of disease progression [2].

Chronic kidney disease (CKD) could be considered a key driver of CKM syndrome, as it is closely associated with hypertension, atherosclerosis, insulin resistance, and systemic inflammation [2, 3]. Renal dysfunction leads to an accumulation of uremic toxins, dysregulation of the renin–angiotensin–aldosterone system (RAAS), and electrolyte imbalances, all of which exacerbate cardiovascular and metabolic derangements. In addition, CKD-induced endothelial dysfunction and

C. Brinza (✉)
Grigore T. Popa University of Medicine and Pharmacy, Iasi, Romania
e-mail: crischentian.brinza@d.umfiasi.ro

A. Covic
Grigore T. Popa University of Medicine and Pharmacy, Iasi, Romania

Nephrology Clinic, Dialysis, and Renal Transplant Center - "C.I. Parhon" University Hospital, Iasi, Romania

A. Burlacu
Grigore T. Popa University of Medicine and Pharmacy, Iasi, Romania

Institute of Cardiovascular Diseases "Prof. Dr. George I.M. Georgescu", Iasi, Romania

M. Floria, D. M. Tanase (eds.), *Cardiovascular-Kidney-Metabolic Syndrome*,
https://doi.org/10.1007/978-3-032-11445-7_12

oxidative stress further contribute to the pathophysiological continuum of CKM syndrome [3–6].

Given the bidirectional relationships between kidney disease, cardiovascular dysfunction, and metabolic disorders, understanding the role of the kidney in CKM syndrome is essential for developing effective preventive and therapeutic strategies. This chapter explores molecular and pathophysiological mechanisms linking renal dysfunction to CKM syndrome, highlights the clinical implications of kidney disease in accelerating cardiovascular and metabolic pathology, and discusses emerging therapeutic approaches for reducing renal and systemic complications.

This chapter integrates current evidence to provide a comprehensive understanding of the kidney's role in CKM syndrome, emphasizing the need for interdisciplinary management strategies to improve patient outcomes.

Pathophysiology of CKM Syndrome and Role of the Kidney

The pathogenesis of CKM syndrome involves a complex interplay between genetic factors and molecular pathways, which affect renal, cardiovascular, and metabolic functions. Understanding these genetic factors and molecular pathways provides insight into CKM syndrome's mechanisms and could inform targeted therapeutic strategies [4].

The development of CKM syndrome involves a convergence of renal, metabolic, and cardiovascular dysfunction, often exacerbated by environmental and dietary factors. In a novel murine model, the combination of moderate chronic renal failure induced by unilateral nephrectomy and prolonged exposure to a Western-type diet (rich in carbohydrates, fat, and salt) resulted in a robust phenotype mimicking the human CKM syndrome. This model led to progressive renal impairment, hypertension, altered glucose metabolism, adipocyte dysfunction, systemic inflammation, and cardiac remodeling [7]. This study provides preclinical evidence for the dual role of the kidney and diet in the pathogenesis of the multisystem deterioration observed in CKM syndrome. Moreover, it supports the role of the kidney as both a target and mediator of metabolic and cardiovascular dysfunction, particularly in dietary excess [7].

Role of Obesity in CKM Syndrome

Obesity represents a state of chronic systemic inflammation that contributes to the pathogenesis of multiple components of the CKM syndrome. Beyond excess energy storage, obesity disrupts immune and metabolic homeostasis, initiating a cascade of molecular events that could promote cardiovascular, renal, and metabolic deterioration. This process is central to remodeling adipose tissue, which becomes immunologically active and a key source of inflammatory mediators [8].

Inflammation—Linking Obesity to CKM Syndrome

A fundamental alteration in obesity pathogenesis is the upregulation of signaling cascades involving tumor necrosis factor (TNF) and other pro-inflammatory cytokines within adipose tissue. These cytokines induce adipocyte apoptosis and facilitate the recruitment of immune cells to the expanding adipose depots. The subsequent elevation of pro-inflammatory cytokine levels contributes to lipotoxicity, glucotoxicity, and the development of insulin resistance. In long-term exposure, these effects promote ectopic lipid deposition in non-adipose tissues, including the liver or skeletal muscle, thereby exacerbating glucose intolerance, systemic metabolic dysfunction, and tissue injury [8–12].

While traditionally viewed as a primary site for energy storage, white adipose tissue (WAT) is now recognized to play an important role in metabolic homeostasis. In addition to adipocytes and preadipocytes, WAT comprises a dynamic population of immune cells, including macrophages, dendritic cells, and lymphocytes, actively modulating adipocyte function and maintaining hormonal responses. However, this complex immunometabolic interaction transitions to a pathological state in the context of obesity. Notably, macrophages, which can constitute a substantial proportion (up to 50%) of the cellular composition of WAT in obese individuals, exhibit a phenotypic polarization toward a pro-inflammatory M1-like state. These M1 macrophages aggregate around apoptotic adipocytes, forming characteristic crown-like structures, a histological feature consistently correlated with insulin resistance in both human and animal studies [8, 13, 14].

Adipose tissue-derived hormones, or adipokines, further mediate the link between obesity and systemic inflammation. Leptin, which increases in obesity, acts as a pro-inflammatory adipokine that also regulates appetite and energy expenditure. Conversely, adiponectin, which is typically reduced in obese individuals, exerts anti-inflammatory and insulin-sensitizing properties by suppressing pro-inflammatory cytokines such as TNF-α, MCP-1, and interleukin-6 (IL-6) [8, 15, 16].

AMP-activated protein kinase (AMPK) serves as a metabolic checkpoint by inhibiting anabolic processes and enhancing catabolic pathways like β-oxidation. While adiponectin stimulates AMPK activation in tissues such as skeletal muscle, the effects of leptin are context-dependent. It activates AMPK peripherally but inhibits it in the hypothalamus, contributing to satiety and reduced food intake. In obesity, the imbalance between leptin and adiponectin disrupts AMPK signaling, reinforcing metabolic derangement [8, 17].

Beyond macrophages, which have been extensively studied in obesity-induced inflammation, other studies have highlighted the critical role of neutrophils as early mediators in adipose tissue immune activation. Neutrophils are the most abundant leukocytes in circulation, yet their presence within adipose tissue is reduced. However, in obesity, neutrophils represent the first wave of immune cell infiltration into the expanding adipose tissue. Some preclinical models have suggested that neutrophil dysfunction in obesity contributes directly to adipose tissue inflammation and the development of insulin resistance, underscoring their role as more than transient responders in innate immunity [18, 19].

In visceral adipose tissue (VAT), neutrophil infiltration is observed remarkably early following the introduction of a high-fat diet (HFD), often preceding any significant weight gain or insulin sensitivity alterations. Murine studies have demonstrated that neutrophil infiltration can be detected as early as 3 days after HFD initiation, with levels declining by the end of the first month, suggesting a temporally restricted but critical window for neutrophil action in initiating tissue inflammation and macrophage recruitment [19, 20].

Taken together, these mechanisms demonstrate that obesity is not merely a comorbidity of CKM syndrome—it is a driving force. Through inflammatory reprogramming of adipose tissue, hormonal dysregulation, and ectopic lipid toxicity, obesity initiates and sustains the pathophysiological progression of cardiovascular, renal, and metabolic injury [21, 22].

Impact of CKD on CKM Syndrome: A Central Driver?

CKD is increasingly recognized as a pivotal contributor to the development and progression of CKM syndrome. The American Heart Association (AHA) has highlighted the intricate interplay between metabolic risk factors, such as obesity and diabetes, CKD, and cardiovascular disease, emphasizing their combined impact on adverse health outcomes [23]. CKD not only exacerbates cardiovascular and metabolic disorders but also introduces unique management challenges, requiring a comprehensive approach to prevention and treatment. Understanding the multifaceted role of CKD within the CKM syndrome is essential for developing effective strategies to mitigate associated risks and improve patient outcomes [23–25].

Given the high global prevalence of CKD, studies have focused on uncovering the mechanisms responsible for the markedly elevated rates of atherosclerosis and cardiovascular disease in this population [26, 27]. While conventional risk factors, such as arterial hypertension, elevated cholesterol levels, and obesity, are prevalent in CKD, they do not fully account for the disproportionately high cardiovascular morbidity and mortality observed in CKD patients. Therefore, the research focus has expanded to encompass nontraditional risk factors potentially contributing to increased cardiovascular risk in CKD. Chronic systemic inflammation and oxidative stress have emerged as key drivers, alongside endothelial dysfunction, vascular calcification, and fluid overload. Among these, inflammation and oxidative stress are receiving increasing validation as central contributors to the pathophysiology of cardiovascular disease in CKD, highlighting the necessity for therapeutic interventions targeting CKD-associated risk factors [26–29].

(a) *Oxidative stress—bridging CKD with cardiometabolic risk*

CKD is characterized by an imbalance between prooxidant and antioxidant activities, leading to oxidative stress. This redox imbalance contributes significantly to the progression of CKD, as well as the development of associated complications, including cardiovascular and metabolic disorders. Furthermore, oxidative stress in

CKD patients is associated with endothelial dysfunction, a precursor to atherosclerosis and cardiovascular disease. Also, the reduced bioavailability of nitric oxide (NO) due to reactive oxygen species (ROS) leads to impaired vasodilation and promotes vascular stiffness. Consequently, the interplay between oxidative stress and inflammation in CKD creates a vicious cycle that accelerates disease progression. Inflammatory cytokines can enhance ROS production, while oxidative stress can activate pro-inflammatory pathways, further damaging renal tissue [26, 30].

Oxidative stress could be regarded as a key contributor to the pathogenesis of CKM syndrome, acting as a molecular bridge between CKD and cardiometabolic dysfunction. In CKD, the balance between ROS production and the antioxidant mechanisms is disrupted, resulting in a prooxidative state. This imbalance promotes the oxidation of lipids, proteins, and nucleic acids, leading to cellular injury and organ dysfunction. Mitochondria are central sources of ROS, with enzymes such as cytochrome P450 playing an important role in ROS generation. These mitochondrial-derived radicals initiate and propagate tissue injury within the kidney and vasculature, exacerbating renal decline and cardiovascular complications [31, 32].

Among the primary ROS species involved, superoxide anions are particularly pathogenic. They are generated predominantly through activation of nicotinamide adenine dinucleotide phosphate (NADPH) oxidases, especially in immune and endothelial cells. In CKD, the expression of NADPH oxidase is significantly upregulated, while antioxidant enzymes like superoxide dismutase (SOD) are downregulated. This imbalance magnifies oxidative stress, contributing to endothelial dysfunction, impaired vasodilatory responses, and the depletion of bioavailable NO, a key regulator of vascular tone [26, 31].

The development of a prooxidative state may occur relatively early in CKD, even at stage 3, as evidenced by increased circulating biomarkers indicative of oxidative stress. This disruption in redox balance contributes to the progression of renal dysfunction through a complex interplay of mechanisms, including promotion of inflammation, activation of nuclear factor kappa B (NF-κB), increased systemic blood pressure, glomerular injury, and the occurrence of renal fibrosis. In individuals requiring dialysis, oxidative stress is often exacerbated, largely due to the potential of bioincompatible materials to stimulate the production of ROS. Also, in dialysis patients, oxidative stress could be exacerbated by the duration of dialysis, antioxidant filtration, and anticoagulant therapy. The mechanisms driving oxidative stress in CKD encompass a combination of factors linked to the uremic environment and dialysis, reflecting the multifactorial nature of this pathological process [33–36].

One of the key contributors to oxidative stress in CKD patients is the accumulation of uremic toxins. Consequently, the uremic environment could stimulate systemic inflammation by activating polymorphonuclear leukocytes and cytotoxic $CD8^+$ T cells, leading to an amplified immune response. Also, studies have demonstrated that baseline serum levels of superoxide anions are significantly elevated in individuals undergoing chronic hemodialysis compared to healthy controls. This sustained production of ROS perpetuates a vicious cycle of inflammation and oxidative injury, reinforcing the deterioration of renal and cardiovascular systems.

Notably, clinical evidence has consistently linked oxidative stress and inflammation with adverse clinical outcomes in CKD patients [35, 37–39].

ROS scavenging of NO could play a significant role in developing vascular endothelial dysfunction, a key initial step in forming atherosclerotic lesions. As these lesions advance, the structural and functional integrity of the endothelium is progressively impaired, contributing to a continuous cycle of vascular damage. Reducing NO bioavailability diminishes endothelium-dependent vasodilation, fostering increased vascular stiffness and inflammation within the vessel walls [40, 41].

Moreover, oxidative stress has an important role in the remodeling and hypertrophy of vascular smooth muscle cells, which contribute significantly to vascular pathology in CKD patients and associated cardiovascular disorders. In addition, ROS serve as important intracellular signaling molecules that can stimulate a cascade of redox-sensitive pathways, promoting vascular smooth muscle cells proliferation and structural alterations. Specifically, ROS are known to activate mitogen-activated protein kinases (MAPKs), and upregulate proto-oncogenes including c-fos, c-myc, and c-jun. Furthermore, ROS alter the extracellular matrix composition through modulation of matrix metalloproteinases (MMP-2 and MMP-9). These enzymatic changes ultimately lead to thickening and structural remodeling of the vascular wall. All these data underscore the pathogenic role of oxidative stress in the vascular complications associated with CKD and CKM syndrome [41–43].

(b) *Inflammation in CKD—an amplifier of cardiovascular and metabolic risk*

A persistent state of low-grade inflammation is a common and important characteristic of CKD, especially in end-stage kidney disease (ESKD) patients and those receiving dialysis. This pro-inflammatory condition occurs through a complex interplay of several contributing factors. These factors include oxidative stress, increased susceptibility to infections, alterations in the gut microbiome (intestinal dysbiosis), metabolic acidosis, and the accumulation of pro-inflammatory cytokines due to impaired renal elimination. The confluence of these elements establishes a systemic inflammatory environment that significantly contributes not only to CKD progression but also to increased risk of cardiovascular events and overall mortality observed in this context [25, 44, 45].

Inflammation and increased cytokine levels have been demonstrated to modulate basal energy expenditure and disrupt endocrine axes in CKD patients. Specifically, inflammatory mediators can suppress signaling pathways involving growth hormone and insulin-like growth factor-1, inhibit anabolic processes, and attenuate the erythropoietic response to erythropoietin. These disruptions contribute to the development of sarcopenia and protein-energy wasting (PEW), a catabolic syndrome marked by skeletal muscle depletion, anorexia, fatigue, and symptoms of depression. Notably, the presence of PEW increases the risk of mortality in patients with CKD [25, 46, 47].

A key contribution to understanding inflammatory biomarkers in CKD progression comes from the Chronic Renal Insufficiency Cohort (CRIC) Study, which is designed to evaluate risk factors for renal function decline in patients with established CKD. In a cohort of 3430 participants followed over a median period of 6.3 years, researchers examined the association between several systemic inflammatory markers, including IL-6, TNF-α, fibrinogen, and high-sensitivity C-reactive protein (hsCRP), and adverse renal outcomes, defined as either a ≥50% reduction in estimated glomerular filtration rate (eGFR) or progression to ESKD. The authors reported that higher circulating concentrations of fibrinogen and TNF-α were independently associated with a more rapid decline in renal function, respectively, HR 1.49, 95% CI: 1.20–1.86 ($P < 0.001$) and HR 1.42, 95% CI: 1.11–1.81 ($P < 0.001$). Notably, reduced serum albumin concentrations were also strongly associated with accelerated CKD progression, with an HR of 1.52, 95% CI: 1.24–1.87 ($P < 0.001$). These findings reinforce the role of systemic inflammation as a nontraditional but relevant determinant of kidney deterioration, and support its inclusion in future risk stratification models and management strategies for patients with CKD [45].

A recent study investigated the association between Systemic Inflammatory Response Index (SIRI) and all-cause mortality and cardiovascular mortality [48]. A total of 9115 patients with CKD were enrolled in this study. SIRI quartiles stratified patients, and outcomes assessed included all-cause and cardiovascular disease-related mortality. Kaplan–Meier survival analysis demonstrated significantly higher mortality rates among individuals in the upper SIRI quartiles. In multivariable Cox regression models adjusted for demographic, clinical, and laboratory variables, each unit increase in SIRI was independently associated with a 20% higher risk of all-cause mortality and a 33% increased risk of cardiovascular mortality. Notably, individuals in the third and fourth quartiles of SIRI exhibited significantly higher risk for both all-cause and cardiovascular mortality compared to those in the lowest quartile. These results highlight the prognostic utility of SIRI in risk stratification among patients with CKD, reflecting underlying inflammatory activity. Given the association between SIRI and adverse outcomes in CKD, inflammatory indices may offer additional insights into disease progression and help identify patients at high risk for cardiovascular events and premature death [48].

Systemic inflammation has emerged as a fundamental contributor to the development and progression of atherosclerotic cardiovascular disease (ASCVD), particularly in individuals with coexisting CKD. A recent population-level study from Spain highlighted the increased prevalence of inflammatory burden in this high-risk group of patients. The analysis included 15,798 patients with established ASCVD and evaluated for systemic inflammation, defined by elevated C-reactive protein (CRP) levels. At the time of initial CRP assessment, over half of the ASCVD cohort had systemic inflammation, with prevalence reaching 65% among CKD patients. Moreover, patients with ASCVD and systemic inflammation had more frequent traditional cardiovascular risk factors such as smoking, obesity, and dyslipidemia. These findings suggest that CKD is an inflammatory amplifier in patients with ASCVD, underscoring the importance of identifying and managing inflammation as a modifiable risk factor [49].

IL-6 has gained increasing attention as a biomarker of both cardiovascular and all-cause mortality in patients with CKD. In a recent meta-analysis focusing on ESKD patients undergoing dialysis, the pooled HR for all-cause mortality was 1.02

per pg/mL increase in IL-6 (95% CI: 1.01–1.03, $P < 0.001$), indicating a consistent, dose-dependent relationship between systemic IL-6 concentration and mortality. These data indicate a consistent, dose-dependent association between systemic IL-6 levels and mortality risk in this population. Consequently, IL-6 may serve as a key inflammatory mediator in CKD, supporting the integration of inflammation-based risk markers into prognostic models for patients receiving renal replacement therapy (RRT) [50].

(c) *Fluid overload—a driver of cardiovascular risk*

In patients with advanced CKD, fluid overload has emerged as an important, yet often underrecognized, determinant of adverse clinical outcomes [25]. An observational study encompassing 478 patients with stages 4–5 CKD investigated the link between fluid overload and adverse clinical outcomes. The fluid status was quantified using the overhydration-to-extracellular water (OH/ECW) ratio, and a value greater than 7% was defined as fluid overload. Over a median follow-up of approximately 23 months, patients with higher OH/ECW values exhibited a significantly increased incidence of a composite outcome comprising all-cause mortality and cardiovascular morbidity. Specifically, patients with OH/ECW >7% had nearly double the risk of combined adverse events, compared to those with OH/ECW below this cut-off (HR 1.93, 95% CI: 1.01–3.69, $P = 0.04$) [51].

Moreover, in CKD patients receiving RAAS inhibitors, adding furosemide may offer benefits beyond blood pressure management [52]. A randomized controlled trial enrolled 40 hypertensive patients with CKD (eGFR ranging between 15 and 60 mL/min/1.73 m^2). The authors reported that adjunctive therapy with furosemide significantly reduced left ventricular mass index (LVMI) over 52 weeks of follow-up compared to the control group receiving non-diuretic antihypertensives ($P = 0.013$), despite achieving similar blood pressure reduction. Notably, structural cardiac improvement was correlated with a measurable reduction in extracellular water, as assessed with bioimpedance analysis. Extracellular volume declined significantly only in patients receiving furosemide, not in the control group. Consequently, the observed regression in LVMI may be closely associated with improved volume status control rather than solely attributable to the blood pressure-lowering effect. Also, these results underscore the critical role of effective fluid volume management in mitigating left ventricular hypertrophy in CKD patients [52].

In ESKD patients, fluid and sodium retention represent hallmark features of progressive volume dysregulation, yet their systemic implications extend beyond a simple hemodynamic compromise [53]. Notably, research has suggested a significant association between salt and water overload and the activation of inflammatory and endothelial injury pathways, highlighting a potential interplay between volume expansion and microvascular dysfunction in this population. In one study that compared ESKD patients to healthy controls, bioimpedance analysis revealed a significant excess of extracellular fluid in the ESKD group. Also, magnetic resonance imaging demonstrated elevated sodium concentrations, particularly within subcutaneous tissues, which were associated with fluid overload [53].

These data underscore the prognostic relevance of volume status assessment in CKD patients. Monitoring and managing subclinical fluid accumulation may represent a valuable target to mitigate cardiovascular complications and premature mortality in this high-risk cohort of patients. Integrating objective volume status assessment tools into routine CKD care pathways may enhance risk stratification and guide therapeutic interventions [25, 51].

(d) *Anemia in CKD—a contributor to cardiovascular morbidity*

Anemia is a prevalent consequence of CKD, resulting from a multifactorial interplay of impaired erythropoietin production, systemic inflammation, disrupted iron homeostasis, and the uremic syndrome. The sustained reduction in systemic oxygen delivery exerts compensatory hemodynamic adaptations, including an elevation in cardiac output, which can progressively induce structural alterations within the myocardium. Specifically, the augmented cardiac workload contributes to the development of left ventricular hypertrophy and promotes maladaptive arterial remodeling. These vascular changes encompass intima-media thickening and arteriosclerosis, both recognized as precursors of cardiovascular morbidity [25].

A comprehensive systematic literature review synthesized findings from 191 studies examining the clinical impact of anemia in CKD patients [54]. Overall, the data consistently demonstrated a strong inverse association between hemoglobin (Hb) levels and cardiovascular risk, with lower Hb levels correlating with a higher incidence of major adverse cardiovascular events and mortality. For CKD patients not on dialysis, those with Hb levels below 10 g/dL exhibited a significantly elevated risk of major adverse cardiovascular events, with a pooled HR of 1.44 (95% CI: 1.17–1.76). Among dialysis-dependent patients, cardiovascular risk was even more significant at low Hb thresholds. Specifically, CKD patients with Hb <10 g/dL had an HR of 2.31 (95% CI: 1.14–4.66) for adverse cardiovascular events, suggesting more than double the risk compared to those with higher Hb levels [54].

In addition, in non-dialysis CKD patients, each 1 g/dL increment in Hb was associated with an 8% relative reduction in the risk of adverse cardiovascular events (HR 0.92, 95% CI: 0.86–0.99). A similar trend was observed in dialysis patients (HR 0.72; 95% CI: 0.21–2.46 per 1 g/dL increase). These findings confirm that anemia is not merely a marker of disease severity but a modifiable cardiovascular risk factor in CKD. Early recognition and individualized management of anemia may therefore be critical for improving quality of life and mitigating cardiovascular risk [54].

Strategies for Kidney Preservation in the Context of CKM Syndrome

Preserving renal function represents a central therapeutic objective in managing patients with CKM syndrome, as the kidney is pivotal in amplifying cardiovascular and metabolic risk. Effective protective strategies must adopt a multifactorial approach, including optimal control of blood pressure, correction of metabolic disturbances such as hyperglycemia and dyslipidemia, and targeted inhibition of neurohormonal pathways that contribute to renal injury and systemic inflammation. Interventions that address these interdependent mechanisms can attenuate disease progression and improve clinical outcomes [25].

Antihypertensive Management in CKD

Current guidelines recommend a blood pressure target of less than 120/80 mmHg for patients with CKD. However, given the complexity and fragility of CKD patients, especially those with multiple comorbidities, a more moderate threshold of <130/80 mmHg is often considered safer and more feasible in clinical practice. For patients with CKD stages 1–4 who have diabetes and albuminuria, treatment with either an angiotensin-converting enzyme inhibitor (ACEi) or an angiotensin receptor blocker (ARB) is recommended. Moreover, in patients with diabetes and CKD but without albuminuria, treatment with ACEi or ARBs is also recommended [25].

Recent evidence from a network meta-analysis evaluating dual renin–angiotensin system inhibitor-based antihypertensive regimens in patients with non-dialysis CKD highlighted the superior cardiovascular and blood pressure benefits of combining an ARB with a calcium channel blocker (CCB) [55]. This regimen was associated with a significantly reduced risk of major cardiovascular events when compared with several other commonly used treatment strategies, including ACEi (monotherapy OR 3.19, 95% CI: 1.25–8.17; $p = 0.0156$) or ARB (monotherapy OR 2.64, 95% CI: 1.18–5.87, $P = 0.0177$) [55].

Concerning blood pressure control, the ARB–CCB combination demonstrated the most pronounced reductions in systolic and diastolic pressures. Compared to ACEi monotherapy, systolic blood pressure was reduced by a standardized mean difference (SMD) of 17.60 (95% CI: 6.96–28.23, $P = 0.0035$) and diastolic blood pressure by 9.40 (95% CI: 2.95–15.86, $P = 0.0043$). Notably, this regimen also outperformed ARB monotherapy (SMD for systolic blood pressure 13.20, 95% CI: 6.44–19.96, $P = 0.0012$ and SMD for diastolic blood pressure 5.00, 95% CI: 0.27–9.73, $P = 0.0382$) and ACEi–CCB therapy (SMD for systolic blood pressure 12.90, 95% CI: 1.44–24.35, $P = 0.0499$ and SMD for diastolic blood pressure 9.90, 95% CI: 2.59–17.22, $P = 0.0080$) [55].

While significant advantages in cardiovascular protection and blood pressure control were observed with ARB–CCB combination therapy, the risks of hyperkalemia, ESKD, and all-cause mortality were similar across most treatment groups. However, ACEi-based therapy combined with spironolactone was associated with a notably higher incidence of hyperkalemia when compared to CCB monotherapy ($P < 0.05$). Regarding overall therapeutic ranking, ARB–CCB dual therapy emerged as one of the most favorable strategies, balancing efficacy in cardiovascular risk reduction and blood pressure lowering, without increasing the likelihood of adverse renal outcomes or electrolyte imbalances [55].

In patients with advanced CKD with eGFR ≤30 mL/min/1.73 m^2, the clinical utility of RAAS inhibition constitutes an area of ongoing evaluation. A recent systematic review and meta-analysis encompassing nine randomized controlled trials with a total of 1150 patients assessed the impact of RAAS blockade on renal and cardiovascular outcomes in this high-risk cohort of patients [56]. The primary finding was a statistically significant reduction in progression to ESKD among patients receiving RAAS inhibitors compared to the control group (placebo or alternative antihypertensive agents), with an RR of 0.84 (95% CI: 0.74–0.96, $P = 0.01$) [56].

In contrast, the benefits of RAAS inhibition were not observed regarding secondary endpoints. The pooled analysis from two randomized controlled trials revealed no statistically significant effect on major adverse cardiovascular events, defined as myocardial infarction, ischemic stroke, or cardiac death, with an RR of 0.87 (95% CI: 0.49–1.57, $P = 0.65$) [56]. Similarly, all-cause mortality was similar between RAAS-treated and control groups (RR 1.02, 95% CI: 0.63–1.65; $P = 0.93$). Findings from this meta-analysis suggest that in carefully selected patients with advanced CKD, RAAS inhibitors may be beneficial for delaying the onset of ESKD. Clinical decisions should weigh individual risk profiles and closely monitor potential adverse effects such as hyperkalemia or kidney function deterioration [56].

The clinical utility of RAAS inhibition in dialysis patients remains uncertain. A meta-analysis synthesizing data from 11 studies involving 1856 patients undergoing dialysis evaluated the effect of ACEi and ARB on cardiovascular events and residual renal function in this population. ARB therapy significantly reduced heart failure risk compared to placebo or other antihypertensive agents (RR 0.67, 95% CI: 0.47–0.93). However, no significant differences were reported between RAAS inhibitors and control groups regarding cardiovascular mortality (RR 0.89, 95%: CI 0.64–1.26), all-cause mortality (RR 0.94, 95% CI: 0.75–1.17), myocardial infarction (RR 1.00, 95% CI: 0.45–2.22), or stroke (RR 1.16, 95% CI: 0.69–1.96). Nevertheless, ACEI and ARB therapies were found to significantly attenuate the decline in kidney function compared to controls [57].

Consequently, while RAAS inhibitors may not confer broad cardiovascular protection in dialysis patients, ARBs could offer selective benefit in reducing heart failure risk. Moreover, both ACEIs and ARBs contribute to preserving residual renal function. These findings support the selective use of RAAS blockade in dialysis patients, with individualized risk-benefit assessment [57].

Dyslipidemia Management in CKD

Statins have long been recognized for their capacity to reduce low-density lipoprotein cholesterol (LDL-C) and the risk of atherosclerotic vascular events in the general population. This relationship between the extent of LDL-C reduction and the proportional decrease in cardiovascular events is well established. However, in patients with CKD, the benefit of LDL-C reduction appears to diminish with advancing kidney impairment [25].

A meta-analysis that included 48 studies assessed the impact of statin therapy on renal outcomes and lipid parameters in individuals with and without CKD at baseline. Statin use was associated with a decline in LDL-C, from a mean of 143 ± 32 mg/dL to 100 ± 21 mg/dL. Notably, statin therapy was associated with a statistically significant increase in eGFR, with a mean difference of 0.067 mL/min/1.73 m^2 (95% CI: 0.055–0.079, $P < 0.00001$), suggesting a beneficial effect on kidney function preservation. In addition, statins significantly reduced proteinuria, with a pooled mean difference of −0.643 ($P < 0.00001$). These findings support a dual cardiometabolic and reno-protective role for statins in the CKD population, though further randomized trials are warranted to establish their efficacy in attenuating renal disease progression as a primary endpoint.

Optimizing Glycemic Control

(a) *Sodium-glucose cotransporter 2 inhibitors*

Sodium-glucose cotransporter 2 (SGLT2) inhibitors exert their nephroprotective effects primarily through inhibition of glucose and sodium reabsorption in the proximal renal tubule. Thus, SGLT2 inhibitors could contribute to long-term preservation of nephron integrity. Several pivotal clinical trials have demonstrated the efficacy of these agents in slowing kidney disease progression, with a consistent 30–40% risk reduction in kidney endpoints. Beyond kidney protection, SGLT2 inhibitors have shown robust improvement in cardiovascular outcomes [25]. In line with their proven reno- and cardioprotective effects, SGLT2 inhibitors are now endorsed by the 2024 European Society of Cardiology (ESC) guidelines on hypertension with class I, level A recommendation for use in patients with CKD and eGFR above 20 mL/min/1.73 m^2 [58].

A meta-analysis of 13 large-scale, double-blind, placebo-controlled trials including 90,409 patients evaluated the renal and cardiovascular effects of SGLT2 inhibitors across populations with and without diabetes. The pooled data demonstrated that SGLT2 inhibitors were associated with a 37% lower risk of kidney disease progression compared to placebo (RR 0.63, 95% CI: 0.58–0.69). This effect was consistent irrespective of diabetic status or underlying kidney pathology. Regarding acute kidney injury, treatment with SGLT2 inhibitors conferred a 23% risk reduction (RR 0.77, 95% CI 0.70–0.84). Moreover, SGLT inhibitors were associated with a lower risk of composite outcome, including cardiovascular death or hospitalization for heart failure (RR 0.77, 95% CI 0.74–0.81). These therapeutic effects were uniform across trials with various baseline eGFR values, emphasizing the broad applicability of SGLT2 inhibitors in mitigating both renal and cardiac risk profiles [59].

(b) *Glucagon-like peptide-1 receptor agonists*

Glucagon-like peptide-1 receptor agonists (GLP-1 RAs) have become integral in the management of patients with CKM syndrome, particularly those with type 2 diabetes, obesity, or associated comorbidities such as hypertension and cardiovascular disease. GLP-1 RAs were approved not only for glycemic control and weight reduction, but also for cardiovascular risk reduction in select high-risk populations. Recent clinical trials highlighted their potential to improve both cardiovascular and kidney outcomes, reinforcing their role in CKM risk modification [60].

A recent meta-analysis of 11 large randomized controlled trials with over 85,000 participants assessed the impact of GLP-1 RAs on cardiovascular and renal outcomes. In patients with type 2 diabetes, GLP-1 RAs significantly reduced the composite renal outcome that included kidney failure, a ≥50% decline in eGFR, or death due to renal causes (HR 0.82, 95% CI: 0.73–0.93). The risk of kidney failure alone was also significantly lower (HR 0.84, 95% CI: 0.72–0.99). Cardiovascular benefit was also reported, with a 13% reduction in major adverse cardiovascular events, encompassing cardiovascular death, nonfatal myocardial infarction, and nonfatal stroke [61].

A meta-analysis of randomized controlled trials focusing on CKD patients evaluated the efficacy of GLP-1 RAs on renal and cardiovascular outcomes [62]. Among 17,996 participants from 12 eligible trials, treatment with GLP-1 RAs was associated with a 15% reduction in the risk of a composite kidney outcome (OR 0.85, 95% CI: 0.77–0.94, $P = 0.001$). All-cause mortality was also reduced in the GLP-1 RAs treatment arm (OR 0.77, 95% CI, 0.60–0.98, $P = 0.03$). Moreover, GLP-1 RA therapy exhibited a reduced risk of composite cardiovascular events (OR 0.86, 95% CI: 0.74–0.99, $P = 0.03$). These findings support the utility of GLP-1 RAs in mitigating progression of renal dysfunction and cardiovascular risk in patients with CKD [62].

Consequently, data from large-scale randomized trials support the integration of GLP-1 RAs as a key therapeutic strategy into the management of patients with CKM syndrome, particularly those with type 2 diabetes and CKD. Beyond their established metabolic benefits, GLP-1 RAs have shown significant reductions in both renal events and cardiovascular morbidity, including kidney failure, major adverse cardiovascular events, and all-cause mortality. These findings reinforce the dual cardiorenal protective role of GLP-1 RAs and provide a strong rationale for their broader implementation in CKM populations at high metabolic and cardiovascular risk [25].

Learning Objectives

- Understand the pathophysiological mechanisms by which chronic kidney disease (CKD) contributes to the development and progression of cardiovascular–renal–metabolic (CKM) syndrome.
- Identify the roles of oxidative stress, inflammation, fluid overload, and anemia as mediators of increased cardiovascular and metabolic risk in CKD patients.
- Recognize the bidirectional relationships between renal impairment and systemic comorbidities such as obesity, diabetes mellitus, and atherosclerotic cardiovascular disease.
- Appraise therapeutic strategies with renal and cardiovascular benefits, including RAAS inhibitors, SGLT2 inhibitors, GLP-1 receptor agonists, and statins.
- Apply current guideline recommendations and evidence-based strategies to the prevention and management of CKM syndrome in clinical practice.

Key Readings

- *The kidney plays a central role* in the pathogenesis of CKM syndrome through interrelated mechanisms of inflammation, oxidative stress, neurohormonal dysregulation, and metabolic alteration.
- *CKD accelerates cardiovascular morbidity* via nontraditional risk factors such as oxidative stress and chronic systemic inflammation, beyond classic contributors like hypertension or dyslipidemia.
- *Mitochondrial dysfunction and increased NADPH oxidase activity in CKD result in excessive reactive oxygen species* (ROS) production, leading to nitric oxide depletion, endothelial dysfunction, and vascular remodeling.
- *Inflammatory indices* such as IL-6 and the Systemic Inflammation Response Index (SIRI) are associated with renal function decline, cardiovascular events, and mortality in the CKD population.
- *Fluid overload in CKD contributes to hypertension and left ventricular hypertrophy*, making volume control a therapeutic priority.
- *CKD-related anemia* promotes maladaptive cardiac remodeling and vascular dysfunction, increasing the risk of adverse cardiovascular events.
- *Pharmacologic strategies* such as SGLT2 inhibitors and GLP-1 receptor agonists provide dual renal and cardiovascular protection.
- *Antihypertensive regimens combining ARBs with calcium channel blockers* show superior cardiovascular and renal benefits compared to monotherapy in CKD patients.
- *Early recognition and individualized intervention targeting renal function preservation are essential* for mitigating the systemic impact of CKM syndrome.

References

1. Ndumele CE, et al. Cardiovascular-kidney-metabolic health: a presidential advisory from the American Heart Association. Circulation. 2023;148(20):1606–35.
2. Ferdinand KC. An overview of cardiovascular-kidney-metabolic syndrome. Am J Manag Care. 2024;30(10 Suppl):S181–8.
3. Kadowaki T, et al. Interconnection between cardiovascular, renal and metabolic disorders: a narrative review with a focus on Japan. Diabetes Obes Metab. 2022;24(12):2283–96.
4. Marassi M, Fadini GP. The cardio-renal-metabolic connection: a review of the evidence. Cardiovasc Diabetol. 2023;22(1):195.
5. Slee AD. Exploring metabolic dysfunction in chronic kidney disease. Nutr Metab. 2012;9(1):36.
6. Prasad GV. Metabolic syndrome and chronic kidney disease: current status and future directions. World J Nephrol. 2014;3(4):210–9.
7. Carvalho LRRA, et al. A novel model of cardiovascular–kidney–metabolic syndrome combining unilateral nephrectomy and high-salt–sugar–fat diet in mice. Lab Anim. 2024;53(11):336–46.
8. Hildebrandt X, Ibrahim M, Peltzer N. Cell death and inflammation during obesity: "know my methods, WAT(son)". Cell Death Differ. 2023;30(2):279–92.
9. Ryden M, Arner P. Tumour necrosis factor-α in human adipose tissue–from signalling mechanisms to clinical implications. J Intern Med. 2007;262(4):431–8.
10. Wen X, et al. Signaling pathways in obesity: mechanisms and therapeutic interventions. Signal Transduct Target Ther. 2022;7(1):298.
11. Diehl AM. Tumor necrosis factor and its potential role in insulin resistance and nonalcoholic fatty liver disease. Clin Liver Dis. 2004;8(3):619–38.
12. Sethi JK, Hotamisligil GS. Metabolic messengers: tumour necrosis factor. Nat Metab. 2021;3(10):1302–12.
13. Cinti S, et al. Adipocyte death defines macrophage localization and function in adipose tissue of obese mice and humans. J Lipid Res. 2005;46(11):2347–55.
14. Murano I, et al. Dead adipocytes, detected as crown-like structures, are prevalent in visceral fat depots of genetically obese mice. J Lipid Res. 2008;49(7):1562–8.
15. Engin A. Adiponectin-resistance in obesity. In: Obesity and lipotoxicity. Cham: Springer; 2017. p. 415–41.
16. Villarreal-Molina M, Antuna-Puente B. Adiponectin: anti-inflammatory and cardioprotective effects. Biochimie. 2012;94(10):2143–9.
17. Kubota N, et al. Adiponectin stimulates AMP-activated protein kinase in the hypothalamus and increases food intake. Cell Metab. 2007;6(1):55–68.
18. Li H, et al. Macrophages, chronic inflammation, and insulin resistance. Cells. 2022;11(19):3001.
19. Savulescu-Fiedler I, et al. The interplay between obesity and inflammation. Life. 2024;14(7):856.
20. Elgazar-Carmon V, et al. Neutrophils transiently infiltrate intra-abdominal fat early in the course of high-fat feeding. J Lipid Res. 2008;49(9):1894–903.
21. Longo M, et al. Adipose tissue dysfunction as determinant of obesity-associated metabolic complications. Int J Mol Sci. 2019;20(9):2358.
22. Hanumegowda SM, et al. Obesity and metabolic syndrome: the repetitious disaster of modern times. In: Body recomposition. CRC Press; 2024. p. 3–42.
23. Ndumele CE, et al. A synopsis of the evidence for the science and clinical management of cardiovascular-kidney-metabolic (CKM) syndrome: a scientific statement from the American Heart Association. Circulation. 2023;148(20):1636–64.
24. Kahn MR, et al. Management of cardiovascular disease in patients with kidney disease. Nat Rev Cardiol. 2013;10(5):261–73.
25. Zoccali C, et al. Cardiovascular complications in chronic kidney disease: a review from the European Renal and Cardiovascular Medicine Working Group of the European Renal Association. Cardiovasc Res. 2023;119(11):2017–32.

26. Podkowińska A, Formanowicz D. Chronic kidney disease as oxidative stress- and inflammatory-mediated cardiovascular disease. Antioxidants (Basel). 2020;9(8):752.
27. Shlipak MG, et al. Cardiovascular mortality risk in chronic kidney disease: comparison of traditional and novel risk factors. JAMA. 2005;293(14):1737–45.
28. Zoccali C. Traditional and emerging cardiovascular and renal risk factors: an epidemiologic perspective. Kidney Int. 2006;70(1):26–33.
29. Norris KC, et al. Current view on CKD risk factors: traditional, noncommunicable diseases—diabetes, hypertension, and obesity. In: Chronic kidney disease in disadvantaged populations. Elsevier; 2017. p. 183–90.
30. Kishi S, et al. Oxidative stress and the role of redox signalling in chronic kidney disease. Nat Rev Nephrol. 2024;20(2):101–19.
31. Ling XC, Kuo K-L. Oxidative stress in chronic kidney disease. Ren Replace Ther. 2018;4(1):53.
32. Addabbo F, Montagnani M, Goligorsky MS. Mitochondria and reactive oxygen species. Hypertension. 2009;53(6):885–92.
33. Tarng D-C, et al. Increased oxidative damage to peripheral blood leukocyte DNA in chronic peritoneal dialysis patients. J Am Soc Nephrol. 2002;13(5):1321–30.
34. Kim HJ, Vaziri ND. Contribution of impaired Nrf2-Keap1 pathway to oxidative stress and inflammation in chronic renal failure. Am J Physiol Renal Physiol. 2010;298(3):F662–71.
35. Daenen K, et al. Oxidative stress in chronic kidney disease. Pediatr Nephrol. 2019;34:975–91.
36. Vida C, et al. Oxidative stress in patients with advanced CKD and renal replacement therapy: the key role of peripheral blood leukocytes. Antioxidants. 2021;10(7):1155.
37. Oberg BP, et al. Increased prevalence of oxidant stress and inflammation in patients with moderate to severe chronic kidney disease. Kidney Int. 2004;65(3):1009–16.
38. Sarnak M, et al. Cardiovascular disease risk factors in chronic renal insufficiency. Clin Nephrol. 2002;57(5):327–35.
39. Kaysen GA. The microinflammatory state in uremia: causes and potential consequences. J Am Soc Nephrol. 2001;12(7):1549–57.
40. Zalba G, et al. Vascular NADH/NADPH oxidase is involved in enhanced superoxide production in spontaneously hypertensive rats. Hypertension. 2000;35(5):1055–61.
41. Higashi Y. Roles of oxidative stress and inflammation in vascular endothelial dysfunction-related disease. Antioxidants. 2022;11(10):1958.
42. Rao GN, Berk BC. Active oxygen species stimulate vascular smooth muscle cell growth and proto-oncogene expression. Circ Res. 1992;70(3):593–9.
43. Rajagopalan S, et al. Reactive oxygen species produced by macrophage-derived foam cells regulate the activity of vascular matrix metalloproteinases in vitro. Implications for atherosclerotic plaque stability. J Clin Invest. 1996;98(11):2572–9.
44. Kadatane SP, et al. The role of inflammation in CKD. Cells. 2023;12(12):1581.
45. Amdur RL, et al. Inflammation and progression of CKD: the CRIC study. Clin J Am Soc Nephrol. 2016;11(9):1546–56.
46. Wing MR, Raj DS, Velasquez MT. Protein energy metabolism in chronic kidney disease. In: Chronic renal disease. Elsevier; 2015. p. 106–25.
47. Slee AD. Exploring metabolic dysfunction in chronic kidney disease. Nutr Metab. 2012;9:1–16.
48. Wei L, et al. Association of systemic inflammation response index with all-cause mortality as well as cardiovascular mortality in patients with chronic kidney disease. Front Cardiovasc Med. 2024;11:1363949.
49. Pesce G, et al. Systemic inflammation prevalence in patients with atherosclerotic cardiovascular disease and chronic kidney disease: a population-based study using a nationwide primary care database in Spain. Front Cardiovasc Med. 2025;12:1538466.
50. Istanbuly O, et al. Estimating the association between systemic Interleukin-6 and mortality in the dialysis population. Re-analysis of the global fluid study, systematic review and meta-analysis. BMC Nephrol. 2023;24(1):312.

51. Tsai YC, et al. Association of fluid overload with cardiovascular morbidity and all-cause mortality in stages 4 and 5 CKD. Clin J Am Soc Nephrol. 2015;10(1):39–46.
52. Zamboli P, et al. Effect of furosemide on left ventricular mass in non-dialysis chronic kidney disease patients: a randomized controlled trial. Nephrol Dial Transplant. 2010;26(5):1575–83.
53. Mitsides N, et al. Salt and water retention is associated with microinflammation and endothelial injury in chronic kidney disease. Nephron. 2019;143(4):234–42.
54. Palaka E, et al. The impact of CKD anaemia on patients: incidence, risk factors, and clinical outcomes-a systematic literature review. Int J Nephrol. 2020;2020:7692376.
55. Cho M, et al. Clinical outcomes of renin angiotensin system inhibitor-based dual antihypertensive regimens in chronic kidney disease: a network meta-analysis. Sci Rep. 2023;13(1):5727.
56. Vendeville N, et al. Clinical outcomes of renin-angiotensin-aldosterone blockade in patients with advanced chronic kidney disease: a systematic review and meta-analysis. Can J Cardiol. 2024;40(9):1718–28.
57. Liu Y, et al. Effects of angiotensin-converting enzyme inhibitors and angiotensin receptor blockers on cardiovascular events and residual renal function in dialysis patients: a meta-analysis of randomised controlled trials. BMC Nephrol. 2017;18(1):206.
58. McEvoy JW, et al. 2024 ESC guidelines for the management of elevated blood pressure and hypertension: developed by the task force on the management of elevated blood pressure and hypertension of the European Society of Cardiology (ESC) and endorsed by the European Society of Endocrinology (ESE) and the European Stroke Organisation (ESO). Eur Heart J. 2024;45(38):3912–4018.
59. Baigent C, et al. Impact of diabetes on the effects of sodium glucose co-transporter-2 inhibitors on kidney outcomes: collaborative meta-analysis of large placebo-controlled trials. Lancet. 2022;400(10365):1788–801.
60. Abasheva D, Ortiz A, Fernandez-Fernandez B. GLP-1 receptor agonists in patients with chronic kidney disease and either overweight or obesity. Clin Kidney J. 2024;17(Suppleme nt_2):ii19–35.
61. Badve SV, et al. Effects of GLP-1 receptor agonists on kidney and cardiovascular disease outcomes: a meta-analysis of randomised controlled trials. Lancet Diabetes Endocrinol. 2025;13(1):15–28.
62. Chen J-Y, et al. Kidney and cardiovascular outcomes among patients with CKD receiving GLP-1 receptor agonists: a systematic review and meta-analysis of randomized trials. Am J Kidney Dis. 2025;85(5):555–569.e1.

Chapter 13
The Role of the Heart in Cardiovascular-Kidney-Metabolic Syndrome

Silviu Stanciu, Sinziana-Andreea Pucerea, and Adrian-Gabriel Florescu

Introduction

Cardiovascular-renal-metabolic syndrome does not represent a novel pathogenic entity, it does constitute an umbrella term meant to raise awareness of the mutual amplification of metabolic, cardiovascular and renal comorbidities, even in the early stages only marked by the presence of risk factors.

Heart disease and cardiovascular mortality represent the main drivers of prognosis in all CKM syndrome comorbidities. Hence, special consideration should be directed toward understanding pathophysiological mechanisms through which all these metabolic risk factors converge toward cardiovascular impairment. Additionally, emphasis should be placed on the early and appropriate initiation of the right medication for the right patient, tailored to the estimated individual risk, particularly concerning the novel drug classes that have demonstrated beneficial effects across all components of the CKM syndrome—GLP1 receptor agonists, SGLT2 inhibitors, and the nonsteroidal mineralocorticoid receptor antagonist finerenone.

This chapter emphasizes the role of the heart in the CKM spectrum, with particular interest in pathophysiological mechanisms, risk stratification, and therapeutic implications.

S. Stanciu (✉) · S.-A. Pucerea
Central Military Emergency University Hospital Carol Davila Bucharest, Bucharest, Romania

University of Medicine and Pharmacy Carol Davila Bucharest, Bucharest, Romania
e-mail: silviu.stanciu@umfcd.ro

A.-G. Florescu
Central Military Emergency University Hospital Carol Davila Bucharest, Bucharest, Romania

M. Floria, D. M. Tanase (eds.), *Cardiovascular-Kidney-Metabolic Syndrome*,
https://doi.org/10.1007/978-3-032-11445-7_13

Mechanisms of Heart Disease in Cardiovascular-Renal-Metabolic Syndrome

Cardiovascular-renal-metabolic syndrome does not represent a novel pathogenic entity, it does constitute an umbrella term meant to raise awareness of the mutual amplification of metabolic, cardiovascular and renal comorbidities, even in the early stages only marked by the presence of risk factors.

In heart failure with preserved ejection fraction (HFpEF), there are comorbidities such as diabetes mellitus, obesity, and hypertension that contribute to a systemic proinflammatory environment. The main pathophysiological feature that links all of these conditions is endothelial dysfunction, which leads to coronary microvasculature inflammation [1].

This chapter emphasizes the role of the heart in renal and metabolic deterioration, pathophysiological mechanisms, risk stratification, and therapeutic implications.

Pathophysiological Mechanisms: Obesity and Heart Failure

Obesity is an independent factor for developing heart failure, and its prevalence is higher in patients with HFpEF. It has been shown that the adipose tissue functions as an endocrine organ and has the capacity to release a variety of bioactive molecules known as adipokines [2]. The adipose tissue is distributed among three main depots: visceral adipose tissue, subcutaneous adipose tissue, and non-storage depots. The most independent risk factor for cardiovascular diseases is visceral adipose tissue [3]. It has been shown that the greater the accumulation of visceral adipose tissue, the lower the levels of adiponectin, a key anti-inflammatory protein secreted by adipose tissue. In obese patients, adipose tissue expands, adipocytes enlarge, and it recruits monocytes from the blood circulation. The dysregulation of adipokine molecules contributes to the initiation and perpetuation of chronic systemic inflammation. These monocytes differentiate into macrophages, which release free fatty acids and activate other inflammatory mediators, such as TNF-α. This inflammatory response leads to a reduction in adiponectin levels, a key anti-inflammatory protein secreted by adipose tissue. The resulting neuroendocrine imbalance sustains a chronic state of systemic inflammation. There are some mechanisms through which obesity is thought to cause heart failure. The accumulation of free fatty acids can lead to impaired insulin-glucose uptake, inducing insulin resistance, which can cause the accumulation of toxic lipids like ceramides. These mechanisms are thought to contribute to cardiac hypertrophy, which is frequently encountered in obese patients and can also lead to systolic dysfunction [4].

Endothelial dysfunction and impaired vascular compliance are other factors that lead to heart failure. Although it was thought that leptin, a protein found in subcutaneous adipose tissue, had a vasodilator effect in high concentrations, actually, because of leptin resistance in obese individuals and low levels of adiponectin, the balance inclines towards increased vasoconstriction. Because of the release of vasoconstrictive mediators by the endothelium, the coronary perfusion can be altered.

There are some significant changes in cardiac hemodynamics caused by obesity, such as an increase in blood volume. A retrospective cohort analysis of 700 patients by Stelfox et al. analyzed the relationship between body mass index (BMI), cardiac output (CO), and stroke volume (SV) during coronary angiography. The study revealed that each 1 kg/m^2 increase in BMI was associated with a 0.08 L/min increase in cardiac output, and regarding the stroke volume, there was a 1.35 mL increase per BMI-unit [5].

Another observation is that left ventricular wall thickening (LVWT) and left ventricular mass rise with BMI and body weight. There was a study conducted on 35 obese patients separated into two categories based on the duration of their obesity, monitored through noninvasive methods, which concluded that LVWT and left ventricular mass increase with obesity duration, particularly when it exceeds 15 years. Also, because of poor left ventricular compliance and myocardial changes, one of the earliest cardiac impairments is diastolic dysfunction [6].

Another phenomenon described is the obesity paradox. This paradox states that individuals with BMI >30 kg/m^2 and cardiovascular diseases had the lowest mortality rate. The ADHERE (Acute Decompensated Heart Failure National Registry) study, conducted between 2001–2004, which included 108,927 hospitalizations, demonstrated that BMI is inversely associated with mortality. Given that the term *obesity paradox* has been applicable in several studies conducted in recent years, the European Society of Cardiology no longer recommends weight loss in heart failure patients, except for those with a BMI greater than 35 kg/m^2 [7].

Heart Failure and Risk Development of Type 2 Diabetes Mellitus

Diabetes mellitus is an independent risk factor for the development of cardiovascular diseases. Type 2 diabetes and heart failure share a bidirectional relationship; while diabetes can lead to heart failure, it is equally important to recognize that heart failure itself can predispose individuals to develop type 2 diabetes through multiple neurohormonal, inflammatory, and metabolic mechanisms. The prevalence of diabetes in patients with chronic heart failure, disregarding the ejection fraction, was around 30%, but this value is influenced by different regions in different countries of Europe or worldwide. For example, a study published in 2001 conducted in England with patients >41 years with heart failure concluded that the prevalence of diabetes mellitus type 2 was 24%, as opposed to patients without heart failure, who had 3% [7].

First, patients with heart failure often experience fatigue and reduced exercise tolerance that can lead to sedentary behavior. This is an independent risk factor for developing diabetes. Skeletal muscle is the largest site for glucose uptake mediated by insulin; after a meal, it disposes of around 70–80% of glucose. Muscle tissue stores glucose as glycogen, but as muscle mass decreases, there will be fewer insulin-sensitive cells available to absorb glucose. This will force the pancreatic cells to produce more insulin because of the hyperglycemia, and insulin resistance will develop over time.

Heart failure activates the renin-angiotensin-aldosterone system (RAAS) and promotes chronic systemic inflammation. Because of Angiotensin II, which binds to receptors in adipose tissue and muscles, a proinflammatory cascade is initiated, leading to impaired glucose uptake in muscle and fat. Also, Angiotensin II damages insulin signalling pathways through the production of reactive oxygen species, further promoting chronic inflammation [8].

Furthermore, some heart failure treatments can increase diabetes risk through altering the glucose tolerance, like beta-blockers (especially older generations) and thiazide diuretics [9].

Right heart failure is another risk factor for developing type 2 diabetes because of the hepatic congestion. In RHF, there is a reduced venous return to the liver and diminished perfusion. The hepatic cells will be less able to filter and degrade insulin, and this will result in hyperinsulinemia and insulin resistance. Due to hypoxia, in time, the liver's ability to respond to insulin properly will alter the main processes of gluconeogenesis and glycogen storage [8].

In general, patients with heart failure (including HFpEF or HFrEF) associated with diabetes mellitus tend to develop earlier in life symptoms of heart failure and a more rapid decline in functional status and a higher mortality rate than patients without diabetes [10, 11]. There are several studies conducted in Europe that compared the long-term mortality after HF-hospitalization, and all patients with associated diabetes mellitus had a higher cardiovascular mortality. There was a randomized control trial, the EVEREST trial, which included 4133 patients hospitalized for heart failure symptoms followed 9.9 months post-discharge. The aim was to evaluate the prevalence of diabetes in this kind of group and how the antidiabetic therapy influences the outcomes after discharge. They concluded that the prevalence of diabetes is higher in patients hospitalized for HF with reduced EF; they have higher cardiovascular morbidity, and antidiabetic therapy didn't impact the post-discharge outcomes [12].

It is known that insulin resistance and hyperglycemia produce oxidative stress, inflammation, and endothelial dysfunction. One of the main problems in patients with heart failure that is associated with diabetes is microvascular dysfunction. Chronic hyperglycemia leads to the formation of advanced glycosylation end products, which disrupt the normal contraction of myocardial proteins [13]. The deposition of AGE in myocardial tissue with consecutive left ventricular remodeling and hypertrophy leads to cardiac steatosis, confirmed by MRI. These further damage the myocardium, leading to myocardial stiffness and diastolic dysfunction. Whether the risk of mortality in patients with HF and diabetes is higher in those correlated with coronary artery disease remains a question. For example, in the CHARM trial study, patients with both heart failure and diabetes exhibited an increased risk of mortality, irrespective of the presence or absence of coronary artery disease [14].

Phenotypes of Cardiomyopathy Related to Type 2 Diabetes Mellitus

The first cardiovascular alteration observed in patients with diabetes is diastolic dysfunction. Usually, the severity correlates with the duration and severity of hyperglycemia [14]. Left ventricular dysfunction is a subtle change that appears before the classical symptoms of heart failure and can appear during physical exercise. More than 50% of individuals with type 2 diabetes and heart failure have HFpEF, which is usually encountered in older patients and females, and it is associated with hypertension [15]. Given the fact that patients may not develop the symptoms at rest, it is important to evaluate them through exercise stress tests and also use biomarkers like natriuretic peptides to diagnose subclinical HF.

Another phenotype of cardiomyopathy associated with type 2 diabetes is HFrEF, which is usually related to coronary artery disease. Patients with heart failure and reduced ejection fractions who have diabetes typically present with diffuse, complex multivessel disease, more severe symptoms, and an increased risk of stroke and all-cause mortality [16, 17].

Heart Failure and Renal Disease

It is well established that the correlation between chronic kidney disease and heart failure is known as cardiorenal syndrome. Kidney dysfunction is a consequence of heart failure, but it is also a trigger that can worsen the progression of heart failure. The connection between these two is linked through inflammatory, neurohormonal, and hemodynamic mechanisms (Fig. 13.1). Sometimes it is hard to distinguish primary organ injuries from secondary ones due to common risk factors and systemic disorders [18, 19].

The hemodynamic changes that appear in heart failure, such as low cardiac output and systemic congestion, cause elevated central pressure, contributing to impaired glomerular filtration. Due to chronic inflammation sustained by both renal and cardiac dysfunction, there is an overproduction of reactive oxygen species (ROS). ROS react with nitric oxide to form peroxynitrite, a toxic compound that reduces the availability of nitric oxide (NO), damaging the endothelial cells. Reduced NO levels impair vasodilation, which worsens organ perfusion, increasing afterload and promoting vascular stiffness [18].

Another important mechanism that leads to the decrease of renal function is the activation of the renin-angiotensin-aldosterone axis. Whenever there is a reduction

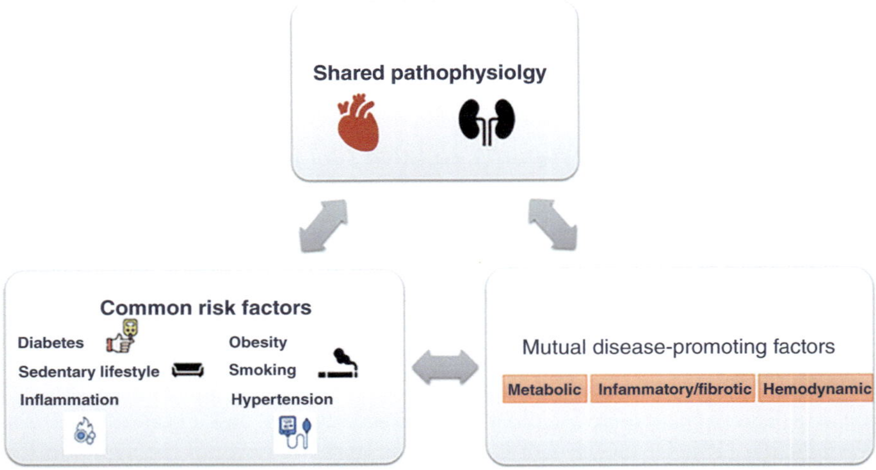

Fig. 13.1 The cardiorenal connection in the context of organ failure

of renal blood flow, due to an episode of decompensated HF, there is vasoconstriction of the efferent arteriole, which tries to maintain the glomerular filtration rate (GFR). At the same time, the activation of the RAAS axis causes the vasoconstriction of the afferent arteriole to ensure the renal blood flow and, consequently, it will cause a reduction in GFR. Also, aldosterone is secreted to maintain effective plasma volumes, reabsorbing the sodium and water in the distal tubules, causing more congestion and oliguria [20].

Due to shared pathophysiological mechanisms, the homeostasis of the cardiovascular and renal systems is interdependent. For instance, patients with heart failure may undergo a decline in GFR mainly because of both reduced cardiac output and systemic congestion, which activate neurohormonal mechanisms and the sympathetic nervous system. As the GFR decreases, a vicious cycle is triggered, leading to worsening fluid retention and systemic vascular congestion, further promoting the deterioration and dysfunction of both organs [18].

In the Swedish Heart Failure Registry, a study of 42,583 patients reported that 23% had heart failure with preserved ejection fraction (HFpEF), 21% had mildly reduced ejection fraction (HFmrEF), and 56% had a reduced ejection fraction (HFrEF). Common comorbidities included type 2 diabetes mellitus (24%), chronic kidney disease (51%), and atrial fibrillation (56%), with 8% of patients presenting with all three conditions. Significant differences were observed among the heart failure subtypes. In HFpEF patients, chronic kidney disease was more prevalent (56%), and non-cardiovascular events were more frequent. Conversely, in HFrEF patients, the prevalence of chronic kidney disease was lower (46%), but cardiovascular events were more common. The prevalence of type 2 diabetes mellitus was similar across all heart failure subtypes, regardless of ejection fraction [21].

Clinical Manifestations of Heart Failure in CKM Syndrome

CKM syndrome has a heterogeneity of clinical manifestations, and when heart failure is present, the symptoms are directly influenced by the interplay between cardiac dysfunction, renal impairment, and metabolic abnormalities like diabetes or anemia.

One of the first clinical manifestations of heart failure is *fatigue and exercise intolerance*. Although fatigue can appear just during exercise, it is important to diagnose subclinical HF. When there is worsening renal function and the onset of anemia, exercise capacity will deteriorate.

Volume overload is a hallmark of heart failure. Physical examination of the patient and clinical symptoms are the first steps in diagnosing HF. *Peripheral edema*, particularly in the lower extremities, is one of the most visible signs indicating fluid redistribution. Pulmonary congestion presents as *dyspnea, orthopnea, or paroxysmal nocturnal dyspnea* and may be accompanied by rales or crackles upon auscultation of the lungs. Jugular venous distension is a key indicator of elevated central venous pressure and can be evaluated with the patient in a semi-recumbent position. In advanced cases, ascites may be present due to hepatic congestion and right heart failure. When examining the patient, S3 is frequently present. There is a protodiastolic gallop associated with heart failure caused by elevated filling pressure or mitral regurgitation.

Another sign is *tachycardia*, a compensatory mechanism to maintain cardiac output. In heart failure, stroke volume is reduced due to high filling pressure and impaired myocardial contractility.

Due to right heart failure progression, there can be hepatic congestion and gut edema, which leads to early satiety, anorexia, and nausea. In the final stages, there is weight loss from cachexia.

When renal dysfunction appears, signs like oliguria and electrolyte disturbances can be present. Uremia can worsen fatigue, dyspnea, and cognitive symptoms, leading to uremic encephalopathy. Also, anemia is present in chronic renal disease, the primary cause being decreased erythropoietin production, and it can consequently aggravate the preexisting symptoms like fatigue and dyspnea.

Frequently, the patient presents clinical signs of dyslipidemia like xanthomas, xanthelasma (around the eyelids), corneal arcus (grey-white ring around the cornea), lipemia retinalis (due to high triglyceride levels), or can be asymptomatic until a complication arises, such as atherosclerotic cardiovascular disease or myocardial infarction [19].

The symptoms of heart failure are directly linked to the stages of CKM syndrome. There are four stages of CKM, based on risk factors and certain parameters, a system designed to classify patients into a specific category to guide early management and prevent the progression of preexisting disease [22]:

Stage 0: Individuals without risk factors, obesity, chronic kidney disease, or clinical/subclinical cardiovascular disease

Stage 1: Overweight individuals or excessive adipose tissue characterized by: waist circumference >88/102 cm in women/men, BMI >25 kg/m^2, or the presence of impaired glucose tolerance (HbA1c >5.7%, no more than 6.4% and fasting plasma glucose >100–125 mg/dl)

Stage 2: Individuals with metabolic risk factors (obesity, diabetes) or CKD

Stage 3: Individuals with obesity who present with subclinical atherosclerotic vessel disease, subclinical heart failure, or other metabolic risk factors:

- Elevated cardiac biomarkers: NT-proBNP >125 pg/mL, high-sensitivity Troponin I >10 ng/L or >12 ng/L in women/men
- Very high-risk CKD, either G4 or G5
- High 10-year predicted cardiovascular risk

Stage 4: Individuals with clinical cardiovascular disease and obesity or chronic renal disease

- Stage 4a: No kidney failure present
- Stage 4b: Kidney failure present [22]

Patients who are classified as stage 0 of CKM without evident risk factors require primary prevention measures, a healthy lifestyle, and annual evaluations to detect subclinical cardiovascular diseases. Starting from stage 1 of CKM, modification of risk factors is required, and lifestyle interventions are necessary. Weight loss is required to achieve a normal BMI <25 kg/m^2. If fasting blood glucose or glycated hemoglobin is elevated (5.7–6.4%), a reduction in carbohydrate intake and avoidance of foods with processed sugars is necessary. This is where the role of a diabetologist comes in, both in regulating diet and taking preventive measures to prevent the development of cardiovascular disease or the progression to chronic kidney disease [23].

From stage 2 of CKM, the disease has progressed and requires more targeted interventions. The patient requires strict monitoring and regular assessments of renal function through monitoring: serum creatinine, glomerular filtration rate, and urine albumin-to-creatinine-ratio to assess the progression of kidney disease, but also routine cardiovascular risk assessment through monitoring blood pressure, lipid profile, ECG, and echocardiogram. Regular monitoring of blood glucose levels and glycated hemoglobin, along with dietary adjustments to ensure a healthy, balanced diet and a normal body weight, is also recommended. Patient education, geared towards managing cardiovascular and kidney risk factors and preventing further progression of the disease, plays a key role. Starting from this stage, a multidisciplinary approach is important for the patient's benefit and for reducing the risk of cardiovascular mortality [23].

Cardiovascular Assessment in Patients with CKM Syndrome

Cardiovascular assessment in patients with CKM is essential to evaluate the extent of cardiovascular involvement, guide management, and reduce the risk of morbidity and mortality. CKM, as a multifactorial syndrome, requires a comprehensive and systematic approach to assess both cardiovascular and renal risk factors. Besides personal medical history and risk factor evaluation, it is important to have a full physical examination. Regular blood pressure measurement is crucial to evaluate hypertension; for all patients, the target for blood pressure is lower than 130/80 mmHg. Laboratory tests like serum lipid profile unravel dyslipidemia and guide the clinician regarding baseline values and the target LDL cholesterol level. Biomarkers like BNP/NT-proBNP can help assess heart failure. Also, measurement of serum creatinine, eGFR, and urine albumin-to-creatinine ratio is a key marker of early kidney dysfunction and is associated with increased cardiovascular risk.

Echocardiography plays a pivotal role in the assessment and management of patients with CKM because there is a high burden of subclinical cardiac abnormalities, and early detection is essential. In the initial stages of CKM, there are structural and functional cardiac changes that are frequently silent.

Left ventricular hypertrophy (LVH) defines a condition where the myocardial wall thickness increases. Various etiologies can lead to the development of LVH, besides the pathophysiological changes that appear in CKM, like hypertension (especially in patients with uncontrolled hypertension) and aortic valve stenosis. This is the compensatory mechanism that results from a contraction of the left ventricle against an elevated afterload. LVH can be discovered through transthoracic or transesophageal echocardiography. Based on the patient's weight and height, the LV mass index can be determined. In the ESC 2015 guidelines for cardiac chamber quantification, left ventricular hypertrophy is defined by: LVMI (left ventricular mass index) >115 g/m^2 in men and >95 g/m^2 in women [24]. In special populations, such as those with obesity or metabolic syndrome, indexing to body surface area can underestimate LVH due to excess body weight. American Society of Echocardiography and European Association of Cardiovascular Imaging guidelines suggest that when diagnosing left ventricular hypertrophy in patients with CKM, it should be indexed to height^2.7. There was a study that included 2213 patients with hypertension in the Evaluation of Target Organ Damage in Hypertension, who were categorized by their body mass index. The prevalence rate of left ventricular hypertrophy based on body mass index was lower than that indexed to height^2.7. This highlights the importance of using this formula to avoid underdiagnosis of LVH [25].

The Role of Echocardiography in the Detection of Subclinical Heart Failure and Diastolic Dysfunction

Diastolic dysfunction is one of the first abnormalities that occurs when the left ventricle becomes stiff or noncompliant. In CKM syndrome, all of the components, like hypertension, type 2 diabetes mellitus, obesity, and chronic kidney disease, contribute to myocardial stiffness, which leads to abnormal relaxation. This impaired relaxation leads to increased filling pressures, which further cause the congestion of lungs and the onset of heart failure even if the left ventricular ejection fraction is preserved. It is frequently underdiagnosed because patients may remain asymptomatic in early stages.

One of the first investigations for detecting diastolic dysfunction is transthoracic echocardiography. Usually, diastolic dysfunction can be determined according to ejection fraction by two main algorithms. One is used for the diagnosis in subjects with normal left ventricular ejection fraction, and one is used for grading diastolic function in patients with low ejection fraction or the presence of myocardial diseases.

In patients with normal ejection fraction, the following parameters are assessed, and the presence of diastolic dysfunction may be established if more than 50% of the evaluated parameters meet the diagnostic criteria:

- Average E/e` >14 describes high left ventricular filling pressures; it is less age dependent, and it is very rarely high in normal individuals.
- Septal e` velocity <7 cm/s or lateral e` velocity <10 cm/s.
- Tricuspid regurgitation velocity >2.8 m/s.
- LA volume index >34 ml/m^2, without chronic atrial arrhythmia, is correlated with left ventricular stiffness and diastolic dysfunction [25, 26].

The proposed algorithm for individuals with low ejection fraction is based on the mitral inflow pattern. It is based on the mitral inflow pattern E and A velocities obtained by PW Doppler at the base of the mitral annulus:

- E/A <0.8 and peak E velocity <50 cm/sec corresponds to normal left atrial pressure and grade I diastolic dysfunction.
- E/A ratio >2 defines increased atrial pressures and diastolic dysfunction grade III.
- E/A ratio is between 0.8–2 or E/A <0.8 and peak E velocity >50 cm/sec. There are other parameters to use to classify diastolic dysfunction: LA volume >34 ml/m^2, tricuspid regurgitation velocity >2.8 m/s by CW Doppler, and E/e` >14 [27].

Cardiac Computer Tomography (CT) Angiography

Cardiac CT angiography is a noninvasive method that is used for the detection of coronary artery anomalies and calcifications. In patients with CKM syndrome due to a high risk for the development of subclinical atherosclerosis, it is important to make an early diagnosis of coronary artery disease to guide appropriate management. This method allows describing not only significant stenosis but also non-obstructive plaques, which are frequent in patients with CKM. It allows the physician to differentiate between plaques with vulnerable components (lipid components or inflammation signs), contributing to risk stratification and optimal preventive treatment.

Because patients with cardiovascular-kidney-metabolic syndrome often present silent myocardial ischemia, coronary CT angiography provides a valuable tool: the calcium score, which aids in the detection of myocardial lesions. The Agatston score is the final score that sums up all of the calcified lesions in the coronary arteries, and it is most useful, especially in asymptomatic patients or those at an intermediate cardiovascular risk:

- Score 0: Suggests low cardiovascular risks in the next 5–10 years
- Score 1–100: Mildly high risk
- Score 101–400: Moderate risk
- Score >400: High risk [28]

Epicardial Fat Correlation with CKM Syndrome

Epicardial fat is an independent marker that may provide additional prognostic information about the cardiovascular risk of an individual. It can be measured by echocardiography, cardiac CT angiography, or MRI. Once the patient presents with comorbidities such as obesity, dyslipidemia, or diabetes, the adipose tissue surrounding the heart begins to secrete proinflammatory cytokines, leading to vascular remodeling in coronary arteries and the development of coronary artery disease. Many studies suggest that cardiac CT angiography has the highest spatial resolution and reproducibility when it comes to describing epicardial fat. A study that included 1379 patients who had been scanned by cardiac CT angiography concluded that diabetic patients had more epicardial fat distributed than other groups of patients [28].

Learning Objectives

- A thorough understanding of the cardiovascular-renal-metabolic (CKM) syndrome concept and its pathophysiological basis, with a particular focus on the cardiovascular component
- The acknowledgement of the central role of the cardiovascular system in the CKM continuum, with bidirectional interactions with renal and metabolic systems
- The understanding of the influence of cardiovascular impairment on CKM progression, with identification of the key mechanisms responsible

Key Reading

- *Cardiovascular disease, namely heart failure and atherosclerotic disease, is a common manifestation in CKM syndrome*, arising from the bidirectional pathophysiological interactions between the cardiovascular, renal, and metabolic systems.
- *At the core of the syndrome's pathophysiology* lies an excessive or metabolically impaired adipose tissue.
- *The adipose tissue* functions as an endocrine organ, with the capacity to release a variety of bioactive molecules known as adipokines. Obesity-related adipokine dysregulation (leptin resistance, low levels of adiponectin) and chronic inflammation promote endothelial dysfunction and neurohormonal activation, pathways known to be crucial in the development of cardiovascular morbidity.
- *Diabetes mellitus* is known to be a main risk factor for the development of heart failure, but the diabetes–heart failure relationship is bidirectional, as the latter can predispose diabetes development through multiple mechanisms: reduced exercise tolerance, which can lead to sedentarism, sarcopenia, and renin-angiotensin-aldosterone system hyperactivation with chronic systemic inflammation, both increasing insulin resistance.
- There is a well-established relationship between chronic kidney disease and heart failure known as cardiorenal syndrome. Kidney dysfunction may be initiated or aggravated by heart failure, but it is also a trigger that can worsen the progression of heart failure. The connection between these two is linked through inflammatory, neurohormonal, and hemodynamic mechanisms. Regarding patient evaluation, this should be performed thoroughly to classify the patient within a specific stage of this syndrome and to estimate their cardiovascular event risk. The purpose of this evaluation is to guide the selection and intensity of therapeutic interventions.
- The management should be comprehensive and patient-centered, based on an individual's risk and needs. The nonpharmacological treatment should include measures to increase one's level of physical activity, improve their diet, reduce their salt and alcohol intake, help them quit smoking, maintain a normal body weight and waist circumference, and increase their sleep quality. In certain cases, more complex strategies, beyond basic lifestyle advice, have demonstrated clinical benefits, including bariatric surgery or continuous positive airway pressure therapy for obstructive sleep apnea.

References

1. Hillege HL, Nitsch D, Pfeffer MA, Swedberg K, McMurray JJV, Yusuf S, et al. Renal function as a predictor of outcome in a broad spectrum of patients with heart failure. Circulation. 2006;113(5):671–8.
2. Badimon L, Bugiardini R, Cenko E, Cubedo J, Dorobantu M, Duncker DJ, et al. Position paper of the European Society of Cardiology–working group of coronary pathophysiology and microcirculation: obesity and heart disease. Eur Heart J. 2017;38(25):1951–8.
3. Rao VN, Zhao D, Allison MA, Guallar E, Sharma K, Criqui MH, et al. Adiposity and incident heart failure and its subtypes. JACC. Heart Fail. 2018;6(12):999–1007.
4. Guarini G, Kiyooka T, Ohanyan V, Pung YF, Marzilli M, Chen YR, et al. Impaired coronary metabolic dilation in the metabolic syndrome is linked to mitochondrial dysfunction and mitochondrial DNA damage. Basic Res Cardiol. 2016;111(3):29.
5. Stelfox HT, Ahmed SB, Ribeiro RA, Gettings EM, Pomerantsev E, Schmidt U. Hemodynamic monitoring in obese patients: the impact of body mass index on cardiac output and stroke volume. Crit Care Med. 2006;34(4):1243–6.
6. Nakajima T, Fujioka S, Tokunaga K, Hirobe K, Matsuzawa Y, Tarui S. Noninvasive study of left ventricular performance in obese patients: influence of duration of obesity. Circulation. 1985;71(3):481–6.
7. Fonarow GC, Srikanthan P, Costanzo MR, Cintron GB, Lopatin M. An obesity paradox in acute heart failure: analysis of body mass index and inhospital mortality for 108927 patients in the Acute Decompensated Heart Failure National Registry. Am Heart J. 2007;153(1):74–81.
8. Palazzuoli A, Iacoviello M. Diabetes leading to heart failure and heart failure leading to diabetes: epidemiological and clinical evidence. Heart Fail Rev. 2022;28(3):585–96.
9. Hall JJ, Eurich DT, Nagy D, Tjosvold L, Gamble JM. Thiazide Diuretic–induced change in fasting plasma glucose: a meta-analysis of randomized clinical trials. J Gen Intern Med. 2020;35(6):1849–60.
10. Kristensen SL, Preiss D, Jhund PS, Squire I, Cardoso JS, Merkely B, et al. Risk related to pre–diabetes mellitus and diabetes mellitus in heart failure with reduced ejection fraction: insights from prospective comparison of ARNI with ACEI to determine impact on global mortality and morbidity in heart failure trial. Circ Heart Fail. 2016;9(1):e002560.
11. Suskin N. Glucose and insulin abnormalities relate to functional capacity in patients with congestive heart failure. Eur Heart J. 2000;21(16):1368–75.
12. Sarma S, Mentz RJ, Kwasny MJ, Fought AJ, Huffman M, Subacius H, et al. Association between diabetes mellitus and post-discharge outcomes in patients hospitalized with heart failure: findings from the EVEREST trial. Eur J Heart Fail. 2013;15(2):194–202.
13. Van Heerebeek L, Hamdani N, Handoko ML, Falcao-Pires I, Musters RJ, Kupreishvili K, et al. Diastolic stiffness of the failing diabetic heart: importance of fibrosis, advanced glycation end products, and myocyte resting tension. Circulation. 2008;117(1):43–51.
14. MacDonald MR, Petrie MC, Varyani F, Ostergren J, Michelson EL, Young JB, et al. Impact of diabetes on outcomes in patients with low and preserved ejection fraction heart failure: an analysis of the Candesartan in Heart failure: Assessment of Reduction in Mortality and morbidity (CHARM) programme. Eur Heart J. 2008;29(11):1377–85.
15. Stahrenberg R, Edelmann F, Mende M, Kockskämper A, Düngen HD, Scherer M, et al. Association of glucose metabolism with diastolic function along the diabetic continuum. Diabetologia. 2010;53(7):1331–40.
16. Gu K, Cowie CC, Harris MI. Mortality in adults with and without diabetes in a National Cohort of the U.S. population, 1971–1993. Diabetes Care. 1998;21(7):1138–45.

17. Kannel WB, McGee DL. Diabetes and glucose tolerance as risk factors for cardiovascular disease: the Framingham Study. Diabetes Care. 1979;2(2):120–6.
18. Méndez AB, Azancot MA, Olivella A, Soler MJ. New aspects in cardiorenal syndrome and HFpEF. Clin Kidney J. 2022;15(10):1807–15.
19. Arnett DK, Blumenthal RS, Albert MA, Buroker AB, Goldberger ZD, Hahn EJ, et al. 2019 ACC/AHA guideline on the primary prevention of cardiovascular disease: a report of the American College of Cardiology/American Heart Association Task Force on Clinical Practice Guidelines. Circulation [Internet]. 2019 [cited 2025 May 17];140(11). Available from: https://www.ahajournals.org/doi/10.1161/CIR.0000000000000678.
20. Lee WL, Cheung AM, Cape D, Zinman B. Impact of diabetes on coronary artery disease in women and men: a meta-analysis of prospective studies. Diabetes Care. 2000;23(7):962–8.
21. Savarese G, Settergren C, Schrage B, Thorvaldsen T, Löfman I, Sartipy U, et al. Comorbidities and cause-specific outcomes in heart failure across the ejection fraction spectrum: a blueprint for clinical trial design. Int J Cardiol. 2020;313:76–82.
22. Ndumele CE, Rangaswami J, Chow SL, Neeland IJ, Tuttle KR, Khan SS, et al. Cardiovascular-kidney-metabolic health: a Presidential Advisory from the American Heart Association. Circulation. 2023;148(20):1606–35.
23. Visseren FLJ, Mach F, Smulders YM, Carballo D, Koskinas KC, Bäck M, et al. 2021 ESC Guidelines on cardiovascular disease prevention in clinical practice. Eur Heart J. 2021;42(34):3227–337.
24. Cuspidi C, Meani S, Negri F, Giudici V, Valerio C, Sala C, et al. Indexation of left ventricular mass to body surface area and height to allometric power of 2.7: is the difference limited to obese hypertensives? J Hum Hypertens. 2009;23(11):728–34.
25. Lang RM, Badano LP, Mor-Avi V, Afilalo J, Armstrong A, Ernande L, et al. Recommendations for cardiac chamber quantification by echocardiography in adults: an update from the American Society of Echocardiography and the European Association of Cardiovascular Imaging. J Am Soc Echocardiogr. 2015;28(1):1–39.e14.
26. Caballero L, Kou S, Dulgheru R, Gonjilashvili N, Athanassopoulos GD, Barone D, et al. Echocardiographic reference ranges for normal cardiac Doppler data: results from the NORRE study. Eur Heart J Cardiovasc Imaging. 2015;16:1031.
27. Nagueh SF, Smiseth OA, Appleton CP, Byrd BF, Dokainish H, Edvardsen T, et al. Recommendations for the evaluation of left ventricular diastolic function by echocardiography: an update from the American Society of Echocardiography and the European Association of Cardiovascular Imaging. J Am Soc Echocardiogr. 2016;29(4):277–314.
28. Division of Radiology, University of Parma, Parma, Italy, Milanese G, Department of Medicine and Surgery, University of Parma, Parma, Italy, Silva M, Division of Radiology, University of Parma, Parma, Italy, Department of Medicine and Surgery, University of Parma, Parma, Italy, et al. Quantification of epicardial fat with cardiac CT angiography and association with cardiovascular risk factors in symptomatic patients: from the ALTER-BIO (Alternative Cardiovascular Bio-Imaging markers) registry. Diagn Interv Radiol. 2019;25(1):35–41.

Chapter 14
Sarcopenia and Muscle Metabolism in Cardiovascular–Kidney–Metabolic Syndrome: Pathophysiology, Clinical Implications, and Therapeutic Strategies

Adina Carmen Ilie, Anca Iuliana Pîslaru, Sabinne-Marie Albişteanu, and Ioana Dana Alexa

Introduction

The frequent overlap between cardiovascular disease, renal disease, and metabolic disorders-accompanied by increased morbidity and mortality and common mechanisms-led to a new conceptual framework. In this context, a recent statement by the American Heart Association (AHA), published in the journal *Circulation*, defines the negative interplay among these conditions as the CKM syndrome (CKM) [1]. Data from the NHANES study indicate that nearly 90% of American adults have the early stages (stage 1 or 2) of the syndrome, highlighting an alarming prevalence and underscoring the need for effective preventive interventions, as also confirmed by other data [2–4].

Sarcopenia is a progressive and generalized muscle disorder and a major geriatric concern, associated with frailty and an increased risk of falls, fractures, functional dependence, and mortality [5]. The most used definition of sarcopenia is proposed by the European Working Group on Sarcopenia in Older People (EWGSOP2). According to this definition, low muscle mass is a key characteristic, and the diagnosis is confirmed by both reduced muscle quantity and quality. Poor physical performance indicates a severe form of sarcopenia. The diagnostic criteria for sarcopenia include the loss of muscle mass, decreased muscle strength, and functional decline-typically assessed through grip strength and gait speed [6].

The clinical relevance of sarcopenia has numerous major concerns related to health and quality of life. Among these are the increased risk of falls, fractures, and immobility, loss of autonomy, with a reduced ability to perform daily activities, association with other conditions (such as cardiovascular disease, respiratory

A. C. Ilie (✉) · A. I. Pîslaru · S.-M. Albişteanu · I. D. Alexa
Grigore T Popa University of Medicine and Pharmacy, Iasi, Romania
e-mail: adina.ilie@umfiasi.ro

M. Floria, D. M. Tanase (eds.), *Cardiovascular-Kidney-Metabolic Syndrome*,
https://doi.org/10.1007/978-3-032-11445-7_14

disorders, and cognitive decline) and the economic impact, including prolonged hospitalizations and the associated healthcare costs [6, 7].

The prevalence of sarcopenia among adults aged 60 and over ranges from 10% to 27%. The incidence of sarcopenia increases with age, particularly affecting individuals over the age of 80 [8, 9]. Other data indicate that sarcopenia affects between 10% and 16% of older adults worldwide [10].

The mechanisms of interaction between the CKM syndrome and muscle metabolism are bidirectional and involve numerous pathways of mutual amplification. Excess visceral adipose tissue and ectopic fat deposition in organs such as the liver, heart, and skeletal muscles are commonly observed in CKM syndrome. These fat accumulations are associated with the development of insulin resistance, systemic inflammation, and oxidative stress, all of which contribute to muscle protein degradation and a reduction in muscle mass [1].

Furthermore, in the context of chronic kidney disease, the inefficient elimination of toxins can lead to the accumulation of substances that negatively affect muscle metabolism, promoting protein catabolism and muscle mass loss [11].

The coexistence of CKM syndrome and sarcopenia amplifies the risk of all-cause mortality and cardiovascular events. A recent study stated that patients with both conditions have a significantly higher risk of mortality, particularly among men and individuals under the age of 60 [12]. Muscle metabolism is recognized for its major implications in ensuring and maintaining metabolic balance within the body. Muscle is a true metabolic organ, contributing 30% of the basal metabolic rate. It is the primary consumer of glucose during physical exercise and of lipids during the postexercise recovery process [13]. This process is stimulated by insulin, thereby playing a crucial role in insulin resistance [14].

Muscles, by modifying their mass and metabolic demands, compensate for the needs of other organs. Additionally, muscles regulate body metabolism through the secretion of muscle-derived factors, known as myokines or myometabolites, which exert autocrine, paracrine, and endocrine effects. The general deficiency of muscle mass in sarcopenia can disrupt inter-tissue communication and the systemic metabolic control exerted by muscles, increasing the risk of developing age-related diseases such as obesity, diabetes, cardiovascular diseases, cancer, and overall mortality [15, 16].

The increasing prevalence of metabolic syndrome (MetS), along with age-related muscle loss, leads to a high prevalence of sarcopenia. A vicious cycle between muscle loss and intramuscular fat accumulation can be associated with MetS through a complex interaction of factors such as nutritional intake, physical activity, body fat percentage, oxidative stress, pro-inflammatory cytokines, insulin resistance, hormonal changes, and mitochondrial dysfunction. Sarcopenia associated with MetS has significant health consequences. Although there is currently no consensus on the treatment of sarcopenia, lifestyle changes, including diet and strength training exercises, appear to be the best option [17, 18].

Pathophysiology of Sarcopenia in Cardiovascular-Kidney-Metabolic Syndrome

Role of Chronic Inflammation and Oxidative Stress

Sarcopenia is essential in the CKM syndrome, as it negatively affects the prognosis of patients through multiple interconnected mechanisms [19– 22].

In the center of the pathogenesis of cardiovascular diseases, diabetes, chronic kidney damage, and even sarcopenia lie two interconnected mechanisms: oxidative stress and inflammation. Oxidative stress occurs when the excessive production of reactive oxygen species (ROS) exceeds the body's ability to neutralize them through its antioxidant systems. Inflammation, on the other hand, is a protective response triggered by tissue injury or infections. Research shows that these processes not only play a crucial role in the onset of these diseases but also contribute to their progression [23].

Sarcopenia and cardiovascular diseases present a bidirectional relationship, maintained by common pathogenic factors such as chronic inflammation, oxidative stress, mitochondrial dysfunction, and hormonal alterations, which affect both the myocardium and skeletal muscle. Cardiac dysfunction promotes muscle atrophy by reducing tissue perfusion, activating catabolic processes, and disrupting muscle regeneration, while sarcopenia worsens the progression of cardiovascular diseases by decreasing exercise tolerance and disrupting the metabolic and endocrine functions of muscle [24].

Chronic inflammation, often associated with aging or metabolic conditions, promotes the release of pro-inflammatory cytokines, which contribute to muscle protein degradation and inhibit cellular repair processes. At the same time, oxidative stress damages cellular structures in muscles, affecting the mitochondria and altering their function in energy production required for muscle contraction. These interconnected processes accelerate muscle mass loss and the decline in muscle strength, essential factors in the development of sarcopenia [23].

Increased oxidative stress and inflammation reinforce each other and manifest in many diseases associated with skeletal muscle loss. Experimental data show a significant negative relationship between muscle protein synthesis rates and circulating concentrations of immune activation markers, such as IL-6 and TNF-α, highlighting the negative impact of inflammatory status on muscle quality and integrity [25, 26]. TNF-α plays a crucial role in triggering cellular apoptosis in muscles, which, along with inflammation and oxidative stress, contributes to the loss of muscle mass and strength. Inflammation negatively affects muscles either directly, through catabolic actions, or indirectly, by reducing levels of growth hormone (GH) and insulin-like growth factor (IGF-1) or inducing anorexia. Moreover, the decline in IGF-1 is correlated with sarcopenia, frailty, and an increased risk of mortality, while the anorexigenic effects of cytokines such as TNF-α underscore the importance of nutrition in the prevention of sarcopenia [25, 26].

NADPH oxidase is the primary source of superoxide anions (·O2−) in cardiovascular tissues, playing a role in endothelial dysfunction and cardiac and renal remodeling. Although reactive oxygen species (ROS) generated by the activity of this enzyme are involved in physiological cellular processes, excessive activation and an imbalance between ROS production and antioxidant systems lead to oxidative stress, negatively impacting cardiac, vascular, and renal function, as well as the integrity of muscle mass. ROS modulate critical signaling pathways, apoptosis, proliferation, and hydro-electrolyte homeostasis. Free radicals such as ·O2−, ClO−, •OH, ONOO−, and oxidized species of proteins and lipids are transient and are neutralized by endogenous antioxidant mechanisms [11].

In the context of obesity, increased exposure to excess fatty acids, angiotensin II, and aldosterone, as well as high salt intake, promotes alterations in signaling pathways, including the functions of ion channels, mitogenic and transcription factors, and tyrosine kinases/phosphatases. The impact of reactive oxygen species (ROS) is influenced by the local balance between pro- and antioxidant mechanisms, whether in the heart, aorta, or kidneys [11, 27].

In sarcopenic obesity and metabolic syndrome, adipocytes undergo hypertrophy and hyperplasia, facilitating the infiltration of adipose tissue with pro-inflammatory macrophages and other immune cells. These cells excessively secrete adipokines and pro-inflammatory cytokines such as leptin, adiponectin, TNF-α, IL-6, and CRP, negatively affecting hypothalamic, hepatic, pancreatic, and muscular functions. Alteration of the adipokine profile may stimulate food intake and reduce insulin sensitivity in skeletal muscles. Additionally, intramuscular lipid deposits contribute to insulin resistance and mitochondrial dysfunction, exacerbating muscle atrophy. These mechanisms, associated with chronic inflammation and metabolic dysfunction, form the basis for the development of sarcopenia in the context of obesity [17].

Oxidative stress and chronic inflammation are implicated in the onset of endothelial dysfunction, which is also considered a precursor to atherosclerosis. Higashi et al. highlighted in their analysis how these processes mutually amplify each other, leading to cardiovascular complications. Oxidative stress, triggered by the activation of NADPH oxidase, xanthine oxidase, and mitochondrial dysfunction, contributes to endothelial damage. At the same time, chronic inflammation supports the progression of atherosclerosis [28].

All of these processes generate reactive oxygen species (ROS), which contribute to endothelial damage and, consequently, to the disruption of blood flow and the supply of oxygen and nutrients to skeletal muscles. At the same time, chronic inflammation plays a crucial role in the progression of atherosclerosis, amplifying vascular damage and reducing the metabolic capacity of muscles.

Role of Endocrine Dysregulation

Insulin resistance represents both a cause and an effect of metabolic syndrome as well as sarcopenia. It promotes hyperglycemia, dyslipidemia, and increased secretion of biliary cholesterol, exacerbating metabolic syndrome. At the muscular level, it stimulates protein degradation, inhibits their synthesis, and activates autophagy through increased expression of FoxO factors. The accumulation of lipids and local inflammation impair insulin signaling, while mitochondrial oxidative stress, through reactive oxygen species (ROS) and nuclear factor kappa B (NF-κB), accelerates muscle atrophy. Chronic low-grade inflammation, pro-inflammatory cytokines, lipotoxicity, and altered muscle fiber composition further contribute to metabolic dysfunction and the progression of insulin resistance [29].

A study that analyzed the association between metabolic syndrome, its components, and sarcopenia using a large sample of nearly 15,000 participants identified a significant association between metabolic syndrome and sarcopenia among men [29]. Additionally, another study stated that insulin resistance is a significant determinant of sarcopenia in the advanced stages of kidney disease, negatively affecting the anabolic response of insulin in skeletal muscle [30].

The primary target organ of insulin is skeletal muscle, which accounts for 40–50% of lean body mass in adults. Insulin resistance refers to the reduced response of skeletal muscle target cells to insulin and the impaired glucose metabolism in cells throughout the body, leading to the development of sarcopenia. It has been confirmed that insulin resistance plays a significant role in the pathogenesis of sarcopenia by inducing muscle atrophy, primarily through the following mechanisms: increased protein catabolism and decreased protein synthesis in skeletal muscles, increased expression of the FoxO family, which reduces muscle mass either directly or by enhancing protein degradation and autophagy in skeletal muscle cells [31].

In individuals with obesity, elevated insulin levels are required to maintain glucose homeostasis and lipid metabolism in insulin-sensitive tissues, such as muscles, liver, and adipose tissue. Additionally, insulin also acts on "nontraditional" tissues, such as the heart, aorta, and kidneys. Insulin resistance is not uniform, selectively affecting tissue responses. The reduced insulin metabolic signaling leads to impaired glucose utilization and vascular dysfunction. This imbalance contributes to altered nitric oxide-mediated vasodilation. In parallel, the hyperactivation of certain insulin pathways stimulates the sympathetic nervous system and the renin-angiotensin-aldosterone system (RAAS). The result is chronic inflammation, oxidative stress, and salt retention. All of these mechanisms promote the development of the CKM syndrome [11, 32].

The exact mechanisms leading to muscle mass loss are not fully understood, but several factors contribute to sarcopenia, sarcopenic obesity, and sarcopenia associated with metabolic syndrome, including changes in circulating steroid hormone levels. There are significant differences between the effects of androgens and estrogens on skeletal muscles, and these effects depend on the expression of muscle receptors and the sensitivity of different muscle types to these hormones [17].

Women, having more adipose tissue and reduced muscle strength, are more predisposed to the loss of muscle function. In men, grip strength declines faster than muscle mass, especially in the upper body. Aging affects muscle quality through the loss of type 2 fibers, increased levels of pro-inflammatory cytokines, and neurogenic changes. The infiltration of adipose tissue into muscles, particularly in the thigh muscle, is a strong predictor of mobility limitations and is correlated with lower muscle mass and reduced muscle strength [17].

Testosterone stimulates protein synthesis and inhibits protein degradation in muscle cells, playing an important role in increasing muscle mass by replicating and activating satellite cells in muscle fibers. After the age of 35–40, circulating testosterone levels decrease by approximately 1–3% per year, and the obvious clinical signs of relative testosterone deficiency in men include decreased muscle and bone strength and mass, as well as increased central body fat. Additionally, testosterone stimulates muscle anabolism by increasing the expression of mRNA for insulin-like growth factor (IGF-1), an important anabolic hormone. A decrease in free testosterone, lack of physical activity, and cardiovascular diseases are significant predictors of sarcopenia. Moreover, estrogens, which are produced through the aromatization of testosterone, may also contribute to sarcopenia, and estradiol (E2) deficiency in older men leads to hypergonadotropism, osteoporosis, and decreased muscle mass [17].

Estrogen plays a protective role in cardiac, smooth, and skeletal muscles, contributing to the maintenance of muscle mass. Although the mechanisms are not fully understood, estrogens exhibit antioxidant activity, stabilize cell membranes, and regulate gene expression through specific receptors. They enhance contractile function by directly activating muscle fibers. The decrease in estrogen levels during menopause leads to accelerated loss of muscle mass and strength. Estrogen deficiency promotes systemic inflammation (CRP, TNF-α, IL-1, IL-6), with catabolic effects on muscle tissue [33].

Growth hormone (GH), essential for muscle mass development, progressively decreases after the age of 30. In older individuals, hormone supplementation has not been shown to be effective against sarcopenia and has had minor adverse effects. In obesity, free fatty acids inhibit GH secretion and reduce IGF-1 levels. A recent study showed lower GH secretion in obese individuals with sarcopenia compared to those without sarcopenia, and a GH receptor analog improved body composition without affecting glucose homeostasis or inducing adverse reactions [17].

The renin-angiotensin system (RAS) is an important regulator of skeletal muscle mass. It includes both the classical axis (angiotensin II, angiotensin-converting enzyme (ACE), AT1 and AT2 receptors) and the nonclassical axis (angiotensin 1–7, ACE2, and the Mas receptor), which are present in skeletal muscles and influence muscle function through the differential expression of the biochemical and metabolic characteristics of muscle fibers. The metabolic effects of RAS on skeletal muscles are multifaceted. Activation of the classical RAS axis has negative effects, such as muscle degradation. In contrast, angiotensin 1–7 has beneficial effects, inhibiting catabolic pathways of sarcomeric proteins and preventing atrophy induced by TGF-β. Treatment with angiotensin 1–7 has demonstrated the maintenance of muscle strength and prevention of reductions in muscle diameter and mass through the activation of IGF-1 and Akt pathways, which can also improve insulin resistance in skeletal muscle. Additionally, angiotensin 1–7 has positive effects on insulin resistance, hypertriglyceridemia, hepatic steatosis, inflammation, obesity, and oxidative stress. As such, some researchers suggest the use of angiotensin-converting enzyme inhibitors to modulate the renin-angiotensin-aldosterone system, promoting the production of angiotensin 1–7, altering body composition, preventing sarcopenia, and metabolic syndrome [17, 34].

Increased levels of aldosterone are correlated with visceral adiposity, and adipose tissue expresses a local renin-angiotensin-aldosterone system (RAAS), suggesting an autocrine-paracrine role. Angiotensin II (Ang II), the main effector of RAAS, acts through AT1R, triggering vasoconstrictive and pro-oxidative effects, partially counterbalanced by AT2R, affecting insulin signaling. Aldosterone has profibrotic, pro-inflammatory, and pro-oxidative effects in the heart, blood vessels, and kidneys, reducing nitric oxide availability and promoting tissue remodeling [34, 35].

Role of Mitochondrial Dysfunction and Impaired Bioenergetics

Mitochondrial oxidative phosphorylation (OXPHOS) represents the primary energy source during intense muscular contractions, especially in oxidative fibers, which are rich in mitochondria. Glycolytic fibers, which are poorer in mitochondria, support short bursts of high-intensity effort. In skeletal muscle, mitochondria form an interconnected network that facilitates the rapid distribution of energy. Various mitochondrial types, strategically located (paravascular, I-band, longitudinal, and transverse), contribute to the efficient production and transport of ATP. Mitochondrial dynamics involve fusion and fission, essential processes for maintaining functionality and removing residual components, thereby ensuring cellular energy homeostasis [15].

Since skeletal muscle is a postmitotic tissue, maintaining mitochondrial function depends on the balance between biogenesis (the formation of new mitochondria), fusion (the integration of new mitochondria into the network), fission (the fragmentation of the network to isolate damaged parts), and mitophagy (the selective removal of defective mitochondria through autophagy). These mechanisms, collectively referred to as mitochondrial dynamics, are essential for the quality of the mitochondrial network. Disruptions in this balance contribute to muscular dysfunction and are implicated in sarcopenia and other associated pathologies [15].

Mitochondrial dysfunction plays a central role in the pathophysiology of the CKM syndrome (CRS), being involved in both heart failure (HF) and chronic kidney diseases (CKD). In fact, in vitro and animal experiments have confirmed this aspect. According to recent data, maintaining mitochondrial homeostasis may be a promising therapeutic strategy to break the vicious cycle between heart failure and acute kidney injury (AKI)/CKD [36].

The loss of mitochondrial integrity affects ATP production, protein balance, calcium handling, oxidative stress levels, and inflammation factors that contribute to aging and CKM syndrome. With aging, the capacity of mitochondria in skeletal muscle to produce energy declines, especially under conditions of maximal effort. This decline is accompanied by an increased production of free radicals (ROS), which further damage mitochondrial DNA and the respiratory chain. In sarcopenia, the calcium exchange between mitochondria and the sarcoplasmic reticulum is reduced, affecting the muscle's energetic response to contractions. Thus, functional mitochondrial decline is closely linked to the loss of muscle strength and a reduction in mitochondrial plasticity over time [15].

Additionally, in healthy cells, the number of mitochondria adapts according to the energy demands through a balance between biogenesis and mitophagy. Mitochondrial biogenesis is regulated by coactivators PGC-1α and PGC-1β, which are activated by stimuli such as physical exercise, fasting, or cold exposure. With aging, the expression of PGC-1α/β decreases, which also contributes to mitochondrial decline [15].

A study shows that in type 4 cardiorenal metabolic syndrome (CRS4), a common complication of chronic kidney disease (CKD), there is a negative regulation of PGC-1α expression in the myocardium. This regulation is mediated by the transcription factor IRF1, which is activated by hyperphosphatemia, a characteristic marker of CKD. By directly binding to the promoter region of PGC-1α, IRF1 inhibits its transcription, thereby affecting mitochondrial biogenesis and myocardial energy metabolism. Restoring PGC-1α expression or inhibiting IRF1 protects the heart from metabolic remodeling and myocardial hypertrophy induced by hyperphosphatemia, suggesting that the IRF1-PGC-1α axis plays a central role in the pathogenesis of CRS4 [37].

A decrease in PGC-1α expression specific to muscle tissue results in an accelerated aging phenotype, characterized by mitochondrial dysfunction, increased inflammation, reduced muscle strength, and impaired motor coordination. In contrast, the overexpression of PGC-1α in muscle tissue delays the aging process and is associated with younger muscle metabolism, such as a favorable transcriptome, optimal mitochondrial function, intact neuromuscular architecture, and efficient calcium homeostasis, contributing even to a moderate extension of lifespan [15].

In the context of mitochondrial stress, skeletal muscle releases two key myomitokines—FGF21 and GDF15—which mediate both local and systemic adaptive responses. These molecules are minimally expressed under normal conditions, but their levels increase significantly in response to stressors such as physical exercise or mitochondrial dysfunction. At moderate levels, FGF21 and GDF15 exert beneficial effects on metabolism, enhance metabolic flexibility, protect against obesity and insulin resistance, and may even contribute to lifespan extension. However, chronically elevated and sustained levels of these myomitokines are associated with age-related chronic diseases, including type 2 diabetes, cardiovascular disease, cancer, and sarcopenia. Thus, they may represent a critical link in the pathophysiology of the CKM syndrome [15, 36].

Mitochondrial diabetes is a genetic defect of pancreatic β-cells characterized by impaired insulin secretion due to insufficient mitochondrial ATP production. Additionally, insulin resistance is recognized as a second major pathophysiological mechanism, closely linked to mitochondrial dysfunction through processes that affect muscle metabolism, as previously mentioned. A decline in the mitochondrial capacity to oxidize NADH leads to an increased NADH/NAD^+ ratio, promoting the formation of reactive oxygen species (ROS) that further compromise mitochondrial function. This imbalance contributes to decreased insulin sensitivity in skeletal muscle by impairing insulin signaling and glucose uptake. Moreover, endoplasmic reticulum stress, inflammation, and insulin receptor dysfunction exacerbate insulin resistance, worsening metabolic disturbances and disrupting muscular energy homeostasis [28, 38].

Role of Autophagy and Proteolytic Pathways in Muscle Degradation

Autophagy is an essential process through which cells degrade damaged proteins and organelles, with skeletal muscles being among the most active tissues in this regard. Although excessive activation can lead to muscle atrophy, both upregulation and downregulation of autophagy affect insulin sensitivity and muscle degradation. Insulin inhibits autophagy by activating mTORC1 and interfering with TFEB, while mTORC2 exerts variable effects depending on the physiological context. FoxO3 induces autophagy by activating the E3 ubiquitin ligase FBXO32, and under nutrient stress, excessive activation of autophagy may contribute to sarcopenia. However, in certain cases, increased autophagy decreases endoplasmic reticulum stress and improves insulin sensitivity. Inhibition of genes such as ATG7 or Atg16l1 has been associated with muscle atrophy and impaired insulin response. Therefore, maintaining autophagic balance is crucial, and the PI3K-AKT-mTORC signaling pathway remains a key regulatory axis in the interaction between insulin and skeletal muscle, offering potential therapeutic targets [31].

Understanding the autophagy-lysosome and ubiquitin-proteasome degradation systems, including their associated signaling pathways such as AKT and its major effectors, mTOR and FoxO3, is essential for elucidating the cellular mechanisms regulating protein homeostasis and stress responses. The critical role of autophagy has been highlighted in maintaining cellular homeostasis, regulating glycogen levels, organelle turnover, and protein quality control. Due to the importance of proteostasis in cell survival, recent research has focused on the involvement of these mechanisms in muscle atrophy. Both excessive activation and significant inhibition of protein degradation can contribute to muscle degeneration through distinct mechanisms [39–41].

The two major protein degradation pathways, the ubiquitin-proteasome system and the autophagy-lysosome system, are activated during muscle atrophy and contribute variably to the loss of muscle mass. These degradation systems are regulated by a transcriptional program that modulates the expression of key enzymes controlling these proteolytic pathways. FoxO transcription factors, which are negatively regulated by the Insulin-Akt signaling pathway, and NF-κB, which is activated by inflammatory cytokines, were among the first identified as critical mediators of the atrophy process [42].

The ubiquitin-proteasome system (UPS) is essential for the degradation of damaged or unnecessary proteins. In the CKM syndrome, oxidative stress and inflammation can impair UPS function, leading to the accumulation of damaged proteins and cellular dysfunction. Activation of the NF-κB pathway, mediated by UPS, is associated with chronic inflammation and impaired cardiac and renal function. Proteasome inhibition has shown protective effects in certain models of heart disease, suggesting a potential therapeutic role for UPS modulation [43].

Evidence from the scientific literature increasingly highlights the involvement of proteotoxicity—defined as the result of impaired protein quality control in the pathophysiology of metabolic disorders and their associated cardiovascular complications. In this context, the ubiquitin-proteasome system (UPS) and the autophagy-lysosomal pathway, two essential but functionally distinct cellular mechanisms, contribute to the maintenance of protein homeostasis. Thus, they can be valuable therapeutic targets in the integrative management of CKMS [44].

Studies over the past two decades have confirmed the important role of the ubiquitin-proteasome system in mediating muscle proteolysis, particularly of myofibrillar proteins. However, recent observations have shown that autophagy, calpains, and caspases also contribute to the turnover of muscle proteins under catabolic states. Furthermore, these diverse proteolytic systems interact with each other at various levels [45]. Calpains, calcium-dependent proteases, play a crucial role in the degradation of muscle proteins under catabolic conditions. In the CKMS, excessive activation of calpains has been associated with the deterioration of cardiac and renal function. For example, in experimental models of diabetes, calpain activation led to the degradation of essential proteins for autophagy, such as Atg5 and LAMP2, exacerbating myocardial damage [46].

The IGF1/AKT pathway plays a crucial role in maintaining muscle mass and preventing atrophy. Studies have shown that activation of this pathway inhibits FOXO transcription factors, reducing the expression of ubiquitin ligases such as MuRF1 and Atrogin-1, which are involved in the degradation of muscle proteins. In nonischemic dilated cardiomyopathy, a decrease in the expression of AKT and FOXO1 has been observed, suggesting dysregulation of this pathway in CKMS [47, 48]. Changes in protein synthesis are evident in animal models and in patients with chronic kidney disease, with the insulin/IGF-1-PI3K-Akt pathway playing a crucial role in stimulating protein synthesis by activating mTOR and inhibiting the FoxO protein. Insulin resistance contributes to muscle atrophy, while treatments with IGF-1 and testosterone can reduce FoxO expression and promote protein synthesis. Therapies targeting these mechanisms, such as metformin, testosterone, selective androgen receptor modulators, and amino acid supplementation, can aid in combating sarcopenia in chronic kidney disease [49].

Myostatin, a member of the TGF-β family, is a potent inhibitor of muscle growth. By activating ActRIIB receptors and the Smad2/3/4 pathway, myostatin suppresses protein synthesis and stimulates muscle protein degradation. In metabolic syndrome, elevated levels of myostatin have been associated with obesity, insulin resistance, and muscle atrophy, indicating a significant role in the pathogenesis of CKMS [47, 50].

In CKDs, uremic toxins accumulate in the blood as renal function declines, playing a central role in the development of sarcopenia associated with chronic kidney disease. Toxins such as p-cresyl sulfate and indoxyl sulfate influence the insulin signaling pathway and promote muscle atrophy by activating factors like myostatin and atrogin-1, while also increasing levels of reactive oxygen species and inflammatory cytokines. Although treatments aimed at eliminating these toxins, such as AST-120, have shown benefits in animal models, clinical studies in humans have not demonstrated significant improvements, highlighting the need for more effective targeted therapies [49].

Clinical Implications of Sarcopenia in CKM Syndrome

Impact on Cardiovascular Health

Cardiometabolic diseases represent an escalating global health problem, slowing down or even reversing the previous decline in cardiovascular disease-related mortality. Scientific evidence highlights a significant interaction between sarcopenia and cardiovascular health in the context of the CKM syndrome, with implications that affect cardiac function, arterial stiffness, and frailty [51].

Sarcopenia is commonly observed in patients with heart failure (both reduced and preserved ejection fraction), coronary artery disease, and peripheral artery disease, as well as in the context of valvuloplasty interventions or cardiac surgery. Sarcopenia exacerbates cardiovascular symptoms through the loss of muscle mass and function, and is closely linked to chronic inflammation, oxidative stress, and malnutrition. It also negatively impacts postoperative recovery [52].

Sarcopenia significantly contributes to the worsening of myocardial remodeling processes and the deterioration of left ventricular function, most likely through mechanisms associated with chronic inflammation and oxidative stress characteristic of the cardiometabolic syndrome. A reduction in muscle mass has been correlated with increased arterial stiffness, which may promote higher systolic blood pressure and an increased incidence of cardiovascular events. Furthermore, the presence of frailty, frequently coexisting with sarcopenia, is associated with an unfavorable cardiovascular prognosis and an increased risk of repeated hospitalizations, creating a pathological cycle where heart failure exacerbates muscle atrophy, and the latter contributes to cardiac function decompensation. These interactions are particularly pronounced in older patients with CKMS, as insulin resistance and chronic systemic inflammation further compromise muscle protein synthesis, thus amplifying the impact of sarcopenia on cardiovascular risk [24].

Sarcopenia is very common among individuals with heart failure, with a prevalence ranging from 10% to 68%, being more frequently observed in men than in women [22]. Although the prevalence of sarcopenia among patients with cardiovascular conditions varies widely, studies show a significantly increased incidence in both acute and chronic heart failure, as well as in arrhythmias, highlighting the importance of recognizing this association in clinical practice [24].

Sarcopenia is common in chronic heart failure and represents an important predictive factor for frailty, reduced survival, and progression to cardiac cachexia. Despite some therapeutic advances based on physical exercise, nutrition, and pharmacological agents under investigation, such as synthetic ghrelin and androgen receptor modulators, cachexia remains a severe and underdiagnosed complication, with a major negative impact on the prognosis of patients with heart failure. Factors such as malnutrition, intestinal congestion, and the cytokine storm exacerbate this condition. Elevated levels of adiponectin indicate changes in body composition and may serve as a biomarker for cachexia and mortality in heart failure [54].

The association between sarcopenia and cardiac dysfunction significantly increases the risk of heart failure, even in young patients with idiopathic dilated cardiomyopathy, where loss of body mass is common, even in the absence of other major comorbidities. In CKMS, the simultaneous deterioration of both cardiac and renal function promotes the onset of cachexia and sarcopenic obesity, phenomena influenced by the activation of the inflammatory, neuroendocrine, and oxidative stress systems [17, 52, 53].

The concomitant presence of metabolic syndrome and sarcopenia is associated with a significantly increased risk of overall and cardiovascular mortality, particularly in men and individuals under the age of 60, compared to the presence of a single condition [12].

Reduced muscle mass, a central component of sarcopenia, has been associated with an unfavorable prognosis in acute coronary syndromes, being identified as a predictor of major cardiovascular events and mortality through indices such as the creatinine/cystatin C ratio and the psoas muscle index [55].

Sarcopenia is associated with an increased risk of atrial fibrillation; the risk is higher in patients with reduced muscle mass and strength, particularly in women, individuals under 65 years of age, and those with valvular diseases. Additionally, sarcopenia may influence the metabolism of direct oral anticoagulants, increasing the risk of bleeding, highlighting the need for evaluating muscle mass in the management of patients with atrial fibrillation [55].

Another data highlight a higher prevalence of sarcopenia in patients with cardiovascular diseases, particularly heart failure and arrhythmias, suggesting common mechanisms that negatively affect their survival and prognosis. Early screening and physical interventions are essential for improving quality of life, and future research should explore the causal relationship between sarcopenia and cardiovascular diseases for more effective treatments [24].

Renal Complications

In chronic kidney disease (CKD), sarcopenia is common and correlated with poor prognosis. Inflammation, metabolic acidosis, and malnutrition play a bidirectional role between sarcopenia and renal impairment.

The prevalence of sarcopenia varies depending on the type of renal treatment, being higher in patients undergoing hemodialysis (5.9–14% in CKD patients without renal replacement therapy; 13.7–42.2% in patients on hemodialysis; 4–15.5% in those on peritoneal dialysis) and significantly impacts physical performance, disability risk, mortality, and cardiovascular events.

Sarcopenia in CKD patients is associated with reduced physical performance, increased risk of disability, hypotension during hemodialysis, increased mortality, and cardiovascular events. Risk factors include malnutrition, low body mass index, age, male sex, diabetes, prolonged dialysis duration, and type of dialysis [49].

Sarcopenia occurs in patients with impaired renal function, characterized by a low glomerular filtration rate and an elevated albumin-to-creatinine ratio. Patients with CKD exhibit significantly lower muscle strength compared to age-matched individuals without renal disease, which is associated with factors such as neurological dysfunction, inflammation, fat infiltration of muscles, and hormonal imbalances. Muscle strength decreases as kidney disease advances, and recovery is more common in the early stages of the disease [49].

Participants with CKD and sarcopenia had a 33% higher risk of mortality and a lower 10-year survival probability. They also had a doubled risk of developing end-stage renal disease. Sarcopenia was associated with advanced age, inflammation, lower renal function, and lower serum albumin, total testosterone, and hemoglobin levels [56, 57].

Sarcopenia in CKD is not only associated with increased mortality but also has multiple other negative consequences. These include reduced functional capacity and quality of life, increased risk of falls and hospitalizations, as well as a decreased ability to tolerate specific treatments, such as dialysis. Furthermore, sarcopenia may contribute to the faster progression of CKD by disrupting metabolic balance, exacerbating systemic inflammation, and reducing the protein reserves necessary to maintain homeostasis [58].

Currently, the scientific literature does not provide direct evidence that sarcopenia significantly contributes to the worsening of metabolic acidosis in patients with CKD. However, there is a pathophysiological hypothesis suggesting that muscle mass loss could reduce the body's ability to buffer excess acids, given that skeletal muscles play a crucial role in maintaining acid-base balance. Thus, in the context of CKD, where the renal excretion of acids is already impaired, sarcopenia could theoretically exacerbate the acid-base imbalance [58].

Sarcopenia and relative sarcopenia are significantly associated with mortality, regardless of the stage of chronic kidney disease. Relative sarcopenia, characterized by the loss of muscle mass and/or strength, but without meeting the strict criteria for complete sarcopenia, is nearly three times more prevalent and increases the risk of mortality. This association is weaker in individuals with a higher body mass index [59].

Metabolic Consequences

In CKMS, sarcopenia favors the development of metabolic complications such as dyslipidemia and hyperglycemia, exacerbating the metabolic imbalance of the CKM syndrome.

Sarcopenia contributes to insulin resistance through mechanisms such as abnormal lipid infiltration into skeletal muscles, lipotoxicity, and a reduction in the proportion of type I fibers. Lipid infiltration activates signaling pathways that inhibit insulin signaling, and intracellular lipid deposits, such as triglycerides and ceramides, play a key role in the development of insulin resistance. These processes are accompanied by muscle inflammation and the production of reactive oxygen species, leading to mitochondrial dysfunction and loss of oxidative capacity. Endoplasmic reticulum stress, activated by lipid accumulation, amplifies these effects and contributes to the progression of insulin resistance [31].

Diabetes is a significant risk factor for kidney disease, and it can worsen type 2 diabetes through mechanisms such as insulin resistance and insulin signaling deficiencies, particularly in skeletal muscles. Chronic inflammation, oxidative stress, metabolic acidosis, and the accumulation of renal toxins contribute to insulin resistance and the deterioration of glucose balance, thereby increasing cardiovascular risk and mortality among patients with chronic kidney disease [60].

Sarcopenia and obesity are both associated with metabolic disorders, and when they coexist, they can have negative effects on metabolic and cardiovascular health, compared to obesity or sarcopenia alone. Observational studies suggest that sarcopenic obesity is linked to metabolic abnormalities, inflammation, and cardiovascular risk factors [61, 62].

Sarcopenic obesity and nonsarcopenic obesity have a similar risk for hypertension, dyslipidemia, and metabolic syndrome, but both obesity groups present a higher risk than those with isolated sarcopenia. Sarcopenic obesity was associated with the highest risk of cardiovascular events and coronary artery disease, compared to obesity or sarcopenia [63].

Regarding type 2 diabetes (T2D), sarcopenia may contribute to its development by impairing glucose management due to reduced muscle mass and local inflammation. One study showed that sarcopenic obesity increases the risk of T2D by nearly 38% compared to isolated obesity or overweight [64].

In patients with type 2 diabetes, sarcopenia is 2–3 times more frequent than in those without diabetes. Furthermore, studies show that sarcopenic obesity is associated with a higher risk of cardiovascular diseases and mortality compared to isolated obesity or sarcopenia. Additionally, sarcopenic obesity is correlated with an increased risk of chronic kidney disease among patients with type 2 diabetes, having a more significant impact on renal function than either sarcopenia or obesity alone [62].

Relationship with Morbidity and Mortality

Epidemiological studies have consistently shown that cardiovascular, renal, and metabolic diseases frequently overlap and coexist in the same individuals. Recent data highlight the significant impact of sarcopenia on morbidity in patients with CKMS. A cohort study revealed that patients with CKD and sarcopenia have a 33% higher risk of mortality and are nearly twice as likely to develop end-stage renal disease (ESRD) compared to those without sarcopenia [56]. Additionally, a meta-analysis identified that sarcopenia increases the risk of mortality by 143% in patients with nondialyzed CKD [65].

Sarcopenic obesity, characterized by the simultaneous presence of reduced muscle mass and excess fat, is associated with additional risks. A Chinese study reported that individuals with sarcopenic obesity have a 78% higher risk of developing CKD and a 79% higher risk of rapid decline in renal function compared to those without this condition [66].

Furthermore, a prospective study showed that, in individuals with type 2 diabetes, sarcopenia is associated with an increased risk of cardiovascular diseases, heart failure, stroke, and myocardial infarction compared to individuals without sarcopenia [67].

Moreover, other recent data highlight that sarcopenic obesity is associated with significantly higher risks of hypertension, dyslipidemia, diabetes, and metabolic syndrome compared to individuals without sarcopenia or obesity [68].

Diagnostic Approaches and Biomarkers

Imaging, functional, and biochemical investigations in patients with sarcopenia and CKMS play crucial roles both in the diagnostic process and in screening and prevention. The diagnosis is under continuous research and requires further refinement through studies. Table 14.1 summarizes the main investigations that are useful, along with their advantages and disadvantages for this vulnerable patient group.

Table 14.1 Diagnostic approaches and biomarkers in patients with sarcopenia and CKMS

Investigation type	Advantages	Disadvantages
DXA (dual-energy X-ray absorptiometry)	Accurately measures lean muscle mass, fat mass, and bone mineral density [62, 69, 70] Particularly useful in patients with chronic kidney disease (CKD) Provides prognostic value in patients with sarcopenia or muscle disorders Radiation free Strong correlation with CT and MRI measurements [71]	High cost Requires trained personnel Cannot be used at the bedside Unable to assess intramuscular fat Inter-device variability Results may be influenced by hydration status in CKD patients
BIA (bioelectrical impedance analysis)	Noninvasive, low cost, and easy to perform at the bedside, including in nephrology or cardiology wards [70] Estimates body composition: Lean mass, fat mass, and total body water-Relevant for monitoring patients with fluid retention or cachexia [69] Useful for tracking muscle changes in chronic cardio-renal diseases Allows for repeated screening, including in outpatient settings Provides indirect data on hydration status, valuable in heart failure and chronic kidney disease	Sensitive to changes in hydration status-a major limitation in patients with heart or kidney failure Requires strict standardization to ensure reliable results Does not assess muscle quality or myosteatosis Less accurate than CT or MRI for muscle mass estimation Inter-device variability-Challenges in comparing results across different centers

(continued)

Table 14.1 (continued)

Investigation type	Advantages	Disadvantages
Ultrasound (sonography)	Non-radiating, low cost, portable-Ideal for repeated use in cardiology or nephrology units [72] Detects muscle fibrosis, inflammation, and intramuscular fat (myosteatosis), relevant in cachexia and chronic low-grade inflammation seen in this syndrome Can be used during hemodialysis, allowing real-time muscle status monitoring Valid alternative to MRI/CT/DXA for assessing muscle mass in patients with fluid shifts due to heart or kidney failure [69] Provides insight into both muscle quantity and quality-Critical in detecting hidden sarcopenia in metabolic or volume-overloaded patients [73, 75] Measurements on the vastus intermedius or diaphragm may predict cardiovascular events or mortality in dialysis patients Minimally affected by fluid retention or removal-Advantageous in managing volume status in heart failure or CKD [70, 73, 74] Useful in early detection and tracking of sarcopenia or sarcopenic obesity, which commonly complicate. CKM conditions [72] Shear wave elastography and panoramic ultrasound allow evaluation of muscle stiffness and microvascular changes, offering added value in identifying muscular and metabolic alterations Supported by the European geriatric medicine society as a predictive tool for sarcopenia and its comorbidities in aging patients with chronic disease burden [69]	Results may vary depending on the operator Lack of widespread standardization Requires training for accurate and reproducible assessments Less commonly used in longitudinal studies Evidence for its diagnostic accuracy in sarcopenia remains limited [71]

(continued)

Table 14.1 (continued)

Investigation type	Advantages	Disadvantages
MRI (magnetic resonance imaging)	Detects microstructural muscle changes, including edema, fibrosis, inflammation, and fatty infiltration, which are common in chronic heart and kidney disease [70, 71] Enables early identification of myosteatosis and sarcopenia, supporting timely interventions in at-risk patients Allows differentiation of muscle hypertrophy from atrophy, aiding in the phenotyping of muscle changes related to metabolic and cardiac conditions [69] Through spectroscopy, assesses biochemical alterations in muscle tissue and intramyocellular lipids, relevant in insulin resistance and metabolic dysfunction [70–72] Provides superior soft-tissue contrast compared to CT, enabling precise evaluation of muscle quality in complex multisystem disorders	High cost, limiting routine use in clinical practice for multimorbid patients Lack of standardized reference values for muscle mass and quality in populations with chronic cardiac and renal disease Requires specialized personnel and expertise, reducing accessibility in non-tertiary care settings
CT (computed tomography)	Detects occult sarcopenia [70] Useful in patients with chronic kidney disease (CKD), as measurements are not influenced by hydration status Considered the reference method for diagnosing abnormal body composition phenotypes, particularly in nutritionally vulnerable patients [69, 70] Measures muscle volume, cross-sectional area, and skeletal muscle index-Parameters strongly associated with patient prognosis	Radiation exposure High cost Not recommended for frequent monitoring Lower accuracy of two-dimensional imaging
Anthropometry (mid-upper arm circumference, triceps skinfold thickness)	Accessible, low cost, and useful in resource-limited settings Indicates muscle mass and nutritional status in the context of CKM syndrome [70, 74, 75]	Less sensitive and specific Depends on the evaluator's experience and hydration status
Calf circumference	Simple, useful as a substitute method for skeletal muscle mass in the absence of other methods; relevant for mobility [70, 75]	High variability between populations Lack of universally applicable standards
Body shape index (BCI)	Integrates waist, BMI, and height; useful in sarcopenic obesity [70]	Does not directly measure muscle mass
Dynamometry (grip strength-Jamar/Smedley)	Reproducible Correlated with mortality and other clinical events [75] Easy to apply in clinical settings [76]	Results vary depending on device and technique

(continued)

Table 14.1 (continued)

Investigation type	Advantages	Disadvantages
Knee extension strength test (KES)	Reflects quadriceps strength; a valid alternative to handgrip strength	Requires specific equipment Not as standardized
Functional tests (5-STS-five times sit-to-stand test, gait speed, SPPB)	Easy to implement [75] Validates physical performance Predictors of sarcopenia severity [75]	Subjective methods Influenced by other comorbidities (e.g., arthritis, neurological disorders)
sEMG (surface electromyography)	Measures neuromuscular activity Can assist in identifying muscle weakness or dysfunction early [69] In conditions like sarcopenia or CKD-related muscle atrophy	Requires technical expertise Complex interpretation
RFD (rate of force development)	A sensitive indicator of early neuromuscular impairment A useful complement to traditional strength tests	Requires specialized equipment and standardized protocols
Serum creatinine	Easily accessible; indirectly reflects muscle mass (in the absence of renal dysfunction) [76]	Nonspecific; influenced by renal function and protein intake
Creatine dilution test	Direct estimation of total muscle mass [76]	Requires labeled creatine Limited clinical availability
Sarcopenia index (creatinine/cystatin C × 100)	Indirect assessment independent of renal function; predictive of mortality [76, 77]	Requires simultaneous measurement of two markers; useful only in patients with normal renal function
Myokines (Activin A, Serpin E1/PAI-1, Irisin)	Reflects muscle atrophy and fibrosis processes; can indicate muscle metabolic activity [78, 79]	Not clinically validated on a large scale; high interindividual variability
Inflammatory markers (IL-6, TNF-α, IL-1β)	Correlated with muscle mass and strength; involved in chronic inflammation (inflamm aging) [78, 79]	Nonspecific; influenced by other systemic inflammatory processes
Markers of mitochondrial dysfunction (GDF15, FGF21)	Reflect altered fatty acid oxidation and muscle energy dysfunction [78, 79]	Not routinely tested in clinical practice; levels show high variability
Extracellular matrix (ECM) and senescence markers (TIMP-1, ICAM-1, Serpin E1)	Correlated with muscle fibrosis and atrophy [78] Provide insights into tissue remodeling [78, 79]	More costly investigations Limited clinical applicability
Serum metabolites (carnosine, branched-chain amino acids, carnitine, etc.)	Identify metabolic alterations relevant to muscle function Can be modulated through nutritional and exercise interventions [79–81]	Require advanced techniques (lipidomics, metabolomics) Not widely validated

(continued)

Table 14.1 (continued)

Investigation type	Advantages	Disadvantages
Specific biomarkers (agrin, P3NP, osteonectin, FABP3, MIF)	Potential for effective screening [79, 80] Relevant for neuromuscular junction and ECM [81]	Not widely validated clinically Requires further research
Systemic inflammatory index (SII)	Strong independent marker Correlated with muscle mass and strength [79–82] Stable and easy to obtain	Not specific to sarcopenia Influenced by general inflammatory conditions

Therapeutic Strategies

Exercise Interventions

The data on the benefits of physical exercise in renal, cardiovascular, and metabolic diseases are significant. A study analyzed the importance of resistance exercises in patients with CKD, showing that, particularly those with progressive intensity and adequate supervision, can improve muscle strength and physical performance [83].

Another prospective observational study investigated a personalized physical activity program tailored to patients with metabolic syndrome. The 6-month intervention, which included moderate-intensity aerobic and resistance training, resulted in significant improvements in cardiorespiratory capacity, lipid profile, and glycemic control, independent of weight loss or dietary changes [84].

Additionally, other findings have demonstrated that physical interventions can mitigate the impact of sarcopenic obesity on cardiovascular disease risk in men. The study showed that physical activity and cardiorespiratory fitness can significantly reduce the risk of cardiovascular diseases in this population [85].

Physical exercise is an important lifestyle factor that contributes to the prevention of sarcopenia, obesity, and sarcopenic obesity. A recent review concluded that physical exercise, particularly resistance training, can improve or maintain physical performance in adults with sarcopenic obesity [86]. In the Louisiana Osteoporosis Study, it was suggested that regular exercise at least three times a week was associated with a lower risk of obesity and sarcopenic obesity in older men and women [62, 87].

Physical activity improves insulin sensitivity and can reduce the risk of type 2 diabetes (T2DM) by up to 44%. However, the application of a standardized exercise protocol for patients with T2DM, without considering the pathophysiological characteristics of muscle metabolism, may not provide optimal benefits. Physical exercise combined with mild caloric restriction reduces symptoms of sarcopenic obesity, contributing to muscle mass gain, strength development, and improvement in functional capacity [17].

Resistance exercise has proven effective in increasing muscle mass, strength, and muscle function in patients with CKMS. It enhances tissue oxygenation, increases muscle perfusion, and stimulates mitochondrial adaptations through the activation of the AMPK-PGC-1α pathway, promoting fatty acid oxidation, glucose uptake, and the removal of dysfunctional mitochondria [24]. It also stimulates mitochondrial biogenesis and increase insulin sensitivity. High-intensity training (HIT) activates key proteins such as PGC-1α, which support the metabolic and functional adaptations of muscles. Additionally, adequate nutritional supplementation combined with physical exercise has led to an increase in muscle mass and a reduction in edema in patients with heart failure [24].

Exercise protocols should include resistance exercises with progressive intensity and a frequency of at least two sessions per week. For severe sarcopenia, it is recommended to start with lower intensity exercises, gradually adjusted based on periodic functional assessments [75]. Guidelines recommend 150–300 min of moderate aerobic activity per week and muscle-strengthening activities at least twice a week to maintain muscle strength and prevent sarcopenia [75].

Resistance training is strongly recommended for improving muscle mass, strength, and physical performance in older adults, with high-quality evidence supporting this. Multiple meta-analyses have shown significant positive effects on lean body mass (e.g., +1.1 kg), muscle strength (24–33% increases in upper and lower limbs), and physical performance (e.g., increases in usual and maximum walking speed by up to 0.26 m/s). The results indicate that higher volume or high-intensity training generates the greatest benefits, and introducing resistance training at a younger age leads to superior outcomes, considering the potential decline in hypertrophic capacity with aging. However, even low-intensity training can be effective. Effective programs involve 1–4 sets of 8–15 repetitions, 2–3 times a week, focusing on large muscle groups in a full-body approach to counteract the generalized effects of sarcopenia on skeletal muscle [88].

Multimodal exercise therapy, which combines resistance training, aerobic exercise, balance, and walking, is recommended for improving muscle mass, strength, and physical function, with demonstrated beneficial effects in both healthy and frail individuals. Blood flow restriction (BFR) training, although less effective than high-load exercises, represents a valid alternative at lower intensities; however, it requires specialized supervision due to potential risks that are insufficiently documented [88].

Physical exercise provides significant functional benefits, including increased muscle mass and strength, improved gait stability, and reduced fall risk, being effective even at low intensities or through alternative methods such as muscle stimulation. In patients with diabetes, positive effects on functional parameters such as chair rise time have been highlighted, but the lack of consistent improvements in muscle strength may be attributed to the methodological limitations of the available studies [89].

Whole-body muscle stimulation has shown limited effects, highlighting the need for further research to validate its efficacy in sarcopenia management [90]. However, resistance training and whole-body muscle electrical stimulation may represent effective interventions for the prevention and treatment of sarcopenia, with both methods showing significant benefits on muscle mass and strength, varying according to the parameters analyzed and individual characteristics. While resistance exercises appear to favorably impact body composition, muscle electrical stimulation has a superior effect on increasing muscle strength, suggesting that a combined, individualized approach could optimize the prevention and treatment of sarcopenia in CKMS [91].

Moreover, increasing recent evidence supports that electrical neuromuscular stimulation has proven to be an effective and complementary method of functional training in older adults. This method appears to be particularly useful for institutionalized older individuals, by improving muscle strength, physical performance, and cardiovascular and inflammatory parameters, without significantly altering body composition. These benefits, attributed to neuromuscular adaptations and positive effects on bone metabolism and arterial stiffness, support the integration of this intervention into personalized multimodal strategies for maintaining functionality in senior individuals with reduced tolerance to conventional physical exercise [92].

Portable devices and digital health platforms are becoming valuable tools for monitoring physical activity and functional capacity. These technologies can track parameters such as walking speed, balance, and overall mobility, providing insights into muscle function and the progression of sarcopenia. Additionally, digital tools can facilitate remote monitoring, allowing healthcare providers to adjust treatment plans based on real-time data and in a personalized manner [93, 94].

Physical exercise and nutritional interventions are the most effective and well-documented strategies for preventing muscle mass loss and functional decline, exerting beneficial molecular effects such as the activation of autophagy, mitophagy, and the regulation of muscle stem cell function. Combining exercise with specific nutrients (e.g., leucine) enhances mitochondrial adaptations, while pharmacological therapies under investigation aim to mimic these effects to combat sarcopenia and age-related degenerative diseases [82].

Nutritional Approaches

Protein-deficient diets have been associated with the development of sarcopenia associated with CKMS, and the Expert Group of the European Society for Clinical Nutrition and Metabolism has recommended a protein intake of 1.0–1.2 g/kg body weight/day to help maintain muscle mass and strength in adults over 65 years of age [95–97].

Other data highlight the benefits of integrating bioactive compounds with antioxidant and anti-inflammatory properties into the diet for improving glycemic control and reducing inflammation in patients with type 2 diabetes. Additionally, the dysregulation of the circadian rhythm, exacerbated with age, has a negative impact on chronic inflammation. In this context, the concept of "inflammaging" becomes crucial in understanding the multiple comorbidities, and nutritional, pharmacological, and lifestyle interventions are promising directions for reducing oxidative stress and systemic inflammation, although further validation through additional studies is needed [23].

A strict diet can exacerbate age-related muscle loss and affect physical function, although weight loss, including the reduction of lean muscle mass, can be an effective intervention for treating sarcopenic obesity. Expert recommendations highlight the benefits of adequate protein intake (25–30 g per meal) and relatively low-carbohydrate diets to optimize muscle protein synthesis and prevent negative impacts on protein metabolism in the older people [17, 75].

Optimizing the diet in chronic inflammatory heart diseases can improve respiratory mechanics, oxygen absorption, and immune system function, while supplementation with leucine may prevent sarcopenia by stimulating muscle protein synthesis and reducing TNF-α levels. Natural antioxidant supplements, such as flavonoids and polyphenols, have beneficial effects on obesity and metabolic syndrome, reducing cardiovascular and neurodegenerative risks, while treatments with resveratrol and quercetin may protect against obesity-induced sarcopenia [17].

Sodium also plays a key role in maintaining blood pressure and fluid-electrolyte balance, being a critical determinant of cardiovascular health. Excessive salt intake is associated with hypertension, vascular damage, and an increased risk of metabolic syndrome. Although its influence on renal function and metabolism is less direct, high sodium consumption contributes to renal impairment and insulin resistance, hence the low sodium diet recommendations. Furthermore, sodium-water imbalance, manifested as mild hyponatremia, may lead to a reduction in skeletal muscle mass, suggesting a role for sodium in the development of sarcopenia within the CKM syndrome [11, 27, 34].

A study evaluated the effects of vitamin D supplementation and physical exercise on physical function, body composition, and metabolic health in overweight or obese older adults with vitamin D deficiency. The results showed significant improvements in physical function and body composition, suggesting a potential benefit of this combined intervention in managing sarcopenia and associated metabolic risks [98].

Another study evaluated the effects of vitamin D supplementation on cardiometabolic parameters in patients with metabolic syndrome. Although significant increases in serum vitamin D levels were observed, the effects on waist circumference, blood glucose, and blood pressure were limited, and the evidence was of low to moderate certainty [99].

The food groups considered myo-protective and cardioprotective include meat, fruits and vegetables, dairy products, whole grains, and fish. Although longitudinal evidence is lacking, some cross-sectional studies suggest that a healthy diet may reduce the risk of sarcopenia through higher consumption of fruits and vegetables, whole grains, and fatty fish. These foods provide essential nutrients for muscle function, such as vitamin D, long-chain polyunsaturated n-3 fatty acids, antioxidants, and proteins. Additionally, recommendations for dietary approaches should focus not only on protein intake but also on healthy fats (such as omega-3 s), hydration, the quality of calories (processed vs. unprocessed), and the potential effects of medication on nutritional intake [75].

An anti-inflammatory diet is essential in the prevention and management of sarcopenia in CKDS, being associated with a reduced risk of muscle mass loss and better functional performance. A pro-inflammatory diet, combined with nutritional deficiencies, significantly contributes to the development of sarcopenia, highlighting the importance of nutritional interventions, supplementation with essential nutrients, and the adaptation of food consistency for improved mastication and swallowing [100].

In another study, the adoption of a pro-inflammatory diet was linked to more severe symptoms of sarcopenia, suggesting that the inflammatory potential of diet may be an important modifiable risk factor in combating the progression of sarcopenia [101].

According to other data, sarcopenia has been associated with increased levels of myostatin, a negative regulator of muscle mass, and with muscle inflammation. It has also been observed in patients with chronic inflammatory conditions, and anti-inflammatory therapy has been shown to reduce inflammation-induced muscle weakness. Diets rich in pro-inflammatory foods, such as those high in sugar, refined grains, red and processed meats, or fried foods, can increase chronic inflammation and contribute to the development of sarcopenia [102].

Personalized nutrition can also target the individual genetic component of each metabolism. Thus, genetic markers related to lipid metabolism, insulin sensitivity, and nutrient absorption can guide personalized dietary interventions, optimizing metabolic outcomes and reducing the risk of sarcopenia. For example, individuals with genetic variants associated with impaired insulin sensitivity may benefit from diets that emphasize low glycemic index foods and increased fiber intake [103, 104].

Pharmacological Interventions

Myostatin Inhibitors

Myostatin (or GDF-8) is a myokine predominantly produced by skeletal muscle, playing a key role in the negative regulation of muscle growth and regeneration. In the context of sarcopenia, elevated levels or excessive activity of myostatin contribute to the loss of muscle mass and function. Inhibiting this pathway represents a promising strategy for combating sarcopenia in the CKM syndrome (CKM), particularly due to its potential impact on muscle mass, insulin sensitivity, and overall metabolic function (Table 14.2).

In this regard, various classes of myostatin inhibitors have been developed, with experimental validation, which are detailed in the following sections:

1. *Monoclonal antimyostatin antibodies*-These antibodies work by directly binding to the myostatin molecule, thereby blocking the activation of the ActRIIB receptor. Among this category, myostatin inhibitors that have demonstrated benefits in sarcopenia within the CKM syndrome include:

Table 14.2 Benefits and limitations of using Myostatin inhibitors in patients with sarcopenia and CKMS

Myostatin inhibitor class	Representatives	Benefits (CKMS & sarcopenia)	Limitations
1. Monoclonal anti-myostatin antibodies	Bimagrumab (BYM338)	Increases muscle mass Reduces fat mass Lowers HbA1c in diabetics Beneficial in CKD and obesity	Limited results on muscle function in certain groups
	Landogrozumab (LY2495655)	Increases lean mass Potential in CKD and sarcopenia	Modest functional efficacy Lack of long-term data
	Trevogrumab (REGN1033)	Good safety profile Theoretical potential in CKM	Modest muscle growth Limited data
	Apitegromab (SRK-015)	Tested in spinal muscular atrophy Possibly transferable to sarcopenia	Indirect evidence Lack of studies dedicated to sarcopenia
	Domagrozumab, Taldefgrobep alfa	Studied in dystrophies Possible muscle growth	Ineffective in clinical studies Development halted
2. Decoy proteins/soluble receptors (ActRIIB)	ACE-031	Modifies lean mass, fat mass, bone density, and 6-min walk test (6MWT) performance	Adverse effects (epistaxis, telangiectasias) Studies discontinued
	ACE-083	Localized muscle hypertrophy Increased muscle volume and function in injected areas	Lack of systemic effects Contradictory results
3. Genetic inhibitors of the MSTN gene	CRISPR/Cas9	Increases muscle mass in animal models Promising in research	Not approved for clinical use Potential teratogenic/ethical concerns
	RNAi/ antisense phosphorodiamidate Morpholino oligomers (PMOs0	Reduces MSTN expression Increases muscle mass	Does not clearly improve glucose metabolism Only experimental
4. Endogenous natural inhibitors	Follistatin (FST344, FST315)	Significant muscle hypertrophy (40–69%) Anabolic potential	Potential negative impact on bone Nonspecific systemic effects
	rAAV1.CMV. huFollistatin344	Improves function in patients with dystrophies Good tolerability	Limited studies on sarcopenia in CKD
	GDF11	Inhibition of it → muscle growth	May negatively affect bone Ambiguous metabolic role

- *Bimagrumab (BYM338)*-it has demonstrated an increase in muscle mass and grip strength, as well as an improvement in mobility in patients with sarcopenia and chronic kidney disease [49]. Additionally, a clinical study highlighted its implications in significantly reducing total fat mass by 20.5%, increasing lean muscle mass by 3.6%, and decreasing HbA1c levels by 0.76 percentage points in patients with type 2 diabetes and obesity over a 48-week period [105]. Bimagrumab stands out due to its combined effects of increasing muscle mass and improving insulin sensitivity, making it a promising candidate for the treatment of sarcopenia within the CKM syndrome.
- *Landogrozumab (LY2495655)*-it has demonstrated increases in lean mass (without fat) and showed a trend toward improvement in functional muscle strength parameters in older patients. The data suggest its potential benefits in sarcopenia associated with chronic kidney disease [49, 106].
- *Trevogrumab (REGN1033)*-it showed a trend of increased muscle mass only in a small group of patients with muscular dystrophy and demonstrated a good safety and tolerability profile. However, there are optimistic views regarding its potential in sarcopenia associated with chronic diseases [49].
- *Apitegromab (SRK-015)*-it has been primarily investigated in spinal muscular atrophy, but it shows transferable potential in secondary sarcopenia [107].
- *Domagrozumab (PF-06252616)* and *Taldefgrobep alfa (BMS 986089)*-Both have been tested in clinical trials for muscular dystrophy, but development was halted due to a lack of significant evidence of efficacy [106].

Thus, it appears that this class of myostatin inhibitors has demonstrated, in the case of certain representatives, the most direct link with the CKM syndrome through combined effects: increased muscle mass and improved insulin resistance.

2. *Decoy proteins/soluble ActRIIB receptors*-these receptors primarily work by mimicking the myostatin receptor, binding to it in circulation, and neutralizing myostatin.

    - *ACE-031*-A soluble ActRIIB receptor; it has shown trends of pharmacodynamic effects on lean mass, fat mass, bone mineral density, and the 6-min walk test (6MWT). Certain adverse events (epistaxis, telangiectasias) contributed to the decision to discontinue the study [108].
    - *ACE-083*-ActRIIB decoy + localized; experimental data are contradictory. Some data attest to benefits in the treatment of sarcopenia through increased local muscle volume and muscle function [109, 110]. Other results indicate a lack of clear evidence regarding these effects [111]. However, all these data agree on the fact that this category of myostatin inhibitors has not demonstrated systemic functional benefits.

3. *Genetic inhibitors of MSTN gene expression*-These inhibitors interfere with the expression of the gene that codes for myostatin.

- *CRISPR/Cas9 anti-MSTN*-it effective in animal models regarding muscle mass, but not recommended for human experiments due to the proven risks of malformations [112, 113].
- *RNAi (RNA interference)*-it reduces MSTN transcript; experimentally used in rare diseases (e.g. muscular dystrophies). In studies on mice with insulin resistance, the administration of antisense oligonucleotides (PMO) reduced MSTN expression and increased muscle mass. However, no significant improvements in glucose uptake were observed, indicating that MSTN inhibition through RNAi may have limited effects on glucose metabolism under certain conditions [114].

4. *Natural myostatin inhibitors*-these are represented by endogenous proteins that act as physiological antagonists of myostatin.

   - *Follistatin (FST344, FST315)*-it is an endogenous protein that inhibits the activity of myostatin and activin A, leading to a significant increase in muscle mass. A study showed that the overexpression of FST-288 and FST-315 in mice resulted in muscle hypertrophy of 40–69% in the injected muscles [115].
   - *rAAV1.CMV.hu Follistatin344*-this gene therapy has been tested in phase I/II clinical trials in patients with Becker muscular dystrophy and sporadic inclusion body myopathy. The treatment led to functional improvements, such as increased distance covered in the 6-min walk test, with no significant adverse effects [116].
   - *GDF11*-it is structurally similar to myostatin. Although it was initially believed to have beneficial effects on muscle regeneration, subsequent results have shown that inhibiting GDF11 can lead to an increase in muscle mass, but also to weakening of the bone structure, suggesting a complex and ambiguous role in muscle and bone metabolism [117, 118].

Thus, this latest class of myostatin inhibitors can be considered relevant for sarcopenia within the CKM syndrome, due to their increased potential for combined therapies with anti-inflammatory and anabolic profiles. Furthermore, all pharmacological interventions targeting sarcopenia are evolving rapidly, with a focus on targeting specific molecular pathways involved in muscle loss.

However, as noted, clinical studies have shown variable results. While some therapies have increased muscle mass, their impact on strength and function has been modest, and long-term safety remains to be evaluated, especially in fragile populations with cardiovascular and renal comorbidities [109, 110, 112, 113, 118].

Thus, myostatin inhibitors represent an innovative therapeutic direction, yet still under validation, which could complement current strategies for the treatment of sarcopenia in the CKM syndrome (Table 14.2).

Anabolic Agents in the Treatment of Sarcopenia Associated with CKMS

Sarcopenia is a central component of the CKM syndrome (CKMS), contributing to the exacerbation of metabolic, cardiovascular, and renal dysfunctions. In this context, anabolic agents substances that stimulate protein synthesis and muscle mass development may offer significant therapeutic benefits, especially when combined with optimized nutrition and resistance exercise (Table 14.3).

Metabolic Modulators

These agents target the optimization of cellular metabolism, particularly mitochondrial function, to support muscle mass and function. In sarcopenia, metabolic modulators may include:

- *Formulas with essential amino acids (EAA),* especially *branched-chain amino acids (BCAA),* which activate the mTORC1 pathway, promoting protein synthesis [119]. Some experimental data conducted on mice have shown that BCAA can counteract the negative effects of the renin-angiotensin system activation on skeletal muscles, alleviating muscle mass loss and improving exercise capacity [120].
- *Cofactors of the Krebs cycle* and *antioxidants* that support mitochondrial quality and reduce oxidative stress. A study demonstrated the effects of vitamin C on mitochondrial dysfunction in type 3 cardiorenal syndrome. The results show that vitamin C can protect mitochondrial function at the cardiac and renal levels, improving mitochondrial dynamics and reducing oxidative stress [121]. An increasing body of evidence supports the benefits of principles based on vitamin C as well as polyunsaturated fatty acids [122].
- *PD-0E7*is an innovative metabolic formula containing essential amino acids (EAA), branched-chain amino acids (BCAA), and cofactors of the Krebs cycle. Experimental results in mice have shown that supplementation with PD-0E7 prevents muscle and cognitive decline associated with aging by improving mitochondrial function and reducing oxidative stress [123].
- *The coactivator PGC-1α* stimulates the secretion of irisin, a myokine with effects on mitochondrial biogenesis and oxidative metabolism. A review article examines the central role of PGC-1α in regulating lipid and energy metabolism, highlighting that PGC-1α induces a significant increase in mitochondrial density and oxidative capacity, both in healthy myocardium and in myocardium affected by disease. These results also suggest that PGC-1α, through irisin, may have a protective role against sarcopenia and metabolic dysfunctions associated with CKM syndrome [124].
- *Metformin* is used in type 2 diabetes, activates AMPK, and has anti-inflammatory effects. A study evaluating the effects of metformin on the risk of sarcopenia in older patients with type 2 diabetes showed that metformin use is associated with a reduced risk of sarcopenia, possibly through mechanisms

Table 14.3 Benefits and limitations of using anabolic agents in patients with sarcopenia and CKMS

Drug class	Representatives	Benefits	Limitations
Metabolic modulators	BCAA, EAA Vitamin C Krebs cofactors PD-0E7 PGC-1α activators Metformin DPP-4 inhibitors	Activates the mTORC1 pathway → protein synthesis Improves mitochondrial dysfunction Reduces oxidative stress Anti-inflammatory effects Increases muscle mass and strength	Partially proven efficacy in animal models Requires extensive clinical validation Some formulations are experimental (e.g., PD-0E7)
Androgens and derivatives	Testosterone SARMs (e.g, ostarine, enobosarm) Nandrolone, Oxymetolone	Stimulation of protein synthesis (Akt/mTORC1) Increase in muscle mass, strength, and performance SARMs: Selective muscle effects Steroids: Increase in strength and muscle mass in patients with CKD	Cardiovascular risk, water–salt retention, prostate impairment (testosterone) SARMs: Hepatotoxic risk Steroids: Limited use
Growth hormone (GH)/ IGF-1	GH IGF-1 MGF	Weak muscle mass increase Stimulates protein synthesis Antioxidant benefits	Modest functional benefits Risk of hyperglycemia, fluid retention, mitogenic effect Limited use in CKD patients with diabetes or cardiovascular conditions
Ghrelin and mimetics	Anamorelin Acylated ghrelin	Stimulates GH, increases lean mass Activates PGC-1α and mitochondrial biogenesis Improves strength and endurance	Minimal effects on muscle strength in human studies Uncertain systemic efficacy, requires further studies
Anabolic beta-agonists	Clenbuterol Terbutaline Salbutamol	Activates cAMP/ PKA → increased protein synthesis Improve glucose tolerance and insulin sensitivity (in animal models)	Limited use in practice due to cardiovascular side effects Lack of clinical validation in humans
Renin-angiotensin system inhibitors	ACE inhibitors (e.g., enalapril) ARBs (angiotensin II receptor blockers) (e.g., losartan)	Reduces cardiovascular damage and progression of kidney disease Reduction of inflammation and oxidative stress	Activation of the RAS system has catabolic effects on skeletal muscle

involving AMPK activation and reduction of chronic inflammation, both essential factors in the pathogenesis of sarcopenia and CKM syndrome. These findings are also supported by previous results [17, 125]. Other data highlight its lipolytic potential and beneficial role in obesity, as well as in sarcopenic obesity, reiterating the advantages of using metformin in patients with chronic diseases [126].
- *Dipeptidyl peptidase-4 inhibitors (DPP-4i)* may improve sarcopenia parameters in older diabetic patients. A prospective study evaluated the effects of DPP-4 inhibitors on sarcopenia parameters in older patients with type 2 diabetes. After 6 months of treatment, significant improvements in muscle mass and muscle strength were observed, suggesting a potential therapeutic role of DPP-4i in managing sarcopenia in this patient group [127, 128].

Thus, therapy with metabolic modulators in sarcopenia aims to counteract anabolic resistance, characterized by a diminished muscle protein synthesis response to stimuli, and is influenced by factors such as insulin resistance, chronic inflammation, and mitochondrial dysfunction. The therapeutic strategies detailed earlier play definitive roles in sarcopenia within the CKM syndrome by improving the anabolic response and reducing muscle mass loss [129].

Testosterone, Androgenic Derivatives, and Anabolic Steroids

- *Testosterone* binds to androgen receptors, activating the Akt/mTORC1 pathways and inhibiting protein degradation by suppressing myostatin expression. It has well-documented anabolic effects on skeletal muscle. In hypogonadal men or those with low testosterone levels due to aging or chronic diseases, therapy can increase muscle mass, strength, and physical performance. However, in CKMS, it must be used cautiously due to risks of water and salt retention, hypertension, cardiovascular impairment, and adverse effects on the prostate. Close monitoring is required, especially in the presence of cardiovascular or renal disease [116, 130, 131].
- *Selective androgen receptor modulators (SARMs)* bind selectively to androgen receptors in muscle tissue, stimulating protein synthesis without significant androgenic effects in other tissues.
- SARMs (e.g., enobosarm, ostarine) offer a selective anabolic profile by activating androgen receptors in muscle tissue, with reduced effects on the prostate and other tissues. Clinical studies have shown moderate increases in muscle mass and, in some cases, improvements in strength or physical performance. Although still in clinical testing phases, SARMs represent a promising therapeutic option for patients with sarcopenia and CKMS, particularly due to their more favorable safety profile compared to testosterone. However, hepatic insufficiency has been reported as a significant adverse effect in this therapeutic class [52, 132].
- *Anabolic steroids*

- *Nandrolone decanoate:* administered intramuscularly, it has demonstrated increases in muscle mass and improvements in functional capacity in hemodialysis patients [133].
- *Oxymetholone:* when administered orally, it has shown increases in lean body mass and improvements in muscle strength in patients with chronic kidney disease [133].

Growth Hormone (GH) and IGF-1

The GH/IGF-1 axis plays a crucial role in maintaining muscle mass. In sarcopenia, the levels of these hormones are often reduced. Administration of GH or IGF-1 can stimulate protein synthesis and increase muscle mass. Preclinical studies conducted on rats have shown that GH, at physiological doses, increases lean muscle mass, stimulates protein synthesis, and reduces oxidative stress, providing clear benefits in sarcopenia prevention. These effects are associated with increased plasma and hepatic IGF-1 levels [134–136].

Another observational study, which included 3276 senior participants, evaluated the relationship between growth hormone (GH) levels, insulin-like growth factor 1 (IGF-1), the mechanical isoform of IGF-1 (MGF), and sarcopenia. The results showed that serum levels of GH, IGF-1, testosterone, and MGF were significantly lower in individuals with sarcopenia compared to those without sarcopenia. Multivariate regression analysis indicated that IGF-1 and MGF are independent predictors of appendicular skeletal muscle mass (ASMI), alongside body mass index (BMI) and gender [137].

However, the functional benefits are modest, and the risks (hyperglycemia, fluid retention, potential mitogenic effects) limit its applicability in CKMS, especially in patients with diabetes or cardiovascular conditions [137].

Ghrelin and Its Mimetics

They bind to ghrelin receptors, stimulating the secretion of growth hormone and promoting muscle mass growth.

Anamorelin has demonstrated increases in lean body mass in clinical studies, although without significant improvements in muscle strength and with systemic effects on other comorbidities, which require further studies [116].

Another study investigated the effects of administering acylated ghrelin to mice with chronic kidney disease (CKD) induced by nephrectomy, a model that exhibits physical decline similar to human sarcopenia. Ghrelin treatment resulted in improvements in muscle strength and exercise endurance, associated with increased muscle mass and mitochondrial content. The proposed mechanism involves demethylation of the PGC-1α promoter, a key regulator of mitochondrial biogenesis, suggesting that ghrelin may alleviate physical decline through mitochondrial activation in muscles [138].

Beta-Agonists with Anabolic Action

Beta-agonists with anabolic action, such as clenbuterol, terbutaline, and salbutamol, activate β2-adrenergic receptors, leading to the activation of the cAMP-PKA pathway. This induces an increase in protein synthesis and inhibits proteolysis.

Research in animal models has shown that the administration of clenbuterol improves glucose tolerance and insulin sensitivity, even in the absence of changes in GLUT4 content. These effects have been attributed to increased muscle mass and alterations in muscle energy metabolism. However, the use of clenbuterol has been associated with cardiac hypertrophy, highlighting the potential cardiovascular risks of beta-agonists [139].

Additionally, a randomized, double-blind, placebo-controlled study investigated the effects of daily inhalation of terbutaline (4 mg/day) for 4 weeks in young, healthy men. The results showed a significant increase in lean body mass (1.1 kg) and a 27% improvement in insulin sensitivity, as measured by the euglycemic-hyperinsulinemic clamp. These findings suggest that the muscle hypertrophy induced by terbutaline may contribute to the improvement of insulin sensitivity [139].

Additionally, beta-agonists can also stimulate the synthesis of IGF-1, an important growth factor in muscle anabolism. Their main actions include: increasing muscle mass, reducing fat mass, and improving physical performance. Although anabolic beta-agonists may provide benefits in increasing muscle mass, their use in CKMS is limited by cardiovascular and metabolic risks. Adverse effects with negative impact on CKMS include tachycardia, hypertension, and metabolic disturbances, particularly those affecting glucose metabolism [139].

Renin-Angiotensin System Inhibitors

These agents improve muscle blood flow, reduce inflammation, and may increase IGF-1 levels, contributing to the maintenance of muscle mass.

According to experimental data, perindopril (an ACE inhibitor) may prevent sarcopenia in patients with CKM diseases by reducing muscle atrophy, improving muscle mass and function, enhancing muscle blood flow, reducing inflammation, and stimulating mitochondria and IGF-1.

Additionally, the same data suggest that losartan (an AT1 receptor antagonist) has beneficial effects in animal models (reducing inflammation and oxidative stress, protecting against atrophy), but clinical studies in humans have yet to demonstrate clear benefits in preventing muscle mass or strength loss [116].

GLP-1 Receptor Agonists

Glucagon-like peptide-1 (GLP-1)-agonists lower blood glucose levels by increasing insulin secretion and decreasing glucagon secretion, while also reducing body weight in patients with type 2 diabetes (T2DM0). In preclinical studies, these agents have improved cardiac function and reduced postischemic ventricular remodeling, possibly through the activation of cell survival pathways (PI3K, AMPK, eNOS) [140].

In clinical studies, liraglutide and semaglutide have reduced cardiovascular mortality and major events in patients with T2DM and increased cardiovascular risk (LEADER and SUSTAIN-6 trials), but they have not improved outcomes in heart failure (HF). Furthermore, liraglutide increased the frequency of adverse events in patients with HFrEF (FIGHT and LIVE trials), with a common adverse effect being an increase in heart rate by approximately 3 beats per minute [140–142].

A recent analysis suggests that GLP-1RAs, such as liraglutide and exenatide, may reduce muscle atrophy by inhibiting the expression of myostatin and atrophy-related factors (MuRF1, MAFbx), while simultaneously activating the Akt/mTOR and PKA/CREB pathways, promoting muscle regeneration and reducing inflammation [143].

An experimental study showed that semaglutide reduces inflammation, improves muscle metabolism, and increases muscle mass in obese mice with sarcopenia. The treatment led to a decrease in the levels of TNF-α, IL-6, and IL-1β, as well as an increase in muscle fiber density and the number of mitochondria [144].

A systematic meta-analysis showed that, although GLP-1RAs reduce fat mass in patients with obesity and type 2 diabetes, the effect on lean mass [including muscle mass] is variable, highlighting the need for further research [145].

A review highlighted that, in addition to glycemic control, GLP-1RAs have anti-inflammatory effects and may reduce inflammation in adipose tissue, contributing to cardiovascular and renal protection. These effects may be beneficial in managing sarcopenia associated with cardio-reno-metabolic syndrome [146].

In a randomized study involving 9650 participants, it was demonstrated that in individuals with type 2 diabetes and atherosclerotic cardiovascular disease, chronic kidney disease, or both, the use of oral semaglutide was associated with a significantly lower risk of major adverse cardiovascular events compared to placebo, without an increase in the incidence of serious adverse events [147].

Additionally, other data show that semaglutide led to significant and consistent reductions in major adverse cardiovascular events, with a larger absolute risk reduction observed over 3 years in patients with a history of coronary artery bypass surgery and obesity, but without diabetes, compared to those without this history. Indirectly, these results reinforce the role of semaglutide in patients with cardiovascular risk factors, who are at risk for sarcopenia and renal complications [148].

Thus, GLP-1 receptor agonists represent a promising therapeutic class in the management of sarcopenia in the context of CKMS, due to their multifactorial action. Beyond the previously documented effects on glycemic control and weight loss, GLP-1RAs positively influence muscle metabolism and reduce systemic inflammation, including in adipose tissue and skeletal muscle. Preclinical studies have confirmed that these molecules can stimulate muscle and mitochondrial regeneration by activating the Akt/mTOR and PKA/CREB pathways and inhibiting myostatin and atrophy factors [147, 148].

Although clinical results remain heterogeneous regarding muscle mass, these mechanisms suggest a genuine potential to intervene in one of the most debilitating aspects of the CKM syndrome—the loss of muscle mass and function. GLP-1RAs are not merely antidiabetic agents but may emerge as true modulators of metabolic and muscular frailty (Table 14.4).

SGLT2 Inhibitors

Sodium-glucose cotransporter-2 inhibitors (SGLT2i) not only control glycemia but also reduce cardiovascular and renal risks. Additionally, these agents enhance hemodynamic, antiatherogenic, and immunomodulatory functions, providing cardiorenal protection. While SGLT2i are already well established in the management of type 2 diabetes (T2D), their benefits are also evident in renal and cardiac conditions, even in the absence of diabetes. The use of glucose-lowering agents and combination therapies with complementary mechanisms may effectively address the spectrum of CKM diseases [60].

Sodium-glucose cotransporter-2 (SGLT2) inhibitors lower blood glucose by blocking the renal reabsorption of glucose in an insulin-independent manner, thereby inducing favorable metabolic and cardiovascular effects, including optimization of myocardial energy substrates and reduction of oxidative stress. Major clinical trials, such as EMPA-REG OUTCOME and CANVAS, have demonstrated significant reductions in cardiovascular mortality and hospitalizations for heart failure, supporting a class effect with broad therapeutic potential in patients with heart failure, regardless of glycemic status [140, 149, 150].

According to additional data, SGLT2 inhibitors have demonstrated efficacy and safety in heart failure, including in the acute phase, through early initiation of therapy, which leads to rapid benefits in decongestion, reduced hospitalizations,

Table 14.4 Benefits and limitations of GLP-1 and SGLT2 use in patients with sarcopenia and CKMS

Drug class	Benefits	Limitations
GLP-1 agonists (Liraglutide, Semaglutide)	Reduces blood glucose, weight, and cardiovascular risk Improves muscle metabolism and mitochondrial function Reduces inflammation and promote muscle regeneration	Variable effects on muscle mass Possible adverse effects, including increased heart rate and digestive symptoms Not effective in severe heart failure
SGLT2 inhibitors (e.g., Empagliflozin)	Reduces blood glucose and improve cardiovascular and renal function Protects muscle mass by reducing inflammation and oxidative stress Benefits in heart failure and CKD	Risks of volume depletion and hyperkalemia Requires strict monitoring of renal function

improved quality of life, and long-term preservation of renal function. More recent clinical trials, such as EMPA-RESPONSE-AHF, EMPULSE, and DICTATE-AHF, support the early use of these agents—even in the presence of chronic kidney disease—without a significant risk of volume depletion or hyperkalemia, confirming their central role in optimizing therapy for heart failure patients. Moreover, SGLT2i treatments reduce levels of pro-inflammatory cytokines and markers of oxidative stress. Since chronic inflammation plays a major role in muscle mass loss, this effect may contribute to the prevention or slowing of sarcopenia progression [151–154].

By rapidly stabilizing cardiac and renal function, SGLT2 inhibitors may prevent the negative metabolic cascade that leads to muscle loss and mitochondrial dysfunction—key aspects in the pathogenesis of sarcopenia. Early administration of these agents has the potential to reduce the acute inflammatory response involved in the activation of muscle catabolic pathways (e.g., NF-κB, myostatin). Through lowering insulin levels, improving insulin sensitivity, and promoting lipid and ketone metabolism, SGLT2 inhibitors may support the preservation of muscle mass and strength during the acute phase of the CKM syndrome [155].

Additional data have shown that SGLT2 inhibitors significantly reduced the recurrence of atrial fibrillation following catheter ablation (CA) in diabetic patients. Moreover, the use of SGLT2 inhibitors has been associated with a lower risk of hospitalization and ischemic stroke [156].

Moreover, recent research indicates that SGLT2 inhibitor therapy initiated after myocardial infarction (MI) may reduce the risk of hospitalization for heart failure and the incidence of major adverse cardiovascular events (MACE), although it appears to have no significant effect on all-cause mortality [157].

Based on the results of the EMPEROR-Preserved trial, empagliflozin, a representative of the SGLT2 inhibitor class, demonstrated significant benefits in heart failure with preserved ejection fraction (HFpEF), regardless of blood pressure control status (controlled, uncontrolled, or resistant). Although the reduction in systolic blood pressure (SBP) was modest (particularly in resistant hypertension) it was sufficient to increase time in the target range and reduce hypertensive emergencies. Importantly, the effects of empagliflozin on clinical outcomes (including renal function and quality of life) were not influenced by hypertension category. In the context of chronic kidney disease (CKD) and the CKM syndrome, these effects may also have positive implications for sarcopenia, as the reduction in cardiovascular stress and improvement in renal function contribute to a more stable metabolic environment, supportive of muscle mass and function preservation. Thus, empagliflozin may indirectly support the prevention or mitigation of sarcopenia by controlling blood pressure, reducing inflammation, and improving overall functional status in patients with HFpEF and CKD [158].

A study investigated the effects of empagliflozin on hepatic and metabolic parameters in patients with type 2 diabetes mellitus (T2DM) and metabolic dysfunction-associated steatotic liver disease (MASLD). Administration of empagliflozin for 6 months resulted in a significant reduction in hepatic steatosis, as assessed by MRI and ultrasound, compared to the control group. The likelihood of steatosis progression was over 48 times higher in the control group, highlighting the notable impact of the treatment.

The intervention was also associated with significant decreases in liver enzyme levels (ALT, AST, ALP), as well as in systolic blood pressure, suggesting concurrent hepatic, metabolic, and cardiovascular benefits. The favorable effects on liver function may be attributed to improved insulin sensitivity, reduced hepatic lipotoxicity, and the anti-inflammatory actions of empagliflozin. Overall, these findings support the potential expansion of empagliflozin's indications to include pathologies with a complex metabolic background [159].

Thus, SGLT2 inhibitors prove to be a promising therapeutic option for patients with CKM syndrome, offering beneficial effects on sarcopenia through the control of inflammation, improvement of metabolism, and protection of cardiac and renal function (Table 14.4).

Emerging Therapies

A study conducted on experimental mice demonstrated the long-term efficacy of AAV-FGF21 gene therapy, which induces sustained production of the FGF21 protein, showing significant beneficial effects in the treatment of metabolic dysfunction-associated steatohepatitis. This therapy led to reductions in steatosis, inflammation, and hepatic fibrosis, as well as preventing progression to liver tumors. Regarding CKMS, it is important to note that steatohepatitis is a liver condition associated with cardiovascular and renal risk factors such as obesity, insulin resistance, and hypertension. Therefore, therapeutic interventions targeting steatohepatitis could also provide indirect benefits for cardiovascular and renal risks. This approach offers advantages over conventional therapies, providing a constant expression of FGF21 protein and better tolerance, with promising results also observed in canine models. Further clinical studies are required to validate these findings in the human population [160].

Other data have highlighted the effectiveness of combining caloric restriction (CR) with inhibition of the myostatin/activin signaling pathway (via sActRIIB) to stimulate muscle growth and improve health in progeroid mice, without negatively affecting other major organs. This approach enhances the outlook on physiological health and may prevent age-associated sarcopenia, even in advanced stages of disease, representing a promising option for antiaging treatments [161].

A recent review examined how histone acetylation modifications regulate skeletal muscle metabolism, highlighting the crucial role of histone acetyltransferases (HATs) and histone deacetylases (HDACs) in maintaining muscle integrity and insulin sensitivity. Advances in epigenomic technologies, such as ChIP-seq and ATAC-seq, provide new insights into these enzymes as therapeutic targets for muscle diseases [162].

Other data have shown that the stimulation of mitophagy (through the expression of PINK1, Parkin, DRP1, or p62 in animal models) improves muscle function and extends lifespan. Additionally, urolithin A, a natural compound from pomegranate seeds, increases mitophagy and mitochondrial respiratory capacity, enhancing muscle strength in mice and mitochondrial gene expression in humans. Physical exercise remains the most effective nonpharmacological method for activating mitophagy and mitochondrial biogenesis via PGC1-α [15].

Supplementation with NAD precursors (such as nicotinamide riboside) successfully prevented muscle stem cell senescence and improved their function in old sarcopenic mice [82].

Stem cell therapy, particularly with mesenchymal stem cells (MSCs) and induced pluripotent stem cells (iPSCs), represents a promising approach in the treatment of sarcopenia, with the ability to regenerate damaged muscle tissue through paracrine mechanisms, immunomodulatory effects, and mitochondrial transfer [163].

Future Directions

Given the diagnostic and therapeutic challenges posed by CKMS in clinical practice, the need for large-scale longitudinal studies to explore their impact on patients is mandatory. Extensive research is also essential to guide therapeutic strategies and prevention methods.

Personalized medicine approaches, including genetic interventions, nutrition, and tailored pharmacology, offer promising strategies for CKMS. Genetic editing technologies, such as clustered regularly interspaced short palindromic repeats (CRISPR) and antisense oligonucleotides, allow for targeting the molecular substrates of sarcopenia. Additionally, pharmacogenomics optimizes pharmacological interventions, while genetic profiling aids in personalizing anabolic treatments, maximizing efficacy, and minimizing adverse effects [164, 165].

Pharmacogenomics plays a crucial role in personalized pharmacology, enabling healthcare providers to tailor medication regimens based on an individual's genetic profile and becoming a fundamental pillar in addressing sarcopenia in senior persons with multiple comorbidities [125, 166].

The gut microbiota plays a crucial role in the pathogenesis of CKMS, influencing metabolism, systemic inflammation, and muscle function through immune and metabolic mechanisms. Intestinal dysbiosis, associated with aging and cardiovascular and renal risk factors, exacerbates inflammation and frailty, thereby contributing to the progression of comorbidities as well as muscle loss. Bacterial imbalance, characterized by the predominance of pro-inflammatory microorganisms, affects the gut-muscle axis and can worsen cardiovascular, renal dysfunctions, and muscle loss. Therefore, dietary and probiotic interventions may help restore microbiotic balance, with the potential to prevent the progression of CKM syndrome and sarcopenia [129, 167–169].

Artificial intelligence plays a crucial role in the diagnosis and management of sarcopenia associated with CKM syndrome, being utilized in imaging for image segmentation, 3D reconstruction, and lesion analysis through machine and deep learning, providing essential information for body composition evaluation. Thus, artificial intelligence enables the automatic segmentation of muscle mass in CT, MRI, and ultrasound images, enhancing diagnostic and prognostic accuracy, as well as treatment recommendations. Dedicated software programs, such as Horos, facilitate 3D analysis and volumetric reconstruction of muscle mass and adipose tissue, while AI-based analyses can contribute to the assessment of associated cardiovascular and renal risks. Recent studies show that these programs can predict responses to neoadjuvant treatments and identify determinants of muscle quality, thus supporting personalized sarcopenia management within the context of CKM syndrome [71, 72].

Learning Objectives

- Describe the key pathophysiological mechanisms of CKM syndrome, including chronic inflammation, oxidative stress, insulin resistance, and hormonal dysregulation.
- Explain how ectopic fat accumulation and mitochondrial dysfunction contribute to metabolic imbalance and multiorgan damage in CKMS.
- Understand the role of muscle metabolism in CKM syndrome progression.
- Discuss the bidirectional relationship between sarcopenia and organ dysfunction (heart, kidney, metabolic).
- Identify clinical consequences of CKM syndrome, such as increased cardiovascular events, heart failure, renal decline, and mortality.
- Recognize sarcopenia as a clinical marker and amplifier of frailty, disability, and adverse outcomes in CKM syndrome.
- Outline evidence-based therapeutic strategies, including exercise, nutritional support, and pharmacologic interventions.

Key Reading

- *Sarcopenia is a key factor in the pathology of CKM syndrome*, having a significant impact on muscle metabolism and being closely linked to chronic inflammation, oxidative stress, and endocrine dysfunctions.
- *Chronic inflammation, oxidative stress, and hormonal dysregulations* (including insulin resistance and alterations in the renin-angiotensin system) contribute to the development and progression of sarcopenia within the CKM syndrome. Additionally, mitochondrial dysfunction and deficiencies in energy metabolism are fundamental mechanisms of muscle degradation.
- *Sarcopenia exacerbates cardiovascular problems*, potentiating the decline in cardiac function and arterial stiffness, with significant muscle mass loss in chronic kidney diseases and metabolic acidosis.

- *Insulin resistance, altered carbohydrate metabolism, and the obesity paradox are closely related to sarcopenia*, and this condition significantly increases morbidity and mortality risks among patients with CKM syndrome.
- *Imaging techniques (DXA, MRI, CT) and functional assessments* (handgrip strength, gait speed, muscle mass indices) *are essential for diagnosing and monitoring sarcopenia*, along with biochemical markers such as myokines and inflammatory markers.
- *Exercise interventions* (resistance training and aerobic exercises), *nutritional approaches* (protein supplements, amino acids, vitamin D), *and pharmacological therapies* (myostatin inhibitors, anabolic agents, SGLT2 inhibitors, GLP-1 agonists) are essential for sarcopenia management. Furthermore, emerging therapies such as gene therapy and stem cell therapy represent interesting and viable directions for future treatments.
- *Large-scale longitudinal studies are needed to better understand the complex relationships between sarcopenia and CKM syndrome*, while personalized treatment approaches and the integration of artificial intelligence in the diagnosis and management of sarcopenia are promising directions.

References

1. Ndumele CE, Rangaswami J, Chow SL, Neeland IJ, Tuttle KR, Khan SS, American Heart Association, et al. Cardiovascular-kidney-metabolic health: a presidential advisory from the American Heart Association. Circulation. 2023;148:1606–35. https://doi.org/10.1161/CIR.0000000000001241.
2. Aggarwal R, Ostrominski JW, Vaduganathan M. Prevalence of cardiovascular-kidney-metabolic syndrome stages in US adults, 2011–2020. JAMA. 2024;331(21):1858–60. https://doi.org/10.1001/jama.2024.6892.
3. Tian Z, Soltani S, Bauersachs J, Schmidt-Ott K, Melk A, Schmidt B. High prevalence of the cardiovascular-kidney-metabolic syndrome among US adults from 1999–2020 – an analysis of the NHANES survey. 2024; https://doi.org/10.1101/2024.03.04.24303751.
4. Cases A, Broseta JJ, Marqués M, Cigarrán S, Julián JC, Alcázar R, Ortiz A. Cardiovascular-kidney-metabolic syndrome definition and its role in the prevention, risk staging, and treatment. An opportunity for the Nephrology. Nefrología (English Edition). 2024 Nov-Dec;44(6):771–83. https://doi.org/10.1016/j.nefroe.2024.11.011.
5. Boccardi V. Sarcopenia: a dive into metabolism to promote a multimodal, preventive, and regenerative approach. Mech Ageing Dev. 2024 Jun;219:111941. https://doi.org/10.1016/j.mad.2024.111941.
6. Cruz-Jentoft AJ, Bahat G, Bauer J, Boirie Y, Bruyère O, Cederholm T, Cooper C, Landi F, Rolland Y, Sayer AA, Schneider SM, Sieber CC, Topinkova E, Vandewoude M, Visser M, Zamboni M. Writing Group for the European Working Group on sarcopenia in older people 2 (EWGSOP2), and the extended group for EWGSOP2. Sarcopenia: revised European consensus on definition and diagnosis. Age Ageing. 2019;48(1):16–31. https://doi.org/10.1093/ageing/afy169.

7. Gao Y, Huang Y, An R, Yang Y, Chen X, Wan Q. Risk factors for sarcopenia in community setting across the life course: a systematic review and a meta-analysis of longitudinal studies. Arch Gerontol Geriatr. 2025;133:105807. https://doi.org/10.1016/j.archger.2025.105807.
8. Petermann-Rocha F, Balntzi V, Gray SR, Lara J, Ho FK, Pell JP, Celis-Morales C. Global prevalence of sarcopenia and severe sarcopenia: a systematic review and meta-analysis. J Cachexia Sarcopenia Muscle. 2022 Feb;13(1):86–99. https://doi.org/10.1002/jcsm.12783.
9. Meng S, He X, Fu X, Zhang X, Tong M, Li W, Zhang W, Shi X, Liu K. The prevalence of sarcopenia and risk factors in the older adult in China: a systematic review and meta-analysis. Front Public Health. 2024;12:1415398. https://doi.org/10.3389/fpubh.2024.1415398.
10. Yuan S, Larsson SC. Epidemiology of sarcopenia: prevalence, risk factors, and consequences. Metabolism. 2023 Jul;144:155533. https://doi.org/10.1016/j.metabol.2023.155533.
11. Workeneh BT, Mitch WE. Review of muscle wasting associated with chronic kidney disease. Am J Clin Nutr. 2010 Apr;91(4):1128S–32S. https://doi.org/10.3945/ajcn.2010.28608B.
12. Huang W, Deng S, Liu S, Ma Q, Cao L, Liu L, Wan H, Shen J. Association of metabolic syndrome and sarcopenia with all-cause and cardiovascular mortality: a prospective cohort study based on the NHANES. Front Endocrinol (Lausanne). 2024;15:1346669. https://doi.org/10.3389/fendo.2024.1346669.
13. Hargreaves M, Spriet LL. Author correction: skeletal muscle energy metabolism during exercise. Nat Metab. 2020 Sep;2(9):990. https://doi.org/10.1038/s42255-020-0251-4.
14. Phielix E, Mensink M. Type 2 diabetes mellitus and skeletal muscle metabolic function. Physiol Behav. 2008;94(2):252–8. https://doi.org/10.1016/j.physbeh.2008.01.020.
15. Romanello V. The interplay between mitochondrial morphology and Myomitokines in aging sarcopenia. Int J Mol Sci. 2021;22:91. https://doi.org/10.3390/ijms22010091.
16. Abi Akar E, Weill L, El Khoury M, Caradeuc C, Bertho G, Boutary S, Bezier C, Clerc Z, Sapaly D, Bendris S, Cheguillaume F, Giraud N, Eid AA, Charbonnier F, Biondi O. The analysis of the skeletal muscle metabolism is crucial for designing optimal exercise paradigms in type 2 diabetes mellitus. Mol Med. 2024;30(1):80. https://doi.org/10.1186/s10020-024-00850-7.
17. Rubio-Ruiz ME, Guarner-Lans V, Pérez-Torres I, Soto ME. Mechanisms underlying metabolic syndrome-related sarcopenia and possible therapeutic measures. Int J Mol Sci. 2019;20(3):647. https://doi.org/10.3390/ijms20030647.
18. Kim SH, Jeong JB, Kang J, Ahn DW, Kim JW, Kim BG, Lee KL, Oh S, Yoon SH, Park SJ, Lee DH. Association between sarcopenia level and metabolic syndrome. PLoS One. 2021;16(3):e0248856. https://doi.org/10.1371/journal.pone.0248856.
19. International Cardiometabolic Working Group, Krentz A, Jacob S, Heiss C, Sattar N, Lim S, Khunti K, Eckel RH. Rising to the challenge of CKM disease in the 21st century: translating evidence into best clinical practice to prevent and manage atherosclerosis. Atherosclerosis. 2024;396:118528. https://doi.org/10.1016/j.atherosclerosis.2024.118528.
20. Kraaijenhof JM, Mol BM, Nurmohamed NS, Dzobo KE, Kroon J, Hovingh GK, Mokry M, de Borst GJ, Stroes ESG, de Kleijn DPV. Plasma C-reactive protein is associated with a pro-inflammatory and adverse plaque phenotype. Atherosclerosis. 2024;396:118532., 398:118610. https://doi.org/10.1016/j.atherosclerosis.2024.118532.
21. Wang K, Liu Q, Tang M, Qi G, Qiu C, Huang Y, Yu W, Wang W, Sun H, Ni X, Shen Y, Fang X. Chronic kidney disease-induced muscle atrophy: molecular mechanisms and promising therapies. Biochem Pharmacol. 2023 Feb;208:115407. https://doi.org/10.1016/j.bcp.2022.115407.
22. Chandrashekhar Iyer L, Vaishali K, Babu AS. Prevalence of sarcopenia in heart failure: a systematic review. Indian Heart J. 2023;75(1):36–42. https://doi.org/10.1016/j.ihj.2022.12.004.
23. Nediani C, Ruzzolini J, Dinu M. Oxidative stress and inflammation as targets for novel preventive and therapeutic approaches in non-communicable diseases III. Antioxidants (Basel). 2024;13(11):1404. https://doi.org/10.3390/antiox13111404.

24. Zuo X, Li X, Tang K, Zhao R, Wu M, Wang Y, Li T. Sarcopenia and cardiovascular diseases: a systematic review and meta-analysis. J Cachexia Sarcopenia Muscle. 2023 Jun;14(3):1183–98. https://doi.org/10.1002/jcsm.13221.
25. Meng SJ, Yu LJ. Oxidative stress, molecular inflammation and sarcopenia. Int J Mol Sci. 2010;11(4):1509–26. https://doi.org/10.3390/ijms11041509.
26. Cheng Y, Lin S, Cao Z, Yu R, Fan Y, Chen J. The role of chronic low-grade inflammation in the development of sarcopenia: advances in molecular mechanisms. Int Immunopharmacol. 2025;147:114056. https://doi.org/10.1016/j.intimp.2025.114056.
27. Otsuka H, Abe M, Kobayashi H. The effect of aldosterone on Cardiorenal and metabolic systems. Int J Mol Sci. 2023;24(6):5370. https://doi.org/10.3390/ijms24065370.
28. Takano C, Ogawa E, Hayakawa S. Insulin resistance in mitochondrial diabetes. Biomolecules. 2023;13(1):126. https://doi.org/10.3390/biom13010126.
29. Li M, Ji R, Liu X, Wu Y. Associations of metabolic syndrome and its components with sarcopenia, and the mediating role of insulin resistance: findings from NHANES database. BMC Endocr Disord. 2024;24(1):203. https://doi.org/10.1186/s12902-024-01736-9.
30. Deger SM, Hewlett JR, Gamboa J, Ellis CD, Hung AM, Siew ED, Mamnungu C, Sha F, Bian A, Stewart TG, Abumrad NN, Ikizler TA. Insulin resistance is a significant determinant of sarcopenia in advanced kidney disease. Am J Physiol Endocrinol Metab. 2018;315(6):E1108–20. https://doi.org/10.1152/ajpendo.00070.2018.
31. Liu ZJ, Zhu CF. Causal relationship between insulin resistance and sarcopenia. Diabetol Metab Syndr. 2023;15(1):46. https://doi.org/10.1186/s13098-023-01022-z.
32. Kosmas CE, Bousvarou MD, Kostara CE, Papakonstantinou EJ, Salamou E, Guzman E. Insulin resistance and cardiovascular disease. J Int Med Res. 2023;51(3):3000605231164548. https://doi.org/10.1177/03000605231164548.
33. Critchlow AJ, Hiam D, Williams R, Scott D, Lamon S. The role of estrogen in female skeletal muscle aging: a systematic review. Maturitas. 2023 Dec;178:107844. https://doi.org/10.1016/j.maturitas.2023.107844.
34. Thuzar M, Abdul Halim M, Stowasser M. The mineralocorticoid system, cardiometabolic health and its interplay with adipose tissue. J Endocrinol. 2024;263(2):e240119. https://doi.org/10.1530/JOE-24-0119.
35. Whaley-Connell A, Sowers JR. Oxidative stress in the cardiorenal metabolic syndrome. Curr Hypertens Rep. 2012 Aug;14(4):360–5. https://doi.org/10.1007/s11906-012-0279-2.
36. Shi S, Zhang B, Li Y, Xu X, Lv J, Jia Q, Chai R, Xue W, Li Y, Wang Y, Wu H, Song Q, Hu Y. Mitochondrial dysfunction: an emerging link in the pathophysiology of Cardiorenal syndrome. Front Cardiovasc Med. 2022 Feb 25;9:837270. https://doi.org/10.3389/fcvm.2022.837270.
37. Huang Y, Wang S, Zhou J, Liu Y, Du C, Yang K, Bi X, Liu M, Han W, Wang K, Xiong J, Wang S, Wang Y, Nie L, Liu C, Zhang D, Gu J, Zeng C, Zhao J. IRF1-mediated downregulation of PGC1α contributes to cardiorenal syndrome type 4. Nat Commun. 2020;11(1):4664. https://doi.org/10.1038/s41467-020-18519-0.
38. Wang J, Wu J, Li W, Wang X, Liu R, Liu T, Xiao J. Linking mitochondrial function to insulin resistance: focusing on comparing the old and the young. Front Nutr. 2022;9:892719. https://doi.org/10.3389/fnut.2022.892719.
39. Sandri M, Coletto L, Grumati P, Bonaldo P. Misregulation of autophagy and protein degradation systems in myopathies and muscular dystrophies. J Cell Sci. 2013;126(Pt 23):5325–33. https://doi.org/10.1242/jcs.114041.
40. Chen K, Gao P, Li Z, Dai A, Yang M, Chen S, Su J, Deng Z, Li L. Forkhead box O signaling pathway in skeletal muscle atrophy. Am J Pathol. 2022 Dec;192(12):1648–57. https://doi.org/10.1016/j.ajpath.2022.09.003.
41. Franco-Romero A, Sandri M. Role of autophagy in muscle disease. Mol Asp Med. 2021 Dec;82:101041. https://doi.org/10.1016/j.mam.2021.101041.

42. Sandri M. Protein breakdown in muscle wasting: role of autophagy-lysosome and ubiquitin-proteasome. Int J Biochem Cell Biol. 2013 Oct;45(10):2121–9. https://doi.org/10.1016/j.biocel.2013.04.023.
43. Zheng Q, Wang X. Autophagy and the ubiquitin-proteasome system in cardiac dysfunction. Panminerva Med. 2010;52(1):9–25. PMID: 20228723; PMCID: PMC2840262
44. Zhang Y, Whaley-Connell AT, Sowers JR, Ren J. Autophagy as an emerging target in cardiorenal metabolic disease: from pathophysiology to management. Pharmacol Ther. 2018 Nov;191:1–22. https://doi.org/10.1016/j.pharmthera.2018.06.004.
45. Wing SS, Lecker SH, Jagoe RT. Proteolysis in illness-associated skeletal muscle atrophy: from pathways to networks. Crit Rev Clin Lab Sci. 2011;48(2):49–70. https://doi.org/10.3109/10408363.2011.586171.
46. Guan L, Yu Z, Che Z, Zhang H, Yu Y, Yang D, Qian D, Chen R, Yu M. Experimental diabetes exacerbates autophagic flux impairment during myocardial I/R injury through calpain-mediated cleavage of Atg5/LAMP2. J Cell Mol Med. 2023 Jan;27(2):232–45. https://doi.org/10.1111/jcmm.17642.
47. Yang M, Liu C, Jiang N, Liu Y, Luo S, Li C, Zhao H, Han Y, Chen W, Li L, Xiao L, Sun L. Myostatin: a potential therapeutic target for metabolic syndrome. Front Endocrinol (Lausanne). 2023;14:1181913. https://doi.org/10.3389/fendo.2023.1181913.
48. Hildebrandt L, Dieterlen M-T, Klaeske K, Haunschild J, Saeed D, Eifert S, Borger MA, Jawad K. Myostatin/AKT/FOXO signaling is altered in human non-ischemic dilated cardiomyopathy. Life. 2022;12(9):1418. https://doi.org/10.3390/life12091418.
49. Kim DW, Song SH. Sarcopenia in chronic kidney disease: from bench to bedside. Korean J Intern Med. 2023;38(3):303–21. https://doi.org/10.3904/kjim.2022.338.
50. Lőrincz H, Somodi S, Ratku B, Harangi M, Paragh G. Crucial regulatory role of Organokines in relation to metabolic changes in non-diabetic obesity. Meta. 2023;13(2):270. https://doi.org/10.3390/metabo13020270.
51. Theodorakis N, Nikolaou M. From cardiovascular-kidney-metabolic syndrome to cardiovascular-renal-hepatic-metabolic syndrome: proposing an expanded framework. Biomolecules. 2025;15(2):213. https://doi.org/10.3390/biom15020213.
52. Damluji AA, Alfaraidhy M, AlHajri N, Rohant NN, Kumar M, Al Malouf C, Bahrainy S, Ji Kwak M, Batchelor WB, Forman DE, Rich MW, Kirkpatrick J, Krishnaswami A, Alexander KP, Gerstenblith G, Cawthon P, deFilippi CR, Goyal P. Sarcopenia and cardiovascular diseases. Circulation. 2023;147(20):1534–53. https://doi.org/10.1161/CIRCULATIONAHA.123.064071.
53. Sato R, Vatic M, da Fonseca GWP, von Haehling S. Sarcopenia and frailty in heart failure: is there a biomarker signature? Curr Heart Fail Rep. 2022;19(6):400–11. https://doi.org/10.1007/s11897-022-00575-w.
54. Lena A, Anker MS, Springer J. Muscle wasting and sarcopenia in heart failure-the current state of science. Int J Mol Sci. 2020;21(18):6549. https://doi.org/10.3390/ijms21186549.
55. Cho HW, Chung W, Moon S, Ryu OH, Kim MK, Kang JG. Effect of sarcopenia and body shape on cardiovascular disease according to obesity phenotypes. Diabetes Metab J. 2021 Mar;45(2):209–18. https://doi.org/10.4093/dmj.2019.0223.
56. Wilkinson TJ, Miksza J, Yates T, Lightfoot CJ, Baker LA, Watson EL, Zaccardi F, Smith AC. Association of sarcopenia with mortality and end-stage renal disease in those with chronic kidney disease: a UK biobank study. J Cachexia Sarcopenia Muscle. 2021 Jun;12(3):586–98. https://doi.org/10.1002/jcsm.12705.
57. Chatzipetrou V, Bégin MJ, Hars M, Trombetti A. Sarcopenia in chronic kidney disease: a scoping review of prevalence, risk factors, association with outcomes, and treatment. Calcif Tissue Int. 2022 Jan;110(1):1–31. https://doi.org/10.1007/s00223-021-00898-1.
58. Tsai C-C, Wang P-C, Hsiung T, Fan Y-H, Wu J-T, Kan W-C, Shiao C-C. Sarcopenia in chronic kidney disease: a narrative review from pathophysiology to therapeutic approaches. Biomedicine. 2025;13(2):352. https://doi.org/10.3390/biomedicines13020352.

59. Ziolkowski SL, Long J, Baker JF, Chertow GM, Leonard MB. Relative sarcopenia and mortality and the modifying effects of chronic kidney disease and adiposity. J Cachexia Sarcopenia Muscle. 2019;10(2):338–46. https://doi.org/10.1002/jcsm.12396.
60. Marassi M, Fadini GP. The CKM connection: a review of the evidence. Cardiovasc Diabetol. 2023 Jul;22(1):195. https://doi.org/10.1186/s12933-023-01937-x.
61. Atkins JL, Wannamethee SG. Sarcopenic obesity in age ing: cardiovascular outcomes and mortality. Br J Nutr. 2020;124:1102–13. https://doi.org/10.1017/S0007114520001782.
62. Wannamethee SG, Atkins JL. Sarcopenic obesity and Cardiometabolic health and mortality in older adults: a growing health concern in an ageing population. Curr Diab Rep. 2023;23(11):307–14. https://doi.org/10.1007/s11892-023-01522-2.
63. Liu C, Wong PY, Chung YL, Chow SK, Cheung WH, Law SW, et al. Deciphering the "obesity paradox" in the elderly: a sys tematic review and meta-analysis of saropenic obesity. Obes Rev. 2023;24:e13534. https://doi.org/10.1111/obr.13534.
64. Khadra D, Itani L, Tannir H, Kreidieh D, El Masri D, Ghoch E. Association between sarcopenic obesity and higher risk of type 2 diabetes in adults: a systematic review and meta-analysis. World J Diabetes. 2019;10:311–23. https://doi.org/10.4239/wjd.v10.i5.311.
65. Santana Gomes T, Espirito Santo Silva DD, Xavier Junior GF, de Farias Costa PR, Gusmão Sena MHL, Barreto Medeiros JM. Sarcopenia and mortality in patients with chronic non-dialytic renal disease: systematic review and meta-analysis. J Ren Nutr. 2022 Mar;32(2):135–43. https://doi.org/10.1053/j.jrn.2021.07.008.
66. Zeng M, Zhou L, Chen X, Chen G, Xiao L. Effects of sarcopenic obesity on incident chronic kidney disease and rapid kidney function decline: evidence from the China health and retirement longitudinal study. Postgrad Med J. 2025:qgaf007. https://doi.org/10.1093/pmj/qgaf007.
67. Boonpor J, Pell JP, Ho FK, Celis-Morales C, Gray SR. In people with type 2 diabetes, sarcopenia is associated with the incidence of cardiovascular disease: a prospective cohort study from the UK biobank. Diabetes Obes Metab. 2024 Feb;26(2):524–31. https://doi.org/10.1111/dom.15338.
68. Mirzai S, Carbone S, Batsis JA, Kritchevsky SB, Kitzman DW, Shapiro MD. Sarcopenic obesity and cardiovascular disease: an overlooked but high-risk syndrome. Curr Obes Rep. 2024 Sep;13(3):532–44. https://doi.org/10.1007/s13679-024-00571-2.
69. Tagliafico AS, Bignotti B, Torri L, Rossi F. Sarcopenia: how to measure, when and why. Radiol Med. 2022 Mar;127(3):228–37. https://doi.org/10.1007/s11547-021-01492-5.
70. Sabatino A, D'Alessandro C, Regolisti G, di Mario F, Guglielmi G, Bazzocchi A, Fiaccadori E. Muscle mass assessment in renal disease: the role of imaging techniques. Quant Imaging Med Surg. 2020 Aug;10(8):1672–86. https://doi.org/10.21037/qims-20-534.
71. Li C, Huang Y, Wang H, et al. Application of imaging methods and the latest progress in sarcopenia. Chin J Acad Radiol. 2024;7:15–27. https://doi.org/10.1007/s42058-024-00142-3.
72. Salaffi F, Carotti M, Di Matteo A, Ceccarelli L, Farah S, Villota-Eraso C, Di Carlo M, Giovagnoni A. Ultrasound and magnetic resonance imaging as diagnostic tools for sarcopenia in immune-mediated rheumatic diseases (IMRDs). Radiol Med. 2022 Nov;127(11):1277–91. https://doi.org/10.1007/s11547-022-01560-y.
73. Yang Q, Zhang C, Zhang Z, Su B. Muscle ultrasound to diagnose sarcopenia in chronic kidney disease: a systematic review and bayesian bivariate meta-analysis. BMC Nephrol. 2024;25(1):12. https://doi.org/10.1186/s12882-023-03445-2.
74. Chatrenet A, Piccoli G, Audebrand JM, Torreggiani M, Barbieux J, Vaillant C, Morel B, Durand S, Beaune B. Analysis of the rate of force development reveals high neuromuscular fatigability in elderly patients with chronic kidney disease. J Cachexia Sarcopenia Muscle. 2023 Oct;14(5):2016–28. https://doi.org/10.1002/jcsm.13280.
75. Lim WS, Cheong CY, Lim JP, Tan MMY, Chia JQ, Malik NA, Tay L. Singapore clinical practice guidelines for sarcopenia: screening, diagnosis, Management and Prevention. J Frailty Aging. 2022;11(4):348–69. https://doi.org/10.14283/jfa.2022.38.

76. Mirzai S, Eck BL, Chen PH, Estep JD, Tang WHW. Current approach to the diagnosis of sarcopenia in heart failure: a narrative review on the role of clinical and imaging assessments. Circ Heart Fail. 2022 Oct;15(10):e009322. https://doi.org/10.1161/CIRCHEARTFAILURE.122.009322.
77. Cesari M, Cherubini A, Guralnik JM, Beresniak A, Rodriguez-Mañas L, Inzitari M, Walston J. Early detection of accelerated aging and cellular decline (AACD): a consensus statement. Exp Gerontol. 2021 Apr;146:111242. https://doi.org/10.1016/j.exger.2021.111242.
78. Picca A, Calvani R, Coelho-Júnior HJ, Marini F, Landi F, Marzetti E. Circulating inflammatory, mitochondrial dysfunction, and senescence-related markers in older adults with physical frailty and sarcopenia: a BIOSPHERE exploratory study. Int J Mol Sci. 2022;23(22):14006. https://doi.org/10.3390/ijms232214006.
79. Hsu WH, Wang SY, Chao YM, Chang KV, Han DS, Lin YL. Novel metabolic and lipidomic biomarkers of sarcopenia. J Cachexia Sarcopenia Muscle. 2024 Oct;15(5):2175–86. https://doi.org/10.1002/jcsm.13567.
80. Qaisar R, Karim A, Muhammad T, Shah I, Khan J. Prediction of sarcopenia using a battery of circulating biomarkers. Sci Rep. 2021;11(1):8632. https://doi.org/10.1038/s41598-021-87974-6.
81. Zhang J, Wang Y, Liu H, Lei Z, Cheng S, Cao H. The association between eight complete blood count-derived inflammatory markers and muscle health. Front Nutr. 2025 Feb;3(12):1498757. https://doi.org/10.3389/fnut.2025.1498757.
82. Picca A, Lozanoska-Ochser B, Calvani R, Coelho-Júnior HJ, Leewenburgh C, Marzetti E. Inflammatory, mitochondrial, and senescence-related markers: underlying biological pathways of muscle aging and new therapeutic targets. Exp Gerontol. 2023 Jul;178:112204. https://doi.org/10.1016/j.exger.2023.112204.
83. Noor H, Reid J, Slee A. Resistance exercise and nutritional interventions for augmenting sarcopenia outcomes in chronic kidney disease: a narrative review. J Cachexia Sarcopenia Muscle. 2021 Dec;12(6):1621–40. https://doi.org/10.1002/jcsm.12791.
84. Braggio M, Dorelli G, Olivato N, Lamberti V, Valenti MT, Dalle Carbonare L, Cominacini M. Tailored exercise intervention in metabolic syndrome: cardiometabolic improvements beyond weight loss and diet – a prospective observational study. Nutrients. 2025;17(5):872. https://doi.org/10.3390/nu17050872.
85. Kim S. Physical activity and cardiorespiratory fitness attenuate the impact of sarcopenic-obesity on cardiovascular disease risk in Korean men: a cross-sectional study. J Men's Health. 2020;16(2):39–49. https://doi.org/10.15586/jomh.v16i2.251.
86. Ghiotto L, Muollo, Tatangelo T, Schena F, Rossi AP. Exercise and physical performance in older adults with sarcopenic obe sity: a systematic review. Front Endocrinol. 2022;13:913953. https://doi.org/10.3389/fendo.2022.913953.
87. Du Y, Xu T, Yin Z, Espinoza S, Xie Y, Gentry C, et al. Associa tions of physical activity with sarcopenia and sarcopenic obe sity in middle-aged and older adults: the Louisana osteoporosis study. BMC Public Health. 2022;22:896. https://doi.org/10.1186/s12889-022-13288-5.
88. Beckwée D, Delaere A, Aelbrecht S, Baert V, Beaudart C, Bruyere O, de Saint-Hubert M, Bautmans I. Exercise interventions for the prevention and treatment of sarcopenia. A systematic umbrella review. J Nutr Health Aging. 2019;23(6):494–502. https://doi.org/10.1007/s12603-019-1196-8.
89. Gao S, Yu L, Yi G, et al. Exercise intervention as a therapy in patients with diabetes mellitus and sarcopenia: a meta-analysis. Diabetes Ther. 2022;13:1311–25. https://doi.org/10.1007/s13300-022-01275-3.
90. Lu L, Mao L, Feng Y, et al. Effects of different exercise training modes on muscle strength and physical performance in older people with sarcopenia: a systematic review and meta-analysis. BMC Geriatr. 2021;21:708. https://doi.org/10.1186/s12877-021-02642-8.
91. Pano-Rodriguez A, Beltran-Garrido JV, Hernandez-Gonzalez V, Nasarre-Nacenta N, Reverter-Masia J. Impact of whole body Electromyostimulation on velocity, power and body

composition in postmenopausal women: a randomized controlled Trial. Int J Environ Res Public Health. 2020;17(14):4982. https://doi.org/10.3390/ijerph17144982.

92. Zarzeczny R, Nawrat-Szołtysik A, Polak A. Effects of 12 weeks of neuromuscular electrical stimulation of the quadriceps muscles on the function and physio-biochemical traits in functionally fit female nursing-home residents aged 75+ years: a pilot study. Eur J Appl Physiol. 2024 Mar;124(3):945–62. https://doi.org/10.1007/s00421-023-05321-1.
93. Ho MH, Peng CY, Liao Y, Yen HY. Efficacy of a wearable activity tracker with step-by-step goal-setting on older adults' physical activity and sarcopenia indicators: clustered trial. J Med Internet Res. 2024;26:e60183. https://doi.org/10.2196/60183.
94. Menassa M, Wilmont I, Beigrezaei S, Knobbe A, Arita VA, Valderrama JF 5th, Bridge L, Verschuren WMM, Rennie KL, Franco OH, van der Ouderaa F. The future of healthy ageing: wearables in public health, disease prevention and healthcare. Maturitas. 2025 May;196:108254. https://doi.org/10.1016/j.maturitas.2024.108254.
95. Goisser S, Kemmler W, Porzel S, Volkert D, Sieber CC, Bol heimer LC, et al. Sarcopenic obesity and complex interventions with nutrition and exercise in community-dwelling older per sons-a narrative review. Clin Interv Aging. 2015;10:1267–82. https://doi.org/10.2147/CIA.S81338.
96. Deutz NE, Bauer JM, Barazzoni R, Biolo G, Boirie Y, Bosy Westphal A, et al. Protein intake and exercise for optimal muscle function with aging: recommendations from the ESPEN Expert Group. Clin Nutr. 2014;33:929–36. https://doi.org/10.1016/j.clnu.2014.04.007.
97. Wannamethee SG, Atkins JL. Sarcopenic obesity and Cardiometabolic health and mortality in older adults: a growing health concern in an ageing population. Curr Diab Rep. 2023 Nov;23(11):307–14. https://doi.org/10.1007/s11892-023-01588-1.
98. Mesinovic J, Rodriguez AJ, Cervo MM, Gandham A, Xu CLH, Glavas C, de Courten B, Zengin A, Ebeling PR, Scott D. Vitamin D supplementation and exercise for improving physical function, body composition and metabolic health in overweight or obese older adults with vitamin D deficiency: a pilot randomized, double-blind, placebo-controlled trial. Eur J Nutr. 2023 Mar;62(2):951–64. https://doi.org/10.1007/s00394-022-03038-z.
99. Aquino S, Cunha A, Gomes Lima J, Sena-Evangelista K, Gouveia Oliveira A, Cobucci RN, Fc Pedrosa L. Effects of vitamin D supplementation on cardiometabolic parameters among patients with metabolic syndrome: a systematic review and GRADE evidence synthesis of randomized controlled trials. Heliyon. 2023;9(11):e20845. https://doi.org/10.1016/j.heliyon.2023.e20845.
100. Bian D, Xuan C, Li X, Zhou W, Lu Y, Ding T, Shen J, Shi Y, Li G. The association of dietary inflammatory potential with sarcopenia in Chinese community-dwelling older adults. BMC Geriatr. 2023;23(1):281. https://doi.org/10.1186/s12877-023-03938-7.
101. Linton C, Wright HH, Wadsworth DP, Schaumberg MA. Dietary inflammatory index and associations with sarcopenia symptomology in community-dwelling older adults. Nutrients. 2022;14(24):5319. https://doi.org/10.3390/nu14245319.
102. Geng J, Deng L, Qiu S, Bian H, Cai B, Jin K, Zheng X, Li J, Liao X, Li Y, Li J, Qin Z, Cao Z, Bao Y, Su B. Dietary inflammatory potential and risk of sarcopenia: data from national health and nutrition examination surveys. Aging (Albany NY). 2020 Dec;13(2):1913–28. https://doi.org/10.18632/aging.202141.
103. Wang F, Zheng J, Cheng J, Zou H, Li M, Deng B, Luo R, Wang F, Huang D, Li G, Zhang R, Ding X, Li Y, Du J, Yang Y, Kan J. Personalized nutrition: a review of genotype-based nutritional supplementation. Front Nutr. 2022;9:992986. https://doi.org/10.3389/fnut.2022.992986.
104. Frydrych A, Kulita K, Jurowski K, Piekoszewski W. Lipids in clinical nutrition and health: narrative review and dietary recommendations. Foods. 2025;14(3):473. https://doi.org/10.3390/foods14030473.
105. Heymsfield SB, Coleman LA, Miller R, Rooks DS, Laurent D, Petricoul O, Praestgaard J, Swan T, Wade T, Perry RG, Goodpaster BH, Roubenoff R. Effect of Bimagrumab vs placebo on body fat mass among adults with type 2 diabetes and obesity: a phase 2 ran-

domized clinical Trial. JAMA Netw Open. 2021;4(1):e2033457. https://doi.org/10.1001/jamanetworkopen.2020.33457.
106. Kwak JY, Kwon KS. Pharmacological interventions for treatment of sarcopenia: current status of drug development for sarcopenia. Ann Geriatr Med Res. 2019 Sep;23(3):98–104. https://doi.org/10.4235/agmr.19.0028.
107. Jang JY, Kim D, Kim ND. Pathogenesis, intervention, and current status of drug development for sarcopenia: a review. Biomedicine. 2023;11(6):1635. https://doi.org/10.1002/mus.25268.
108. Campbell C, McMillan HJ, Mah JK, Tarnopolsky M, Selby K, McClure T, Wilson DM, Sherman ML, Escolar D, Attie KM. Myostatin inhibitor ACE-031 treatment of ambulatory boys with Duchenne muscular dystrophy: results of a randomized, placebo-controlled clinical trial. Muscle Nerve. 2017 Apr;55(4):458–64. https://doi.org/10.1002/mus.25268.
109. Glasser CE, Gartner MR, Wilson D, Miller B, Sherman ML, Attie KM. Locally acting ACE-083 increases muscle volume in healthy volunteers. Muscle Nerve. 2018 Jun;57(6):921–6. https://doi.org/10.1002/mus.26113.
110. Pearsall RS, Davies MV, Cannell M, Li J, Widrick J, Mulivor AW, Wallner S, Troy ME, Spaits M, Liharska K, Sako D, Castonguay R, Keates S, Grinberg AV, Suragani RNVS, Kumar R. Follistatin-based ligand trap ACE-083 induces localized hypertrophy of skeletal muscle with functional improvement in models of neuromuscular disease. Sci Rep. 2019;9(1):11392. https://doi.org/10.1038/s41598-019-47818-w.
111. Thomas FP, Brannagan TH 3rd, Butterfield RJ, Desai U, Habib AA, Herrmann DN, Eichinger KJ, Johnson NE, Karam C, Pestronk A, Quinn C, Shy ME, Statland JM, Subramony SH, Walk D, Stevens-Favorite K, Miller B, Leneus A, Fowler M, van de Rijn M, Attie KM. Randomized phase 2 study of ACE-083 in patients with Charcot-Marie-tooth disease. Neurology. 2022;98(23):e2356–67. https://doi.org/10.1212/WNL.0000000000200241.
112. Guo R, Wan Y, Xu D, Cui L, Deng M, Zhang G, Jia R, Zhou W, Wang Z, Deng K, Huang M, Wang F, Zhang Y. Generation and evaluation of Myostatin knock-out rabbits and goats using CRISPR/Cas9 system. Sci Rep. 2016 Jul;15(6):29855. https://doi.org/10.1038/srep29855.
113. Dilger AC, Chen X, Honegger LT, et al. The potential for gene-editing to increase muscle growth in pigs: experiences with editing myostatin. CABI Agric Biosci. 2022;3:36. https://doi.org/10.1186/s43170-022-00106-6.
114. Eilers W, Cleasby M, Foster K. Development of antisense-mediated myostatin knockdown for the treatment of insulin resistance. Sci Rep. 2021;11(1):1604. https://doi.org/10.1038/s41598-021-81222-7.
115. Chan ASM, McGregor NE, Poulton IJ, Hardee JP, Cho EH, Martin TJ, Gregorevic P, Sims NA, Lynch GS. Bone geometry is altered by Follistatin-induced muscle growth in young adult male mice. JBMR Plus. 2021;5(4):e10477. https://doi.org/10.1002/jbm4.10477.
116. Feike Y, Zhijie L, Wei C. Advances in research on pharmacotherapy of sarcopenia. Aging Med (Milton). 2021;4(3):221–33. https://doi.org/10.1002/agm2.12168.
117. McPherron AC. Metabolic functions of myostatin and GDF11. Immunol Endocr Metab Agents Med Chem. 2010 Dec;10(4):217–31. https://doi.org/10.2174/187152210793663810.
118. Suh J, Kim NK, Lee SH, Eom JH, Lee Y, Park JC, Woo KM, Baek JH, Kim JE, Ryoo HM, Lee SJ, Lee YS. GDF11 promotes osteogenesis as opposed to MSTN, and follistatin, a MSTN/GDF11 inhibitor, increases muscle mass but weakens bone. Proc Natl Acad Sci USA. 2020 Mar;117(9):4910–20. https://doi.org/10.1073/pnas.1913500117.
119. Zuo X, Zhao R, Wu M, Wang Y, Wang S, Tang K, Wang Y, Chen J, Yan X, Cao Y, Li T. Multiomic profiling of sarcopenia identifies disrupted branched-chain amino acid catabolism as a causal mechanism and therapeutic target. Nat Aging. 2025 Mar;5(3):419–36. https://doi.org/10.1038/s43587-024-00797-8.
120. Yamanashi K, Kinugawa S, Fukushima A, Kakutani N, Takada S, Obata Y, Nakano I, Yokota T, Kitaura Y, Shimomura Y, Anzai T. Branched-chain amino acid supplementation ameliorates angiotensin II-induced skeletal muscle atrophy. Life Sci. 2020;250:117593. https://doi.org/10.1016/j.lfs.2020.117593.

121. Neres-Santos RS, Junho CVC, Panico K, Caio-Silva W, Pieretti JC, Tamashiro JA, Seabra AB, Ribeiro CAJ, Carneiro-Ramos MS. Mitochondrial dysfunction in Cardiorenal syndrome 3: Renocardiac effect of vitamin C. Cells. 2021;10(11):3029. https://doi.org/10.3390/cells10113029.
122. Affourtit C, Carré JE. Mitochondrial involvement in sarcopenia. Acta Physiol Oxf. 2024;240(3):e14107), (Gonzalez A, Simon F, Achiardi O, Vilos C, Cabrera D, Cabello-Verrugio C. The Critical Role of Oxidative Stress in Sarcopenic Obesity. Oxid Med Cell Longev. 2021 Oct 12; 2021:4493817. https://doi.org/10.1111/apha.14107.
123. Brunetti D, Bottani E, Segala A, Marchet S, Rossi F, Orlando F, Malavolta M, Carruba MO, Lamperti C, Provinciali M, Nisoli E, Valerio A. Targeting multiple mitochondrial processes by a metabolic modulator prevents sarcopenia and cognitive decline in SAMP8 mice. Front Pharmacol. 2020 Jul;31(11):1171. https://doi.org/10.3389/fphar.2020.01171.
124. Cheng C-F, Ku H-C, Lin H. PGC-1α as a pivotal factor in lipid and metabolic regulation. Int J Mol Sci. 2018;19(11):3447. https://doi.org/10.3390/ijms19113447.
125. Hu Y, Lu S, Xue C, Hu Z, Wang Y, Zhang W, Wang D, Wang J, Ding G, Yu J, Hu Y, Liu Y. Exploring the protective effect of metformin against sarcopenia: insights from cohort studies and genetics. J Transl Med. 2025;23(1):356. https://doi.org/10.1186/s12967-025-06357-x.
126. Lyu Q, Wen Y, He B, Zhang X, Chen J, Sun Y, Zhao Y, Xu L, Xiao Q, Deng H. The ameliorating effects of metformin on disarrangement ongoing in gastrocnemius muscle of sarcopenic and obese sarcopenic mice. Biochim Biophys Acta Mol basis Dis. 2022;1868(11):166508. https://doi.org/10.1016/j.bbadis.2022.166508.
127. Sencan C, Dost FS, Ates Bulut E, Isik AT. DPP4 inhibitors as a potential therapeutic option for sarcopenia: a 6-month follow-up study in diabetic older patients. Exp Gerontol. 2022 Jul;164:111832. https://doi.org/10.1016/j.exger.2022.111832.
128. Bayanati M, Ismail Mahboubi Rabbani M, Sirous Kabiri S, Mir B, Rezaee E, Tabatabai SA. Dipeptidyl Peptidase-4 inhibitors: a systematic review of structure-activity relationship studies. Iran J Pharm Res. 2024 Oct 29;23(1):e 151581. https://doi.org/10.5812/ijpr-151581.
129. Cacciatore S, Calvani R, Esposito I, et al. Emerging targets and treatments for sarcopenia: a narrative review. Nutrients. 2024 Sep;16(19):3271. https://doi.org/10.3390/nu16193271.
130. Parahiba SM, Ribeiro ÉCT, Corrêa C, Bieger P, Perry IS, Souza GC. Effect of testosterone supplementation on sarcopenic components in middle-aged and elderly men: a systematic review and meta-analysis. Exp Gerontol. 2020 Dec;142:111106. https://doi.org/10.1016/j.exger.2020.111106.
131. Dos Santos MR, Storer TW. Testosterone treatment as a function-promoting therapy in sarcopenia associated with aging and chronic disease. Endocrinol Metab Clin N Am. 2022 Mar;51(1):187–204. https://doi.org/10.1016/j.ecl.2021.11.007.
132. Kwak JY, Kwon KS. Pharmacological interventions for treatment of sarcopenia: current status of drug development for sarcopenia. Ann Geriatr Med Res. 2019 Sep;23(3):98–104. https://doi.org/10.4235/agmr.19.0022.
133. Cha RH. Pharmacologic therapeutics in sarcopenia with chronic kidney disease. Kidney Res Clin Pract. 2024 Mar;43(2):143–55. https://doi.org/10.23876/j.krcp.22.265.
134. Brioche T, Kireev RA, Cuesta S, Gratas-Delamarche A, Tresguerres JA, Gomez-Cabrera MC, Viña J. Growth hormone replacement therapy prevents sarcopenia by a dual mechanism: improvement of protein balance and of antioxidant defenses. J Gerontol A Biol Sci Med Sci. 2014 Oct;69(10):1186–98. https://doi.org/10.1093/gerona/glu040.
135. Poudel SB, Dixit M, Neginskaya M, Nagaraj K, Pavlov E, Werner H, Yakar S. Effects of GH/IGF on the aging mitochondria. Cells. 2020;9(6):1384. https://doi.org/10.3390/cells9061384.
136. Mohammadjafari H, Arazi H, Nemati N, Bagherpoor T, Suzuki K. Acute effects of resistance exercise and the use of GH or IGF-1 hormones on oxidative stress and antioxidant markers in bodybuilders. Antioxidants. 2019;8(12):587. https://doi.org/10.3390/antiox8120587.
137. Bian A, Ma Y, Zhou X, Guo Y, Wang W, Zhang Y, Wang X. Association between sarcopenia and levels of growth hormone and insulin-like growth factor-1 in the elderly. BMC Musculoskelet Disord. 2020;21(1):214. https://doi.org/10.1186/s12891-020-03258-2.

138. Hagiwara A, Wakino S, Inoue H, Fujii K, Fujii C, Endo S, Uto A, Mitsuishi M, Sato M, Doi T, Itoh H. Ghrelin treatment improves physical decline in sarcopenia model mice through muscular enhancement and mitochondrial activation. Endocr J. 2017;64(Suppl):S47-S51. https://doi.org/10.1507/endocrj.EJ17-0305.
139. Jessen S, Baasch-Skytte T, Onslev J, Eibye K, Backer V, Bangsbo J, Hostrup M. Muscle hypertrophic effect of inhaled beta2 -agonist is associated with augmented insulin-stimulated whole-body glucose disposal in young men. J Physiol. 2022 May;600(10):2345–57. https://doi.org/10.1113/JP282501.
140. Heymans S. Heart failure and diabetes: metabolic alterations and therapeutic interventions: a state-of-the-art review from the translational research Committee of the Heart Failure Association-European Society of cardiology. Eur Heart J. 2018;39(48):4243–54. https://doi.org/10.1093/eurheartj/ehy596.
141. Marso SP, Daniels GH, Brown-Frandsen K, Kristensen P, Mann JF, Nauck MA, Nissen SE, Pocock S, Poulter NR, Ravn LS, Steinberg WM, Stockner M, Zinman B, Bergenstal RM, Buse JB, LEADER Steering Committee; LEADER Trial Investigators. Liraglutide and cardiovascular outcomes in type 2 diabetes. N Engl J Med. 2016;375(4):311–22. https://doi.org/10.1056/NEJMoa1603827.
142. Marso SP, Bain SC, Consoli A, Eliaschewitz FG, Jódar E, Leiter LA, Lingvay I, Rosenstock J, Seufert J, Warren ML, Woo V, Hansen O, Holst AG, Pettersson J, Vilsbøll T, SUSTAIN-6 Investigators. Semaglutide and cardiovascular outcomes in patients with type 2 diabetes. N Engl J Med. 2016;375(19):1834–44. https://doi.org/10.1056/NEJMoa1607141.
143. Zhao X, Liu Y, Wang D, Li T, Xu Z, Li Z, Bai X, Wang Y. Role of GLP-1 receptor agonists in sepsis and their therapeutic potential in sepsis-induced muscle atrophy (review). Int J Mol Med. 2025 May;55(5):74. https://doi.org/10.3892/ijmm.2025.5135.
144. Ren Q, Chen S, Chen X, Niu S, Yue L, Pan X, Li Z, Chen X. An effective glucagon-like Peptide-1 receptor agonists, Semaglutide, improves Sarcopenic obesity in obese mice by modulating skeletal muscle metabolism. Drug Des Devel Ther. 2022;16:3723–373. https://doi.org/10.2147/DDDT.S380493.
145. Karakasis P, Patoulias D, Fragakis N, Mantzoros CS. Effect of glucagon-like peptide-1 receptor agonists and co-agonists on body composition: systematic review and network meta-analysis. Metabolism. 2025 Mar;164:156113. https://doi.org/10.1016/j.metabol.2024.156113.
146. D'Marco L, Morillo V, Gorriz JL, Suarez MK, Nava M, Ortega Á, Parra H, Villasmil N, Rojas-Quintero J, Bermúdez V. SGLT2i and GLP-1RA in Cardiometabolic and renal diseases: from glycemic control to adipose tissue inflammation and senescence. J Diabetes Res. 2021;2021:9032378. https://doi.org/10.1155/2021/9032378.
147. McGuire DK, Marx N, Mulvagh SL, Deanfield JE, Inzucchi SE, Pop-Busui R, Mann JFE, Emerson SS, Poulter NR, Engelmann MDM, Ripa MS, Hovingh GK, Brown-Frandsen K, Bain SC, Cavender MA, Gislum M, David JP, Buse JB, SOUL Study Group. Oral Semaglutide and cardiovascular outcomes in high-risk type 2 diabetes. N Engl J Med. 2025; https://doi.org/10.1056/NEJMoa2307565.
148. Verma S, Emerson S, Plutzky J, Kahn SE, Stensen S, Weeke PE, Musinga D, Poirier P, Lingvay I, Lincoff AM. Semaglutide improves cardiovascular outcomes in patients with history of coronary artery bypass graft and obesity. J Am Coll Cardiol. 2025;85(5):541–5. https://doi.org/10.1016/j.jacc.2024.11.030.
149. Zinman B, Wanner C, Lachin JM, Fitchett D, Bluhmki E, Hantel S, Mattheus M, Devins T, Johansen OE, Woerle HJ, Broedl UC, Inzucchi SE, EMPA-REG OUTCOME Investigators. Empagliflozin, Cardiovascular outcomes, and mortality in type 2 diabetes. N Engl J Med. 2015;373(22):2117–28. https://doi.org/10.1056/NEJMoa1504720.
150. Perkovic V, Jardine MJ, Neal B, Bompoint S, Heerspink HJL, Charytan DM, Edwards R, Agarwal R, Bakris G, Bull S, Cannon CP, Capuano G, Chu PL, de Zeeuw D, Greene T, Levin A, Pollock C, Wheeler DC, Yavin Y, Zhang H, Zinman B, Meininger G, Brenner BM, Mahaffey KW, CREDENCE Trial Investigators. Canagliflozin and renal outcomes in type

2 diabetes and nephropathy. N Engl J Med. 2019 Jun 13;380(24):2295–306. https://doi.org/10.1056/NEJMoa1811744.
151. Damman K, Beusekamp JC, Boorsma EM, Swart HP, Smilde TDJ, Elvan A, van Eck JWM, Heerspink HJL, Voors AA. Randomized, double-blind, placebo-controlled, multicentre pilot study on the effects of empagliflozin on clinical outcomes in patients with acute decompensated heart failure (EMPA-RESPONSE-AHF). Eur J Heart Fail. 2020 Apr;22(4):713–22. https://doi.org/10.1002/ejhf.1710.
152. Ponikowski P, Biegus J. Empagliflozin in patients hospitalized for acute heart failure. Eur Heart J. 2022;43(41):4219–21. https://doi.org/10.1093/eurheartj/ehac557.
153. Cox ZL, Collins SP, Hernandez GA, McRae AT 3rd, Davidson BT, Adams K, Aaron M, Cunningham L, Jenkins CA, Lindsell CJ, Harrell FE Jr, Kampe C, Miller KF, Stubblefield WB, Lindenfeld J. Efficacy and safety of Dapagliflozin in patients with acute heart failure. J Am Coll Cardiol. 2024;83(14):1295–306. https://doi.org/10.1016/j.jacc.2024.02.009.
154. Merlo A, D'Elia E, Di Odoardo L, Sciatti E, Senni M. SGLT2 inhibitors and new frontiers in heart failure treatment regardless of ejection fraction and setting. Eur Heart J Suppl. 2025;27(Suppl 1):i137–40. https://doi.org/10.1093/eurheartjsupp/suae117.
155. Mazzotta R, Garofalo M, Salvi S, Orlandi M, Marcaccini G, Susini P, Checchi L, Palazzuoli A, Di Mario C, Pieroni M, Beltrami M. Early administration of SGLT2 inhibitors in hospitalized patients: a practical guidance from the current evidence. ESC Heart Fail. 2025;12(4):2631–42. https://doi.org/10.1002/ehf2.14867.
156. Abdelhadi NA, Ragab KM, Elkholy M, Koneru J, Ellenbogen KA, Pillai A. Impact of sodium-glucose co-transporter 2 inhibitors on atrial fibrillation recurrence post-catheter ablation among patients with type 2 diabetes mellitus: a systematic review and meta-analysis. J Cardiovasc Electrophysiol. 2025 Mar;36(3):673–82. https://doi.org/10.1111/jce.16544.
157. Hu S, Tang T, Yu Q, Tong X, You Y, Zhang S, Chen C, Tang J, Wang C, Wang H, Fu X, Chen J, Zhang X, Wang M, Liu L. Cardiovascular Outcome of the SGLT2 inhibitor in acute myocardial infarction: a meta-analysis. Rev Cardiovasc Med. 2025;26(2):26136. https://doi.org/10.31083/RCM26136.
158. Böhm M, Butler J, Coats A, Lauder L, Mahfoud F, Filippatos G, Ferreira JP, Pocock SJ, Brueckmann M, Hauske SJ, Schueler E, Wanner C, Verma S, Zannad F, Packer M, Anker SD. Empagliflozin in resistant hypertension and heart failure with preserved ejection fraction: the EMPEROR-preserved trial. Eur Heart J. 2025;46(14):1304–17. https://doi.org/10.1093/eurheartj/ehad123.
159. Shojaei F, Erfanifar A, Kalbasi S, Nikpour S, Gachkar L. The effect of empagliflozin on non-alcoholic fatty liver disease-related parameters in patients with type 2 diabetes mellitus: a randomized controlled trial. BMC Endocr Disord. 2025;25(1):52. https://doi.org/10.1186/s12902-025-01882-8.
160. Jimenez V, Sacristan V, Jambrina C, Jaen ML, Casana E, Muñoz S, Marcó S, Molas M, Garcia M, Grass I, León X, Elias I, Ribera A, Elias G, Sanchez V, Vilà L, Casellas A, Ferre T, Rodó J, Carretero A, Pumarola M, Navarro M, Andaluz A, Moll X, Añor S, Franckhauser S, Vergara M, Caixàs A, Bosch F. Reversion of metabolic dysfunction-associated steatohepatitis by skeletal muscle-directed FGF21 gene therapy. Mol Ther. 2024;32(12):4285–43. https://doi.org/10.1016/j.ymthe.2024.10.023.
161. Vermeij WP, Alyodawi K, van Galen I, von der Heide JL, Birkisdóttir MB, Van't Sant LJ, Ozinga RA, Komninos DSJ, Smit K, Rijksen YMA, Brandt RMC, Barnhoorn S, Jaarsma D, Vaiyapuri S, Ritvos O, Huber TB, Kretz O, Patel K. Improved health by combining dietary restriction and promoting muscle growth in DNA repair-deficient progeroid mice. J Cachexia Sarcopenia Muscle. 2024 Dec;15(6):2361–74. https://doi.org/10.1002/jcsm.13570.
162. Xu J, Li C, Kang X. The epigenetic regulatory effect of histone acetylation and deacetylation on skeletal muscle metabolism-a review. Front Physiol. 2023 Dec;8(14):1267456. https://doi.org/10.3389/fphys.2023.1267456.

163. Najm A, Niculescu A-G, Grumezescu AM, Beuran M. Emerging therapeutic strategies in sarcopenia: an updated review on pathogenesis and treatment advances. Int J Mol Sci. 2024;25(8):4300. https://doi.org/10.3390/ijms25084300.
164. Gellhaus B, Böker KO, Schilling AF, Saul D. Therapeutic consequences of targeting the IGF-1/PI3K/AKT/FOXO3 Axis in sarcopenia: a narrative review. Cells. 2023 Dec 7;12(24):2787. https://doi.org/10.3390/cells12242787.
165. Arora Y, Priya, Kumar M, Kumar D. Current approaches in CRISPR-Cas system for metabolic disorder. In: Prog Mol Biol Transl Sci, vol. 210; 2025. p. 1–19. https://doi.org/10.1016/bs.pmbts.2024.10.001.
166. Lu Y, Li T, Shu Y, Lu C, Luo Z, Wang J, Xiong H, Li W. Lipid peroxidation and sarcopenia: molecular mechanisms and potential therapeutic approaches. Front Med (Lausanne). 2025;12:1525205. https://doi.org/10.3389/fmed.2025.1525205.
167. Kanbay M, Ozbek L, Guldan M, Abdel-Rahman SM, Narin AE, Ortiz A. Ultra-processed foods and cardio-kidney-metabolic syndrome: a review of recent evidence. Eur J Intern Med. 2025;136:4–18. https://doi.org/10.1016/j.ejim.2025.03.003.
168. Chew W, Lim YP, Lim WS, Chambers ES, Frost G, Wong SH, Ali Y. Gut-muscle crosstalk. A perspective on influence of microbes on muscle function. Front Med (Lausanne). 2023;9:1065365. https://doi.org/10.3389/fmed.2022.1065365.
169. Sattar N, McMurray J, Borén J, Rawshani A, Omerovic E, Berg N, Halminen J, Skoglund K, Eliasson B, Gerstein HC, McGuire DK, Bhatt D, Rawshani A. Twenty years of cardiovascular complications and risk factors in patients with type 2 diabetes: a Nationwide Swedish Cohort Study. Circulation. 2023;147(25):1872–86. https://doi.org/10.1161/CIRCULATIONAHA.122.063374.

Chapter 15
Sleep Disorders and Circadian Sleep Disruption in Cardiovascular–Kidney–Metabolic Syndrome

Radu Crisan Dabija and Andreea Zabara Antal

Introduction

Sleep and circadian rhythms are pivotal in regulating cardio-metabolic and renal physiology. Disruption of these systems, through sleep disorders such as insomnia or obstructive sleep apnea (OSA), shift work, or environmental misalignment, has been strongly linked to the development and progression of cardiovascular, metabolic, and kidney diseases. This chapter explores the molecular architecture of the circadian clock, individual variation in chronotype, and the complex interplay between circadian misalignment and systemic disease. Insomnia contributes to metabolic dysfunction via sympathetic overactivity, inflammation, and impaired glucose metabolism. Likewise, OSA is implicated in the pathogenesis of hypertension, insulin resistance, and chronic kidney disease through intermittent hypoxia, oxidative stress, and fluid shifts. Both conditions amplify the pathophysiological burden of the recently defined cardiovascular–kidney–metabolic (CKM) syndrome. Therapeutic strategies discussed include cognitive behavioral therapy for insomnia (CBT-I), continuous positive airway pressure (CPAP) therapy for OSA, and novel chronotherapeutic interventions such as timed light exposure, time-restricted feeding, and chrono-pharmacology. This approach aims to restore circadian alignment, improve sleep quality, and mitigate cardio-metabolic risk. A multidisciplinary, chronobiology-informed approach integrating sleep assessment into routine care can improve long-term health outcomes and reduce disease burden across interconnected systems.

R. C. Dabija
Grigore T. Popa University of Medicine and Pharmacy, Iasi, Romania

Clinical Hospital of Pulmonary Diseases, Iasi, Romania

A. Z. Antal (✉)
Grigore T. Popa University of Medicine and Pharmacy, Iasi, Romania

M. Floria, D. M. Tanase (eds.), *Cardiovascular-Kidney-Metabolic Syndrome*,
https://doi.org/10.1007/978-3-032-11445-7_15

Circadian Rhythms and Their Clinical Implications: From Molecular Mechanisms to Disease Risk

Overview of Circadian Rhythms and the Molecular Components of the Circadian Clock

Circadian rhythms are innate. There are approximately 24-hour cycles in biological processes synchronized with the Earth's rotation and the light–dark cycle. These rhythms are found in almost all living organisms, including animals, plants, fungi, and bacteria [1].

The daily rhythms are ruled by an internal timekeeping system known as the circadian clock, which helps coordinate physiological processes to ensure alignment between internal functions and external environmental cues. The biological clock regulates various processes, including intracellular signaling, DNA damage response and repair, angiogenesis, cell proliferation, metabolic balance, redox homeostasis, and immune and inflammatory responses across various organs and tissues. The master circadian clock is located in the suprachiasmatic nucleus (SCN) of the hypothalamus, while peripheral clocks operate in tissues such as muscle, adipose tissue, liver, and pancreas. Light is the most potent environmental cue (or *Zeitgeber)* that synchronizes the clock. Light signals are detected by the retina and transmitted via the retinohypothalamic tract to the SCN, thereby setting the circadian phase [1, 2].

At the molecular level, both central and peripheral clocks are regulated by transcriptional–translational feedback loops. Key molecular components of this system include neuronal PAS domain protein 2 (NPAS2), brain and muscle ARNT-like 1 (BMAL1), period genes (PER1, PER2, PER3), cryptochrome genes (CRY1, CRY2), nuclear receptor genes (NR1D1 and NR1D2), and retinoic acid-related orphan receptors (RORα, RORβ, and RORγ). Systemic synchronization between the central clock and peripheral tissues is determined by a network of neural, hormonal, thermal, and behavioral signals, enabling coordinated physiological function throughout the body [2].

Animal and human studies have demonstrated that genetic variation can influence circadian timing, contributing to significant differences in the intrinsic circadian period among individuals. In humans, the sleep–wake cycle follows a predictable developmental pattern, delaying progressively during adolescence and peaking around the age of 20, gradually advancing across the adult lifespan [2]. Considering that circadian rhythm is part of a complex biological cycle, regulated by interactions between intracellular mechanisms, physiological processes, individual behavior, and environmental factors, there is increasing evidence that its dysregulation contributes to the development of cardiovascular pathologies, chronic kidney disease, and metabolic dysfunctions [3].

Chronotype: Individual Variation in Circadian Phase and Metabolic Health

The individual's daily rhythm of sleep and activity, known as the *chronotype*, reflects differences in the circadian clock's phase angle of entrainment and intrinsic circadian period. Both environmental influences and biological age shape chronotype. It can be evaluated subjectively using validated questionnaires, such as the Morningness–Eveningness Questionnaire (MEQ), which assesses preferred behavioral timing, or the Munich Chronotype Questionnaire (MCTQ), which analyzes differences in sleep patterns between workdays and free days. Objective assessment is achieved through wrist actigraphy, a wearable accelerometer worn on the nondominant wrist, which allows for long-term, noninvasive tracking of sleep–wake cycles and circadian rhythm patterns. Individuals with an early chronotype tend to wake up and perform optimally in the morning, while those with a late chronotype prefer evening activity and show a delayed sleep phase. Although the precise mechanism underlying chronotype variation remains unclear, lifestyle and behavioral factors are thought to play a significant role [4].

Research has consistently shown that late chronotypes increase risk for cardiometabolic disorders, such as elevated fasting blood glucose, HbA1c, triglycerides, and low-density lipoprotein (LDL) cholesterol. A higher body mass index (BMI) is associated with a late chronotype among women. A key feature of the late chronotype is social jet lag, the misalignment between endogenous circadian timing and externally imposed schedules (e.g., work or school). This mismatch leads to chronic circadian disruption and has been linked to reduced glucose tolerance and an increased risk of type 2 diabetes mellitus. Longitudinal studies suggest that individuals maintain a relatively stable chronotype ranking across their lifespan compared to peers in similar geographic settings. Sex-based differences in chronotype expression also emerge with age: younger women more commonly exhibit early chronotypes, but this pattern frequently reverses after age 40 [5]. Findings from the Study of Women's Health Across the Nation (SWAN) cohort indicate that perimenopausal women with greater variability in bedtime have higher BMI, increased body fat percentage, and lower lean mass percentage. Moreover, social jet lag is associated with elevated cholesterol levels in younger women, a pattern not observed in men [6].

Circadian Control of Glucose and Cardiovascular Physiology

Glucose homeostasis is tightly regulated by clock-controlled mechanisms in metabolic organs, including the pancreas, liver, muscle, and adipose tissue. These systems work together to align blood glucose levels with the circadian phase. Glycemia typically peaks at the start of the active phase, regardless of food intake, under the regulation of the central brain clock. This master clock also modulates the expression of glucose transporters, glucagon receptors, and enzymes involved in gluconeogenesis. Critically, glucose tolerance is highest in the early active phase and gradually declines throughout the day. Therefore, eating at biologically inappropriate times, such as late at night, can result in misaligned insulin release, leading to postprandial hyperglycemia and metabolic dysregulation [7]. Each metabolic organ possesses a functional circadian clock, underscoring its coordinated role in glucose regulation. Numerous studies have shown that early chronotypes tend to have a lower risk of developing type 2 diabetes mellitus [8]. Experimental studies conducted under controlled laboratory conditions have demonstrated that circadian misalignment impairs glucose metabolism. For example, healthy individuals working simulated night shifts exhibited increased postprandial glucose levels due to reduced β-cell responsiveness. Similar effects have been observed in individuals with impaired glucose tolerance or type 2 diabetes mellitus [9]. Morris et al. demonstrated a 6% increase in postprandial glucose levels under conditions of circadian misalignment. In another study [10], Bescós found a decrease in insulin sensitivity following four consecutive simulated night shifts in healthy participants [11]. Prospective cohort studies, including data from the American Nurses Health Study, have confirmed a dose–response relationship between shift work duration and the risk of developing type 2 diabetes mellitus, independent of BMI [12].

Circadian Impact on Cardiovascular Risk

Of further relevance, cardiovascular events exhibit marked diurnal variation, with incidence peaks observed around 9:00 AM and again at 8:00 PM, underscoring the physiological importance of circadian timing in cardiovascular health. Cardiovascular outcomes are also adversely affected; data from the EARLY-MYO-CMR registry indicated that shift workers with ST-elevation myocardial infarction (STEMI) had larger post-reperfusion infarct sizes and, over a median follow-up of 5 years, a higher incidence of major adverse cardiovascular events [13]. Mechanistic studies suggest that circadian disruption can induce inflammatory pathways, such as interleukin-6 (IL-6) signaling, contributing to vascular dysfunction. Structural indicators, like increased carotid intima-media thickness, have been observed in night shift workers. Elevated sympathetic tone and reduced cardioprotective parasympathetic activity during misaligned sleep–wake cycles may further exacerbate cardiovascular risk [14]. Epidemiological data reveal that shift workers regularly experience elevated systolic and diastolic blood pressures. A systematic review of 45 studies confirmed significantly higher blood pressure among shift workers. In a US cohort study involving 2151 manufacturing workers, individuals engaged in predominantly night work with frequent schedule rotations had a fourfold increased risk of hypertension. The highest hypertension rates were noted among those working 95–100% night shifts [15].

Circadian Rhythm Sleep–Wake Disorders (CRSWDs)

Circadian rhythm sleep–wake disorders (CRSWDs) are characterized by a misalignment between an individual's endogenous circadian timing system and the external environment. This discordance between internal biological rhythms and the sleep–wake schedule demanded by societal, occupational, or personal obligations often leads to sleep disturbances or impairments in daytime functioning. CRSWDs are broadly classified into intrinsic and extrinsic types. Intrinsic disorders originate from internal alterations of the circadian timing system, while environmental or behavioral factors primarily induce extrinsic disorders [16].

Advanced sleep-wake phase disorder (ASWPD) is defined by habitual sleep and wake times several hours earlier than socially conventional. Individuals typically report difficulty staying awake in the evening and waking up excessively early. While the precise etiology remains poorly understood, diagnosis necessitates carefully excluding other primary sleep disorders, particularly insomnia [16].

Non-24–hour sleep–wake rhythm disorder is mostly seen in totally blind individuals. This disorder results from a failure of the circadian pacemaker to entrain the 24-hour light–dark cycle. Affected individuals exhibit a free-running rhythm, with sleep and wake times progressively delaying each day. Although rare in sighted individuals, it may occur in the context of psychiatric comorbidities [16].

Irregular sleep–wake rhythm disorder is characterized by the absence of a well-defined circadian sleep–wake pattern. Individuals with this condition experience multiple short periods of sleep and wakefulness throughout the 24-hour day. This leads to fragmented sleep, excessive daytime sleepiness, and impaired social and occupational functioning [16].

Extrinsic circadian rhythm sleep–wake disorders include shift work disorder and jet lag disorder [16].

Health Impacts of Shift Work and Jet Lag

In contemporary society, shift work is prevalent across sectors such as healthcare, transportation, emergency services, and manufacturing. According to European Working Conditions Survey data, only 43% of workers maintain regular schedules, while 21% work rotating or permanent shifts, and 19% engage in night work [16]. Such schedules often lead to a misalignment between internal circadian rhythms and externally imposed work times, resulting in chronic sleep deprivation, fatigue, and adverse health outcomes [17].

Jet lag disorder arises following rapid trans-meridian travel, which causes a temporary mismatch between the circadian clock and the destination's local time. Typically, symptoms include insomnia, daytime sleepiness, impaired cognitive performance, and gastrointestinal disturbances [15].

Shift work has been associated with a host of adverse health outcomes, including increased risks for cardiovascular disease, metabolic syndrome, gastrointestinal dysfunction, mood disturbances, and cancer. The International Agency for Research on Cancer (IARC) has classified night shift work involving circadian disruption as "probably carcinogenic to humans" (Group 2A) [18]. Disruption of circadian rhythms due to shift work may lead to hormonal imbalances, elevated blood pressure, immune dysfunction, and altered metabolic profiles. Numerous studies have reported a strong association between shift work and obesity. A meta-analysis of 28 studies concluded that night shift workers are significantly more likely to be overweight or obese compared to day workers. The intensity, duration, and frequency of night shift exposure are critical determinants of this risk [19].

The Interconnected Web: Insomnia's Role in Metabolic and Cardiovascular Health

Understanding Sleep Disorders: Classification, Criteria, and the Case of Chronic Insomnia

Sleep is a fundamental biological process essential in maintaining physical, mental, and cognitive health. Increasing evidence indicates that approximately 30–40% of adults fail to obtain the recommended minimum 7 hours of nightly sleep. The National Sleep Foundation (NSF) recommends a sleep duration of 7–9 hours per night for adults aged 18–64 years. Both short sleep duration (6 hours or less) and long sleep duration (10 hours or more) have been associated with adverse effects on health and well-being [20, 21].

Sleep disorders encompass a group of medical conditions that disrupt the usual pattern, quality, timing, or duration of sleep. Consequently, in addition to impairing physical, mental, and emotional functioning, sleep disorders can significantly impact an individual's overall health status [22].

The *International Classification of Sleep Disorders, Third Edition* (ICSD-3), published by the American Academy of Sleep Medicine, provides a comprehensive taxonomy of sleep disorders and detailed diagnostic criteria aligned with ICD-11 guidelines [23].

One such disorder is *chronic insomnia,* characterized by persistent difficulty initiating or maintaining sleep and experiencing non-restorative sleep despite adequate opportunity and appropriate conditions. To meet diagnostic criteria, these symptoms must occur at least three nights per week and persist for over 3 months. Chronic insomnia typically results in significant distress or daytime impairment, including fatigue, mood disturbances or irritability, general malaise, and cognitive difficulties such as reduced concentration or memory [23].

Insomnia-Induced Metabolic Disturbances: From Sympathetic Overactivation to Gut Microbiota Alterations

Insomnia significantly contributes to glycemic disturbances through interconnected pathophysiological mechanisms that impair glucose metabolism and reduce insulin sensitivity. A central feature of insomnia is chronic sleep deprivation, which leads to sustained activation of the sympathetic nervous system and a corresponding reduction in parasympathetic activity. The autonomic imbalance induces insulin secretion that promotes hepatic gluconeogenesis. These processes foster insulin resistance and set the stage for broader metabolic dysfunction. Sleep disturbances are associated with elevated levels of pro-inflammatory cytokines, particularly interleukin-6 (IL-6) and tumor necrosis factor-alpha (TNF-α). These cytokines interfere with insulin signaling pathways, reducing insulin sensitivity and impairing glucose uptake in peripheral tissues [24].

Metabolic syndrome (MetS) is a group of simultaneous disorders including central obesity, hypertension, increased fasting glucose levels, higher triglyceride levels, or low high-density lipoprotein (HDL) levels. The prevalence data range from 20% to 45% in the global population, from 20% to 30% among different ethnicities in the United States, and is approximately 24% in Asia [25]. A systematic review and meta-analysis incorporating 27 cross-sectional and nine prospective studies, encompassing over 235,000 participants, found that short sleep duration is significantly associated with an increased risk of metabolic syndrome. Specifically, individuals with insufficient sleep exhibited a 15% higher likelihood of developing this cluster of cardio-metabolic risk factors than those with adequate sleep duration [26].

A recent clinical investigation examined the relationship between insomnia symptoms and metabolic syndrome in a cohort of 272 patients diagnosed with severe psychiatric disorders at the Shantou University Mental Health Centre. Utilizing the Pittsburgh Sleep Quality Index (PSQI >7) to define insomnia, the study found that 34.6% of patients exhibited clinically significant insomnia symptoms. Notably, this subgroup displayed a markedly higher prevalence of metabolic syndrome (23.4% vs 12.4%, $p = 0.019$) and hypertriglyceridemia (30.9% vs. 19.1%, $p = 0.029$), along with marginally elevated indices of fasting insulin, insulin resistance (HOMA-IR), and prevalence of insulin resistance. Multivariate logistic regression analyses revealed that individuals experiencing insomnia symptoms had significantly increased odds of meeting diagnostic criteria for key metabolic disturbances. Specifically, they were nearly three times more likely to have metabolic syndrome (OR = 2.99; 95% CI: 1.25–7.14), over three times more likely to present with central obesity (OR = 3.02), and more than twice as likely to exhibit hypertriglyceridemia (OR = 2.46), even after adjusting for potential confounding variables [27].

The gut microbiota, comprising thousands of microbial species encountered in the human gastrointestinal tract, is an essential player in digestion and regulating the host's immune response, metabolic activity, and neural function. Research data support the significance of the "gut–brain axis," a complex, bidirectional communication system linking the gastrointestinal tract and the central nervous system, in modulating emotional responses, mood, and sleep cycles [28]. Certain gut bacteria can produce neurotransmitters such as serotonin and gamma-aminobutyric acid (GABA), influencing sleep quality and emotional well-being. Notably, individuals with insomnia often exhibit reduced gut microbiota diversity, which has been associated with impaired stress regulation and emotional dysregulation. Specific bacterial genera, including *Faecalibacterium* and *Bifidobacterium*, have been positively linked to better sleep outcomes [29]. A recent study by Xie et al. [30] used a two-sample Mendelian randomization approach to investigate the causal relationship between gut microbial metabolic pathways and insomnia. Drawing on genetic data from the Openwas and FinnGen databases, the study found that specific microbial pathways, particularly those involved in carbohydrate metabolism, such as gluconeogenesis and the tricarboxylic acid (TCA) cycle VII acetate producers (PWY.7254), were positively associated with insomnia risk. Conversely, the hexitol fermentation to lactate, formate, ethanol, and acetate pathway (P461. PWY) demonstrated a protective effect. Multivariable MR analyses confirmed these associations as robust and independent, without evidence of pleiotropy or heterogeneity [30].

The Cardiovascular Burden of Insomnia: Neuroendocrine Mechanisms, Inflammation, and Mortality Risk

Disruptions in sleep duration and quality have been increasingly recognized as significant risk factors for cardiovascular disease, primarily through mechanisms involving immune alteration, elevated sympathetic nervous system activity, chronic activation of the endocrine stress response, and endothelial dysfunction. The hypothalamic–pituitary–adrenal (HPA) axis is related to this response, a key neuroendocrine system closely synchronized with circadian rhythms. Dysregulation of the HPA axis due to poor sleep contributes to physiological stress, increased heart rate, reduced heart rate variability, and elevated catecholamine secretion. After just a few nights of restricted sleep, limited to 3–4 hours per night, hormonal alterations occur, resulting in a marked decrease of approximately 30% in morning cortisol levels and an increase of approximately 40% in afternoon cortisol concentrations [31].

The physiological circadian rhythm directly regulates immune cells and inflammatory cytokines, including tumor necrosis factor (TNF-α) and interleukins: IL-1, IL-2, IL-6, and IL-10. The Cleveland Family Study showed that each hour less of sleep recorded via specific means was associated with an 8% increase in TNF-α [32]. Elevated high-sensitivity C-reactive protein (CRP), which plays a crucial role in opsonizing low-density lipoprotein cholesterol by macrophages in atherosclerotic plaque, has been linked with decreased sleep duration, especially in women

[31]. A recent meta-review and Mendelian randomization (MR) meta-analysis published in 2023 has provided robust evidence linking insomnia to an increased risk of cardiovascular diseases (CVDs). By synthesizing results from both observational and genetic studies, the research confirms that insomnia is not merely a symptom but a potential causal contributor to conditions such as coronary artery disease, atrial fibrillation, heart failure, hypertension, and ischemic stroke. Specifically, MR findings, which offer stronger causal inference, demonstrated that genetic predisposition to insomnia significantly raises the odds of developing coronary artery disease (OR = 1.14), hypertension (OR = 1.16), and other major CVDs. These associations persisted even after accounting for common confounders, suggesting the link is biologically grounded rather than behavioral. No causal association was found for cardio-embolic or small vessel stroke subtypes. This body of evidence emphasizes the clinical importance of early insomnia diagnosis and intervention to improve sleep. This is a strategic component of cardiovascular disease prevention [32].

An assessment of the risk in cardiovascular events and mortality, via a comprehensive meta-analysis of 21 studies, found that people with insomnia face a 53% higher risk of cardiovascular mortality and a 48% increased likelihood of experiencing a myocardial infarction. Furthermore, the analysis indicates a 31% rise in all-cause mortality and a 14% greater incidence of cardiovascular disease among individuals affected by insomnia [33]. A recent study combining observational cohort data with Mendelian randomization analyses demonstrated that sleep disturbances, particularly insomnia and short sleep duration, are associated with an increased risk of atrial fibrillation (AF). Using data from the UK Biobank and the Trondelag Health Study (HUNT2), researchers found that individuals with a genetic predisposition to insomnia symptoms had a 14% higher risk of AF. At the same time, those predisposed to short sleep duration (≤6 hours) showed a similarly elevated risk. Notably, participants genetically predisposed to both insomnia and short sleep exhibited the most significant AF risk, and the effects were additive rather than synergistic. While findings in the HUNT2 cohort were less consistent, this study highlights the potential cardiovascular consequences of poor sleep and supports targeting sleep traits in AF prevention strategies [34].

The Interwoven Pathophysiology and Socioeconomic Burden of Obstructive Sleep Apnea (OSA) Within the Framework of Cardio–Kidney–Metabolic (CKM) Syndrome

Global Epidemiology, Economic and Societal Burden of OSA

Sleep is a key regulator of several physiological processes associated with regulating cardio-metabolic function. Insufficient or poor-quality sleep alters glucose metabolism, facilitates insulin resistance, and contributes to weight gain through increased energy intake, thereby amplifying the risk of obesity and related metabolic disorders. Moreover, long-term sleep deprivation is directly associated with elevated blood pressure, systemic inflammation, and oxidative stress, all being key drivers in the pathogenesis of hypertension, atherosclerosis, and major adverse cardiovascular events [35].

The first study incorporating global epidemiological data on obstructive sleep apnea (OSA) was published in 2019. It is estimated that approximately 936 million individuals (95% CI: 903–970 million), aged between 30 and 69 years, are affected by OSA worldwide when applying an apnea–hypopnea index (AHI) threshold of 5 events/hour [36]. When the diagnostic threshold is increased to 15 events/hour, the number of affected individuals in the same age group decreases to 425 million (95% CI: 399–450 million). The highest national prevalence rates were recorded in China, followed by the United States and Brazil [37]. OSA is more prevalent in men than in women, with estimated rates ranging from 13% to 33% in men and from 6% to 19% in women in the general adult population. This sex-based disparity narrows after menopause [38]. Several physiological factors contribute to the higher prevalence in men, including greater upper airway collapsibility, heightened chemoreceptor sensitivity, and a diminished ventilatory response to carbon dioxide. In contrast, women with OSA tend to exhibit shorter apneic episodes, a higher frequency of hypopneas rather than apneas, and a greater predominance of rapid eye movement (REM)-related OSA, with fewer cases of supine-predominant OSA compared to men [39].

The economic cost of OSA is due mainly to the high prevalence of underdiagnosed cases and poor adherence among diagnosed patients. It includes a broad spectrum of expenses in the healthcare system and a social burden that arises from its association with various comorbidities and complications. These health complications increase healthcare expenditures, including diagnosis, treatment, hospitalization, and long-term comorbidity management. There is also an economic impact: more visits to the doctor, as well as higher costs for medical treatment and medications for comorbid conditions affected by OSA. There are substantial indirect costs of sleep apnea and narrow direct medical costs. These involve the reduced work efficiency associated with excessive daytime sleepiness (EDS), cognitive dysfunction, and mood disorders such as depression, which are heightened by poor sleep quality from OSA [40]. For companies, the implications can manifest as increased absenteeism and reduced work performance, negatively affecting economic productivity. OSA can contribute to a higher rate of sick leave, absenteeism, and diminished workplace effectiveness due to its impact on cognitive function and overall well-being [41, 42]. Sleep disorders are associated with increased workplace accidents [35]. It is also linked to poor learning skills, memory, executive function, attention, cognition, work limitations, and absenteeism. Other nonfinancial costs are derived from the loss of life quality and premature death [43].

A European Union multicenter study involving 2008 eligible patients reported that OSA patients with concomitant excessive daytime sleepiness (EDS) required significantly more healthcare provider interactions and emergency department visits, leading to decreased productivity at work and at home. Additionally, these patients reported substantially impaired health-related quality of life compared to OSA patients without EDS [44]. Some symptoms of EDS, which can have significant functional consequences, include lack of attention, lapses in judgment, impaired concentration, reduced social interaction, and the tendency to fall asleep during day-to-day activities.

Furthermore, the presence of OSA has been linked to an increase in motor vehicle crashes; the social costs of such events represent an additional aspect of social cost, underscoring the importance of timely diagnosis and treatment [45]. EDS is also recognized as a contributing factor to motor vehicle accidents (MVAs) [46].

A study of the Australian population estimated that individuals with sleep apnea collectively experienced 193.7 million years of life lost and 182.7 million PALYs (productivity-adjusted life-years) over their lifetimes. If there is a 10% reduction in OSA and comorbid conditions, the potential incremental gains in life years and PALYs could be 45,401 and 150,950, respectively. From an economic perspective, this health gain was estimated to produce more than AU$25 billion in extra GDP among the working-age population. In addition, this intervention could prevent an estimated 116,701 deaths and 47,542 cardiovascular events, as well as reduce the incidence of type 2 diabetes mellitus (T2DM) and the associated healthcare expenditures [47]. The expanding research landscape in sleep apnea generates accumulating evidence that underscores not only the cardio-metabolic implications of OSA but also its broader systemic effects [48]. In some studies, OSA was evaluated, whereas in other studies, the concept of sleep apnea (SA) was used, referring also to central sleep apnea (CSA) and mixed sleep apnea (MSA).

Pathophysiological Mechanism, Clinical Manifestations, and Diagnostic Criteria of OSA

Obstructive sleep apnea is defined by intermittent events of complete or partial upper airway obstruction during the night that result in arousal from sleep and/or a decrease in oxyhemoglobin saturation (SpO_2). Obstructive apnea is defined as an at least 90% reduction in airflow for at least 10 s in the presence of inspiratory efforts of the upper airway muscles against the occluded airway. Hypopnea is a reduction of at least 30% in airflow for at least 10 s associated with a 3% or more drop in SpO_2 levels and/or arousal. We can also report hypopneas using a definition requiring an associated ≥4% desaturation [1, 3]. Obstructive sleep apnea diagnosis is based on the number of apneas and hypopneas per sleep hours, defined as an apnea–hypopnea index (AHI). According to the International Classification of Sleep Disorders-Third edition published in 2014 (ICSD-3), OSA is defined as: (1) having an AHI of 5 events/hour or more on polysomnography (PSG) or home sleep apnea test (HSAT) associated with typical symptoms of OSA, or comorbid conditions (hypertension, coronary artery disease, stroke); or (2) having an AHI of at least 15 events/hour in the absence of symptoms or comorbidities [49, 50].

The American Academy of Sleep Medicine (AASM) Task Force has established severity criteria for obstructive sleep apnea (OSA) based on daytime sleepiness and the frequency of respiratory events during the night. OSA severity is classified according to the number of obstructive breathing events per hour of sleep: mild (5–15 events/hour), moderate (>15–30 events/hour), and severe (more than 30 events/hour) [51]. Edwards et al. attempted to provide a new perspective on the definition and diagnostic criteria of obstructive sleep apnea syndrome, establishing some OSA phenotypes with particular signs and symptoms, each with different prognoses and management recommendations adapted to the patient's needs. In this context, they proved that out of the three predominant phenotypes, the disturbed sleep group, the minimally symptomatic group, and the excessive daytime sleepiness group, the minimally symptomatic group showed a significantly high association with comorbidities like hypertension, diabetes, and cardiovascular pathology. This fact further highlights the high frequency of OSA in those with associated cardiometabolic disease [52].

OSA is a multifactorial disorder, with a pathogenesis influenced by anatomical, neuromuscular, and physiological factors. During sleep, nasal breathing is often impaired due to increased mucosal congestion in the supine position and circadian fluctuations in nasal resistance [53, 54]. Elevated nasal resistance encourages mouth breathing [55], raising upper airway resistance by as much as 2–2.5 times. This mechanism may contribute to pharyngeal lumen narrowing and an increased frequency of obstructive events [56]. Another contributing mechanism involves the nasal ventilatory reflex, which posits that reduced nasal airflow leads to diminished stimulation of nasal receptors, thereby decreasing pharyngeal muscle tone and central respiratory drive, factors that exacerbate apneic episodes [57, 58]. Studies have demonstrated that the pharyngeal lumen in individuals with OSA and habitual snorers often exhibits an elliptical shape, with the long axis oriented in the anterior–posterior direction. This contrasts with the lateral orientation seen in individuals without OSA and may reflect lateral wall collapse [59, 60]. Contributing factors to this collapse include vascular congestion or chronic inflammation resulting from repetitive trauma due to snoring vibrations [61]. Additional anatomical variations, such as soft palate thickening, uvular hypertrophy, and enlarged tonsils, are also associated with increased OSA severity [62]. Craniofacial abnormalities significantly influence OSA susceptibility. Structural features such as increased lower facial height, a shortened mandible, a more obtuse cranial base angle, macroglossia, and inferior displacement of the hyoid bone are all implicated. These may be further compounded by deleterious oral habits (e.g., thumb sucking), aberrant tongue posture, chronic mouth breathing, tumorous growths, or endocrine disorders [63, 64]. Neuromuscular tone is essential for maintaining upper airway patency during sleep. In individuals with OSA, the genioglossus muscle, a key upper airway dilator, displays a predominance of fast-twitch fibers and a relative deficit in slow-twitch fibers, leading to reduced tonic activity during the transition to sleep. An overly sensitive ventilatory control system, characterized by elevated loop gain, can induce exaggerated oscillatory responses from the brainstem, reducing arterial partial pressure of carbon dioxide ($PaCO_2$) below the apnea threshold [65]. In addition, a low respiratory arousal threshold may predispose individuals to obstructive events by triggering premature awakenings before compensatory upper airway muscle activation can occur [66].

A strong and well-documented relationship exists between elevated body mass index (BMI) and the risk of developing obstructive sleep apnea (OSA). Approximately 40% of adults with obesity suffer from severe OSA, and more than 70% of patients diagnosed in sleep clinics are classified as obese [67]. Prospective population studies indicate that a 10% increase in body weight is associated with a sixfold increase in the risk of developing OSA. Conversely, a 10% weight reduction can lead to a 26% improvement in the severity of OSA [68]. The mechanisms underlying this association include fat accumulation around the upper airway, which compromises airway patency, alterations in the drive-to-load balance of ventilation, reduced lung volumes, and elevated leptin levels that may influence respiratory control [69]. Lifestyle factors also contribute to OSA risk. Cigarette smoking is known to increase upper airway inflammation and promote the collapsibility of airway structures, thereby raising the likelihood of obstructive events [70]. Similarly, alcohol consumption, particularly in the evening, has been shown to impair the function of pharyngeal dilator muscles and reduce the arousal response to apneic episodes. These effects are dose-dependent and significantly influence OSA severity [71].

Genetics also plays a significant role in OSA susceptibility. Heritability studies estimate familial factors, such as shared obesity, may account for up to one-third of the apnea–hypopnea index (AHI) variability. Moreover, non-obesity-related genetic influences, including craniofacial morphology, variations in soft-tissue structure, and specific genetic polymorphisms, further contribute to OSA risk [72–74].

Cardiovascular–Kidney–Metabolic (CKM) Syndrome: Interconnected Pathologies

In 2023, the American Heart Association proposed the concept of cardiovascular–kidney–metabolic (CKM) syndrome, defining it as a health disorder involving the physiological processes of obesity, diabetes, chronic kidney disease, and cardiovascular disease (CVD) [75].

Cardio–kidney–metabolic (CKM) syndrome is an important clinical and pathophysiological concept. Being a significant connection between these three medical entities, it has been defined in the last few years. The similar pathophysiological basis of these diseases has implied the requirement for uniformly dealing with them, thus conditioning a sophisticated integrated diagnostic and therapeutic approach designed explicitly on the patient's profile. CKM is a syndrome in which metabolic risk factors, chronic kidney disease, and the cardiovascular system are interconnected. If, on the one hand, patients with CKD frequently express metabolic risk factors that contribute to the establishment of cardiovascular pathology, patients with preexisting cardiovascular pathology frequently exhibit metabolic risk factors, which, in turn, favor the installation or progression of the renal damage [75].

The CKM syndrome is a progressive condition, as it evolves through specific stages: Stage 0 occurs when no CKM risk factors are present; stage 1 is characterized by abnormal or excessive adiposity; stage 2 includes additional metabolic risk factors such as hypertension, diabetes, metabolic syndrome or moderate-to-high risk for CKD; stage 3 includes evidence of subclinical CVD or equivalent predicted high cardiovascular risk in those with abnormal/excessive adiposity, other metabolic risk factors or CKD; stage 4 is the onset of clinical CVD, being divided into its substages that include or do not include kidney failure. The staging emphasizes the value of early CKM syndrome detection to prevent further complications [75].

Table 15.1 provides a detailed overview of the staging system for cardiovascular–kidney–metabolic (CKM) syndrome as proposed by the American Heart Association in 2023. This progressive classification reflects the continuum of interrelated pathophysiological changes between metabolic dysfunction, cardiovascular disease, and chronic kidney disease (CKD). Each stage integrates clinical markers and risk factors, including anthropometric measures (such as body mass index and waist circumference), metabolic parameters (e.g., blood pressure, glucose, lipid profile), renal function (eGFR, albuminuria), and cardiovascular risk or disease (ASCVD risk score, subclinical atherosclerosis, cardiovascular events).

Table 15.1 Overview of the staging system for cardiovascular–kidney–metabolic (CKM) syndrome

Stage	Description	Key features
Stage 0	No CKM risk factors	Normal BMI (18.5–24.9 kg/m^2) Normal blood pressure (<120/80 mmHg) Fasting glucose <100 mg/dL – eGFR ≥90 mL/min/1.73 m^2 with no markers of kidney damage
Stage 1	Abnormal or excessive adiposity	BMI ≥25 kg/m^2 (overweight) BMI ≥30 kg/m^2 (obesity) Waist circumference > 102 cm (men), >88 cm (women)
Stage 2	Metabolic risk factors and/or moderate-to-high CKD risk	*Hypertension:* ≥130/80 mmHg or need for antihypertensive use *Type 2 diabetes mellitus:* Fasting glucose ≥126 mg/dL or HbA1c ≥6.5% *Dyslipidemia:* TG ≥150 mg/dL, HDL <40 mg/dL (men) / <50 mg/dL (women) *CKD risk:* eGFR 60–89 mL/min/1.73 m^2 with albuminuria (ACR ≥30 mg/g) or other structural abnormalities
Stage 3	Subclinical CVD or high predicted cardiovascular risk	*Coronary artery calcium score > 100* *LV hypertrophy or diastolic dysfunction on imaging* *high 10-year ASCVD risk* (≥7.5–20% depending on guideline) *Elevated carotid intima-media thickness*
Stage 4	Clinical CVD (± kidney failure)	*MI, angina, heart failure, stroke, PAD* *eGFR < 60 mL/min/1.73 m^2* or *kidney failure (eGFR < 15 or dialysis)* *Albuminuria ≥ 300 mg/g* (severe)

The pathophysiological consequences of CKM syndrome result from recurrent interactions between metabolic risk factors, chronic kidney disease, and cardiovascular physiology. Abdominal obesity, abnormal glucose metabolism, dyslipidemia, and hypertension, components of metabolic syndrome (MetS), are among the most significant features of the CKM syndrome. Excess secretion or dysfunction of adipose tissue, specifically in the visceral compartment, is recognized to be a source of pro-inflammatory and pro-oxidative mediators that cause structural and functional modifications in vascular, myocardial, and renal tissues. These inflammatory pathways impair insulin sensitivity and alter glucose metabolism [76]. Moreover, metabolic dysfunction-associated steatotic liver disease (MASLD, previously called nonalcoholic fatty liver disease) exacerbates systemic inflammation and insulin resistance. Various inflammatory and oxidative mediators released in the systemic circulation aggravate atherosclerosis, myocardial injury, glomerular sclerosis, tubular inflammation, and kidney fibrosis. Apart from the systemic contributions, ectopic adipose tissue, namely pericardial, epicardial, and perirenal, releases local factors contributing to local pressure elevation. In consequence, arrhythmia and myocardial dysfunction can develop along with coronary artery disease. Type 2 diabetes (T2D), the most frequent complication of MetS, appears as a consequence of sustained insulin resistance and pancreatic beta-cell dysfunction, ultimately leading to increased renal and vascular complication risk [75].

In the CKM syndrome, vascular, myocardial, and kidney injury include the interactions between four predominant pathways: hemodynamic, metabolic, inflammatory, and fibrotic. Glomerular hyperfiltration and intraglomerular hypertension, two well-known hemodynamic phenomena that were found to participate in the onset of kidney disease, are due to hyperglycemia. These processes not only have a role in obesity and systemic hypertension, but they also both contribute to increased endothelial stress and vascular injury, leading to atherosclerosis and glomerulosclerosis. Hypertension and adipose tissue are essential mediators of left ventricular hypertrophy and heart failure. In T2D, prolonged hyperglycemia induces intracellular signaling programs. It leads to tissue destruction in the shape of inflammation and fibrosis, as well as the extent of advanced glycation end products (AGEs) and reactive oxygen species (ROS) levels. These molecular events eventually lead to chronic inflammation, immune cell influx, and fibrogenic signaling [77].

Over time, the CKM syndrome will become increasingly common since the number of people affected by these mutually reinforcing conditions increases. Results from SIMETAP, a cross-sectional observational multicentric study in which 6588 subjects aged 18.0 to 102.8 years (55.9% females) were enrolled, showed that almost two-fifths of MetS patients are at moderate, high, or very high risk of CKD, and four-fifths are at high or very high cardiovascular risk [78].

Despite the definition that describes the CKM syndrome as a dysfunction caused by the interactions between cardiovascular, renal, and metabolic systems, its clinical and biological complexity implies that it is not just an exclusive result of the pathophysiological mechanisms of these axes and opens up a wide field of research on the influence of other pathologies, such as hepatic or pulmonary, on the genesis and progression of the CKM syndrome. In this regard, some scientific projects are actively proposing the conceptual expansion to "Cardiovascular–Renal–Hepatic–Metabolic Syndrome" [79] while pointing out the need to investigate the added value of sleep disturbances, such as obstructive sleep apnea and insomnia, and circadian rhythm disturbances, common among patients with a severe degree of metabolic dysfunction [79].

Emerging evidence highlights the central role of sleep disorders and circadian rhythm disruption in the pathophysiology of the cardio-kidney-metabolic syndrome. In addition to metabolic and hemodynamic perturbations, degraded sleep patterns and circadian regulatory systems are, more than ever, recognized as potent determinants of the systemic inflammatory response, neurohormonal dysregulation, and sympathetic impairment. These amplifiers are involved in endothelial dysfunction and progressive tissue injury and act as second messengers within the network of cardiovascular, renal, and metabolic disorders. The nature of these interactions is bidirectional, mirroring a cycle in which disrupted sleep impairs existing comorbidities while simultaneously advancing the development of new dysfunctions [78].

Hong et al. showed that the pathophysiological mechanisms of sleep disruption causing metabolic dysfunction include circadian rhythm modification and alterations in glucose and lipid metabolism. It activates inflammatory pathways and modulates the gut genome. The molecular mechanisms linking these processes involve intricate interactions between core clock genes and metabolic regulators, such as AMPK (5′ adenosine monophosphate-activated protein kinase), pro-inflammatory mediators including NF-kB (nuclear factor kappa B), and the NLRP3 (nucleotide-binding domain, leucine-rich–containing family, pyrin domain–containing-3) inflammasome, along with hormonal changes like leptin resistance, high ghrelin levels, cortisol dysregulation, melatonin disruptions, and fluctuations in the composition of the gut microbiota, such as microbial dysbiosis, increased intestinal barrier permeability, and endotoxin translocation [80].

Obstructive Sleep Apnea and Chronic Kidney Disease: A Bidirectional Nexus with Cardiometabolic Consequences

Chronic kidney disease (CKD) is associated with an increased risk of cardiovascular events, which is independent of traditional cardiovascular risk factors, albuminuria, and low GFR, being directly related to the risk of atherosclerotic events, heart failure, and cardiovascular death. A comprehensive systematic review and meta-analysis involving over 26 million participants demonstrated that patients diagnosed with OSA had higher levels of albuminuria than those without OSA [81].

The risk of CKD, metabolic diseases such as diabetes, dyslipidemia, ischemic heart disease, and total CVD was significantly higher among OSA patients ($n = 103{,}785$) compared with controls in a large ($n = 311{,}355$) nationwide cohort in South Korea. Furthermore, they demonstrated an increased susceptibility to metabolic syndrome-related disorders, potentially driven by OSA-induced systemic inflammation and subsequent vascular endothelial damage, which, in some instances, progressed to insulin resistance, glucose intolerance, and the onset of metabolic disorders [82].

New data suggest that sleep-disordered breathing and, in particular, OSA also constitute an additional risk factor for cardiovascular and metabolic dysfunction in patients with CKD [83].

The intermittent hypoxia and disturbed sleep fragmentation that accompany OSA induce sympathetic overactivity, increased oxidative stress, and systemic inflammation, a range of mechanisms that substantially overlap with the ones that characterize CKM syndrome [83]. Excessive reactive oxygen species (ROS) production under intermittent hypoxia results in oxidative stress and inflammation. This process affects the vascular endothelium and, together with metabolic dysfunction, induces atherosclerosis development [84]. OSA can activate the renin–angiotensin–aldosterone system (RAAS), resulting in sodium and water retention, an increase in plasma volume, arterial hypertension, and heart overload, leading to the development of heart failure [85]. In patients with some degree of renal dysfunction, cyclical hypoxia and arousal-induced elevated blood pressure may increase glomerular injury and lower eGFR [86]. CKD may also contribute to the development or aggravation of the sleep disease through upper airway narrowing caused by fluid retention and redistribution, impaired chemoreceptor sensitivity, and the accumulation of uremic toxins, which can diminish pharyngeal muscle tone as well as contribute to uremia-induced neuropathy or myopathy [87]. This evidence suggests that OSA not only accelerates the progression of existing CKD but may also confer risk for new-onset renal injury. On the other hand, CKD can predispose to the development or worsening of OSA, creating a mutually reinforcing cycle that complicates the clinical course of both conditions [88].

It is well established that patients with reduced kidney function are at greater risk of developing OSA, and evidence suggests a high prevalence of OSA among individuals with CKD: 67–94% in non-dialyzed patients and 40–80% in those undergoing dialysis [88].

OSA itself has also been linked to insulin resistance and glucose dysregulation and may accelerate the transition from MetS to T2D in CKD patients [89, 90]. Diabetes and CKD of any cause are significant risk factors for the leading causes of mortality in the diabetic population, since <10% of diabetic patients with CKD survive long enough to require dialysis. Among adults with T2D, the high burden of CKD is demonstrated in the prevalence estimates from NHANES 2007–2014: approximately 18% of adults with T2D have CKD of any kind, with stage 3a (10.4%) and stage 3b (5.4%) being the most common categories, indicating moderate reduction in kidney function. The proportion of diabetics with kidney damage declines markedly during more advanced stages: only 1.8% have stage 4, and 0.4% have stage 5 (end-stage) [91]. The majority of diabetic patients with CKD have moderate-stage kidney damage, and a minority develop advanced-stage kidney damage. These data open a critical therapeutic window in which practitioners can intervene with the hope of slowing disease progression and avoiding end-stage renal failure. Besides the cardiovascular consequences of OSA, recent work increasingly highlights its interaction with renal function. In this context, the concept of a renal-sleep axis has emerged, highlighting that OSA and renal function are linked in a bidirectional and pathophysiologically intertwined manner [83]. In the context of OSA-related renal injury, intermittent hypoxemia triggers ischemia–reperfusion damage, sympathetic activation, and oxidative stress, collectively contributing to various detrimental renal mechanisms. Furthermore, hypervolemia, increased chemosensitivity, and uremic neuropathy/myopathy contribute to rostral fluid shift, ventilatory instability, and increased airway collapsibility, thereby promoting the development and aggravation of OSA [92].

Although we cannot precisely explain the bidirectional pathophysiological mechanisms that connect the kidneys with the heart, we do know that many of the risk factors are common. Both diabetes and CKD are related to a pro-inflammatory phenotype with increased plasma levels of circulating inflammatory mediators, causally associated with the occurrence of major cardiovascular events. Vascular calcification is a common feature in CKD and results in ischemic heart disease and peripheral vascular disease [93]. Patients with diabetes and CKD also have an increased prevalence of infra-popliteal peripheral artery disease (with minimal revascularization possibilities and a significant ischemic burden) [94]. CKD aggravates anemia and mineral-bone conditions that consequently worsen heart disease, lower oxygen carriage, and increase strain on the coronary arteries. Therefore, heart failure is established as a contributor to CKD because of diminished renal perfusion related to lower cardiac output, elevated venous pressures, and neurohormonal activation. From this point of view, lower eGFR worsens volume overload and venous congestion and leads to a vicious cycle of organ dysfunction influencing one another. Atherosclerotic stenosis of the renal arteries can also cause substantial ischemia, which promotes the development of treatment-resistant hypertension and renal failure [95].

While OSA is marked by intermittent nocturnal hypoxia, in CKD, the "chronic hypoxia hypothesis" proposes that ongoing renal hypoxia, driven by inflammation, microvascular dysfunction, glomerular injury, and tubulointerstitial fibrosis, plays a key role in progressive renal impairment. OSA also promotes a chronic systemic inflammatory state, which may further contribute to renal injury. Within the framework of this bidirectional relationship, OSA can contribute to renal function decline through multiple pathways: intermittent hypoxia leading to renal hypoxia, sympathetic activation, circadian rhythm disruption, and mitochondrial dysfunction, leading to decreased kidney function and accelerating CKD progression [96]. Metabolic acidosis alters chemoreflex responses, leading to ventilatory instability, hyperventilation, and hypercapnia, all of which contribute to the development of OSA. Additionally, fluid overload causes a rostral fluid shift, and uremic myopathy impairs pharyngeal muscle function, both of which further promote the onset of OSA [97].

Unfortunately, the association between OSA and CKD is linked to increased mortality and worse morbidity, underscoring the critical need for systematic screening, early identification, and prompt initiation of CPAP [90].

Current Therapeutic Strategies in the Management of Sleep and Circadian Disorders

Evidence-Based Behavioral Strategies for Circadian Rhythm Restoration and Sleep Enhancement

Several healthy lifestyle habits can be employed to correct various disturbances in circadian rhythms and improve sleep quality. Maintaining a consistent sleep schedule, aiming for 7–8 hours of sleep per night, going to bed and waking up at the same time each day, including weekends, is essential for regulating the body's internal clock and enhancing sleep quality [98].

Creating a sleep-conducive environment is equally important. This includes sleeping in a calm, quiet, and dark room. Minimizing exposure to artificial blue light hours before bedtime has enhanced melatonin secretion [99].

Morning exposure to natural sunlight is critical in resetting the circadian clock. Spending time outdoors during the first part of the day is highly recommended. In addition, aligning peripheral clocks through consistent meal timing is beneficial for metabolic health and weight management. In contrast, late-night eating has been associated with increased body fat and impaired glucose metabolism [100].

Regular physical activity, particularly in the morning or afternoon, contributes to regulating circadian rhythms and supports better sleep patterns. However, engaging in vigorous exercise close to bedtime may interfere with sleep onset and should be avoided.

Caffeine and alcohol consumption can negatively affect sleep quality and circadian timing. Research indicates that consuming caffeine up to 6 hours before bedtime can significantly impair sleep [101]. Similarly, alcohol use, particularly in the evening, can disrupt sleep architecture and reduce overall sleep quality [102].

Cognitive Behavioral Therapy for Insomnia (CBT-I) and Digital Innovations in Treatment Delivery

Cognitive Behavioral Therapy for Insomnia (CBT-I) is widely regarded as the first-line, non-pharmacological treatment for insomnia. It effectively addresses maladaptive sleep behaviors and dysfunctional cognitions contributing to poor sleep quality, typically through guidance provided by trained therapists. In developed countries, CBT-I is considered the treatment of choice and is often referred to as the "gold standard" for insomnia care [103].

CBT-I integrates multiple sleep-focused psychoeducational components. These include stimulus control, the development of healthier attitudes toward sleep, and techniques for cognitive restructuring. Therapists conduct a comprehensive assessment of cognitive patterns, psychological stressors, and beliefs that may contribute to insomnia. They work with patients through discussion, cognitive monitoring, and behavioral experiments. Behavioral components of CBT-I include relaxation strategies, physical activity recommendations, and techniques aimed at reducing sleep-related anxiety and improving overall sleep hygiene [103].

According to recent literature, five key components define the structure of CBT-I: (1) sleep restriction, (2) cognitive strategies, (3) mindfulness, (4) behavioral strategies, and (5) psychoeducation [103].

Concurrently, artificial intelligence (AI) is gaining prominence in healthcare. It has the potential to revolutionize early diagnosis and treatment across a broad spectrum of diseases, thereby improving the quality of care and patient outcomes. Machine-learning algorithms can detect patterns in complex datasets and autonomously adjust their predictive models without human input. A subset of machine learning, deep learning, processes vast amounts of data to identify intricate patterns through neural networks. These technological advances, such as dynamic model selection and optimized integration of deep-learning architectures, offer a promising framework for enhancing AI-driven cognitive behavioral therapy systems. AI-enabled systems could support adaptive learning and deliver more precise, individualized therapy, potentially expanding access to CBT-I and improving its effectiveness for different patient populations [104].

The United Kingdom's National Institute for Health and Care Excellence (NICE) recommends the Sleepio program, a digital cognitive behavioral therapy for insomnia (CBT-I) intervention, as an effective alternative to pharmacological treatments. Sleepio is a fully automated digital therapeutic that delivers a 6-week, self-guided CBT-I program. It aims to identify and address the thoughts, emotions, and behaviors contributing to insomnia. A randomized controlled trial published in the journal *Sleep* reported that 76% of participants using Sleepio improved clinically significantly in insomnia symptoms [105].

Chronotherapeutic Strategies: Targeting and Modulating the Circadian System to Enhance Health Outcomes

Adopting specific lifestyle interventions can serve as a non-pharmacological, evidence-based foundation for maintaining circadian health and optimal sleep hygiene. On the other hand, chronotype involves using biological clocks as modulators, aligning the timing of medication administration with endogenous rhythms of circadian clocks to enhance therapeutic efficacy and reduce adverse effects [106].

As previously discussed, the circadian system consists of the central (brain) clock and multiple peripheral clocks. These can be synchronized through various environmental and systemic cues, including light exposure, feeding patterns, hormonal signals, and physical activity. By adjusting these *zeitgebers* (time-giving cues), we can enhance the function of the body's internal clocks, improve circadian rhythmicity, and potentially reduce vulnerability to diseases, particularly those sensitive to circadian misalignment [106].

Chronotherapeutic strategies are generally categorized into two domains: (1) clocks as targets and (2) clocks as modulators [106].

In this framework, circadian rhythms or components are directly manipulated using either pharmaceutical or non-pharmaceutical interventions. Chrono-phototherapy, for instance, primarily involves exposure to morning light. Extensive clinical trials have demonstrated that light therapy significantly improves mood and insulin sensitivity in individuals with major depressive disorder and type 2 diabetes mellitus [107]. Bright light therapy is emerging as a valuable chronotherapeutic tool for alleviating motor disturbances, sleep/wake cycle alterations, anxiety, and depression in patients with neurodegenerative diseases [107]. Furthermore, experimental human studies simulating night shift conditions have shown that bright light exposure can rapidly and thoroughly reset peripheral clocks, suggesting that phototherapy may serve as a viable non-pharmacological intervention against the deleterious effects of shift work or jet lag [106].

Chrono-nutrition, such as time-restricted feeding (TRF), involves limiting food intake to specific windows of time each day to synchronize peripheral clocks. Typically, animals exhibit circadian rhythms in feeding, but these are disrupted when food intake is unrestricted. Evidence indicates that early TRF, restricting food intake to a 6-hour daily window followed by an 18-hour fast, improves insulin sensitivity, blood pressure, and oxidative stress in prediabetic men, even without weight loss [108]. Additional studies involving overweight or obese men have shown that short-term TRF (8-hour daily feeding windows) enhances the rhythmicity of serum and muscle metabolites and gene expression related to amino acid transport, without disrupting core clock gene expression. Intermittent fasting, a dietary approach alternating between fasting and non-fasting periods, seems to inhibit tumor growth and enhance antitumor immune responses in preclinical and clinical settings [109].

Chrono-exercise, or timed physical activity, is also gaining attention as a potential chronotherapeutic intervention for preventing and managing various diseases. Both animal and human studies have demonstrated that scheduled exercise can mitigate age-related morbidity by stabilizing circadian rhythms [110]. Time-of-day-dependent effects have been observed, particularly in metabolically compromised individuals. For example, afternoon exercise significantly improved blood glucose levels in patients with type 2 diabetes, whereas morning exercise had adverse effects [111]. Similarly, in men at risk of or diagnosed with type 2 diabetes, afternoon training improved insulin-stimulated glucose disposal, reduced fat mass and body fat percentage, enhanced physical performance, and lowered hepatic glucose output compared to morning exercise [112].

Melatonin, synthesized and secreted by the pineal gland under the control of the suprachiasmatic nucleus (SCN), plays a central role in circadian synchronization and sleep initiation. Various melatonin and melatonin-receptor agonist regimens have been developed to treat circadian and sleep disorders, especially those related to shift work or jet lag. A systematic review and meta-analysis found that melatonin and its analogs effectively resynchronize circadian rhythms and alleviate depressive symptoms [113].

In many clinical settings, medication is administered without regard to timing. However, circadian transcriptomic studies have shown that most drug targets are rhythmically expressed in various tissues, indicating that the timing of drug administration significantly influences therapeutic outcomes. Pharmacokinetics, absorption, distribution, metabolism, and excretion are also regulated by both central and peripheral clocks [114].

Numerous medications exhibit chrono-pharmacological profiles. Clinical trials have demonstrated that evening administration of simvastatin, one of the most prescribed statins for hypercholesterolemia, hyperlipidemia, and coronary artery disease, is more effective than morning dosing. It is, therefore, recommended to take simvastatin "once daily at night" [115].

Because blood pressure tends to rise in the early morning, administering antihypertensive medications at night is more effective. Various classes of antihypertensive and vasodilatory drugs, including calcium channel blockers, β-adrenoceptor antagonists, ACE inhibitors, and angiotensin II receptor blockers, have demonstrated improved efficacy when taken at bedtime [116]. In patients with chronic kidney disease, nighttime administration of one or more antihypertensives significantly reduced nocturnal blood pressure and restored a healthy "dipping" pattern in the 24-hour blood pressure cycle [117].

Anti-thrombotic drugs are also more effective when administered at bedtime, likely because this timing optimizes platelet inhibition during the high-risk morning hours. For example, bedtime administration of rivaroxaban was associated with reduced thrombin levels and a lower incidence of thrombotic events during early morning hours [117, 118].

Targeting Circadian Disruption in the Management of CKM Syndrome: The Role of Light Exposure and Chronotherapy

A recent cross-sectional study, and the first one which investigated whether circadian rhythm imbalances have an impact on CKM development, showed that among 7493 participants, those with the shortest overlap between light exposure and activity cycles exhibited a 61% higher risk of developing the CKM syndrome (OR = 1.61), with an 84% increased risk of all-cause mortality and a 110% greater risk of cardiovascular mortality, over a median follow-up of 6.83 years. The results greatly emphasize the importance of considering circadian rhythm abnormalities as a modifiable risk factor in the CKM syndrome [3]. In this line, research published by Fernández et al. [119] indicates that exposure to artificial light, particularly at night, may disrupt metabolic balance through the circadian regulation of homeostasis. Artificial Light at Night (ALAN) contributes to environmental conditions that disturb circadian homeostasis and drive the internal body clock to become misaligned from the natural time of light and darkness. Even weak light at night, such as in everyday life (e.g., hospitals, night work, trans-meridian flights across several time zones), affects clock gene expression and temporal coordination and leads to systemic dysregulation. Persistent ALAN, in the absence of excessive caloric intake or activity changes, favors altered metabolism, increased adiposity, and altered glucose homeostasis. As a result, ALAN reduces insulin sensitivity and glucose tolerance in humans and animals by modulating thermogenesis and the β3-adrenergic pathways. In this way, it disrupts the energy balance. Furthermore, ALAN disrupts the HPA (hypothalamic–pituitary–adrenal) axis, which elevates glucocorticoid levels when exposed to some types of light. It may also affect the secretion of melatonin, the primary hormone that influences the 24-hour cycle and is particularly sensitive to light intensity, duration, and wavelength. Melatonin suppression is disruptive not only to the architecture of sleep but also to immune function and oxidative stress responses, as well as the endocrine axes of other glands, including the thyroid, adrenal, and reproductive glands. The results reveal the intricate perturbations in the circadian disruption caused by light and the associated neuroendocrine and cardiometabolic imbalances [119].

Bridging Sleep and Kidney Health: Therapeutic Perspectives in Comorbid OSA and CKD

Given the high prevalence of kidney dysfunction among individuals with OSA and the significant occurrence of OSA in patients with CKD, we emphasize the importance of a multidisciplinary approach that incorporates routine sleep assessments, early detection, and appropriate management. Clear evidence indicates that CPAP therapy contributes to a decrease in morbidity and mortality in this patient population. Also, CPAP reduces cardiovascular morbidity and mortality, potentially through its modulation of sympathetic nervous system hyperactivity, inflammation, endothelial dysfunction, and lipid metabolism [120]. Optimal OSA management requires a multifaceted approach, strongly supported by evidence, that integrates CPAP therapy with lifestyle interventions, such as prioritizing sleep hygiene, managing stress, increasing physical activity, a healthy diet, weight management, substance avoidance, and the routine integration of sleep assessment [121].

There is evidence that adherence to CPAP therapy in patients with OSA can slow the progression of CKD, with significant improvements in intrarenal hemodynamics observed after CPAP initiation. This therapy may help stabilize, or at least partially prevent, further decline in renal function [122], and it also appears to offer some protection against hypoxic injury to kidney tissues [123]. Benefits from CPAP therapy were quantified through eGFR and albuminuria measurements, with greater improvements observed in patients demonstrating higher compliance [65].

The neuromuscular dysfunction has become an important therapeutic target. Different interventions, such as pharmacological modulation and hypoglossal nerve stimulation, as a treatment for sleep apnea, are under investigation in order to confirm their long-term efficacy and safety. An overly sensitive ventilatory control system, characterized by elevated loop gain, can induce exaggerated oscillatory responses from the brainstem, reducing arterial partial pressure of carbon dioxide ($PaCO_2$) below the apnea threshold [66]. In addition, a low respiratory arousal threshold may predispose individuals to obstructive events by triggering premature awakenings before compensatory upper airway muscle activation can occur [65].

An overview of therapeutic strategies targeting circadian and sleep disorders in managing the CKM syndrome is presented in Table 15.2.

Table 15.2 Overview of therapeutic strategies targeting circadian and sleep disorders in managing cardiovascular–kidney–metabolic syndrome

Therapeutic strategy	Target	CKM-related impact
Cognitive behavioral therapy for insomnia (CBT-I)	Cognitive and emotional sleep disruptions	Improves sleep quality, reduces stress-related metabolic dysregulation
AI-enhanced digital CBT-I (e.g., Sleepio)	Insomnia symptoms via digital delivery	Expands access to effective insomnia treatment, supports glycemic control
Chrono-phototherapy (bright light therapy)	Circadian desynchronization and metabolic balance	Improves insulin sensitivity and mood, counteracts circadian misalignment
Chrono-nutrition (time-restricted feeding)	Peripheral clock alignment and metabolic regulation	Improves insulin sensitivity, glucose tolerance, and weight control
Chrono-exercise (timed physical activity)	Circadian stabilization and metabolic health	Improves glucose metabolism, reduces cardiovascular risk
Melatonin and melatonin agonists	Circadian phase alignment and sleep initiation	Supports circadian alignment, reduces inflammation, and oxidative stress
Chrono-pharmacology (time-based drug administration)	Enhanced drug efficacy and reduced side effects	Optimizes cardiovascular, renal, and metabolic treatment outcomes
CPAP therapy for OSA	OSA-related hypoxia and systemic inflammation	Reduces cardiovascular and renal morbidity in OSA–CKD patients
Hypoglossal nerve stimulation	Neuromuscular control of upper airway	Improves upper airway patency, reduces AHI, enhances OSA outcomes

Learning Objectives

- To elucidate the foundational principles and characteristics of major sleep disorders, fostering a comprehensive understanding of their importance.
- To evaluate the systemic effects of circadian rhythm disruptions, emphasizing their profound influence across the human body.
- To delineate the critical interplay between sleep disorders and associated metabolic, renal, and cardiovascular imbalances, underscoring their clinical significance and implications for holistic health management.

Key Reading

- *Cardiovascular–kidney–metabolic (CKM) syndrome* describes a pathophysiological continuum in which metabolic disorders, CKD, and cardiovascular disease interact synergistically. Emerging evidence suggests that circadian rhythm disruption, sleep disorders like OSA and insomnia, and hormonal dysregulation significantly contribute to CKM pathogenesis.
- *Circadian rhythms* are 24-hour cycles that regulate physiological functions such as metabolism, immunity, and hormone secretion. Individual variation in circadian phase, known as chronotype, influences behavioral patterns and metabolic outcomes.
- *Insomnia* is characterized by difficulty initiating or maintaining sleep, often leading to daytime dysfunction. Chronic sleep deprivation disrupts the hypothalamic–pituitary–adrenal (HPA) axis, alters cortisol rhythms, and increases cardiovascular stress. Insomnia is now recognized as an independent contributor to metabolic syndrome and cardiovascular pathology.
- *Obstructive sleep apnea* is a sleep-related breathing disorder defined by recurrent upper airway obstructions during sleep, resulting in intermittent hypoxia and fragmented sleep. These disturbances promote oxidative stress, inflammation, and activation of the renin–angiotensin–aldosterone system (RAAS), contributing to hypertension, insulin resistance, and vascular injury.
- *Behavioral interventions*, such as maintaining a consistent sleep schedule, limiting evening light exposure, and aligning meals with the biological day, can reinforce internal rhythms. *Cognitive behavioral therapy for insomnia (CBT-I)*, including digital tools like Sleepio, has proven effective in improving sleep quality and metabolic outcomes. *Chronotherapy approaches* such as bright light therapy, time-restricted feeding, and appropriately timed exercise enhance circadian stability and insulin sensitivity. Moreover, CPAP therapy in OSA–CKD patients significantly improves renal function and reduces cardiovascular morbidity.

Acknowledgments The authors express their profound gratitude to the Pulmonology Clinic team, for their dedicated involvement in finalizing this chapter, in alphabetical order: Dr. Adriana Loredana Pintilie, Dr. Ruxandra Stirbu, Dr. Raluca Tiron, and Dr. David Toma.

References

1. Fagaini F, Di Marino D, et al. Molecular regulations of circadian rhythm and implications for physiology and disease. Signal Transduct Target Ther. 2022;7:41. https://doi.org/10.1038/s41392-022-00899-y.
2. Catalano F, de Vito F, Cassano V, et al. Circadian clock desynchronization and insulin resistance. Int J Environ Res Public Health. 2023;20:29. https://doi.org/10.3390/ijerph20010029.
3. Bolin L, Xinping K, Yushan L, et al. Cross-sectional and longitudinal associations between circadian alignment and cardiovascular-kidney-metabolic syndrome in US adults. medRxiv. 2025:03.25.25323796. https://doi.org/10.1101/2025.03.25.25323796.
4. Marhefkova N, Sládek M, Sumova´ A, Dubsky M. Circadian dysfunction and cardiometabolic disorders in humans. Front Endocrinol. 2024;15:1328139. https://doi.org/10.3389/fendo.2024.1328139.
5. Nicholas WG, Liza HA, Ying-Hui F, et al. Human circadian variations. J Clin Invest. 2021;131(16):e148282. https://doi.org/10.1172/JCI148282.
6. Sojeong Kim, Heon-Jeong Lee. Sleep and circadian rhythm disturbances in eating disorders. Chronobiol Med. 2020;2(4):141–7. https://doi.org/10.33069/cim.2020.0027.
7. Sowers MF, Crawford SL, Sternfeld B, Morganstein D, Gold EB, Greendale GA, et al. Design, survey sampling, and recruitment methods of SWAN: a multicenter, multiethnic, community-based cohort study of women and the menopausal transition. Semin Reprod Med. 2000;18(1):11–27. https://doi.org/10.1055/s-2000-7703.
8. Oosterman JE, Wopereis S, et al. The circadian clock, shift work, and tissue specific insuline resistance. Endocrinology. 2020;161(12) https://doi.org/10.1210/endocr/bqaa180.
9. Sharma A, Laurenti MC, et al. Glucose metabolism during rotation shift–work in healthcare workers. Diabetologia. 2017;60:1483–149. https://doi.org/10.1007/s00125-017-4317-0.
10. Morris CJ, Purvis TE, Mistretta J, Scheer FAJL. Effects of the internal circadian system and circadian misalignment on glucose tolerance in chronic shift workers. J Clin Endocrinol Metab. 2016;101(3):1066–74. https://doi.org/10.1210/jc.2015-3924.
11. Bescós R, Boden MJ, Jackson ML, Trewin AJ, Marjot EC, Levinger I, et al. Four days of simulated shift work reduces insulin sensitivity in humans. Acta Physiol (Oxf). 2018;222(4):e13039. https://doi.org/10.1111/apha.13039.
12. Pan A, Schernhammer ES, Sun Q, Hu FB. Rotating night shift work and risk of type 2 diabetes: two prospective cohort studies in women. PLoS Med. 2011;8(12):e1001141. https://doi.org/10.1371/journal.pmed.1001141.
13. Fishbein AB, Kuntson KL, Zee PC. Circadian disruption and human health. J Clin Invest. 2021;131(19):e148286. https://doi.org/10.1172/JCI148286.
14. Valerie Ansu Baidoo, Kristen L. Knutson. Association between circadian disruption and cardiometabolic disease risk: a review. Obesity (Silver Spring). 2023;31:615–24. https://doi.org/10.1002/oby.2366.
15. Ferguson JM, Costello S, Neophytou AM. Night rotational work exposure within the last 12 months and risk of incident hypertension. Scand J Work Environ Health. 2019;45(3):256–66. https://doi.org/10.5271/sjweh.3788.
16. Sack R, Auckley D, Auger RR, Carskadon MA, Wright KP, Viti-ello MV, Zhdanova IV. Circadian rhythm sleep disorders: part II, advanced sleep phase disorder, delayed sleep phase disorder, free-running disor-der, and irregular sleep-wake rhythm. Sleep. 2007;30(11):1484–501.
17. Silva I, Costa D. Consequences of shift work and night work: a literature review. Healthcare. 2023;11:1410. https://doi.org/10.3390/healthcare11101410.
18. International Agency for Research on Cancer – World Health Organization – IARC Monographs Meeting 124: Night Shift Work (4–11 June 2019).
19. Sun M, Feng W, Wang F, et al. Meta – analysis on shift work and risks of specific obesity type. Obes Rev. 2018;19(1):28–40. https://doi.org/10.1111/obr.12621.

20. Hirshkowitz M, Whiton K, Albert SM, Alessi C, Bruni O, DonCarlos L, et al. National Sleep Foundation's sleep time duration recommendations: methodology and results summary. Sleep Health. 2015;1(1):40–3. https://doi.org/10.1016/j.sleh.2014.12.010.
21. Centers for Disease Control and Prevention (CDC). Adults who report fewer than 7 hours of sleep per night. CDC; 2022. https://www.cdc.gov/sleep/data-research/facts-stats/adults-sleep-facts-and-stats.html.
22. Kocevska D, Lysen TS, Dotinga A, et al. Sleep characteristics across the lifespan in 1.1 million people from The Netherlands, United Kingdom and United States: a systematic review and meta-analysis. Nat Hum Behav. 2021;5:113–22. https://doi.org/10.1038/s41562-020-00965-x.
23. Charles M. Morin, Daniel J Buysee. Management of Insomnia. N Engl J Med. 2024;391:247–58. https://doi.org/10.1056/NEJMcp2305655.
24. Irwin MR. Why sleep is important for health: a psychoneuroimmunology perspective. Annu Rev Psychol. 2015;66:143–72. https://doi.org/10.1146/annurev-psych-010213-115205.
25. Hua J, Jiang H, Wang H, Fang Q. Sleep duration and the risk of metabolic syndrome in adults: a systematic review and meta-analysis. Front Neurol. 2021;12:635564. https://doi.org/10.3389/fneur.2021.635564.
26. Li R, Li W, Lun Z, Huiping, et al. Prevalence of metabolic syndrome in mainland china: a meta –analysis of published studies. BMC Public Health. 2016;16:296. https://doi.org/10.1186/s12889-016-2870-y.
27. Zhang W, Sun Q, Chen B, Basta M, Xu C, Li Y. Insomnia symptoms are associated with metabolic syndrome in patients with severe psychiatric disorders. Sleep Med. 2021;83:168–74. https://doi.org/10.1016/j.sleep.2021.04.031.
28. Fan S, Guo WW, et al. Microbiota-gut-brain axis drives overeating disorders. Cell Metab. 35:2011–202. https://doi.org/10.1016/j.cmet.2023.09.005.
29. Zhu R, Fang Y, Li H, Liu Y, Wei J, Zhang S, Wang L, Fan R, Wang L, Li S, Chen T. Psychobiotic Lactobacillus plantarum JYLP-326 relieves anxiety, depression, and insomnia symptoms in test anxious college via modulating the gut microbiota and its metabolism. Front Immunol. 2023;14:1158137. https://doi.org/10.3389/fimmu.2023.1158137.
30. Xie F, Feng Z, Xu B. Metabolic characteristics of gut microbiota and insomnia: evidence from a Mendelian randomization analysis. Nutrients. 2024;16(17):2943. https://doi.org/10.3390/nu16172943.
31. Jaspan VN, Greenberg GS, et al. The role of sleep in cardiovascular disease. Curr Atheroscler Rep. 2024;26(7):249–62.
32. Patel SR, Zhu X, Storfer-Isser A, Mehra R, Jenny NS, Tracy R, Redline S. Sleep duration and biomarkers of inflammation. Sleep. 2009;32(2):200–4. https://doi.org/10.1093/sleep/32.2.200.
33. Li J, Huang Y, Zhang X, Fan J, Li L, Wang Y. Associations of insomnia with cardiovascular disease and all-cause mortality: a systematic review and meta-analysis of cohort studies. PLoS One. 2023;18(10):e0291859. https://doi.org/10.1371/journal.pone.0291859.
34. Knutson KL, Jones SE, Huang Y, Rea MS, Scheer FAJL, Dashti HS, et al. Sleep traits and risk of atrial fibrillation: a study combining observational cohort and Mendelian randomization analyses. J Clin Sleep Med. 2023;19(10):1817–25. https://doi.org/10.5664/jcsm.11326.
35. Da Silva L, St-Onge MP, Tasali E, Gozal D, Brum M. Sleep and cardiometabolic risk: mechanistic insights and clinical implications. Sleep Med Rev. 2024;71:101872. https://doi.org/10.1016/j.smrv.2024.101872.
36. Benjafield AV, Ayas NT, Eastwood PR, et al. Estimation of the global prevalence and burden of obstructive sleep apnoea: a literature-based analysis. Lancet Respir Med. 2019;7(8):687–98. https://doi.org/10.1016/S2213-2600(19)30198-5.
37. Tishler PV, Larkin EK, Schluchter MD, Redline S. Incidence of sleep-disordered breathing in an urban adult population: the relative importance of risk factors in the development of sleep-disordered breathing. JAMA. 2003;289(17):2230–7. https://doi.org/10.1001/jama.289.17.2230.

38. Bonsignore MR, Saaresranta T, Riha RL. Sex differences in obstructive sleep apnoea. Eur Respir Rev. 2019;28(154) https://doi.org/10.1183/16000617.0030-2019.
39. Malhotra A, Huang Y, Fogel RB, et al. The male predisposition to pharyngeal collapse: importance of airway length. Am J Respir Crit Care Med. 2002;166(10):1388–95. https://doi.org/10.1164/rccm.2112072.
40. Reichert CF, Simon M, Liedtke C, Fritschi C, Bloch KE. Health-related quality of life and costs in patients with suspected sleep apnea: a decision analysis. Lung. 2015;193(6):1037–44. https://doi.org/10.1007/s00408-015-9687-9.
41. Wickwire EM, Geiger-Brown J, Scharf SM, Drake CL. Shift work and shift work sleep disorder: clinical and organizational perspectives. Chest. 2017;151(5):1156–72. https://doi.org/10.1016/j.chest.2016.12.027.
42. Hafner M, Stepanek M, Taylor J, Troxel WM, van Stolk C. Why sleep matters — the economic costs of insufficient sleep: a cross-country comparative analysis. Rand Health Q. 2017;6(4):11.
43. Ramar K, Malhotra RK, Carden KA, Martin JL, Abbasi-Feinberg F, Aurora RN, et al. Sleep is essential to health: an American Academy of Sleep Medicine position statement. J Clin Sleep Med. 2021;17(10):2115–9. https://doi.org/10.5664/jcsm.9476.
44. Lechat B, Naik G, Reynolds A, Adams R, Grunstein R, Huggins CE, et al. Health-related quality of life in obstructive sleep apnea patients with excessive daytime sleepiness: The European Sleep Apnea Database (ESADA) cohort. Sleep Med. 2022;91:102–9. https://doi.org/10.1016/j.sleep.2021.09.007.
45. Tregear S, Reston J, Schoelles K, Phillips B. Obstructive sleep apnea and risk of motor vehicle crash: systematic review and meta-analysis. J Clin Sleep Med. 2009;5(6):573–81. PMID: 19494476
46. Sullivan SS, Barger LK, Rajaratnam SMW, Czeisler CA, Wang W, Lockley SW. A systematic review of motor vehicle crash risk and drowsy driving prevention strategies among people with obstructive sleep apnea. Sleep Health. 2022;8(6):634–49. https://doi.org/10.1016/j.sleh.2022.04.003.
47. Hillman DR, Lack LC, Seale JP, D'Rozario AL, Sweetman AM, Smith SS, et al. Economic value of sleep health interventions: a modelling analysis. J Sleep Res. 2022;31(6):e13748. https://doi.org/10.1111/jsr.13748.
48. Badr MS, Ayas NT, Easty A, Fox N, Fox K, Malhotra RK, Owens RL, Patel SR, Watson NF, Weiss JW, Chesson AL. Impact of treatment of obstructive sleep apnea on the risk of adverse cardiovascular events: comparative effectiveness review. J Clin Sleep Med. 2021;17(6):1199–207. https://doi.org/10.5664/jcsm.9218.
49. Sateia MJ. International classification of sleep disorders-third edition: highlights and modifications. Chest. 2014;146(5):1387–94. https://doi.org/10.1378/chest.14-0970.
50. Javaheri S, Barbe F, Campos-Rodriguez F, et al. Sleep apnea: types, mechanisms, and clinical cardiovascular consequences. J Am Coll Cardiol. 2017;69(7):841–58. https://doi.org/10.1016/j.jacc.2016.11.069.
51. Berry RB, Budhiraja R, Gottlieb DJ, et al. Rules for scoring respiratory events in sleep: update of the 2007 AASM Manual for the Scoring of Sleep and Associated Events. Deliberations of the sleep apnea definitions task force of the American Academy of Sleep Medicine. J Clin Sleep Med. 2012;8(5):597–619. https://doi.org/10.5664/jcsm.2172.
52. Edwards BA, Redline S, Sands SA, et al. More than the sum of the respiratory events: personalized medicine approaches for obstructive sleep apnea. Am J Respir Crit Care Med. 2019;200(6):691–703. https://doi.org/10.1164/rccm.201901-0014TR.
53. Desfonds P, Planes C, Fuhrman C, Foucher A, Raffestin B. Nasal resistance in snorers with or without sleep apnea: effect of posture and nasal ventilation with continuous positive airway pressure. Sleep. 1998;21(6):625–32.
54. Craig TJ, Ferguson BJ, Krouse JH. Sleep impairment in allergic rhinitis, rhino sinusitis, and nasal polyposis. Am J Otolaryngol. 2008;29(3):209–17.
55. Meurice JC, Marc I, Carrier G, Series F. Effects of mouth opening on upper airway collapsibility in normal sleeping subjects. Am J Respir Crit Care Med. 1996;153(1):255–9.

56. Fitzpatrick MF, McLean H, Urton AM, Tan A, O'Donnell D, Driver HS. Effect of nasal or oral breathing route on upper airway resistance during sleep. Eur Respir J. 2003;22(5):827–32.
57. McNicholas WT, Coffey M, Boyle T. Effects of nasal airflow on breathing during sleep in normal humans. Am Rev Respir Dis. 1993;147(3):620–3.
58. Berry RB, Kouchi KG, Bower JL, Light RW. Effect of upper airway anesthesia on obstructive sleep apnea. Am J Resp Crit Care. 1995;151(6):1857–61.
59. Bradley TD, Brown IG, Grossman RF, et al. Pharyngeal size in snorers, non snorers, and patients with obstructive sleep apnea. N Engl J Med. 1986;315(21):1327–31.
60. Rodenstein DO, Dooms G, Thomas Y, et al. Pharyngeal shape and dimensions in healthy subjects, snorers, and patients with obstructive sleep apnoea. Thorax. 1990;45(10):722–7.
61. Bradley TD, Rutherford R, Grossman RF, et al. Role of daytime hypoxaemia in the pathogenesis of right heart failure in the obstructive sleep apnea syndrome. Am Rev Respir Dis. 1985;131(6):835–9.
62. Ingman T, Nieminen T, Hurmerinta K. Cephalometric comparison of pharyngeal changes in subjects with upper airway resistance syndrome or obstructive sleep apnoea in upright and supine positions. Eur J Orthod. 2004;26(3):321–6.
63. Riha RL, Brander P, Vennelle M, Douglas NJ. A cephalometric comparison of patients with the sleep apnea/hypopnea syndrome and their siblings. Sleep. 2005;1(28):315–20.
64. Lavie P, Rubin AE. Effects of nasal occlusion on respiration in sleep. Evidence of inheritability of sleep apnea proneness. Acta Otolaryngol. 1984;97:127–30.
65. Wellman A, Jordan AS, Malhotra A, et al. Ventilatory control and airway anatomy in obstructive sleep apnea. Am J Respir Crit Care Med. 2004;170(11):1225–32. https://doi.org/10.1164/rccm.200404-510OC.
66. White DP, Younes MK. Obstructive sleep apnea. Compr Physiol. 2012;2(4):2541–94. https://doi.org/10.1002/cphy.c110064.
67. Young T, Peppard PE, Gottlieb DJ. Epidemiology of obstructive sleep apnea: a population health perspective. Am J Respir Crit Care Med. 2002;165(9):1217–39. https://doi.org/10.1164/rccm.2109080.
68. Peppard PE, Young T, Palta M, Skatrud J. Prospective study of the association between sleep-disordered breathing and hypertension. N Engl J Med. 2000;342(19):1378–84. https://doi.org/10.1056/NEJM200005113421901.
69. Sands SA, Alex RM, Mann D, et al. Pathophysiology underlying demographic and obesity determinants of sleep apnea severity. Ann Am Thorac Soc. 2023;20(3):440–9. https://doi.org/10.1513/AnnalsATS.202203-271OC.
70. Wetter DW, Young TB, Bidwell TR, Badr MS, Palta M. Smoking as a risk factor for sleep-disordered breathing. Arch Intern Med. 1994;154(19):2219–24. https://doi.org/10.1001/archinte.1994.00420190121014.
71. Issa FG, Sullivan CE. Alcohol, snoring and sleep apnea. J Neurol Neurosurg Psychiatry. 1982;45(4):353–9. https://doi.org/10.1136/jnnp.45.4.353.
72. Redline S, Tishler PV, Tosteson TD, et al. The familial aggregation of obstructive sleep apnea. Am J Respir Crit Care Med. 1995;151(3 Pt 1):682–7. https://doi.org/10.1164/ajrccm/151.3_Pt_1.682.
73. Carmelli D, Colrain IM, Swan GE, Bliwise DL. Genetic and environmental influences in sleep-disordered breathing in older male twins. Sleep. 2004;27(5):917–22. https://doi.org/10.1093/sleep/27.5.917.
74. Kadotani H, Kadotani T, Young T, et al. Association between apolipoprotein E epsilon4 and sleep-disordered breathing in adults. JAMA. 2001;285(22):2888–90. https://doi.org/10.1001/jama.285.22.2888.
75. Ndumele CE, Neeland IJ, Tuttle KR, Chow SL, Mathew RO, Khan SS, et al. A synopsis of the evidence for the science and clinical management of cardiovascular-kidney-metabolic (CKM) syndrome: a scientific statement from the American Heart Association. Circulation. 2023;148(20):1636–64. https://doi.org/10.1161/CIR.0000000000001186.
76. Wu M, Shu Y, Wang L, et al. Metabolic syndrome severity score and the progression of CKD. Eur J Clin Invest. 2022;52:e13646. https://doi.org/10.1111/eci.13646.

77. Sebastian SA, Padda I, Johal G. Cardiovascular-kidney-metabolic (CKM) syndrome: a state-of-the-art review. Curr Probl Cardiol. 2024;49(2):102344.
78. Ruiz-García A, Arranz-Martínez E, Serrano-Cumplido A, Cinza-Sanjurjo S, Escobar-Cervantes C, Polo-García J, Pallarés-Carratalá V. From metabolic syndrome to cardio-kidney-metabolic syndrome in the SIMETAP study: prevalence rates of metabolic syndrome and its independent associations with cardio-renal-metabolic disorders other than its defining criteria. Biomedicine. 2025;13:590. https://doi.org/10.3390/biomedicines13030590.
79. Theodorakis N, Nikolaou M. From cardiovascular-kidney-metabolic syndrome to cardiovascular-renal-hepatic-metabolic syndrome: proposing an expanded framework. Biomolecules. 2025;15:213. https://doi.org/10.3390/biom15020213.
80. Hong S, Lee D-B, Yoon D-W, Yoo S-L, Kim J. The effect of sleep disruption on cardiometabolic health. Life. 2025;15:60. https://doi.org/10.3390/life15010060.
81. Tsao CW, Aday AW, Almarzooq ZI, Anderson CAM, Arora P, Avery CL, et al. Heart disease and stroke statistics—2023 update: a report from the American Heart Association. Circulation. 2023;147(8):e93–e621. https://doi.org/10.1161/CIR.0000000000001123.
82. Kim J, Lee J, Kim J, Yook S, Lee S, Park Y, et al. Risk of chronic kidney disease, metabolic disease, ischemic heart disease, and cardiovascular disease in patients with obstructive sleep apnea: a nationwide cohort study. J Clin Med. 2024;13(2):337. https://doi.org/10.3390/jcm13020337.
83. Kalkat RK, Pannu AK, Kaur S, Sekhon MS, Bansal S, Kaur R, et al. Obstructive sleep apnea and chronic kidney disease: a pathophysiological insight and future directions. Sleep Med Rev. 2024;73:101891. https://doi.org/10.1016/j.smrv.2024.101891.
84. Nicholl DD, Hanly PJ. Pathophysiology of renal disease in obstructive sleep apnea: is there a renal–sleep axis? Sleep Med Clin. 2021;16(3):409–20. https://doi.org/10.1016/j.smrv.2021.05.019.
85. Kim JS, Hwang HS. Vascular calcification in chronic kidney disease: distinct features of pathogenesis and clinical implication. Korean Circ J. 2021 Dec;51(12):961–82. https://doi.org/10.4070/kcj.2021.0995.
86. Alghanimi IA, Al-Sharydah AM, Alqutub AA, Zeidan N, Bukhamseen F, Alradhi A, Al-Aftan MS. Anatomical distribution patterns of peripheral arterial disease according to patient characteristics: a unicentral cohort study. Vasc Health Risk Manag. 2023;19:447–57. https://doi.org/10.2147/VHRM.S416967.
87. Marassi M, Fadini GP. The cardio-renal-metabolic connection: a review of the evidence. Cardiovasc Diabetol. 2023;22:195. https://doi.org/10.1186/s12933-023-01937-x.
88. Kalkat RK, Sekhon MS, Pannu AK, Aggarwal N, Kaur S, Bansal S, et al. The bidirectional interaction between obstructive sleep apnea and chronic kidney disease: a clinical perspective. Sleep Med Rev. 2024;73:101898. https://doi.org/10.1016/j.smrv.2024.101898.
89. Huang Z, Zhu T, Xu W, Li Y, Chen X, Liu Y, et al. Association between obstructive sleep apnea and progression of chronic kidney disease: a systematic review and meta-analysis. Sleep Med. 2024;112:1–9. https://doi.org/10.1016/j.sleep.2024.03.010.
90. Taddei S, Montagnani A, Grassi G. Obstructive sleep apnea syndrome and chronic kidney disease: new insights into a dangerous liaison. Sleep Med. 2022;91:151–8. https://doi.org/10.1016/j.sleep.2021.11.023.
91. Chen YT, Hsieh MH, Hsu CY, Chien WC. Risk of obstructive sleep apnea in patients with chronic kidney disease: a nationwide population-based cohort study. Sleep Med. 2024;112:1–7. https://doi.org/10.1016/j.sleep.2024.03.009.
92. Shiina K. Obstructive sleep apnea -related hypertension: a review of the literature and clinical management strategy. Hypertens Res. 2024;47:3085–98. https://doi.org/10.1038/s41440-024-01852-y.
93. Lavalle S, Masiello E, Iannella G, Magliulo G, Pace A, Lechien JR, Calvo-Henriquez C, Cocuzza S, Parisi FM, Favier V, et al. Unraveling the complexities of oxidative stress and inflammation biomarkers in obstructive sleep apnea syndrome: a comprehensive review. Life. 2024;14:425. https://doi.org/10.3390/life14040425.

94. Xu H, Liang C, Zou J, et al. Interaction between obstructive sleep apnea and short sleep duration on insulin resistance: a large-scale study. Respir Res. 2020;21:151. https://doi.org/10.1186/s12931-020-01416-x.
95. Michalek-Zrabkowska M, Macek P, Martynowicz H, Gac P, Mazur G, Grzeda M, Poreba R. Obstructive sleep apnea as a risk factor of insulin resistance in nondiabetic adults. Life. 2021;11:50. https://doi.org/10.3390/life11010050.
96. Loh HH, Lim QH, Chai CS, Goh SL, Lim LL, Yee A, Sukor N. Influence and implications of the renin-angiotensin-aldosterone system in obstructive sleep apnea: An updated systematic review and meta-analysis. J Sleep Res. 2023;32(1):e13726. https://doi.org/10.1111/jsr.13726. Epub 2022 Sep 14. PMID: 36104933; PMCID: PMC10078316
97. Hui L, Benca R. The bidirectional relationship between obstructive sleep apnea and chronic kidney disease. J Stroke Cerebrovasc Dis. 2021;30(9):105652. https://doi.org/10.1016/j.jstrokecerebrovasdis.2021.105652.
98. Mendoza J. Circadian clocks: setting time by food. Clocks Sleep. 2023;5(3):363–72. https://doi.org/10.3390/clockssleep5030034.
99. Gooley JJ, Chamberlain K, Smith KA, Khalsa SBS, Rajaratnam SMW, Van Reen E, et al. Exposure to room light before bedtime suppresses melatonin onset and shortens melatonin duration in humans. J Clin Endocrinol Metab. 2011;96(3):E463–72. https://doi.org/10.1210/jc.2010-2098.
100. Yuan Y, Song Y, Wang X, Wang Y, Zhao J. Chrononutrition: a review of circadian rhythms and diet from the perspectives of chronobiology and endocrinology. Int J Mol Sci. 2023;24(4):3392. https://doi.org/10.3390/ijms24043392.
101. Drake C, Roehrs T, Shambroom J, Roth T. Caffeine effects on sleep taken 0, 3, or 6 hours before going to bed. J Clin Sleep Med. 2013;9(11):1195–200.
102. Roehrs T, Roth T. Sleep, sleepiness, and alcohol use. Sleep Med Rev. 2001;5(4):287–97. https://doi.org/10.1053/smrv.2001.0162.
103. Furukawa TA, Efthimiou O, Salanti G, Cipriani A, Zhou X, Weitz ES, et al. Cognitive behavioral therapy for insomnia: a systematic review and network meta-analysis. JAMA Psychiatr. 2024;81(1):27–36. https://doi.org/10.1001/jamapsychiatry.2023.5060.
104. Zhang C, Luo Z, Lu L, He H, Zhang Y, Xu W, et al. Artificial intelligence–driven cognitive behavioral therapy for insomnia: development and usability study. J Clin Med. 2023;12(7):2265. https://doi.org/10.3390/jcm12072265. https://www.mdpi.com/2077-0383/12/7/2265
105. National Institute for Health and Care Excellence (NICE). Sleepio to treat insomnia and insomnia symptoms [Internet]. London: NICE; 2022 [cited 2025 May 9]. Available from: https://www.nice.org.uk/guidance/mtg70
106. Kervezee L, Cuesta M, Cermakian N, Boivin DB. The phase-shifting effect of bright light exposure on circadian rhythmicity in the human transcriptome. J Biol Rhythms. 2019;34(1):84–97. https://doi.org/10.1177/0748730418821776.
107. Brouwer A, van Raalte DH, Nguyen H-T, Rutters F, van de Ven PM, Elders PJM, Moll AC, Van Someren EJW, Snoek FJ, Beekman ATF, Bremmer MA. Effects of light therapy on mood and insulin sensitivity in patients with type 2 diabetes and depression: results from a randomized placebo-controlled trial. Diabetes Care. 2019;42(4):529–38. https://doi.org/10.2337/dc18-1732.
108. Sutton EF, Beyl R, Early KS, Cefalu WT, Ravussin E, Peterson CM. Early time-restricted feeding improves insulin sensitivity, blood pressure, and oxidative stress even without weight loss in men with prediabetes. Cell Metab. 2018;27(6):1212–1221.e3. https://doi.org/10.1016/j.cmet.2018.04.010.
109. Zhao X, Yang J, Huang R, Guo M, Zhou Y, Xu L. The role and its mechanism of intermittent fasting in tumors: friend or foe? Cancer Biol Med. 2021;18(1):63–73. https://doi.org/10.20892/j.issn.2095-3941.2020.0250.
110. Minuzzi LG, Rama L, Chupel MU, Rosado F, Dos Santos JV, Simões HG, Teixeira AM. Lifelong training improves the immune system in older adults: a cross-sectional study. Life Sci. 2020;256:118453. https://doi.org/10.1016/j.lfs.2020.118453.

111. Savikj M, Gabriel BM, Alm PS, Smith JAB, Caidahl K, Björnholm M, Fritz T, Krook A, Zierath JR, Wallberg-Henriksson H. Afternoon exercise is more efficacious than morning exercise at improving blood glucose levels in individuals with type 2 diabetes: a randomized crossover trial. Diabetologia. 2019;62(2):233–7. https://doi.org/10.1007/s00125-018-4767-z.
112. Mancilla R, Brouwers B, Schrauwen P, Hesselink MKC, Hoeks J, van Marken Lichtenbelt WD. Time-of-day-dependent effects of exercise training on metabolic outcomes in men with type 2 diabetes: a randomized controlled trial. Physiol Rep. 2020;8(18):e14669. https://doi.org/10.14814/phy2.14669.
113. Walker WH II, Walton JC, DeVries AC, Nelson RJ. Circadian rhythm disruption and mental health. Transl Psychiatry. 2020;10(1):28. https://doi.org/10.1038/s41398-020-0694-0.
114. Bicker J, Alves G, Falcão A, Fortuna A. Timing in drug absorption and disposition: the past, present, and future of chronopharmacokinetics. Br J Pharmacol. 2020;177(10):2215–39. https://doi.org/10.1111/bph.15017.
115. Petroff E. Finding the location of a fast radio burst. Science. 2019;365(6453):546–7. https://doi.org/10.1126/science.aay4330.
116. Bowles NP, Thosar SS, Herzig MX, Shea SA. Chronotherapy for hypertension. Curr Hypertens Rep. 2018;20(11):97. https://doi.org/10.1007/s11906-018-0897-4.
117. Hermida RC, Ayala DE, Smolensky MH, Mojón A, Fernández JR, Crespo JJ, Moyá A, Ríos MT, Portaluppi F. Chronotherapy improves blood pressure control and reduces vascular risk in CKD. Nat Rev Nephrol. 2013;9(6):358–68. https://doi.org/10.1038/nrneph.2013.79.
118. Brunton LL, Hilal-Dandan R, Knollmann BC. Comparison between the impact of morning and evening doses of rivaroxaban on coagulation parameters in healthy subjects. J Thromb Haemost. 2015;13(3):396–405. https://doi.org/10.1111/jth.13213.
119. Meléndez-Fernández OH, Liu JA, Nelson RJ. Circadian rhythms disrupted by light at night and mistimed food intake alter hormonal rhythms and metabolism. Int J Mol Sci. 2023;24(4):3392. https://doi.org/10.3390/ijms24043392.
120. McNicholas WT. Cardiovascular outcomes of CPAP therapy in obstructive sleep apnea syndrome. Am J Physiol Regul Integr Comp Physiol. 2007;293(5):R1666–70. https://doi.org/10.1152/ajpregu.00401.2007.
121. Meng F, Ang GY, Chang RRY, Lee CP, Tan KB, Abisheganaden JA. Cost-effectiveness analysis of continuous positive airway pressure treatment for obstructive sleep apnea in Singapore from a health system perspective. J Sleep Res. 2025;34(2):e14326. https://doi.org/10.1111/jsr.14326.
122. Rosenzweig I, Glasser M, Polsek D, Leschziner GD, Williams SCR. Emerging co-morbidities of obstructive sleep apnea. J Thorac Dis. 2016;8(9):E902–12. https://doi.org/10.21037/jtd.2016.09.23.
123. Sircu V, Colesnic S-I, Covantsev S, Corlateanu O, Sukhotko A, Popovici C, Corlateanu A. The burden of comorbidities in obstructive sleep apnea and the pathophysiologic mechanisms and effects of CPAP. Clocks & Sleep. 2023;5(2):333–49. https://doi.org/10.3390/clockssleep5020025.

Chapter 16
Hematological Impact of Cardiovascular–Kidney–Metabolic Syndrome

Claudia Cristina Tărniceriu, Loredana Liliana Hurjui, and Lacrămioara Ionela Şerban

Introduction

The cardiovascular–kidney–metabolic (CKM) syndrome has a systemic impact, contributing to the appearance of clinical and biological manifestations that influence the quality of life of these patients, such as a hypercoagulable state—an acquired form of thrombophilia—as well as an anemic syndrome. This chapter explores the epidemiological, pathophysiological, clinical, and paraclinical details and the therapeutic strategy of thrombophilia and anemic syndrome in the context of CKM syndrome.

Thrombophilia is a condition that involves abnormal coagulation, which increases the risk of thrombosis. Similar terms for thrombophilia are prothrombotic state or hypercoagulable state. The term "thrombophilia" was first used by Nygaard and Brown in 1937, when they described the sudden occlusion of large arteries [1]. Two types of thrombophilia are described—inherited and acquired. Inherited thrombophilia involves two categories of factors: defects/deficiencies of natural anticoagulant proteins or genetic mutations that result in an increased tendency for thrombosis. The first group includes deficiencies of the antithrombin III, protein C, and protein S, and the second group includes activated protein C resistance, factor V Leiden, and prothrombin gene variant [2, 3]. Inherited thrombophilias are

C. C. Tărniceriu (✉) · L. L. Hurjui
Morphofunctional Science I Department, Grigore T. Popa University of Medicine and Pharmacy, Iasi, Romania

Saint Spiridon Emergency Hospital, Iasi, Romania
e-mail: claudia.tarniceriu@umfiasi.ro

L. I. Şerban
Morphofunctional Science II Department, Grigore T. Popa University of Medicine and Pharmacy, Iasi, Romania

M. Floria, D. M. Tanase (eds.), *Cardiovascular-Kidney-Metabolic Syndrome*,
https://doi.org/10.1007/978-3-032-11445-7_16

well-established predisposing factors for venous thromboembolism [2, 3], but their role in arterial thrombosis, such as arterial ischemic stroke, was demonstrated through a meta-analysis by Chiasakul and colab [4]. Acquired conditions can increase the risk of thrombosis, such as antiphospholipid syndrome, acquired abnormalities in coagulation factors and natural anticoagulants (elevated levels of factor VIII and factor IX, and deficiencies of protein C and antithrombin III) or certain diseases (solid cancer, myeloproliferative disorder, paroxysmal nocturnal hemoglobinuria, liver cirrhosis) [5]. Acquired characteristics such as hormone therapy, pregnancy, smoking, obesity, and increasing age also increase the risk of thrombosis [6]. Thromboembolic disease and ischemic stroke are frequently associated with increased mortality and morbidity, which is why understanding the mechanisms that lead to their occurrence in CKM is essential. Thrombophilia in CKM syndrome is an acquired form that involves vascular endothelium, homocysteine, fluid-coagulant system, and platelets. There is also a risk of an association between the two forms of thrombophilia, which requires increased attention in assessing thromboembolic and ischemic risk.

Anemia is a major health problem, with an estimated one-third of the worlds population suffering from it in 2010 [7, 8]. According to the World Health Organization (WHO), anemia is defined as a medical condition in which the total number of red blood cells or their oxygen-carrying capacity is insufficient to meet the physiological needs of the body. It is usually defined by a decrease in total circulating hemoglobin: Hb <13 g/dL in men, Hb <12 g/dL in women, and Hb <11 g/dL in pregnant women [7, 8]. Anemia is often associated with metabolic syndrome (obesity, diabetes mellitus), chronic kidney disease, and cardiovascular diseases. The mass of circulating red blood cells reflects a dynamic balance between their proliferation, influenced by various factors, and their loss/destruction. The pathophysiological changes that are secondary to CKM syndrome lead to the destruction of this balance between the production of erythrocytes and their lifespan, which results in the development of the anemic syndrome. Anemic syndrome is considered a prognostic factor in CKM syndrome, contributing to the decrease in the quality of life of these patients.

The management of these patients with hypercoagulable status and anemia in the context of CKM syndrome most often requires a multidisciplinary approach. The need for multidisciplinary approaches to management is further highlighted by the interorgan crosstalk/interactions that are evident in CKM syndrome and associated comorbidities [9].

Thrombophilia in CKM Syndrome

Venous thromboembolism and atherosclerosis may share common risk factors, including hypertension, diabetes, obesity, and hyperlipidemia [10]. Data published in the literature showed that metabolic syndrome may play a pathogenetic role in idiopathic venous thromboembolism [11]. Another study showed that metabolic syndrome increases the risk of venous thromboembolism recurrence after acute deep vein thrombosis [12]. Some studies have established that the cardiovascular risk factors are associated with venous thromboembolism [13, 14]. Experimental and clinical studies have shown an association between heart failure and a prothrombotic state, and that patients with heart failure experience an increased incidence of stroke and other thromboembolic events, even when they are in sinus rhythm. In patients with heart failure, low cardiac output and cardiac dilatation predispose to thrombus formation [15]. Various factors, including different stages of chronic kidney disease, play significant roles in thrombosis development among these patients [16]. Compared to the general population, individuals with chronic kidney disease are at significantly higher risk of cardiovascular events, including coronary heart disease, stroke, and heart failure [17].

Pathophysiological Mechanisms Underlying Thrombophilia in Cardiovascular–Kidney–Metabolic Syndrome

The normal process of hemostasis mainly involves vascular endothelium, platelets, and coagulation factors. A prothrombotic state occurs because of the disruption of the balance between procoagulant and anticoagulant factors. A series of processes contribute to its occurrence, which lead to the impairment of primary hemostasis, secondary hemostasis, and the fibrinolytic system. Thrombosis is a complex process influenced by a combination of these factors, known as Virchow's triad: endothelial damage, hypercoagulability, and circulatory stasis/turbulence. Virchow's triad and factors involved in CKM syndrome are illustrated in Fig. 16.1, which reveals the multiple etiopathogeneses of the thrombosis process.

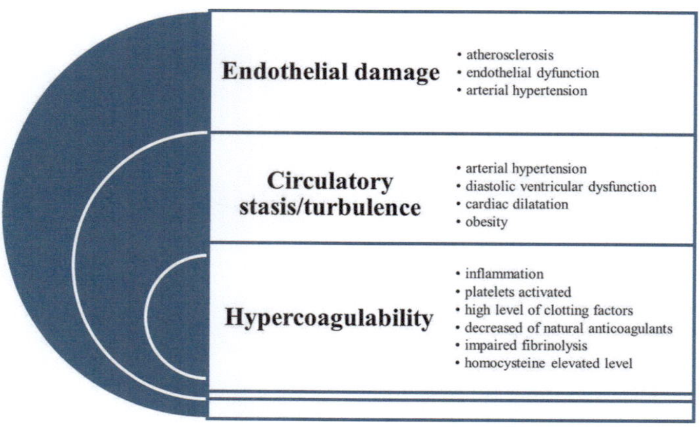

Fig. 16.1 Virchow's triad and factors involved in thrombosis related to CKM syndrome

The Role of the Vascular Endothelium

In cardiovascular–renal–metabolic syndrome (CKD), the vascular endothelium plays a crucial role in the development of thrombophilia, defined as a predisposition to blood clots. Endothelial dysfunction is a condition in which the endothelium does not maintain its normal functions, a situation in which the balance between pro- and anticoagulant factors is disturbed, which ultimately may result in an increased risk of thrombosis [18].

Endothelial cells are found at the interface between the circulating blood and the arterial wall. They act as true sensors and transmitters of signals in the circulating environment and are important in maintaining vascular homeostasis during the production of factors regulating vascular tone, coagulation, lipid transport, and cellular proliferative responses [19, 20]. The vascular endothelium can produce a wide variety of molecules that act as agonists or antagonists, including vasodilators (NO, prostacyclin, EDHF) and vasoconstrictors (endothelin-1, angiotensin-converting enzyme AII, thromboxane A2), procoagulants (thromboxane A2) and anticoagulants (thrombomodulin), inflammatory and anti-inflammatory substances, fibrinolytic and antifibrinolytic agents, and oxidants and antioxidants [21, 22]. In 1980, Furchgott and Zawadzki [23] described an endothelium-derived factor that induces arterial relaxation in response to acetylcholine, later identified as nitric oxide (NO) [24]. The imbalance between procoagulant and anticoagulant factors of endothelial origin that leads to the procoagulant status is illustrated in Fig. 16.2.

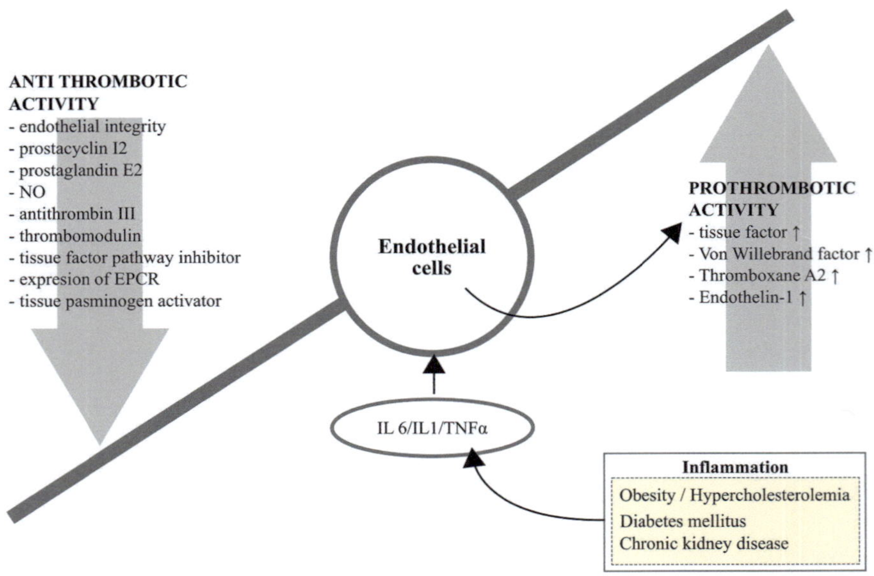

Fig. 16.2 Role of vascular endothelium in CKM syndrome

In addition to its vasodilatory role, NO has antiatherogenic properties, inhibiting platelet aggregation and adhesion, smooth muscle cell proliferation, and having a role in vascular permeability and inflammatory processes [25]. The classical model of NO bioactivity involves its binding to the heme group of guanylate cyclase in target cells (platelets, smooth muscle cells) to increase cellular cGMP and activate cGMP-dependent protein kinase, thus influencing NO-mediated vasodilation and platelet inhibition [25–27].

Regarding the antithrombotic role of the endothelium [28], it is manifested by the presence of glycocalyx (negatively charged protein), synthesis of platelet aggregation inhibitors (PGI2, NO), synthesis of antithrombotic proteins (antithrombin III, thrombomodulin), and synthesis of tPA (tissue plasminogen activator).

A series of evidence indicates the existence, besides NO and prostacyclin, of a third vasodilator pathway mediated by endothelium-derived hyperpolarizing factor (EDHF) [29]. EDHF is a major determinant of vascular tone in small resistance vessels. It acts predominantly by activating calcium-dependent potassium (KCa) channels, the resulting hyperpolarization causing relaxation of vascular smooth myocytes because of a decrease in voltage-dependent calcium influx [30]. In general, the contribution of EDHF to endothelium-dependent vasodilation is assessed by monitoring the response to an endothelium-dependent agonist during combined blockade of NOS and cyclooxygenase. In small resistance vessels, the EDHF pathway appears to be even more important than NO in mediating endothelium-dependent vasodilation. Hyperreactive oxygen species have also been considered for the role of EDHF. Endothelial Cu, Zn-type superoxide dismutase, plays an important role in the EDHF component of endothelium-dependent relaxation in both human and mouse mesenteric arteries [30, 31].

Various studies have demonstrated the essential role played by endothelial dysfunction in the pathophysiology of various cardiovascular diseases. Thus, in stage I of essential arterial hypertension, approximately 60% of patients present inadequate vasodilation on subcutaneous gluteal biopsy [32]. The same phenomenon has been described in type 1 or type 2 diabetes mellitus [33], coronary artery disease [34], peripheral arterial disease, and renal failure. Moreover, endothelial dysfunction can be evidenced in asymptomatic subjects who are at risk for cardiovascular disease, thus demonstrating its role in the diagnosis of subclinical atherosclerosis, in the assessment of cardiovascular prognosis in the medium or long term, and in the choice of an optimal therapeutic approach [35]. The precipitation of acute vascular events in atherosclerosis involves processes that go beyond the vulnerability and rupture of the atheromatous plaque. A whole series of studies confirms that local homeostatic processes in the arterial wall are abnormal in both patients with obvious atherosclerosis and those with risk factors for atherosclerosis.

Circulatory Stasis/Turbulence

In the cardiovascular system the fluid flow is laminar, meaning that each layer passes smoothly over the adjacent layer with little or no mixing resulting, that the velocity of blood flow is highest in the central layers and slowest in peripheral layers. This laminar flow ensures a specific localization of the different components of the blood flow passing through the vessel. Thus, blood cells are in the center of the blood flow, and at the periphery are the plasma components. The presence of the plasma component at the periphery of the blood flow prevents direct interaction between platelets and the vascular endothelium.

In some cardiovascular diseases, laminar flow is replaced by turbulent flow, which leads to mixing of blood flow components and interaction with the vascular wall, increasing the risk of thrombosis. Turbulence blood flow is a factor that contributes to the development of atherosclerosis. Experimental studies have demonstrated that the combination of turbulent blood flow and low wall shear stress, in the presence of hypercholesterolemia and oxidative stress, creates conditions for the formation of incipient atherosclerotic lesions [36]. High blood pressure has an impact on the vascular wall and causes structural and functional alterations, including endothelial dysfunction, oxidative stress, and excessive collagen deposition [37, 38]. All these structural remodeling of the vascular wall as well as endothelial dysfunction contribute to the appearance of a turbulent flow, which, in turn, contributes to thrombosis. Animal models of obesity and metabolic syndrome support the concept of impaired blood flow regulation [39]. Increased sympathetically mediated vasoconstriction significantly impacts local blood flow regulation in obese adults and adults with metabolic syndrome and may have important implications for the thrombosis [40].

On the other hand, circulatory stasis, especially in the lower limbs, and venous insufficiency in obese people contribute to the development of deep venous thrombosis [40].

Platelets in CKM Syndrome

It is well known that platelets play an important role in both hemostasis and the thrombosis process. They are unnucleated cells that are produced in bone marrow from cytoplasmic fragmentation of megakaryocytes [41]. Data published in the literature show that platelets are actively involved in CKM syndrome, leading to the activation of prothrombotic status. Platelets are involved in the production of thrombocytosis, platelet activation, and the release of activated microparticles. All these aspects are highlighted in Fig. 16.3.

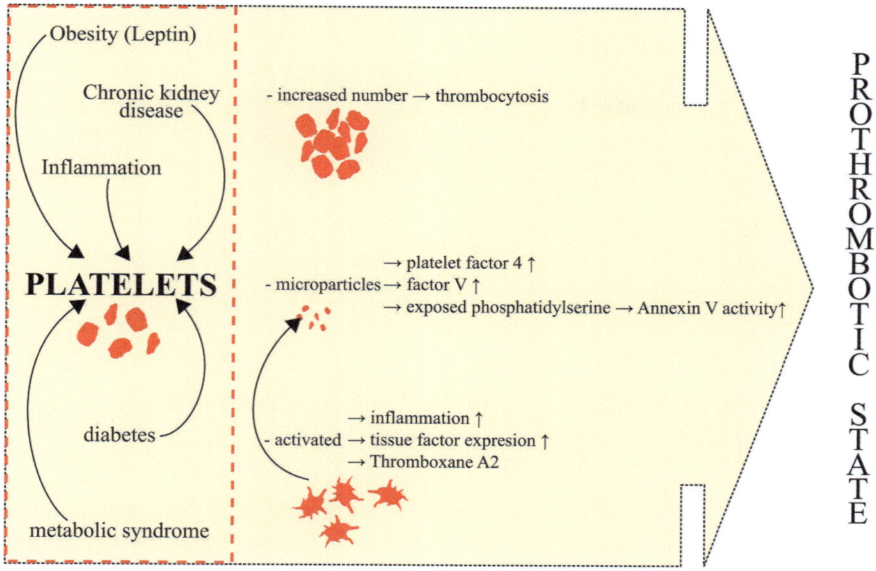

Fig. 16.3 Platelets in CKM syndrome

Obesity and inflammation are associated with an increased platelet number. Platelet counts have been found to be increased in obese individuals compared to nonobese controls [42]. Starting from the idea that obesity is a pro-inflammatory state, the increase in platelet count can be explained by the increased secretion of IL-6, which acts at the bone marrow level by increasing the secretion of thrombopoietin, which stimulates megakaryocytopoiesis [43]. Obesity and metabolic syndrome are also associated with activated platelets [44]. Platelets contain granules (alpha granules, dense granules, lysosomal granules) and cytosol, which have different classes of substances that can promote thrombosis. Factors released during platelet activation that promote thrombosis are illustrated in Table 16.1.

Platelets release small membrane microparticles (MPs) that contain active proteins and are associated with a pro-thrombotic state in CKM syndrome. In 2019, Grand et al. studied the number, size, and proteome of MPs generated in vitro in response to thrombin from platelets of obese women and their matched lean controls [45]. They found that MPs have greater heterogeneity in size distribution and reduced levels of pyruvate kinase, which is a regulator of mitophagy [45]. A defect in the mitophagy response of platelets has also been described in diabetes mellitus [46] and can promote thrombosis as a response to oxidative stress. MPs contain factor V and play an important role in pro-thrombotic state through their profound influence on the production of thrombin [45].

Table 16.1 Factors released during platelet activation that promote thrombosis

Coagulation factors	Cytokines and chemokines	Antifibrinolytic molecules	Adhesion molecules
Factor V	Interleukin 1	Thrombin	Factor von Willebrand
Factor von Willebrand	Platelets factor 4	α2-antiplasmin	P-selectin
Factor XIII		Inhibitor, plasminogen activator inhibitor-1	Fibronectin
Fibrinogen			
Kininogen			

Interplay Between Inflammation, Adipokines, Hemostasis, and Fibrinolysis

Data from the literature suggests that there is a strong association between systemic immune-inflammation index and cardiovascular–kidney–metabolic syndrome inflammation [47], with a key role in prothrombotic state [47, 48]. There is strong evidence that obesity and metabolic syndrome are inflammatory diseases [42]. Adipocytes secrete inflammatory cytokines, especially IL-1, IL-6, TNF-α, leading to the accumulation of macrophages in adipose tissue. Macrophages are activated and present a pro-inflammatory phenotype, playing an important role in interactions with adipocytes and in stimulating the secretion of inflammatory cytokines, thereby contributing to the maintenance of a systemic inflammatory state [42]. Unexplained leukocytosis has been observed in obese patients, especially due to an increase in the number of neutrophils. This increase in the number of neutrophils without an infectious cause is attributed to the effects of inflammatory cytokines secreted by adipose tissue on granulocytopoiesis [42, 43]. Other studies have shown that animal models fed high-fat diets develop myeloid hyperplasia, especially in the granulocytic compartment [43].

Adipose tissue secretes a category of substances that are named adipokines. Some of these adipokines have a prothrombotic role, while others have an antithrombotic role, practically breaking this balance leads to the occurrence of thrombosis, as exemplified in Fig. 16.4.

Adipokines with a pro-thrombotic role include leptin, PAI-1, resistin, and visfatin, whereas anti-thrombotic adipokines include adiponectin and apelin [42].

Chronic inflammation and adipokines contribute to thrombosis through dysfunction of vascular endothelium, activation of platelets, upregulation of hemostasis, and impaired fibrinolysis. Over the past century, several models have attempted to explain the mechanism of coagulation, but the coagulation cascade model has been the most widely accepted. This original model, presented as a Y-shaped diagram, shows two separate pathways: the extrinsic pathway and the intrinsic pathway, which converge on a common pathway that begins with the formation of the

Fig. 16.4 Adipokines and their role in thrombosis

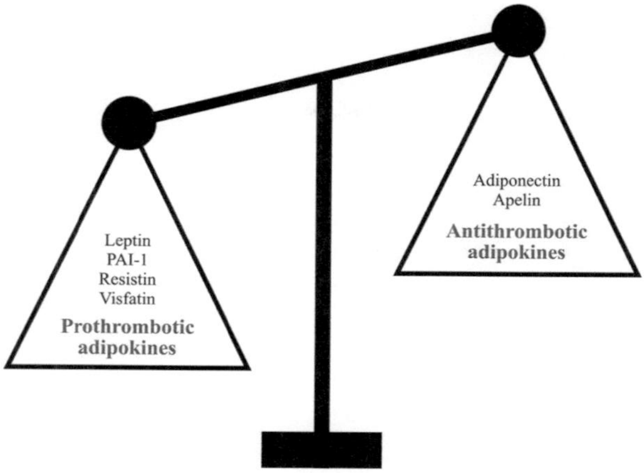

FXa–FVa complex [49]. Extrinsic pathway—It involves the interaction between tissue factor, also called tissue thromboplastin or FIII, and factor VII. Tissue factor is an integral membrane protein expressed in tissues outside the vessels that functions as a receptor for plasma FVII that will activate it. The complex formed by tissue factor and FVIIa will form a complex that will activate FXa then follow the common pathway [49, 50]. Intrinsic pathway—It begins with the activation of factor XII by the negatively charged surface of activated platelet membranes, vascular lesions, or exposed collagen, with high molecular weight kininogen (HMWK) acting as a cofactor. Subsequently, through a positive feedback mechanism, FXIIa will convert prekallikrein to kallikrein, which, in turn, will activate FXII at a much higher rate. Subsequently, a series of cascade reactions will initially cause FXIIa to act enzymatically on FXI to activate it. FXIa together with Ca^{2+} will act enzymatically to activate FIX, and then FIXa together with FVIIIa, platelet phospholipids, and Ca^{2+} will activate FX [50]. Common pathway—once FXa is formed, whether by the intrinsic, extrinsic, or both pathways, it forms, together with FVa and in the presence of tissue phospholipids and Ca^{2+}, the prothrombinase complex, which will convert prothrombin into thrombin. With the help of thrombin, fibrinogen is converted into fibrin, thus strengthening the clot [49, 50].

The cellular model of hemostasis involves three phases: initiation, amplification, and propagation [51, 52]. Tissue factor-bearing cells and platelets are the two essential cellular components, while fibrinogen and thrombin are coagulation proteins that interact with cellular components to achieve hemostasis. In the first phase, when blood is exposed to extravascular cells carrying tissue factor on the membrane surface, hemostasis is initiated at the site of injury. Tissue factor (TF) is commonly present on the surface of smooth muscle cells, and fibroblasts at the subendothelial level, but under conditions of inflammation, it has also been observed inside endothelial cells, macrophages, and blood platelets. Blood that presents coagulation factors, including FVII, binds to TF, being a receptor and cofactor for it, will activate it, thus forming the TF-FVIIa complex, also called the extrinsic tenase complex.

This complex formed at the injury level will catalyze two reactions: FX activation and FIX activation. FXa will form with partially active FV released by activated thrombocytes adhering to the lesion site, forming the prothrombinase complex, which will generate small amounts of thrombin (also called the thrombin spark) at the surface of TF-bearing cells. Any FXa that is dissociated from the cellular level is rapidly inactivated by tissue factor pathway inhibitor (TFPI) and/or antithrombin III so that the initiation phase remains localized to the lesion [52, 53]. Amplification phase—this phase occurs predominantly at the platelet surface. Thrombin formed in the initiation phase is transferred to platelets, where the initial hemostasis signal is amplified by further activation of platelets and cofactors. At the platelet level, thrombin can bind to two membrane receptors: Glycoprotein Ib (GpIb) and protease-activated receptor 1 (PAR1). Binding thrombin to PAR1 will cause platelet activation and binding to GpIb will activate FVIII, partially activated FV/FV (released by activated platelets) and FXI [52, 53]. Propagation phase—FIXa formed during the initiation phase is available despite plasma levels of antithrombin III because its half-life is approximately 1 h in plasma. It will bind to FVIIIa present on the platelet surface to form the intrinsic tenase complex, which will activate FX at a rate 50 times greater than the extrinsic tenase complex. Consequently, thrombin production will be amplified, also called the thrombin burst [52, 53]. Pro-inflammatory cytokines secreted by the adipose tissue lead to an upregulation of clotting factors and downregulation of natural anticoagulants, with an important impact on the hemostasis process. Expression of the tissue factor that initiates coagulation is high on the macrophages, endothelial cells in obese individuals being one of the pathways that lead to the acceleration of the thrombosis process [49]. Finally, chronic inflammatory conditions such as obesity are associated with elevated plasma levels of coagulation factors, such as factor VIII, fibrinogen and von Willebrand factor [54]. These effects are likely mediated by actions of pro-inflammatory cytokines on liver and vascular endothelium that increase secretion of these clotting factors, acting at the same time as inflammatory proteins [54] (Fig. 16.5).

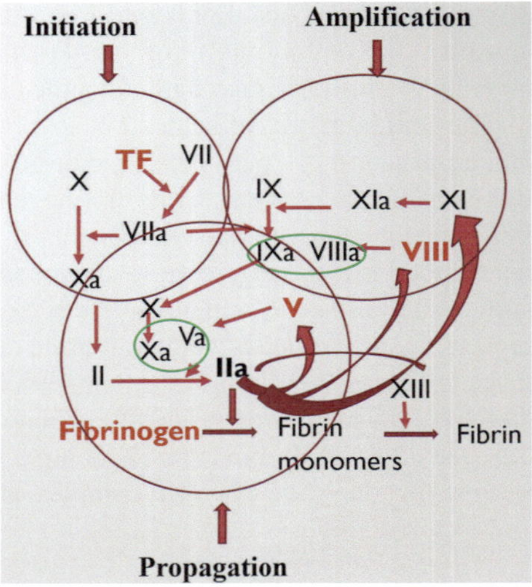

Fig. 16.5 Cellular model of hemostasis. In red, elevated levels of TF—tissue factor, VIII, and fibrinogen, associated with chronic inflammation in CKM syndrome

Chronic inflammation is associated with downregulation of antithrombotic mechanisms, such as protein C anticoagulation system, antithrombin, and tissue factor pathway inhibitor, producing an imbalance between procoagulants factors and anticoagulant proteins [49] (Fig. 16.6).

Fibrinolysis is a central mechanism with an important role in preventing excessive coagulation. The main event of this process is the conversion of plasminogen to plasmin. This, in turn, cleaves coagulation factors V, VIII, von Willebrand, and a complex located on the surface of platelets. The fibrin degradation products resulting from this process have an inhibitory role in fibrin formation. The initial step in the formation of plasmin from plasminogen is stimulated by the action of tissue plasminogen activator, which is secreted by endothelial cells, or by urokinase plasminogen activator, secreted by macrophages/monocytes. The entire fibrinolysis process is regulated and controlled by a series of serine protease inhibitors: plasminogen-activated inhibitor (PAI-1, PAI-2), anti-plasmin, and thrombin-activated fibrinolysis inhibitor (TAFI) [55]. PAI-1 inhibits tissue plasminogen activator and urokinase plasminogen activator. Expression of PAI-1 is elevated in fat tissue in obese patients or in those with metabolic syndrome [56]. Plasma levels of PAI-1 are also elevated in patients with diabetes mellitus, obesity, or metabolic syndrome [57] (Fig. 16.7).

The main effects of chronic inflammation and obesity associated with CKM syndrome on the fluid-coagulant system are summarized in Table 16.2.

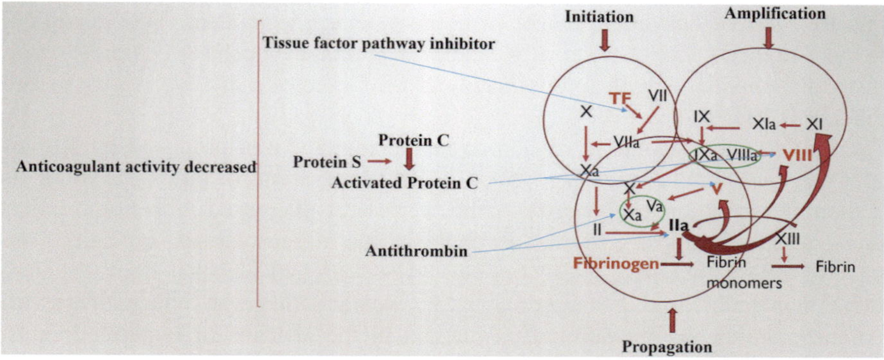

Fig. 16.6 Cellular model of hemostasis. Blue arrows: decreased activity of natural anticoagulants, associated with chronic inflammation in CKM syndrome

Fig. 16.7 Impaired fibrinolysis in CKM syndrome

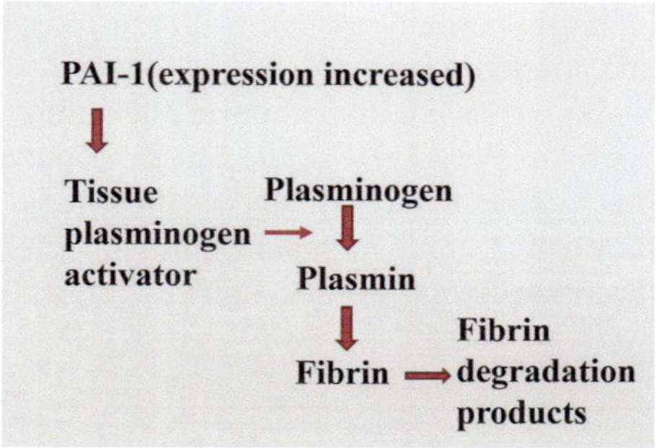

Table 16.2 The main effects of chronic inflammation and obesity on the fluid-coagulant system in CKM syndrome

Procoagulant factor activity increased	Anticoagulant activity decreased	Impaired fibrinolysis
Factor VIII	Tissue factor pathway inhibitor	PAI-1 expression increased
Factor V	Antithrombin	
Fibrinogen	Protein C system	
Factor von Willebrand		

Homocysteine and Its Impact on Hemostasis Process

The current scientific interest in homocysteine primarily stems from its recognition as an independent risk factor for cardiovascular disease (CVD). Homocysteine (2-amino-4-mercaptobutyric acid), a sulfur-containing amino acid closely related to methionine and cysteine, was first described by Butz and du Vigneaud in 1932 [58].

In 1962, Carson and Neil reported an association between elevated homocysteine levels and pathological conditions. They observed increased homocysteine concentrations in the urine of children with intellectual disabilities, later determined to be due to a severe enzymatic defect in homocysteine metabolism. This condition, homocystinuria, was subsequently linked to premature occlusive cardiovascular disease in childhood, with approximately 25% of affected individuals dying before the age of 30 [59].

The vascular hypothesis of homocysteine toxicity was proposed by Kilmer McCully over three decades ago [58, 59]. His observations of infants as young as 2 months old dying from stroke—who were later diagnosed with homocystinuria—revealed extensive arterial thrombosis and atherosclerosis, typically seen only in elderly patients. These findings suggested that elevated homocysteine, rather than methionine, was responsible for vascular damage, as some patients with homocystinuria had hyperhomocysteinemia in the absence of hypermethioninemia. McCully thus proposed that homocysteine was a causal factor in atherosclerotic vascular disease. The term "homocysteine" broadly refers to a plasma pool that includes homocysteine, homocystine (its oxidized dimer), and thiolactone–homocysteine. Subsequent research has confirmed McCully's hypothesis, establishing hyperhomocysteinemia as an independent risk factor for both atherosclerosis and atherothrombosis [60].

While severe hyperhomocysteinemia is rare, moderate elevation occurs in approximately 5–7% of the general population. Individuals with moderate hyperhomocysteinemia are usually asymptomatic until their third or fourth decade, when they may develop premature coronary artery disease and recurrent arterial or venous thromboembolic events. Epidemiological studies have consistently demonstrated that even moderate elevations in homocysteine are independently associated with coronary, cerebral, and peripheral vascular atherosclerosis [61]. Although the exact molecular mechanisms through which homocysteine contributes to atherothrombosis remain unclear, the epidemiological link is well established.

Extensive experimental research has explored possible mechanisms of homocysteine-induced vascular damage [62]. Proposed mechanisms include endothelial surface injury, protein modification via disulfide bond formation, platelet activation, altered monocyte function, upregulation of vascular adhesion molecules, and oxidative stress through reactive oxygen species [63].

A particularly noteworthy mechanism involves homocysteine's effect on methylation pathways. The interconversion of S-adenosylhomocysteine (SAH) and homocysteine, catalyzed by SAH hydrolase, favors SAH formation under physiological conditions. When homocysteine metabolism is impaired—due to genetic mutations, vitamin B deficiencies, or other causes—intracellular levels of both homocysteine and SAH increase. Elevated SAH is a potent feedback inhibitor of S-adenosylmethionine (SAM)-dependent methylation reactions, thereby potentially disrupting numerous cellular functions and contributing to vascular pathology [64].

Another critical area of interest is the interaction between homocysteine, nitric oxide (NO), and endothelial function. Homocysteine has been shown to inhibit nitric oxide synthase (NOS), thereby impairing NO-mediated vasodilation. This contributes to endothelial dysfunction, a key early event in atherogenesis [65].

Hyperhomocysteinemia is also a risk factor for the occurrence of venous thrombosis. A lot of studies have shown that the mean plasma Hcy level and the prevalence of hyperhomocysteinemia were higher in the group of patients with deep vein thrombosis than in controls [66].

In summary, while the precise mechanisms by which homocysteine promotes vascular disease are still under investigation, current evidence suggests that multiple synergistic pathways are involved. These include impaired methylation, oxidative stress, endothelial dysfunction, and inflammation—all of which support the role of hyperhomocysteinemia as a significant contributor to cardiovascular pathology [67]. Studies published in the literature have shown a statistically significant increase in homocysteine levels in individuals with metabolic syndrome [68]. Hyperhomocysteinemia is a predictive marker for the development of cardiovascular disease in young obese people [69]. Also, hyperhomocysteinemia is a significant feature of chronic kidney disease, people with high Hcy levels were more likely to suffer from chronic kidney disease than people with normal Hcy levels [70]. Hyperhomocysteinemia has an impact on both primary and secondary hemostasis and the fibrinolysis process, contributing to the production of a procoagulant status. Thus, it produces endothelial dysfunction and a direct toxic effect on the vascular endothelium as well as platelet activation. Regarding secondary hemostasis, it is associated with increased levels of coagulation factors, to which is added the impairment of the fibrinolysis process. All these aspects are systematically exposed in Fig. 16.8.

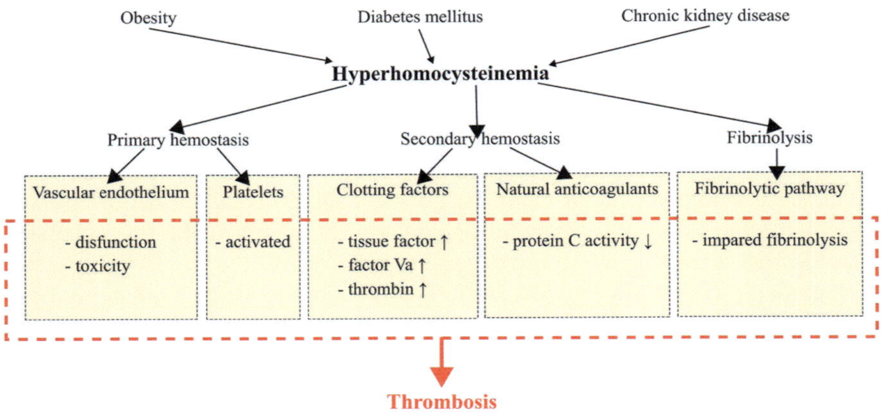

Fig. 16.8 Hyperhomocysteinemia in CKM syndrome and its effect on the hemostasis process

Laboratory Investigation of Thrombosis and Hemostasis in Cardiovascular–Kidney–Metabolic Syndrome

Complete Blood Count

A complete blood count (CBC) can reveal important clues about the body's tendency to form blood clots, a condition known as thrombophilia. This is especially relevant in individuals with cardiovascular, kidney, or metabolic disorders [71]. Within the CBC, certain platelet-related markers—such as the number of platelets, their average size (known as mean platelet volume or MPV), and the ratio of platelets to lymphocytes (PLR)—can indicate increased clotting risk. Research has shown that higher platelet counts and elevated PLR levels are linked to a greater likelihood of developing cardiovascular disease and type 2 diabetes. These findings suggest that the risk of thrombophilia may play a role in the development or progression of these chronic conditions [72]. Clinically, the WBC count is valuable for monitoring treatment responses in infectious or inflammatory conditions [73].

Given the link between WBC elevation and chronic inflammation, this parameter is increasingly recognized as a potential marker for cardiovascular disease (CVD) and metabolic disorders [74]. CBC-derived WBC data, including differential counts, provide an accessible and efficient means of identifying and tracking systemic inflammation and associated disease risks. Elevated white blood cell counts (WBC), particularly the neutrophil-to-lymphocyte ratio (NLR), can indicate systemic inflammation, a key factor in cardiovascular–kidney–metabolic (CKM) syndrome progression. On the other hand, red blood cell parameters like red cell distribution width (RDW) and mean corpuscular volume (MCV) can offer information about inflammation and the overall hemodynamic state [75, 76]. All the aspects that are associated with thrombophilia in CKM syndrome are summarized in Table 16.3.

Table 16.3 Complete blood count and the main markers that show an increased risk of thrombosis in CKM syndrome

Platelets	White blood cells	Erythrocytes
Numberincreased	Neutrophils increased	Hemoglobin decreased
MPV (mean platelet volume) increased	NLR (neutrophils to lymphocytes ratio) increased	RDW (red cell distribution) increased
PLR (platelets-to- lymphocytes ratio) increased		MCV (mean corpuscular volume) variable
Thrombocytosis	***Neutrophilia- inflammation***	***Inflammatory anemia***

Coagulation Profile

Pre-analytical factors can significantly impact the accuracy of routine coagulation tests, which are commonly used in diagnosing thrombophilia. These factors include how the blood sample is collected, handled, transported, processed, and stored [77].

For clot-based functional assays, venous blood should be drawn into tubes containing 3.2% trisodium citrate at a ratio of one part citrate to nine parts blood. Proper technique during collection is essential, including correct order of draw and minimal use of the tourniquet to avoid affecting results. After collection, the samples should be kept at room temperature and ideally analyzed within 4 h [78]. All the laboratory investigations of coagulation profile associated with thrombotic risk are summarized in Table 16.4.

Activated Partial Thromboplastin Time (aPTT)

aPTT is a functional test that evaluates the "intrinsic" (prekallikrein, high molecular weight kininogen—HK, factors XII, XI, IX, VIII) and "common" (factors X, V, II, I) coagulation pathways.

In vivo, the contact system is involved when blood interacts with a foreign surface, such as cardiopulmonary bypass. The zymogen FXII, the first protein in the series, binds to negatively charged surfaces (kaolin, dextran sulfate, sulfatides), causing self-activation and action on the substrates, prekallikrein and FXI, with the formation of kallikrein and FXIa. Kallikrein cleaves HK with the release of bradykinin and kinin-free kininogen (activated HK)—Table 16.4 [79].

While aPTT is not specific to chronic kidney disease (CKD) or cardiovascular–kidney–metabolic (CKM) syndrome, it plays a supportive role in monitoring and managing patients with CKM, a condition defined by the interplay between cardiovascular disease, CKD, and metabolic risk factors [80].

Some clinical applications of aPTT in CKM syndrome can be mentioned such as monitoring bleeding risk, assessing anticoagulant therapy, and detecting coagulation factor deficiency.

Monitoring bleeding risk—CKM patients may have impaired coagulation due to CKD or other metabolic disturbances. A prolonged aPTT can indicate a higher risk of bleeding, making it important to monitor these patients regularly [81].

Table 16.4 Coagulation profile in CKM syndrome

	Increased	Decreased	Clinical application
aPTT	Factor XII, XI, IX, VIII, X, V, II acquired deficiencies Lupic anticoagulant	Hypercoagulability	Intrinsic and common pathways clotting factor deficiencies Monitoring therapy (heparine) Monitoring bleeding risk
PT	Factor II, VII, IX, and X acquired deficiencies Vitamin K deficiency	Hypercoagulability	Extrinsec and common pathways clotting factor deficiencies Monitoring therapy (warfarine) Monitoring bleeding risk
TCT	Fibrinogen deficiency	Hypercoagulability	Fibrinogen deficiency Monitoring therapy (dabigatran)
Fibrinogen	Inflammation–hypercoagulability	Hypocoagulability	Monitoring fibrinogen level
TEG	MA- hypercoagulability R- hypocoagulability		Risk stratification Monitoring therapy Guiding interventions Investigation of hemostasis and fibrinolysis
Clotting factor activity	Factor VIII, V, von Willebrand—hypercoagulability	Hypocoagulability	Evaluation of inflammation Measuring of level of clotting factor
Natural anticoagulant activity		Protein C, S, antithrombin III-hypercoagulability	Measuring of anticoagulants level
D dimers	Hypercoagulability		Measuring of fibrinolytic activity

Assessing anticoagulant therapy—The aPTT test is essential for monitoring the effects of unfractionated heparin, commonly used in CKM patients at increased risk for thrombosis. It helps adjust heparin dosage safely and effectively [82].

Detecting coagulation factor deficiencies—CKM syndrome, particularly when associated with uremia, can cause deficiencies in clotting factors. aPTT can help identify such deficiencies or the presence of coagulation inhibitors [83].

Evaluating underlying systemic conditions—Abnormal aPTT results can reflect broader systemic issues, including kidney dysfunction, liver disease, or autoimmune conditions, all of which may be present in CKM [84].

Since the etiology of thrombosis is multifactorial, the presence of a thrombotic defect is only one of many elements that determine risk. Therefore, the usefulness of thrombophilia testing to inform prevention and treatment decisions is controversial. The tests have been suggested to aid in secondary prevention (determining the duration of anticoagulation following a thrombotic event) and, for hereditary conditions, to aid in primary prevention in relatives of affected patients [85].

Prothrombin Time (PT)

Prothrombin time (PT) is a critical laboratory test that assesses the extrinsic and common pathways of the coagulation cascade. In patients with chronic kidney disease (CKD), PT values can be altered due to various factors, including uremic toxins, vitamin K deficiency, and the use of anticoagulant medications [86].

Patients with CKD, particularly those with end-stage renal disease (ESRD), often exhibit prolonged PT values. This prolongation can be attributed to several mechanisms [86]: uremic toxins (accumulation of uremic toxins in CKD impairs hepatic synthesis of clotting factors, leading to extended PT), vitamin K deficiency (CKD patients may experience vitamin K deficiency due to dietary restrictions and malabsorption, affecting the synthesis of vitamin K-dependent clotting factors II, VII, IX, and X), anticoagulant therapy (the use of anticoagulants, such as warfarin, is common in CKD patients to prevent thrombotic events) (Table 16.4). However, these medications can further prolong PT, necessitating careful monitoring.

Finally, the prolongation of PT in CKD patients has significant clinical implications, such as bleeding risk (extended PT indicates a higher risk of bleeding, which is particularly concerning during surgical procedures or invasive interventions), monitoring anticoagulation (regular assessment of PT is essential for CKD patients on anticoagulant therapy to balance the risks of thrombosis and bleeding), dialysis considerations (hemodialysis can influence coagulation parameters). Studies suggest that dialysis may exacerbate coagulation abnormalities, emphasizing the need for vigilant monitoring [86].

Thrombin Clotting Time

Thrombin clotting time (TCT), similar to thrombin time (TT), is a laboratory assay that measures the time it takes for thrombin to convert fibrinogen into fibrin, forming a blood clot [87]. This test is particularly sensitive to abnormalities in fibrinogen concentration or function and to the presence of thrombin inhibitors. In patients with chronic kidney disease (CKD), various factors can influence TCT, reflecting the complex interplay between renal dysfunction and coagulation pathways [88].

CKD patients often exhibit both qualitative and quantitative fibrinogen abnormalities due to chronic inflammation and uremic toxins. These alterations can prolong TCT, indicating a hypocoagulable state (Table 16.4). Accumulation of endogenous thrombin inhibitors, such as fibrin degradation products, is common in CKD and can lead to extended TCT values, reflecting impaired clot formation [89]. TCT is highly sensitive to direct thrombin inhibitors (e.g., dabigatran) and heparin. In CKD patients, especially those on dialysis, monitoring anticoagulant therapy using TCT can be challenging due to altered drug clearance and increased sensitivity to these agents. Hemodialysis can influence coagulation parameters. The use of heparin during dialysis sessions can prolong TCT, necessitating careful monitoring to balance the risks of thrombosis and bleeding [90].

Fibrinogen

Fibrinogen, a glycoprotein involved in coagulation and an acute-phase reactant, plays a pivotal role in the pathogenesis and progression of CKM syndrome. Elevated plasma fibrinogen levels have been consistently associated with an increased risk of cardiovascular disease (CVD). High fibrinogen concentrations contribute to a prothrombotic state by enhancing blood viscosity, promoting platelet aggregation, and facilitating fibrin formation, thereby accelerating atherogenesis and increasing the likelihood of thrombotic events (Table 16.4). For instance, a study demonstrated that elevated fibrinogen levels were significantly associated with long-term all-cause and cardiac mortality in patients with coronary artery disease undergoing percutaneous coronary intervention [91].

In CKD patients, fibrinogen levels are often elevated due to reduced renal clearance and a persistent inflammatory state. This elevation is linked to an increased risk of cardiovascular complications, which are the leading cause of morbidity and mortality in this population. A review highlighted that high plasma concentrations of fibrinogen are accompanied by an increased risk for cardiovascular complications in patients with renal disease [92].

Metabolic syndrome, characterized by insulin resistance, hypertension, dyslipidemia, and central obesity, is associated with elevated fibrinogen levels. This elevation reflects a state of chronic low-grade inflammation and contributes to the prothrombotic milieu observed in metabolic disorders. Studies have shown that participants with metabolic syndrome had higher fibrinogen concentrations compared to those without the syndrome [93]. Fibrinogen plays a central role in the pathophysiology of CKM syndrome by linking inflammation, coagulation, and vascular dysfunction. Elevated fibrinogen levels are associated with increased risks of cardiovascular events, progression of kidney disease, and metabolic complications. Monitoring fibrinogen levels in patients with CKM syndrome may aid in risk stratification and guide therapeutic strategies aimed at reducing inflammation and thrombosis [93].

Thromboelastography (TEG)

Thromboelastography (TEG) is a viscoelastic hemostatic assay that provides a dynamic assessment of the entire coagulation process, including clot initiation, formation, strength, and dissolution [94]. In patients with CKD, TEG has emerged as a valuable tool to assess the complex hemostatic alterations that are often inadequately captured by conventional coagulation tests such as prothrombin time (PT) and activated partial thromboplastin time (aPTT). In the context of cardiovascular–kidney–metabolic (CKM) syndrome—a complex disorder involving interrelated cardiovascular disease, chronic kidney disease, type 2 diabetes, and obesity—TEG offers valuable insights into the hemostatic alterations that may occur [95]

CKM syndrome is characterized by a pro-inflammatory and prothrombotic state due to the interplay of its constituent conditions. Traditional coagulation tests, such as prothrombin time (PT) and activated partial thromboplastin time (aPTT), often fail to capture the nuanced coagulation abnormalities present in CKM patients. TEG, by contrast, assesses the viscoelastic properties of whole blood, providing a comprehensive evaluation of hemostasis [96].

Studies have demonstrated that TEG can detect hypercoagulable states in patients with cardiovascular diseases. For instance, increased maximum amplitude (MA) values, indicative of enhanced clot strength, have been observed in such patients, suggesting a heightened thrombotic risk. Similarly, in patients with end-stage renal disease (ESRD), TEG has revealed prolonged reaction time (R), reflecting delayed clot initiation, while MA values remained comparable to controls, highlighting the complex coagulation dynamics in CKD (Table 16.4) [97].

In CKM syndrome, TEG has several clinical implications, such as risk stratification (TEG can identify patients at increased risk of thrombotic events by detecting hypercoagulable states not apparent in conventional tests), therapeutic monitoring (TEG allows for real-time monitoring of anticoagulant therapy efficacy, facilitating individualized treatment adjustments), guiding interventions (in surgical or invasive procedures, TEG can inform decisions regarding the need for blood product transfusions or antifibrinolytic therapy).

By providing a holistic view of the coagulation process, TEG aids in the comprehensive management of CKM patients, addressing both thrombotic and bleeding risks. Its ability to detect subtle changes in clot formation and stability enables clinicians to better stratify risk, monitor therapy, and guide interventions, ultimately improving patient outcomes [98].

Clotting Factors Activity, Natural Anticoagulants Activity, and Fibrinolytic Activity

Increased activity of clotting factors such as factor VIII, factor V, von Willebrand factor is associated with CKM syndrome [54]. Measuring the activity of these coagulation factors can provide additional information regarding the risk and prothrombotic status. Thus, factor VIII is also an inflammatory protein and has increased activity in CKM syndrome. Studies have shown that increasing BMI leads to increased factor VIII activity, thus potentiating prothrombotic risk [54, 99].

Protein S is a vitamin K-dependent glycoprotein synthesized in the liver, endothelial cells, and megakaryocytes. Approximately 60% of the circulating amount of protein S is bound to the complement C4b-binding protein. The remainder of the protein is found in a free form, capable of acting as a nonenzymatic cofactor of activated protein C. Protein S enhances the inactivation of factors Va and VIIIa at phospholipid surfaces and also plays a role in the fibrinolytic effect of activated protein C. Studies indicate a possible involvement of the bound fraction of protein S in the anticoagulant activity independent of activated protein C [100, 101]. Protein C is activated by thrombin; the activation rate is accelerated by the formation of a complex between thrombin and endothelial cell thrombomodulin. Activated protein C degrades factors Va and VIIIa by selective proteolytic cleavage, leading to a reduction in the procoagulant activity of plasma. For the inactivation of coagulation factors, the presence of a cofactor—protein S—is required along with calcium ions and a phospholipid membrane surface. Activated protein C is neutralized by specific inhibitors, alpha2-antiplasmin and alpha2-macroglobulin [100, 101]. Antithrombin III is a potent inhibitor of the reactions in the coagulation cascade. Although the name antithrombin implies action only at the level of thrombin, this natural anticoagulant inhibits all coagulation enzymes to some extent. The main enzymes inhibited are factors Xa, IXa, and thrombin (factor IIa), as well as factors XIIa, Xia, and the factor VIIa-tissue factor complex [100, 101]. Antithrombin may be the link between obesity and poorer prognosis [102].

D-dimers are specific fibrin degradation products. They result from the degradation of stabilized, cross-polymerized fibrin by plasmin (unlike PDF, which represents degradation products of both fibrin and fibrinogen). D-dimers are an indicator of coagulation activity [103]. In principle, increased levels of these fragments characterize conditions associated with hypercoagulability or excessive fibrinolysis [103]. The test is used in the diagnosis and monitoring of conditions predisposing to hypercoagulability and thromboembolism (Table 16.4).

Elevated D-dimer levels can be found in all conditions with increased coagulation activation, such as CKM syndrome [104, 105].

Other Biochemical Markers with Impact on Hemostasis and Thrombosis in CKM Syndrome

Inflammatory Markers in Thrombophilia and CKM Syndrome

Chronic inflammation plays a central role in the development and progression of cardiovascular–kidney–metabolic (CKM) syndrome. Individuals with CKM commonly exhibit elevated levels of pro-inflammatory cytokines, such as interleukin-6

(IL-6) and tumor necrosis factor-alpha (TNF-α), indicating a persistent inflammatory state that promotes endothelial dysfunction and accelerates atherosclerosis [106]. Another biomarker of systemic inflammation is high-sensitivity C-reactive protein (hs-CRP), an acute-phase reactant produced by the liver in response to IL-6, which has been associated with increased cardiovascular risk in CKM patients. Elevated CRP levels, especially hs-CRP, are strongly associated with endothelial dysfunction, atherosclerosis, and increased cardiovascular morbidity and mortality [107].

Recent studies have also highlighted the significance of the Systemic Inflammatory Response Index (SIRI) as a prognostic marker. Elevated SIRI levels have been associated with increased risks of all-cause and cardiovascular mortality, particularly in younger adults with advanced CKM stages [108, 109].

Elevated levels of inflammatory cytokines contribute to this hypercoagulable state by upregulating tissue factor expression and suppressing natural anticoagulant mechanisms, particularly the protein C pathway.

In CKM syndrome, the close relationship between inflammation and thrombophilia underscores the need for an integrated management strategy. Anti-inflammatory therapies—particularly statins—have shown effectiveness in lowering high-sensitivity C-reactive protein (hs-CRP) levels and reducing the incidence of cardiovascular events [110]. In addition, novel agents targeting specific inflammatory mediators, such as interleukin-1β (IL-1β) and interleukin-6 (IL-6) inhibitors, are being actively investigated for their potential to reduce inflammation-induced thrombosis [111]. For patients with an elevated thrombotic risk profile, anticoagulant therapy may be warranted; however, careful consideration of bleeding risks remains essential [112, 113].

In CKM syndrome, chronic systemic inflammation plays a central role in connecting metabolic dysfunction with cardiovascular and renal complications, while simultaneously promoting a prothrombotic state. Recognizing the significance of inflammatory markers in contributing to thrombophilia is essential for effective risk stratification and for guiding the development of targeted therapeutic interventions aimed at mitigating the overall impact of CKM syndrome.

Homocysteine

Elevated plasma homocysteine levels are associated with a significantly increased risk of coronary artery disease, myocardial infarction, peripheral occlusive disease, and cerebral and retinal occlusive diseases [114, 115]. Homocysteine levels should be assessed in patients with CKM syndrome, given the direct correlation between thrombotic risk and its level.

Symptoms of Thrombophilia and Thrombotic Risk Assessment in CKM Syndrome

Thrombophilia does not cause specific symptoms, but only the occurrence of thrombotic events leads to the appearance of symptoms depending on the territory where the thromboses are located (arterial, systemic venous, splanchnic). Thrombosis is a condition characterized by the formation of a blood clot (thrombus) within a vein, which can partially or completely obstruct blood flow [116]. These clots develop due to abnormalities in the blood coagulation process [117].

While thrombi can form in various parts of the circulatory system, they most commonly develop in the deep veins of the lower limbs, where blood flow is more prone to stagnation. Although clots can also occur in superficial or upper veins, these are typically less serious and respond well to treatment [118]. A significant danger arises when a thrombus is loosely attached to the vessel wall and becomes dislodged. The resulting embolus travels through the bloodstream and may lodge in a narrower vessel, obstructing blood flow and leading to an embolism. In many cases, emboli originating from leg veins travel to the lungs via the heart, causing a potentially life-threatening condition known as pulmonary embolism [119].

Recognizing the symptoms of thrombosis is essential to prevent serious complications. Common signs include swelling, redness, warmth, and tenderness in the affected limb—typically around the foot, ankle, or thigh. The swelling results from fluid accumulation (edema), which, if untreated, may progress to ulceration [120].

A series of tools are currently used in clinical practice to assess the risk of thrombosis, especially venous, to initiate thromboprophylaxis. Various risk scores have been developed to help clinicians predict venous thromboembolism in patients with certain medical conditions [121]. The most important prediction scores for the occurrence and recurrence of thromboembolic disease are presented in Table 16.5. Some of these scores include, among the items used, markers of CKM syndromes—obesity or homocysteine levels (Table 16.5).

Starting from these scores that evaluate thromboembolic risk, as well as the fact that CKM syndrome is a form of acquired thrombophilia, we found it useful to consider the following factors in the evaluation of thromboembolic risk: patient-related factors, acquired thrombophilia, congenital thrombophilia, treatments associated with thrombotic risk, pregnancy, and other intercurrent factors (Table 16.6).

Thromboprophylaxis must be personalized according to the patient's status. It remains unclear which thromboprophylaxis regimen is ideal, and local traditions and preferences might affect the physician's choice to a certain extent. Low-molecular-weight heparin (LMWH), warfarin, and direct oral anticoagulants have been shown to prevent thrombosis. Aspirin has also been used for thromboprophylaxis in CKM syndrome. Nonpharmacological methods of thromboprophylaxis, such as weight loss and regular physical activity, can help reduce the risk of thromboembolic disease.

Table 16.5 Risk score for prediction of thromboembolic disease used in clinical practice

Tools	Markers of CKM syndrome	Items number	Clinical application
PADUA score	Yes—BMI	11	Thromboembolic risk for hospitalized patients
CAPRINI score	Yes—BMI Elevated serum of homocysteine	14	Thromboembolic risk in surgical patients
TESS scale	Yes—BMI Chronic kidney disease Heart failure	23	Thromboembolic risk in trauma patients
RAPT scale	No	6	Thromboembolic risk in trauma patients
GENEVA score	No	8	Pulmonary embolism
PERC score	No	8	Pulmonary embolism
YEARS score	No	4	Pulmonary embolism
WELLS score	No	10	Clinical criteria for deep venous thrombosis
IMPROVE VTE	No	7	Thromboembolic risk for hospitalized patients
ROGERS score	No	7	Thromboembolic risk in surgical patients
WOTTAWA score	No	5	Venous thrombosis recurrence for Cancer patients
DAMOVES score	Yes—obesity	7	Venous thrombosis recurrence
DASH score	No	4	Venous thrombosis recurrence
HERDOO2 score	Yes—BMI	4	Venous thrombosis recurrence—women
VIENNA score	No	3	Venous thrombosis recurrence
HESTIA score	No	11	PE severity
FAST score	No	3	PE severity
BOVA score	No	4	PE severity
PESI score	No	11	PE severity

Anemia in CKM Syndrome

According to literature data, anemia is frequently associated with chronic kidney disease, cardiovascular disease, and metabolic syndrome. The Chronic Kidney Disease Prognosis Consortium observed that anemia was twice as prevalent in chronic kidney disease patients as in the general population [122]. Anemia is a condition that is frequently associated with chronic diseases like chronic heart failure and is an independent risk factor for cardiac morbidity and mortality [123]. Anemia is often found in patients with coronary artery disease and is related to disease severity [124]. Anemia is estimated to be prevalent in approximately 30–70% of patients with heart failure and 10–43% of patients with coronary artery disease

Table 16.6 Thromboembolic risk for patients with CKM syndrome

Patient-related factors
Age
Sex
History of thrombosis
Smoking
Acquired thrombophilia
Myeloproliferative disorders
Paroxysmal nocturnal hemoglobinuria
Cancer
Liver disorders
Nephrotic syndrome
Inflammatory systemic diseases
CKM syndrome
Antiphospholipid syndrome
Inherited thrombophilia
Positive Factor V Leiden
Positive prothrombin 20210A
Elevated serum homocysteine
Inherited deficiencies of protein C, S antithrombin III
Treatment that increases thrombotic risk
Corticosteroids
Chemotherapy
Hormonotherapy
Intercurrent factors
Surgical intervention
Acute infections/sepsis
Immobilization
Trauma
Central venous catheters
Pregnancy/postpartum status
Increased activity of clotting factors: VII, VIII, IX, X, XII, and von Willebrand
Decreased activity of natural anticoagulants: protein C, S, antithrombin III
Decreased activity of fibrinolysis: PAI-2 increased
D-Dimers increased

[125, 126]. Obesity in the general population is an important public health problem and an independent risk factor for many complications such as anemia. It has been demonstrated that anemia and obesity are physiologically connected, and a significant association has been reported between kidney functions, body mass index, and anemia [127].

Pathophysiological Mechanisms Underlying Anemia in Cardiovascular–Kidney–Metabolic Syndrome

The anemic syndrome occurs because of the installation of an imbalance between the destruction/loss and production of red blood cells, in which a series of etiological factors intervene as a consequence of the installation of the cardiovascular–kidney–metabolic syndrome. The pathophysiological mechanisms underlying the occurrence of anemia in cardiovascular–kidney–metabolic syndrome are multiple, which leads to the existence of several types of anemia (Fig. 16.9).

Impaired Erythropoiesis with the Production of an Insufficient Number of Red Blood Cells

Iron Deficiency

The cardiovascular and renal systems require iron to maintain their high energy demands and metabolic activity. Iron plays an important role in oxygen transport and storage, mitochondrial function, and enzyme activities. Two types of iron deficiency are described: absolute deficiency and functional deficiency.

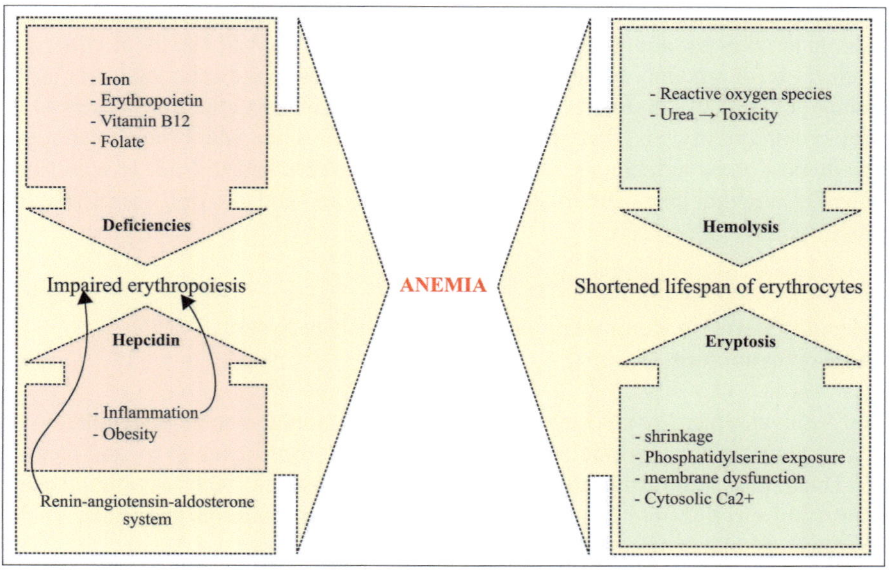

Fig 16.9 Pathophysiological mechanisms underlying anemia in cardiovascular–kidney–metabolic syndrome

Absolute iron deficiency is defined by a decrease in iron and ferritin levels and the appearance of a microcytic hypochromic hyporegenerative anemia. The mechanism responsible for absolute iron deficiency in cardiovascular diseases involves multiple components: nutritional deficiency, intestinal wall edema specific to advanced stages of heart disease that decreases absorption of iron, anomalies of the intestinal wall (increases bacterial concentration and adherence to the intestinal epithelium), and chronic treatment with antiaggregant/anticoagulant agents that lead to microvascular bleeding [128, 129]. The same mechanisms are involved in the absolute iron deficiency of chronic kidney disease, adding the intradialytic blood loss [130]. There is a well-established link between obesity and gastroesophageal reflux disease in individuals with obesity and type 2 diabetes mellitus that can lead to erosive esophagitis with absolute iron deficiency [131].

Interplay Between Inflammation, Hepcidin, and Erythropoiesis

Inflammatory cytokines—IL1, IL-6, TNF-α, interferon gamma, and TGF-β secreted during chronic inflammation in CKM syndrome have a medullary inhibitory role. Erythropoietin level is low—its synthesis being inhibited by inflammatory cytokines, to which is added a decreased erythropoietic response at the medullary level.

The functional deficit of iron is another pathway that interferes with erythropoiesis. Specifically, chronic cytokines TNF-α and IL-6 increase the liver's hepcidin production [132]. Hepcidin controls intestinal iron absorption, the release of iron from macrophages, and the release of iron from the liver. Adipose tissue may also produce small amounts of hepcidin, which contributes to the functional iron deficiency [131]. It was found that high concentrations of hepcidin were observed in people with obesity, and that iron deficiency might be a hepcidin-related phenomenon in most obese individuals, as iron absorption is decreased and, due to sequestration of iron within the macrophages, more iron is stored and less iron is available for erythropoiesis [131, 132].

Interplay Between Renin–Angiotensin–Aldosterone System and Erythropoiesis

The renin–angiotensin–aldosterone system appears to intervene in the regulation of erythropoiesis through stimulating the production of erythropoietin by angiotensin II. Thus, the administration of pharmacological agents such as angiotensin-converting enzyme inhibitors or angiotensin receptor inhibitors may lead to the development of a centrally induced anemic syndrome [133].

Erythropoietin and Other Deficiencies with an Impact on the Erythropoiesis

Erythropoietin is a glycoprotein that is produced by the peritubular cells of the renal cortex and stimulates the proliferation and differentiation of erythrocyte precursors in the bone marrow. Erythropoietin is produced in response to hypoxia. Its mechanism of action occurs at the level of erythropoietic progenitors that present receptors for erythropoietin and determine their division, proliferation, and differentiation through the mediation of cell signaling pathways—JAK-STAT pathway (JAK2 and STAT5) and others [134]. The pro-inflammatory cytokines secreted in increased quantities in the context of CKM syndrome lead to decreased erythropoietin production on the one hand, and on the other hand, renal damage also contributes to the appearance of low erythropoietin levels [134].

Vitamin B12 and folate are essential for erythropoiesis. They are crucial for DNA synthesis, which is vital for the proliferation and differentiation of erythroblasts. Deficiencies of vitamin B12 and folate can lead to ineffective erythropoiesis and centrally induced anemic syndrome where there is a nucleocytoplasmic maturation asynchrony [135]. The relationship between CKM syndrome and deficiencies of folic acid and vitamin B12 has been the subject of many studies. Several studies have reported a positive association between the supplementation of vitamin B12 and folate and their effectiveness in reducing insulin resistance and cardiovascular disease [136, 137].

Shortened Lifespan of Erythrocytes in CKM Syndrome

In CKM syndrome, the lifespan of erythrocytes is often shortened. Two mechanisms are cited that lead to a decrease in the lifespan of erythrocytes: hemolysis and eryptosis. Hemolysis, particularly when combined with chronic kidney disease and heart failure, may lead to anemia. Reactive oxygen species and toxins such as urea can lead to hemolysis and secondary anemia in CKM syndrome. Eryptosis, a form of apoptosis, is associated with hyperlipemia, insulin resistance, obesity, and arterial hypertension. Eryptosis is determined by oxidative stress, energy depletion, and calcium influx [138]. The hallmarks of eryptosis are cell shrinkage, membrane dysfunction, and exposure of phosphatidylserine on the cell membrane [138].

Symptoms, Laboratory Markers, and Therapeutic Strategy of Anemia in CKM Syndrome

Anemia is a major health problem, with an estimated one-third of the world's population suffering from anemia in 2010 [7, 8]. According to the World Health Organization (WHO), anemia is defined as a medical condition in which the total number of red blood cells or their oxygen-carrying capacity is insufficient to meet the physiological needs of the body. It is usually defined by a decrease in total circulating hemoglobin: Hb <13 g/dL in men, Hb <12 g/dL in women, Hb <11 g/dL in pregnant women [7, 8].

The symptoms of anemia are determined by the decrease in the ability of red blood cells to transport oxygen to tissues (physical asthenia/fatigue, apathy/agitation, headache, dizziness, sclero-tegumentary pallor, coldness of the extremities) and signs determined by compensatory mechanisms secondary to tissue hypoxia—cardiovascular hyperkinetic syndrome (tachycardia, palpitations, systolic heart murmurs, capillary pulse), coronary hypoperfusion syndrome and insufficient cardiac output (angina, progressive exertional dyspnea, heart failure), and respiratory (tachypnea, dyspnea).

Understanding the laboratory markers associated with anemia in CKM syndrome is crucial for early diagnosis, risk stratification, and management. Anemia is a prevalent complication within this syndrome, contributing significantly to morbidity and mortality. Several laboratory markers are indicated in the literature such as hemoglobin concentration, hematocrit level, iron concentration, ferritin, hepcidin, erythropoietin level, reticulocyte hemoglobin content, soluble transferrin receptor, and cystatin C.

Hemoglobin Concentration and Hematocrit Levels

These markers are primary indicators for diagnosing anemia [139]. In CKM syndrome, anemia is often normocytic and normochromic, primarily due to decreased erythropoietin production in CKD and chronic inflammation [140].

Investigation of Iron Metabolism

Serum ferritin reflects iron stores, while transferrin saturation (TSAT) indicates the availability of iron for erythropoiesis. In CKM syndrome, inflammation can elevate ferritin levels independently of iron status, potentially masking iron deficiency. Therefore, assessing both ferritin and TSAT provides a more accurate evaluation of iron status [141]. Investigation of iron metabolism can differentiate between absolute iron deficiency and functional iron deficiency (Table 16.7).

Table 16.7 Investigation of iron metabolism in CKM syndrome

Iron deficiency	Mechanism	Iron level	Ferritin level	Hemogram
Absolute	Nutritional intestinal wall abnormalities that decrease absorption Microvascular bleedings	Decreased	Decreased	Microcytic hypochromic hyporegenerative anemia
Functional	Inflammation—sequestration of iron in macrophages	Decreased	Increased	Microcytic hypochromic hyporegenerative anemia

Erythropoietin (EPO)

It is produced by the kidneys and stimulates red blood cell production. In CKD, reduced EPO synthesis leads to anemia. Measuring EPO levels can help differentiate between anemia due to EPO deficiency and other causes [142].

Inflammation Markers

Chronic inflammation in CKM syndrome contributes to anemia by impairing iron metabolism and erythropoiesis. Elevated C-reactive protein (CRP) and interleukin-6 (IL-6) levels are common and correlate with anemia severity. These markers can help assess the inflammatory component of anemia [143].

Hepcidin

It is a liver-derived hormone that regulates iron homeostasis. Inflammation increases hepcidin levels, reducing iron absorption and release, leading to functional iron deficiency. Assessing hepcidin can provide insights into iron-restricted erythropoiesis in CKM syndrome [144].

Reticulocyte Hemoglobin Content (CHr)

It measures the hemoglobin content of reticulocytes, offering real-time information on iron availability for erythropoiesis. It is a sensitive marker for detecting functional iron deficiency before changes in Hb levels occur [145].

Soluble Transferrin Receptor (sTfR)

Its levels reflect cellular iron demand and erythropoietic activity. Unlike ferritin, sTfR is less influenced by inflammation, making it a valuable marker for assessing iron deficiency in CKM patients [146].

Cystatin C

Although cystatin C is primarily used to estimate glomerular filtration rate (GFR), elevated levels have also been linked to anemia and heightened cardiovascular risk in patients with CKM syndrome. It serves as a useful alternative to creatinine-based assessments, particularly in individuals with altered muscle mass [147].

Therapeutic Strategy

Finally, anemia in CKM syndrome is multifactorial, involving decreased erythropoietin production, iron dysregulation, and chronic inflammation. A comprehensive evaluation using a panel of laboratory markers—including Hb, ferritin, TSAT, EPO, inflammatory markers, hepcidin, CHr, sTfR, and cystatin C—facilitates accurate diagnosis and guides targeted therapy. Early identification and management of anemia can improve clinical outcomes and quality of life in patients with CKM syndrome. Several therapeutic options are cited in the literature—blood transfusion, iron supplements, erythropoietin, drugs that interfere with hepcidin and inflammation.

Blood transfusions are recommended in severe symptomatic anemia; a liberal transfusion strategy (trigger threshold of Hb 7–8 g/dL) is recommended in patients with heart disease and chronic kidney disease [148].

Parenteral iron therapy in patients with chronic kidney disease and heart failure has been shown to improve quality of life and exercise capacity of these patients [149].

Erythropoietin-stimulating agent therapy is beneficial in many patients, but a substantial proportion of those with CKM syndrome have resistance to this therapy, likely because of antagonism of EPO by pro-inflammatory cytokines, and do not achieve improvements in hemoglobin levels [149].

New treatment options for anemia management target the inhibition of hepcidin, the hypoxia pathway, and the EPO receptor.

Learning Objectives

- Understand and define acquired thrombophilia in CKM syndrome.
- Explain the interrelated pathophysiological mechanisms linking obesity, type 2 diabetes, hypertension, chronic kidney disease, and thrombophilia.
- Identify and interpret the main laboratory investigations of hemostasis and thrombosis in CKM syndrome.
- Evaluate the risk of thromboembolic disease in patients with CKM syndrome.
- Understand and define anemia in CKM syndrome.
- Explain the interrelated pathophysiological mechanisms linking obesity, type 2 diabetes, hypertension, chronic kidney disease, and anemia
- Identify and interpret the main laboratory investigation of anemia in CKM syndrome.
- Understand the importance of personalized therapy for thromboprophylaxis and anemia in CKM syndrome.

Key Reading

- **Acquired thrombophilia** in CKM syndrome is a prothrombotic state that is not related to genetic predisposition, and its pathophysiological mechanisms include endothelial dysfunction, platelet activation, increased clotting factor activity, decreased natural anticoagulant activity, and impaired fibrinolysis.
- **Obesity and adipokines** are primary drivers of CKM syndrome, promoting chronic inflammation, oxidative stress, and insulin resistance that lead to acquired thrombophilia and increase the risk of thrombosis.
- **Chronic inflammation and oxidative stress** promote acquired thrombophilia and inflammatory anemia in CKM syndrome, with a negative impact on quality of life.
- **Risk score of thromboembolic disease in CKM syndrome** considers the following factors: patient-related factors, congenital thrombophilia, other associated acquired thrombophilia, treatments with thrombotic risk, pregnancy, and intercurrent factors.
- **Functional iron deficiency in CKM syndrome** occurs when chronic inflammation and hepcidin lead to storage of iron in macrophages with secondary impaired erythropoiesis.
- **Hepcidin in CKM syndrome** is a hormone produced by the liver and adipose tissue that interferes with iron metabolism and causes functional iron deficiency. Inflammation increases the secretion of hepcidin. Visceral

fat increases hepcidin expression. Insulin resistance is linked to impaired hepcidin regulation.

- **Eryptosis in CKM syndrome** is an apoptotic process of erythrocytes that is caused by oxidative stress and inflammation and can lead to anemia through the shortened lifespan of erythrocytes.
- **Impaired erythropoiesis in CKM syndrome** occurs when chronic inflammation exerts a direct inhibitory effect on erythropoiesis and decreases the erythropoietin levels secreted by renal cells, with a negative impact on differentiation of erythropoietic progenitor cells.

References

1. Nygaard KK, Brown GE. Essential thrombophilia. Arch Intern Med (Chic). 1937;59(1):82–106. https://doi.org/10.1001/archinte.1937.00170170088006.
2. Coppens M, van de Poel MH, Bank I, Hamulyak K, van der Meer J, Veeger NJ, Prins MH, Buller HR, Middeldorp S. A prospective cohort study on the absolute incidence of venous thromboembolism and arterial cardiovascular disease in asymptomatic carriers of the prothrombin 20210A mutation. Blood. 2006;108:2604–7. https://doi.org/10.1182/blood-2006-04-016527.
3. Khider L, Gendron N, Mauge L. Inherited thrombophilia in the era of direct oral anticoagulants. Int J Mol Sci. 2022;23(3):1821. https://doi.org/10.3390/ijms23031821.
4. Chiasakul T, De Jesus E, Tong J, Chen Y, Crowther M, Garcia D, Chai-Adisaksopha C, Messe SR, Cuker A. Inherited thrombophilia and the risk of arterial ischemic stroke: a systematic review and meta-analysis. JAHA. 2019:119. https://doi.org/10.1161/JAHA.119.012877.
5. Stevens SM, Woller SC, Bauer KA, et al. Guidance for the evaluation and treatment of hereditary and acquired thrombophilia. J Thromb Thrombolysis. 2016;41:154–64. https://doi.org/10.1007/s11239-015-1316-1.
6. Heit JA. The epidemiology of venous thromboembolism in the community. Arterioscler Thromb Vasc Biol. 2008;28:370–2. https://doi.org/10.1161/ATVBAHA.108.162545.
7. Newhall DA, Oliver R, Lugthart S. Anaemia: a disease or symptom. Neth J Med. 2020;78(3):104–10.
8. Chaparro CM, Suchdev PS. Anemia epidemiology, pathophysiology, and etiology in low- and middle-income countries. Ann N Y Acad Sci. 2019;1450(1):15–31. https://doi.org/10.1111/nyas.14092.
9. Angelidi AM, Sanoudou D, Hill MA, Mantzoros CS. Management of patients with the cardio renal liver metabolic syndrome: the need for a multidisciplinary approach in research, education and practice. Metabolism. 2024;159:155997. https://doi.org/10.1016/j.metabol.2024.155997.
10. Ageno W, Becattini C, Brighton T, Selby R, Kamphuisen PW. Cardiovascular risk factors and venous thromboembolism: a meta-analysis. Circulation. 2008;117:93–102. https://doi.org/10.1161/CIRCULATIONAHA.107.709204.
11. Moon JJ, Won-il C, Soo-Mee B, Taeseung L, Yeo-Kyeoung K, Walter A, Doyeun O. Metabolic syndrome is associated with venous thromboembolism in the Korean population. Arterioscler Thrombosis Vasc Biol. 2009;29(3):311–5. https://doi.org/10.1161/ATVBAHA.109.184085.

12. Stewart LK, Kline JA. Metabolic syndrome increases risk of venous thromboembolism recurrence after acute deep vein thrombosis. Blood Adv. 2020;4(1):127–35. https://doi.org/10.1182/bloodadvances.2019000561.
13. Gong W, Liu TT, Zheng Y. Relationship between venous thromboembolism and cardiovascular disease risk factors. Zhonghua Xin Xue Guan Bing Za Zhi. 2018;46(5):407–10. https://doi.org/10.3760/cma.j.issn.0253-3758.2018.05.017.
14. Wattanakit K, Lutsey PL, Bell EJ, Gornik H, Cushman M, Heckbert SR, Rosamond WD, Folsom AR. Association between cardiovascular disease risk factors and occurrence of venous thromboembolism. A time-dependent analysis. Thromb Haemost. 2012;108(3):508–15. https://doi.org/10.1160/TH11-10-0726.
15. Lin A, Dinatolo E, Metra M, et al. Thromboembolism in heart failure patients in sinus rhythm: epidemiology, pathophysiology, clinical trials, and future direction. J Am Coll Cardiol HF. 2021;4:243–53. https://doi.org/10.1016/j.jchf.2021.01.009.
16. Zaikina MP, Tkachev MI, Kogaj VV, et al. Implication of cardiovascular pathology on the risks of thromboembolic complications in cancer patients. Complex Issues Cardiovasc Dis. 2025;14(1):169–79. https://doi.org/10.17802/2306-1278-2025-14-1-169-179.
17. Go AS, Chertow GM, Fan D, et al. Chronic kidney disease and the risks of death, cardiovascular events, and hospitalization. N Engl J Med. 2004;351(13):1296–305. https://doi.org/10.1056/NEJMoa041031.
18. Cases A, Broseta JJ, Marqués M, Cigarrán S, Julián JC, Alcázar R, Ortiz A. Cardiovascular-kidney-metabolic syndrome definition and its role in the prevention, risk staging, and treatment. An opportunity for nephrology. Nefrologia (Engl Ed). 2024;44(6):771–83. https://doi.org/10.1016/j.nefroe.2024.11.011.
19. Ross R. Atherosclerosis – an inflammatory disease. N Engl J Med. 1999;340:115–26. https://doi.org/10.1056/NEJM199901143402.
20. Rubanyi GM. The role of endothelium in cardiovascular homeostasis and diseases. J Cardiovasc Pharmacol. 1993;22:S1–S14. https://doi.org/10.1097/00005344-199322004-00002.
21. Esper RJ, Nordaby RA, Vilariño JO, et al. Endothelial dysfunction: a comprehensive appraisal. Cardiovasc Diabetol. 2006;5:4. https://doi.org/10.1186/1475-2840-5-4.
22. Vanhoutte PM. How to assess endothelial function in human blood vessels. J Hypertens. 1999;17:1047–58. https://doi.org/10.1097/00004872-199917080-00001.
23. Furchgott RF, Zawadzki JV. The obligatory role of endothelial cells in the relaxation of arterial smooth muscle by acetylcholine. Nature. 1980;288:373–6. https://doi.org/10.1097/00004872-199917080-00001.
24. Ignarro LJ, Buga GM, Wood KS, Byrns RE, Chaudhuri G. Endothelium-derived relaxing factor produced and released from artery and vein is nitric oxide. Proc Natl Acad Sci U S A. 1987;84:9265–9. https://doi.org/10.1073/pnas.84.24.9265.
25. Loscalzo J, Welch G. Nitric oxide and its role in the cardiovascular system. Prog Cardiovasc Dis. 1995;38:87–104. https://doi.org/10.1016/S0033-0620(05)80001-5.
26. Ignarro LJ. Haem-dependent activation of guanylate cyclase and cyclic GMP formation by endogenous nitric oxide: a unique transduction mechanism for transcellular signaling. Pharmacol Toxicol. 1990;67:1–7. https://doi.org/10.1111/j.1600-0773.1990.tb00772.x.
27. Ignarro LJ, Burke TM, Wood KS, Wolin MS, Kadowitz PJ. Association between cyclic GMP accumulation and acetylcholine-elicited relaxation of bovine intrapulmonary artery. J Pharmacol Exp Ther. 1984;228:682–90. https://doi.org/10.1016/S0022-3565(25)21916-4.
28. Magda B, Mariana R. Bohotin Catalina – Fiziopatologie Generala. Iasi: Editura Cantes; 2000. p. 396–40.
29. Sandow SL. Factors, fiction and endothelium-derived hyperpolarizing factor. Clin Exp Pharmacol Physiol. 2004;31:563–70. https://doi.org/10.1111/j.1440-1681.2004.04048.x.
30. Morikawa K, Fujiki T, Matoba T, Kubota H, Hatanaka M, Takahashi S. Shimokawa H Important role of superoxide dismutase in EDHF-mediated responses of human mesenteric arteries. J Cardiovasc Pharmacol. 2004;44(5):552–6. https://doi.org/10.1097/00005344-200411000-00006.

31. Knock GA. NADPH oxidase in the vasculature: expression, regulation and signalling pathways; role in normal cardiovascular physiology and its dysregulation in hypertension. Free Rad Biol Med. 2019;145:385–427. https://doi.org/10.1016/j.freeradbiomed.2019.09.029.
32. Prasad A, Tupas-Habib T, Schenke WH, et al. Acute and chronic angiotensin-1 receptor antagonism reverses endothelial dysfunction in atherosclerosis. Circulation. 2000;101:2349. https://doi.org/10.1161/01.cir.101.20.2349.
33. Flaherty JD, Davidson CJ. Diabetes and coronary revascularization. JAMA. 2005;293:1501–8. https://doi.org/10.1001/jama.293.12.1501.
34. Mancini GBJ, Henry GC, Macaya C, et al. Angiotensin-converting enzyme inhibition with quinqpril improves endothelial vasomotor dysfunction in patients with coronary artery disease. The TREND (Trial on Reversing Endothelial Dysfunction) Study. Circulation. 1996;94:258. https://doi.org/10.1161/01.cir.94.3.258.
35. Suwaidi JA, Hamasaki S, Higano S, et al. Long term follow up of patients with mild coronary artery disease and endothelial dysfunction. Circulation. 2000;101:1899. https://doi.org/10.1161/01.CIR.101.9.94.
36. Prado CM, Ramos SG, Elias J Jr, Rossi MA. Turbulent blood flow plays an essential localizing role in the development of atherosclerotic lesions in experimentally induced hypercholesterolaemia in rats. Int J Exp Pathol. 2008;89(1):72–80. https://doi.org/10.1111/j.1365-2613.2007.00564.x.
37. Durante A, Mazzapicchi A, Baiardo RM. Systemic and cardiac microvascular dysfunction in hypertension. Int J Mol Sci. 2024;25(24):13294. https://doi.org/10.3390/ijms252413294.
38. Santamaría R, González-Álvarez M, Delgado R, Esteban S, Arroyo AG. Remodeling of the microvasculature: may the blood flow be with you. Front Physiol. 2020;11:586852. https://doi.org/10.3389/fphys.2020.586852.
39. Frisbee JC, Delp MD. Vascular function in the metabolic syndrome and the effects on skeletal muscle perfusion: lessons from the obese Zucker rat. Essays Biochem. 2006;42:145–61. https://doi.org/10.1042/bse0420145.
40. Limberg JK, Morgan BJ, Schrage WG. Peripheral blood flow regulation in human obesity and metabolic syndrome. Exerc Sport Sci Rev. 2016;44(3):116–22. https://doi.org/10.1249/jes.0000000000000083.
41. Scridon A. Platelets and their role in hemostasis and thrombosis-from physiology to pathophysiology and therapeutic implications. Int J Mol Sci. 2022;23(21):12772. https://doi.org/10.3390/ijms232112772.
42. Raghavan V, Gunasekar D, Rao KR. Relevance of haematologic parameters in obese women with or without metabolic syndrome. J Clin Diagn Res. 2016;10(5):EC11–6. https://doi.org/10.7860/jcdr/2016/18779.7732.
43. Purdy JC, Shatzel JJ. The hematologic consequences of obesity. Eur J Haematol. 2021;106(3):306–19. https://doi.org/10.1111/ejh.13560.
44. Das D, et al. Endothelial dysfunction, platelet hyperactivity, hypertension, and the metabolic syndrome: molecular insights and combating strategies. Front Nutr. 2023;10:1221438. https://doi.org/10.3389/fnut.2023.1221438.
45. Grande R, Dovizio M, Marcone S, Szklanna PB, Bruno A, Ebhardt HA, Cassidy H, Ní Áinle F, Caprodossi A, Lanuti P, Marchisio M, Mingrone G, Maguire PB, Patrignani P. Platelet-derived microparticles from obese individuals: characterization of number, size, proteomics, and crosstalk with cancer and endothelial cells. Front Pharmacol. 2019;10:7. https://doi.org/10.3389/fphar.2019.00007.
46. Park S, Choi SG, Yoo SM, Nah J, Jeong E, Kim H, et al. Pyruvate stimulates mitophagy via PINK1 stabilization. Cell Signal. 2015;27:1824–30. https://doi.org/10.1016/j.cellsig.2015.05.020.
47. Gao C, Gao S, Zhao R, et al. Association between systemic immune-inflammation index and cardiovascular-kidney-metabolic syndrome. Sci Rep. 2024;14:19151. https://doi.org/10.1038/s41598-024-69819-0.

48. Stark K, Massberg S. Interplay between inflammation and thrombosis in cardiovascular pathology. Nat Rev Cardiol. 2021;18:666–82. https://doi.org/10.1038/s41569-021-00552-1.
49. Blokhin IO, Lentz SR. Mechanisms of thrombosis in obesity. Curr Opin Hematol. 2013;20(5):437–44. https://doi.org/10.1097/MOH.0b013e3283634443.
50. Romney G. An updated concept of coagulation with clinical implications. J Am Dental Assoc. 2009;140(5):567–74. https://doi.org/10.14219/jada.archive.2009.0227.
51. Palta S, Saroa R, Palta A. Overview of the coagulation system. Indian J Anaesth. 2014;58(5):515–23. https://doi.org/10.4103/0019-5049.144643.
52. Bijak M, Rzeźnicka P, Saluk J, Nowak P. Cellular model of blood coagulation process. Pol Merkur Lekarski. 2015;39(229):5–8.
53. Sucker C, Zotz RB. The cell-based coagulation model. In: Marcucci C, Schoettker P, editors. Perioperative hemostasis. Berlin/Heidelberg: Springer; 2015. https://doi.org/10.1007/978-3-642-55004-1_1.
54. Tichelaar YI, Kluin-Nelemans HJ, Meijer K. Infections and inflammatory diseases as risk factors for venous thrombosis. A systematic review. Thromb Haemost. 2012;107:827–37. https://doi.org/10.1160/th11-09-0611.
55. Singh R, Gautam P, Sharma C, Osmolovskiy A. Fibrin and fibrinolytic enzyme cascade in thrombosis: unravelling the role. Life. 2023;13(11):2196. https://doi.org/10.3390/life13112196.
56. Ouchi N, Parker JL, Lugus JJ, Walsh K. Adipokines in inflammation and metabolic disease. Nat Rev Immunol. 2011;11:85–97. https://doi.org/10.1038/nri2921.
57. Alessi MC, Nicaud V, Scroyen I, et al. Association of vitronectin and plasminogen activator inhibitor-1 levels with the risk of metabolic syndrome and type 2 diabetes mellitus. Results from the D.E.S.I. R. prospective cohort. Thromb Haemost. 2011;106:416–22. https://doi.org/10.1160/th11-03-0179.
58. McCully KS. Homocysteine and the pathogenesis of atherosclerosis. Exp Rev Clin Pharmacol. 2015;8(2):211–9. https://doi.org/10.1586/17512433.2015.1010516.
59. McCully KS. Homocysteine metabolism, atherosclerosis, and diseases of aging. Comprehens Physiol. 2016;6(1):471–505. https://doi.org/10.1002/j.2040-4603.2016.tb00682.x.
60. Smith AD, Refsum H. Homocysteine–from disease biomarker to disease prevention. J Intern Med. 2012;290(4):826–54. https://doi.org/10.1111/joim.13279.
61. Yuan D, Chu J, Lin H, Zhu G, Qian J, Yu Y. Mechanism of homocysteine-mediated endothelial injury and its consequences for atherosclerosis. Front Cardiovasc Med. 2023;9:1109445. https://doi.org/10.3389/fcvm.2022.1109445.
62. Lentz SR. Mechanisms of homocysteine-induced atherothrombosis. J Thrombosis Haemost. 2005;3(8):1646–54. https://doi.org/10.1111/j.1538-7836.2005.01364.x.
63. Esse R, Barroso M, Tavares de Almeida I, Castro R. The contribution of homocysteine metabolism disruption to endothelial dysfunction: state-of-the-art. Int J Mol Sci. 2019;20(4):867. https://doi.org/10.3390/ijms20040867.
64. James SJ, et al. Elevation in S-adenosylhomocysteine and DNA hypomethylation: potential epigenetic mechanism for homocysteine-related pathology. J Nutr. 2002;132(8):2361S–6S. https://doi.org/10.1093/jn/132.8.2361S.
65. Janaszak-Jasiecka A, Płoska A, Wierońska JM, Dobrucki LW, Kalinowski L. Endothelial dysfunction due to eNOS uncoupling: molecular mechanisms as potential therapeutic targets. Cell Mol Biol Lett. 2023;28(1):21. https://doi.org/10.1186/s11658-023-00423-2.
66. Ben Salah R, Boudaya M, Fendri S, Marrekchi R, Bahloul Z, Jamoussi K. Hyperhomocysteinemia prevalence among patients with venous thromboembolism. Fut Sci OA. 2024;10(1):2430417. https://doi.org/10.1080/20565623.2024.2430417.
67. Ganguly P, Alam SF. Role of homocysteine in the development of cardiovascular disease. Nutr J. 2015;14:1–10. https://doi.org/10.1186/1475-2891-14-6.
68. Shih YL, Shih CC, Huang TC, Chen JY. The relationship between elevated homocysteine and metabolic syndrome in a community-dwelling middle-aged and elderly population in Taiwan. Biomedicines. 2023;11(2):378. https://doi.org/10.3390/biomedicines11020378.

69. Touzani A, et al. Hyperhomocysteinemia and risk factors of metabolic syndrome in obese children. Cases. 2022;1(1):4. https://doi.org/10.35702/cases.10004.
70. Chen W, Feng J, Ji P, et al. Association of hyperhomocysteinemia and chronic kidney disease in the general population: a systematic review and meta-analysis. BMC Nephrol. 2023;24:247. https://doi.org/10.1186/s12882-023-03295-y.
71. An S, Che W, Gao Y, Duo X, Li X, Li J. Predictive value of complete blood count indicators for short-term mortality in patients with combined coronary artery disease and chronic kidney disease. Int J Nephrol Renovasc Dis. 2025;18:113–22. https://doi.org/10.2147/IJNRD.S508019.
72. Song Y, Lin Z, He J, Cui K, Song C, Zhang R, Liu Z, An T, Gao G, Gao Y, Dou K. Association of platelet-to-lymphocyte ratio levels with the risk of cardiac adverse events in people with type 2 diabetes undergoing percutaneous coronary intervention: a large-scale prospective cohort study. Diabetes Metab Syndr. 2024;18(3):102987. https://doi.org/10.1016/j.dsx.2024.102987.
73. Foy BH, Sundt T, Carlson JCT, Aguirre AD, Higgins JM. White blood cell and platelet dynamics define human inflammatory. Nat Commun. 2022;13(1):4705. https://doi.org/10.1101/2021.06.19.21259181.
74. He Y, Li L, Zhou T, Yang H, Liu T, Hu H. Association between inflammation indices derived from complete blood count and coronary artery calcification. J Inflamm Res. 2025;18:3807–16. https://doi.org/10.2147/JIR.S501429.
75. Seo IH, Lee YJ. Usefulness of Complete Blood Count (CBC) to assess cardiovascular and metabolic diseases in clinical settings: a comprehensive literature review. Biomedicines. 2022;10(11):2697. https://doi.org/10.3390/biomedicines10112697.
76. Marra A, Bondesan A, Caroli D, Sartorio A. Complete Blood Count (CBC)-derived inflammation indexes are useful in predicting metabolic syndrome in adults with severe obesity. J Clin Med. 2024;13(5):1353. https://doi.org/10.3390/jcm13051353.
77. Kitchen S, Adcock DM, Dauer R, Kristoffersen AH, Lippi G, Mackie I, Nair S. International Council for Standardisation in Haematology (ICSH) recommendations for collection of blood samples for coagulation testing. Int J Lab Hematol. 2021;43(4):571–80. https://doi.org/10.1111/ijlh.13702.
78. Gosselin RC, Bowyer A, Favaloro EJ, Johnsen JM, Lippi G, Marlar RA, Rollins-Raval MA. Guidance on the critical shortage of sodium citrate coagulation tubes for hemostasis testing. J Thrombosis Haemost. 2021;19(11):2857–61. https://doi.org/10.1111/jth.15514.
79. Park S, Park JK. Back to basics: the coagulation pathway. Blood Res. 2024;59(1):35. https://doi.org/10.1007/s44313-024-00040-8.
80. Saeed Z, Sirolli V, Bonomini M, Gallina S, Renda G. Hallmarks for thrombotic and hemorrhagic risks in chronic kidney disease patients. Int J Mol Sci. 2024;25(16):8705. https://doi.org/10.3390/ijms25168705.
81. Abdelmaguid A, Roberts LN, Tugores L, Joslin JR, Hunt BJ, Parmar K, Nebres D, Naga SS, Khalil ES, Bramham K. Evaluation of novel coagulation and platelet function assays in patients with chronic kidney disease. J Thromb Haemost. 2022;20:845–56. https://doi.org/10.1111/jth.15653.
82. Arachchillage DJ, Kitchen S. Pleiotropic effects of heparin and its monitoring in the clinical practice. Semin Thromb Hemost. 2024;50(8):1153–62. https://doi.org/10.1055/s-0044-1786990.
83. Santos García A, Millán del Valle I, Cruzado Vega L, Ruiz Ferrús R, Tordera Fuentes D, Sabater Belmar A, et al. Tiempo parcial de tromboplastina activado prolongado sin coagulopatía subyacente en diálisis peritoneal. Nefrologia. 2019;39:210–1. https://doi.org/10.1016/j.nefro.2018.07.006.
84. Zaidi A, Green L. Physiology of haemostasis. Anaesth Intens Care Med. 2022;23(2):111–7. https://doi.org/10.1016/j.mpaic.2021.10.023.

85. Mohamed M, Tabel AM, Abdelmoneim AA, Ibrahem WA, El-Aziz AM. Epidemiological aspects and genetic study of hereditary thrombophilia in Egyptian population. Benha Med J. 2025;42(1):1–11. https://doi.org/10.21608/bmfj.2024.155560.1639.
86. Pavlou EG, Georgatzakou HT, Fortis SP, Tsante KA, Tsantes AG, Nomikou EG, Kapota AI, Petras DI, Venetikou MS, Papageorgiou EG, et al. Coagulation abnormalities in renal pathology of chronic kidney disease: the interplay between blood cells and soluble factors. Biomolecules. 2021;11(9):1309. https://doi.org/10.3390/biom11091309.
87. Ignjatovic V. Thrombin clotting time. In: Haemostasis: methods and protocols. Totowa: Humana Press; 2013. p. 131–8. https://doi.org/10.1007/978-1-62703-339-8_10.
88. Tarandovskiy ID, Surov SS, Parunov LA, Liang Y, Jankowski W, Sauna E, Ovanesov MV. Investigation of thrombin concentration at the time of clot formation in simultaneous thrombin and fibrin generation assays. Sci Rep. 2024;14(1):9225. https://doi.org/10.1038/s41598-023-47694-5.
89. Oe Y, Takahash N. Tissue factor, thrombosis, and chronic kidney disease. Biomedicines. 2022;10(11):2737. https://doi.org/10.3390/biomedicines10112737.
90. Wallisch WJ, Kidd B, Shen L, Hammer R, Siscel J. Coagulopathy and emergent reversal of anticoagulation. Anesthesiol Clin. 2023;41(1):249–61. https://doi.org/10.1016/j.anclin.2022.10.006.
91. Xu Z, Liu H, Zhu M, Huang Y. The inverted U-shaped association between blood fibrinogen and rehospitalization risk in patients with heart failure. Sci Rep. 2024;14(1):15060. https://doi.org/10.1038/s41598-024-66002-3.
92. Raimundo M, Lopes JA. Metabolic syndrome, chronic kidney disease, and cardiovascular disease: a dynamic and life-threatening triad. Cardiol Res Pract. 2011;1:747861. https://doi.org/10.4061/2011/747861.
93. Xie E, Wu Y, Ye Z, Gao Y, Zheng J. High fibrinogen levels with diabetes mellitus are associated with all-cause and cardiovascular mortality in patients with end-stage renal disease and acute coronary syndrome. J Inflamm Res. 2024:7409–22. https://doi.org/10.2147/jir.s483001.
94. Faraoni D, DiNardo JA. Viscoelastic hemostatic assays: update on technology and clinical applications. Am J Hematol. 2021;96(10):1331–7. https://doi.org/10.1002/ajh.26285.
95. Jan MY, Patidar KR, Ghabril MS, Kubal CA. Optimization and protection of kidney health in liver transplant recipients: intra-and postoperative approaches. Transplantation. 2025;109(6):938–44. https://doi.org/10.1097/TP.0000000000005252.
96. Hartmann J, Mason D, Achneck H. Thromboelastography (TEG) point-of-care diagnostic for hemostasis management. Point of Care. 2018;17(1):15–22. https://doi.org/10.1097/POC.0000000000000156.
97. Darlington A, Ferreiro JL, Ueno M, Suzuki Y, Desai B, Capranzano P, Capodanno D, Tello-Montoliu A, Bass TA, Nahman NS, Angiolillo DJ. Haemostatic profiles assessed by thromboelastography in patients with end-stage renal disease. Thromb Haemost. 2011;106(1):67–74. https://doi.org/10.1160/th10-12-0785.
98. Maier CL, Brohi K, Curry N, Juffermans NP, Miquel LM, Neal MD, Helms J. Contemporary management of major haemorrhage in critical care. Intens Care Med. 2024; https://doi.org/10.1007/s00134-023-07303-5.
99. Abdollahi M, Cushman M, Rosendaal FR. Obesity: risk of venous thrombosis and the interaction with coagulation factor levels and oral contraceptive use. Thromb Haemost. 2003;89:493–8. https://doi.org/10.1055/s-0037-1613379.
100. Mehic D, et al. Activated protein C and free protein S in patients with mild to moderate bleeding disorders. Thrombosis Res. 2024;235:98–106. https://doi.org/10.1016/j.thromres.2024.01.018.
101. Jennings I, Cooper P. Screening for thrombophilia: a laboratory perspective. În BO'Donnell JS, O'Sullivan JM, Preston RJS. Advances in understanding the molecular mechanisms that maintain normal haemostasis. Br J Haematol. 2019;186(1):24–36. https://doi.org/10.1080/09674845.2003.11783675.

102. Gazzaruso C, Paolozzi E, Valenti C, Brocchetta M, Naldani D, et al. Association between antithrombin and mortality in patients with COVID-19. A possible link with obesity. Nutr Metab Cardiovasc Dis. 2020;30(11):1914–9. https://doi.org/10.1016/j.numecd.2020.07.040.
103. Favresse J, Lippi G, Roy PM, Chatelain B, Jacqmin H, Ten Cate H, Mullier F. D-dimer: preanalytical, analytical, postanalytical variables, and clinical applications. Crit Rev Clin Lab Sci. 2018;55(8):548–77. https://doi.org/10.1080/10408363.2018.1529734.
104. Hansen ES, Rinde FB, Edvardsen MS, Hindberg K, Latysheva N, Aukrust P, Ueland T, Michelsen AE, Hansen JB, Brækkan SK, Morelli VM. Elevated plasma D-dimer levels are associated with risk of future incident venous thromboembolism. Thromb Res. 2021;208:121–6. https://doi.org/10.1016/j.thromres.2021.10.020.
105. Gaugler JO, Righini M, Robert-Ebadi H, Sanchez O, Roy PM, Verschuren F, Miranda S, Delluc A, Le Gal G, Tritschler T. Obesity as a Predictor for pulmonary embolism and performance of the age-adjusted D-dimer strategy in obese patients with suspected pulmonary embolism. Thromb Haemost. 2024;124(1):49–57. https://doi.org/10.1055/s-0043-57018.
106. Marchiori GN, Defagó MD, Baraquet ML, Del Rosso S, Perovic NR, Soria EA. Interleukin-6, tumor necrosis factor-α, and high-sensitivity C-reactive protein for optimal immunometabolic profiling of the lifestyle-related cardiorenal risk. Diagnosis. 2024;11(1):82–90. https://doi.org/10.1515/dx-2023-0159.
107. Iacoviello M, Gori M, Grandaliano G, Minutolo R, Pitocco D, Trevisan R. A holistic approach to managing cardio-kidney metabolic syndrome: insights and recommendations from the Italian perspective. Front Cardiovasc Med. 2025;12:1583702. https://doi.org/10.3389/fcvm.2025.1583702.
108. Cao Y, Wang W, Xie S, Xu Y, Lin Z. Joint association of the inflammatory marker and cardiovascular-kidney-metabolic syndrome stages with all-cause and cardiovascular disease mortality: a national prospective study. BMC Public Health. 2025;25(1):10. https://doi.org/10.1186/s12889-024-21131-2.
109. Mutruc V, Bologa C, Şorodoc V, Ceasovschih A, Morăraşu BC, Şorodoc L, Catar OE, Lionte C. Cardiovascular–kidney–metabolic syndrome: a new paradigm in clinical medicine or going back to basics? J Clin Med. 2025;14(8):2833. https://doi.org/10.3390/jcm14082833.
110. Denegri A, Boriani G. High sensitivity C-reactive protein (hsCRP) and its implications in cardiovascular outcomes. Curr Pharmaceut Desig. 2021;27(2):263–75. https://doi.org/10.2174/1381612826666200717090334.
111. Tu Z, Zhong Y, Hu H, Shao D, Haag R, Schirner M, Leong KW. Design of therapeutic biomaterials to control inflammation. Nat Rev Mater. 2022;7(7):557–74. https://doi.org/10.1038/s41578-022-00426-z.
112. Capodanno D, Angiolillo DJ. Antithrombotic therapy in patients with chronic kidney disease. Circulation. 2012;125(21):2649–61. https://doi.org/10.1161/circulationaha.111.084996.
113. Martens KL, Dekker SE, Crowe M, DeLoughery TG, Shatzel JJ. Challenging clinical scenarios for therapeutic anticoagulation: a practical approach. Thrombosis Res. 2022;218:72–82. https://doi.org/10.1016/j.thromres.2022.08.015.
114. Zhang Z, Gu X, Fang X, Tang Z, Guan S, Liu H, Wu X, Wang C, Zhao Y. Homocysteine and the risk of cardiovascular events and all-cause death in elderly population: a community-based prospective cohort study. Ther Clin Risk Manag. 2020;16:471–81. https://doi.org/10.2147/tcrm.s239496.
115. Haloul M, Vinjamuri SJ, Naquiallah D, Mirza MI, Qureshi M, Hassan C, Masrur M, Bianco FM, Frederick P, Cristoforo GP, et al. Hyperhomocysteinemia and low folate and Vitamin B12 are associated with vascular dysfunction and impaired nitric oxide sensitivity in morbidly obese patients. Nutrients. 2020;12(7):2014. https://doi.org/10.3390/nu12072014.
116. Li P, Ma X, Huang G. Understanding thrombosis: the critical role of oxidative stress. Hematology. 2024;29(1):2301633. https://doi.org/10.1080/16078454.2023.2301633.
117. Alamin AA, Yahia AI, Hm H. Red blood cells in thrombosis: active participants in clot formation and stability: a systematic review. In: Seminars in thrombosis and hemostasis. Thieme Medical Publishers; 2025. https://doi.org/10.1055/a-2552-9525.

118. Safgöl Ö, Erbaş O. Diseases predisposing to thrombosis. Demiroglu Sci Univ Florence Nightingale J Med. 2023;9(2):095–107. https://doi.org/10.5606/fng.btd.2023.127.
119. Mahani S, DiCaro MV, Tak N, Hartnett S, Cyrus, & TaknT. Venous thromboembolism: current insights and future directions. Int J Angiol. 2024; https://doi.org/10.1055/s-0044-1787652.
120. Appelboom Y, Leers MPG, Schoenmakers T, van Twist DJL. Cell population data in venous thrombo-embolism and erysipelas: a potential diagnostic tool? Clin Chem Lab Med. 2024;63(4):e108–12. https://doi.org/10.1515/cclm-2024-1050.
121. Xiong W, Cheng Y, Zhao Y. Risk scores in venous thromboembolism guidelines of ESC, ACCP, and ASH: an updated review. Clin Appl Thrombosis Hemost. 2024:30. https://doi.org/10.1177/10760296241263856.
122. Inker LA, Grams ME, Levey AS, Coresh J, Cirillo M, Collins JF, Gansevoort RT, Gutierrez OM, Hamano T, Heine GH, Ishikawa S, Jee SH, Kronenberg F, Landray MJ, Miura K, Nadkarni GN, Peralta CA, Rothenbacher D, Schaeffner E, Sedaghat S, Shlipak MG, Zhang L, van Zuilen AD, Hallan SI, Kovesdy CP, Woodward M, Levin A, CKD Prognosis Consortium. Relationship of estimated GFR and albuminuria to concurrent laboratory abnormalities: an individual participant data meta-analysis in a Global Consortium. Am J Kidney Dis. 2019;73(2):206–17. https://doi.org/10.1053/j.ajkd.2018.08.013.
123. Turner SJ, Ketch TR, Gandhi SK, Sane DC. Routine hematologic clinical tests as prognostic markers in patients with acute coronary syndromes. Am Heart J. 2008;155(5):806–16. https://doi.org/10.1016/j.ahj.2007.11.037.
124. Lanser L, Fuchs D, Scharnagl H, Grammer T, Kleber ME, März W, Weiss G, Kurz K. Anemia of chronic disease in patients with cardiovascular disease. Front Cardiovasc Med. 2021:8. https://doi.org/10.3389/fcvm.2021.666638.
125. Tang Y-D, Katz SD. Anemia in chronic heart failure. Circulation. 2006;113(20):2454–61. https://doi.org/10.1161/circulationaha.105.583666.
126. Stucchi M, Cantoni S, Piccinelli E, Savonitto S, Morici N. Anemia and acute coronary syndrome: current perspectives. Vasc Health Risk Manag. 2018;14:109–18. https://doi.org/10.2147/vhrm.s140951.
127. Fathi AE, Shahwan M, Hassan N, Abdulrahman A, Shahwan M. Prevalence of Anemia in Type 2 diabetic patients and correlation with body mass index and kidney function in Palestine. Diabetes Metab Syndr Obes. 2024;17:2293–301. https://doi.org/10.2147/DMSO.S454916.
128. Savarese G, von Haehling S, Butler J, Cleland JGF, Ponikowski P, Anker SD. Iron deficiency and cardiovascular disease. Eur Heart J. 2023;44(1):14–27. https://doi.org/10.1093/eurheartj/ehac569.
129. Sîrbu O, Floria M, Dascalita P, Stoica A, Adascalitei P, Sorodoc V, Sorodoc L. Anemia in heart failure – from guidelines to controversies and challenges. Anatol J Cardiol. 2018;20:52–9. https://doi.org/10.14744/anatoljcardiol.2018.08634.
130. Tsukamoto T, Matsubara T, Akashi Y, Kondo M, Yanagita M. Annual iron loss associated with hemodialysis. Am J Nephrol. 2016;43(1):32–8. https://doi.org/10.1159/000444335.
131. Saad RA, Qutob HM. The relationship between anemia and obesity. Exp Rev Hematol. 2022;15(10):911–26. https://doi.org/10.1080/17474086.2022.2131521.
132. Verga Falzacappa MV, Vujic Spasic M, Kessler R, et al. STAT3 mediates hepatic hepcidin expression and its inflammatory stimulation. Blood. 2007;109(1):353–8. https://doi.org/10.1182/blood-2006-07-033969.
133. Jonaitienė N, Ramantauskaitė G, Laukaitienė J. Anaemia in heart failure patients, associated with angiotensin – renin – aldosterone system altering medications. Heart Views. 2021;22(3):196–200. https://doi.org/10.4103/heartviews.heartviews_211_20.
134. Jelkmann W. Physiology and pharmacology of erythropoietin. Transfus Med Hemother. 2013;40(5):302–9. https://doi.org/10.1159/000356193.

135. Bellazzi F, Bertolaso M. Emergence in complex physiological processes: the case of Vitamin B12 functions in erythropoiesis. Systems. 2024;12(4):131. https://doi.org/10.3390/systems12040131.
136. Kataria N, Yadav P, Kumar R, Kumar N, Singh M, Kant R, Kalyani V. Effect of vitamin B6, B9, and B12 supplementation on homocysteine level and cardiovascular outcomes in stroke patients: a meta-analysis of randomized controlled trials. Cureus. 2021:13. https://doi.org/10.7759/cureus.14958.
137. Satapathy S, Bandyopadhyay D, Patro BK, Khan S, Naik S. Folic acid and vitamin B12 supplementation in subjects with type 2 diabetes mellitus: a multi-arm randomized controlled clinical trial. Complement Ther Med. 2020;53:102526. https://doi.org/10.1016/j.ctim.2020.102526.
138. Restivo I, Attanzio A, Tesoriere L, Allegra M. Suicidal erythrocyte death in metabolic syndrome. Antioxidants. 2021;10(2):154. https://doi.org/10.3390/antiox10020154.
139. Tvedten H. Classification and laboratory evaluation of anemia. Schalm's Vet Hematol. 2022:198–208. https://doi.org/10.1002/9781119500537.ch25.
140. Díez SC, de Las Cuevas Allende R, García EC. Anemia of inflammation and iron metabolism in chronic diseases. Revista Clínica Española. 2024; https://doi.org/10.1016/j.rceng.2024.09.002.
141. DePalma RG, Hayes VW, O'Leary TJ. Optimal serum ferritin level range: iron status measure and inflammatory biomarker. Metallomics. 2021;13(6) https://doi.org/10.1093/mtomcs/mfab030.
142. Hain D, Bednarski D, Cahill M, Dix A, Foote B, Haras MS, Gutiérrez OM. Iron-deficiency anemia in CKD: a narrative review for the kidney care team. Kidney Med. 2023;5(8):100677. https://doi.org/10.1016/j.xkme.2023.100677.
143. Badura K, Janc J, Wąsik J, Gnitecki S, Skwira S, Młynarsk E, Franczyk B. Anemia of chronic kidney disease – a narrative review of its pathophysiology, diagnosis, and management. Biomedicines. 2024;12(6):1191. https://doi.org/10.3390/biomedicines12061191.
144. Zhou Y, Li X, Wang J. From cardiovascular-kidney-metabolic syndrome to anemia: the role of inflammation and oxidative stress. Biomolecules. 2023;15(2):213. https://doi.org/10.3390/biom15050670.
145. Choorapoikayil S, Kotlyar MJ, Kawohl L, Pratz PP, Mehic D, Kranke P, Meybohm P. Reticulocyte hemoglobin content: a new frontier in iron deficiency diagnostics for major surgical patients. BMC Anesthesiol. 2025;25(1):1–9. https://doi.org/10.1186/s12871-025-02905-6.
146. Suárez-Ortegón MF, Arbeláez A, Moreno-Navarrete JM, Ortega-Ávila JG, Mosquera M, Fernández-Real JM. Soluble transferrin receptor, antioxidant status and cardiometabolic risk in apparently healthy individuals. Antioxidants. 2022;12(1):19. https://doi.org/10.3390/antiox12010019.
147. Song X, Xiong L, Guo T, Chen X, Zhang P, Zhang X, Liang Z. Cystatin C is a predictor for long-term, all-cause, and cardiovascular mortality in US adults with metabolic syndrome. J Clin Endocrinol Metab. 2024;109(11):2905–19. https://doi.org/10.1210/clinem/dgae225.
148. Hollenberg SM, Warner Stevenson L, Ahmad T, Amin VJ, Bozkurt B, Butler J, et al. 2019 ACC expert consensus decision pathway on risk assessment, management, and clinical trajectory of patients hospitalized with heart failure: a report of the American College of Cardiology Solution Set Oversight Committee. J Am Coll Cardiol. 2019;74:1966–2011. https://doi.org/10.1016/j.jacc.2019.08.001.
149. McCullough PA. Anemia of cardiorenal syndrome. Kidney Int Suppl. 2011;11(1):35–45. https://doi.org/10.1016/j.kisu.2020.12.001.

Chapter 17
Prevention and Treatment Strategies in Cardiovascular–Renal–Metabolic Syndrome

Daniela Maria Tanase, Ioana Bianca Anton, and Evelina Maria Gosav

Introduction

The greatest risk of premature mortality is posed by cardiovascular disease (CVD) and all its phenotypes, such as atrial fibrillation, coronary artery disease, stroke, peripheral artery disease, heart failure, and sudden cardiac death. Associations with comorbidities such as renal disease and type 2 diabetes mellitus (T2DM) increase the risk of major adverse cardiovascular events (MACE) and all-cause mortality. Due to its complex associations, an interdisciplinary approach to CKM syndrome is recommended, considering different common medications and strategies. Prevention strategies implemented early and correct management decrease the risk of CVD events and complications [1].

Lifestyle Changes

Lifestyle modification is a pivotal factor in managing CKM syndrome. It is mainly represented by the weight-loss program that involves dietary changes, increased moderate physical activity, smoking cessation, moderate alcohol consumption, and reduced salt intake. This complex disorder requires major long-term changes to delay its progression and improve patients' overall quality of life [2].

D. M. Tanase · I. B. Anton · E. M. Gosav (✉)
Grigore T. Popa University of Medicine and Pharmacy, Iasi, Romania

Saint Spiridon Emergency Hospital, Iasi, Romania
e-mail: evelina.maria.gosav@umfiasi.ro

M. Floria, D. M. Tanase (eds.), *Cardiovascular-Kidney-Metabolic Syndrome*,
https://doi.org/10.1007/978-3-032-11445-7_17

Dietary Recommendations

Medical nutrition therapy (MNT) is an evidence-based process designed to manage a disease through nutrition, playing a crucial role in the CKM syndrome therapy. The purpose of MNT is to support the shift toward a balanced diet through the adoption of healthy eating patterns, to achieve and maintain individualized weight objectives, and to reach personalized targets for hemoglobin A1c (HbA1c), lipid panel, blood glucose, blood pressure, urine albumin-creatinine ratio, and other laboratory tests. A healthy dietary pattern is represented by fruits, vegetables, low-fat or fat-free dairy, whole grains, brown rice, nuts, fish, and lean chicken while paying attention to portion sizes [3].

Low-carbohydrate diet (LCD) is a dietary strategy proposed by the American Diabetes Association (ADA) that has drawn a lot of attention in recent years as a potential plan of action for weight management and glycemic control. It is represented by a restriction of carbohydrate intake, with only 26–45% of total daily caloric intake, derived from carbohydrate sources, along with a concomitant increase in protein and fat consumption. This approach aims to promote the induction of nutritional ketogenesis, causing the body to shift from glucose metabolism to another metabolic state, where ketone bodies, produced in liver cells by breaking down fatty acids, can serve as an alternative source of energy. This strategy is efficient in reducing appetite, losing weight while also maintaining lean mass and resting metabolic rate (RMR), improving lipid profiles, decreasing insulin requirements in type 2 diabetes, and reducing systemic inflammation [4, 5].

By minimizing carbohydrate intake and consuming more high-fat foods, LCD can modify the lipid panel, with a reduction in plasma triglycerides and total LDL-C, accompanied by an increase in high-density lipoprotein-cholesterol (HDL-C). LDL particles can also be influenced by this dietary regimen, with an increase in peak particle size that can be linked to decreased atherogenicity, resulting in reduced levels of small, dense LDL and a lower risk of cardiovascular disease. It has been argued that dietary carbohydrates' quality, assessed by their complexity and glycemic index, might be responsible for the distribution of different LDL particle subclasses, with no regard to the quantity of carbohydrates that has been ingested [6].

As for the impact of LCD on metabolic risk factors, this diet has been demonstrated to reduce HbA1c, improve insulin resistance, and diminish glucose level fluctuations, with a better outcome as regards metabolic syndrome (Met-S), due to optimal glycemic control. Naturally, a lower carbohydrate intake will decrease both blood glucose and insulin levels, thus forcing the body to redirect lipids from storage to oxidation. Furthermore, ketone bodies, especially β-hydroxybutyrate, offer protection against oxidative stress via inhibition of the NOD-like receptor protein 3 (NLRP3) inflammasome, hence reducing the release of pro-inflammatory cytokines, which maintain a systemic inflammatory status that can result in impaired insulin sensitivity and disorders of lipid metabolism [4].

The effect of a ketogenic diet on the microbiome is related to the benefits observed after prebiotic food consumption, which include complex carbohydrates, polyphenols, oligosaccharides, galactans, fructans, and starch. Consequently, in the colon, there will be a significant increase in *Bifidobacteria*, a type of lactic acid bacteria with beneficial weight-reducing and lipid-lowering effects. Thus, *Bifidobacterium longum* may exert hypocholesterolemic effects via the inhibition of enzymes involved in the cholesterol pathway by the fermentation products of these bacteria. The ingestion of nuts, leafy greens, fruit, and vegetables may provide the bacterial diversity required to maintain a healthy gut microbiome, mainly characterized by a low ratio of *Firmicutes* to *Bacteroides*, the latter having a beneficial effect on improving obesity. The *Firmicutes* phylum is positively correlated with obesity, and the mechanism behind this association may be related to its ability to enhance energy extraction from the respective diet [7, 8].

Interestingly, a ketogenic diet may prove to be useful as an adjuvant cancer therapy, besides standard radio-chemotherapy. Cancer cells exhibit enhanced glucose metabolism, which appears as a compensatory mechanism due to defective mitochondrial respiration, caused by numerous DNA mutations in the mitochondria. As a result, cancer cells produce an increased amount of reactive oxygen species (ROS), which leads to the need for malignant cells to consume more glucose, even in the presence of oxygen. Another benefit of this regimen would be related to decreased levels of insulin resulting from the process of nutritional ketogenesis, with a consequent reduction in insulin-like growth factor levels responsible for cancer proliferation. Hyperinsulinemia, which appears in the context of insulin resistance, a main component of metabolic syndrome, is strongly associated with a risk of developing cancer, because of insulin's both antiapoptotic and pro-mitotic activity that may be linked to tumor progression [9].

However, despite all these potential benefits of a low-carbohydrate diet, this therapeutic dietary regimen can also be associated with several adverse health effects. A commonly discussed effect of this diet is the so-called keto flu, which is a cluster of symptoms usually manifested within the first weeks after the implementation of this regimen that usually includes nausea, fatigue, headache, dizziness, halitosis, gastrointestinal discomfort due to the excessive fat content, and sometimes heartbeat alterations and muscular weakness. LCD may also be associated with a delay in ventricular repolarization, expressed by QT prolongation in an electrocardiograph (ECG), thus emphasizing the risk of developing *torsades de pointes* and sudden cardiac death. From a nutritional point of view, vitamin and mineral deficiencies are long-term adverse effects that may occur after ketogenic diets. Selenium, calcium, phosphorus, and magnesium are some of the elements that seem to decrease after LCD, alongside a decrease in vitamin A and an increase in vitamin E (circulating fat-soluble vitamins). Regarding the metabolism of vitamin D, it has been demonstrated that an acidotic state, determined by ketone bodies, prevents kidney hydroxylases from exerting their effects, thus blocking the conversion of vitamin D to an active form. Thus, progressive skeletal demineralization, along with decreased bone mineral density and growth retardation, defined by altered linear growth, has been observed in patients who adopted a ketogenic diet, especially in children. This imbalanced mineral homeostasis appears secondary to decreased bone remodeling, characterized by a rate of bone resorption much higher than the rate of bone formation. Furthermore, this step-by-step demineralization is also associated with hypercalciuria, an important risk factor in nephrolithiasis development [10, 11].

Physical Activity

Aerobic activity, also known as endurance activity, is a form of exercise meant to improve cardiovascular health, and it represents an attractive strategy to prevent the progression of the CKM syndrome. Resistance exercise, characterized by any kind of exercise that determines muscles to contract against external resistance, has been proven to enhance physical function, reduce blood pressure, increase insulin sensitivity, improve endothelial function, and reduce systemic inflammation. Other positive effects include a decrease in waist circumference and body fat mass, thus preventing a further increase in the body mass index (BMI), defined by a calculated measure of weight to height. The American Physical Activity Guidelines suggest approximately 150–250 min of moderate-intensity physical activity every week or 75 min per week of vigorous physical activity, to improve cardiopulmonary function and ensure the primary prevention of obesity. The recommended duration of physical activity for weight loss is from 225 to 420 min per week, whereas, for successfully maintaining the new weight, a period of 200–300 min every week is highly recommended. Along with certain dietary adjustments, this comprehensive plan of action, whose main target is healthy weight loss, will help reduce the progression of the CKM syndrome and improve the overall quality of life [12, 13].

Cognitive-Behavioral Therapy (CBT)

This structured, goal-oriented therapy has proven to be an effective approach for obesity, targeting the switch from problematic eating patterns to a balanced, healthy diet. CBT may serve as a valuable treatment option in changing lifestyle behaviors, thus alleviating the burden of patients who suffer from this complex syndrome. Healthcare providers should focus their attention on building strong relationships with patients and keeping tabs on their medical condition, lifestyle, long-term goals, and level of knowledge so that the counseling process would be suitable and adapted to the needs of each patient. This type of therapy is useful in addressing behavioral patterns that are usually developed throughout the teen years and tend to carry on during adulthood, thus highlighting the influence of environmental factors on personal habits and way of living. The main goals of cognitive-behavioral therapy regarding the treatment of obesity are to help patients achieve and maintain a healthy weight loss, commit to a new lifestyle that aids weight control, and adopt a mindset that will encourage this difficult transition [14].

Medical Therapy

In emergencies, a multidisciplinary therapeutic approach is highly recommended to address this complex condition, which significantly impacts global morbidity and mortality. The need for interdisciplinary care is paramount, necessitating the development of a well-structured team that includes a CKM coordinator and representatives from primary care and various subspecialties, such as nephrology, cardiology, endocrinology, nursing, and pharmacy, alongside support from social workers, patient navigators, and community health workers. Therefore, effective integrated team care is essential when CVD, CKD, or diabetes are present to ensure the proper application of existing protocols and guidelines and to implement effective screening methods for this syndrome [1].

Sodium–Glucose Cotransporter-2 (SGLT2) Inhibitors

SGLT2 inhibitors (SGLT2i) are antihyperglycemic agents that exert their effects on the SGLT-2 transport proteins found in the proximal convoluted tubules, with their effectiveness related to the ability to lower blood sugar levels independently of insulin activity. Originally developed as antidiabetic drugs, they have also demonstrated pleiotropic effects (Fig. 17.1), including a reduction in Major Adverse Cardiovascular Events (MACE) such as nonfatal stroke or nonfatal myocardial infarction, along with lowering blood pressure, decreasing body weight, improving cardiovascular outcomes, reducing rates of heart failure (HF) hospitalizations, and preserving kidney function [1].

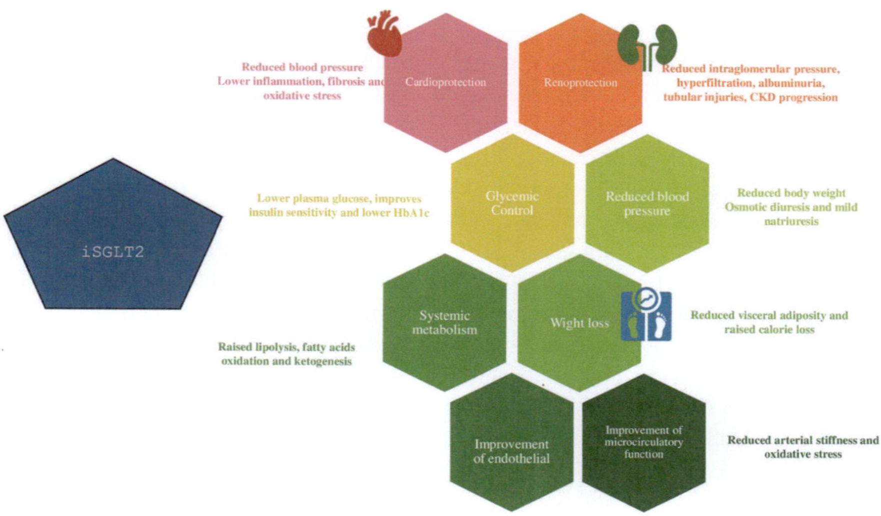

Fig. 17.1 Summary of SGLT2 inhibitors and their pleiotropic effects

These glucose-lowering drugs are derived from phlorizin, a natural dihydrochalcone discovered in 1835 when it was isolated from the root bark of apple trees, where it was initially used to treat malaria and other infections. This nonspecific sodium–glucose cotransporter inhibitor can lower blood glucose levels by inducing glycosuria, without affecting insulin secretion. Besides its antidiabetic purpose, this flavonoid glycoside has also shown neuromodulatory, antioxidant, and anti-inflammatory effects. Phlorizin has limited bioavailability due to its rapid metabolization by lactase-phlorizin hydrolase and reduced absorption in the small intestine. Therefore, more potent and selective phlorizin analogs, such as Dapagliflozin, Canagliflozin, Empagliflozin, and Ertugliflozin, have emerged and are currently approved by the Food and Drug Administration (FDA) and the European Medicines Agency (EMA) [1].

Under normal physiological circumstances, kidneys maintain glucose homeostasis by filtering and reabsorbing up to 180 g of glucose per day, thus leaving no trace of it in the urine. This reabsorption is facilitated by two sodium-dependent glucose cotransporter proteins, SGLT1 and SGLT2, which can transport glucose into the cell via a sodium concentration gradient across the cell membrane, determined by a Na^+/K^+ ATPase pump. SGLT2, a low-affinity high-capacity transporter abundantly found on the luminal side of the S1 and S2 segments of proximal convoluted tubules, is responsible for the reabsorption of 80–90% of filtered glucose. SGLT1, expressed in the S3 segment of the proximal tubule, is responsible for the reabsorption of the remaining 10–20%, thus ensuring that the glucose that may avoid the reabsorption by SGLT2 will be later drawn back into more distal segments. Whereas SGLT1s are located in the small intestine, heart, lungs, skeletal muscles, and to a lesser extent in kidneys, SGLT2s are only limited to the renal cortex [15].

The mechanism of action of SGLT2 inhibitors is represented by the blockade of sodium and glucose reabsorption in the proximal convoluted tubule of the kidney, with an increase in distal tubular sodium, thus resulting in glycosuria and natriuresis. Consequently, an increased sodium chloride delivery to the macula densa activates tubule-glomerular feedback, a major component of renal autoregulation. The result of this mechanism is represented by vasoconstriction of the afferent arteriole and vasodilatation of the efferent arteriole, therefore exerting a nephroprotective effect by reducing hyperfiltration, with a concomitant decrease in the estimated glomerular filtration rate (eGFR) and a reduction of albuminuria. Lowered GFR and glomerular capillary pressure (PGC) alleviate the physical stress exerted on glomerular capillaries, with a consequent decline in the glomerular filtration of compounds known to be toxic for tubular cells, such as albumin, with a positive impact on tubular growth and renal inflammation. In addition, a reduced GFR could lower the tubular transport work, thus decreasing the oxygen demand of the renal cortex, further contributing to a delayed progression of CKD [16].

SGLT2i are also responsible for a rapid, yet modest, contraction of plasma volume, which leads to a reduction in effective circulating volume and a lowering of ventricular filling pressure, thereby improving the preload of the left ventricle through mild natriuresis and osmotic diuresis. Consequently, a reduction in blood pressure (BP) by approximately 3–5 mmHg is observed upon treatment with

SGLT2i, which may be caused by a modest but persistent decrease in plasma volume. Other mechanisms that may provide an explanation for the antihypertensive effects of SGLT2i include body weight reduction and improvements in arterial stiffness and endothelial dysfunction, through nitric oxide (NO) production and inhibition of intracellular and mitochondrial reactive oxygen species (ROS) production. SGLT2i have been demonstrated to possess anti-inflammatory effects, as well as antifibrotic properties, mediated by the inhibition of tumor growth factor-1 (TGF-1) receptors. Besides, the combined effects of BP lowering and amelioration of vascular dysfunction will result in a reduction in afterload, with the potential to prevent further HF events [17, 18].

The inhibition of SGLT2 is also linked to a slight early weight loss, which varies between 2% and 4% of initial body weight. In the beginning, this reduction in body weight is caused by the excretion of fluid via osmotic diuresis and a loss of approximately 240–320 kcal per day as a consequence of induced glycosuria. It is argued that the intensity of glycosuria per nephron is possibly responsible for the initiation of lipolysis and weight decrease. This important drop in plasma glucose levels will lead to lower levels of plasma insulin and decreased insulin/glucagon ratio, with a succeeding boost in hepatic glycogenolysis and gluconeogenesis. Following diminished insulin secretion, lipolytic activity is enhanced, whereas lipogenesis is inhibited, thus resulting in elevated levels of free fatty acids (FFAs). Through decreased lipid deposition in visceral fat, SGLT2i exert their benefits in weight loss and body fat reduction, which involves visceral and subcutaneous fat [17].

SGLT2 inhibitors lead FFAs to undergo oxidation to fulfill the energetic requirements, and thus avoid their amassing in adipose tissue. The beta-oxidation of FFAs generates ketone bodies, primarily β-hydroxybutyrate, which constitute a better energetic substrate in comparison to FFAs, due to higher ATP production, accompanied by lower oxygen consumption, this being the main reason why they are regarded as "super fuel." As a result, in case of oxygen deprivation that accompanies heart failure, ketones seem to be a better option for ATP production in cardiomyocytes. Apart from their participation in energy metabolism, they also exhibit a notable decrease in inflammation and oxidative stress, due to the positive effect of β-hydroxybutyrate on redox homeostasis [19].

In all patients with heart failure, both with preserved ejection fraction (HFpEF) and with reduced ejection fraction (HFrEF), an SGLT2 inhibitor should be administered no matter the status of diabetes, to reduce cardiovascular mortality and the rate of HF hospitalization. The same dose of 10 mg per day should be prescribed for both Dapagliflozin (marketed as *Farxiga*®) and Empagliflozin (marketed as *Jardiance*®). Regarding the treatment of CKD, SGLT2i can be initiated in patients with type 2 diabetes and eGFR ≥20 mL/min/1.73 m^2, but this therapy can be continued in the event of even lower levels of eGFR. Canagliflozin and Dapagliflozin are the two therapeutic agents preferred in this case, with corresponding doses of 100 mg per day and 10 mg per day, respectively. Therefore, a modest drop in eGFR, of approximately 3–4 mL/min/1.73 m^2, is expected after beginning the treatment with these inhibitors [16].

Regarding their pharmacokinetics, SGLT2 inhibitors can be administered once a day, due to their reasonably long half-life, between 5 and 20 hours, in the form of oral tablets. They are properly absorbed in the gastrointestinal tract, thus demonstrating exceptional oral bioavailability. Other characteristics that display their valuable pharmacokinetic profile include a low accumulation index, dose–exposure linearity, relatively low renal excretion, and the absence of active metabolites. There is little to no interference with food ingestion, except for Canagliflozin, but to avoid postprandial glucose elevation in plasma, caused by the delayed absorption of glucose in the intestine, SGLT2 inhibitors should be administered before eating any meal. A potential risk of these inhibitors is represented by drug–drug interactions, with significant clinical implications. An increased risk of severe hypoglycemia is observed when SGLT2i are administered concomitantly with insulin or insulin-secreting drugs, such as sulfonylureas, but mainly in the case of Glibenclamide. As for Canagliflozin, when used at a maximum dose of 300 mg per day, at the same time as Digoxin, it has proven to increase the latter's peak drug concentration, thus requiring careful monitoring of Digoxin blood levels and further dose adjustments. During this treatment, the evaluation of certain parameters is required: complete blood count (CBC), hematocrit, hemoglobin, basic metabolic panel (BMP), lipid panel, HbA1c, serum creatinine, serum electrolytes, eGFR, blood urea nitrogen (BUN), LDL cholesterol, and serum bicarbonate. Moreover, volume status monitoring is extremely important, since these drugs may have an impact on the intravascular volume, with a potential symptomatic decrease in blood pressure [20].

Despite the numerous benefits of this safe and effective class of drugs, there is a series of notable adverse effects that may be taken into careful consideration. The most frequent ones are genital mycotic infections and urinary tract infections (UTIs). Genital mycotic infections, which usually include vulvovaginitis and vulval abscess, have an increased incidence among postmenopausal women and women with prior antecedents of UTIs. These could be easily prevented through an adequate local hygiene routine, and mild-to-moderate infections can be cured with topical antifungal treatment, such as Clotrimazole or Miconazole, and sometimes oral administration of Fluconazole. UTIs may be associated with the use of SGLT2i because of their ability to induce glycosuria, thus creating favorable conditions for bacterial growth, besides poor local hygiene, obesity, and insufficient liquid intake, which can also contribute to the genesis of these infections [16]. In extremely rare cases, increased glucose levels in the urine and immunosuppression could promote the development of Fournier gangrene, a necrotizing fasciitis that occurs in the perineal and genito-urinary region. This life-threatening infection expands at a fast pace and involves the tissues close to the muscles, blood vessels, fat, and nerves of the perineum, leading to multi-organ dysfunction and septic shock. Fournier gangrene is usually polymicrobial; the incriminating pathogenic agents are *Staphylococcus aureus*, *Escherichia coli*, *Klebsiella pneumoniae*, and *Bacteroides fragilis*. The symptoms associated with this aggressive infection could be itching, localized tenderness and swelling in the perineal area, lethargy, fever, tachycardia, subcutaneous crepitation, and possibly purulent drainage. Another possible risk linked to the consumption of SGLT2i is bladder cancer. This correlation is still being researched, but several cases have been reported, especially with the use of Dapagliflozin. Persistent induced glycosuria and recurrent UTIs may serve as the main risk factors responsible for the tumor growth process [21]. Thus, it is strongly advised that Dapagliflozin should be cautiously used in patients with hematuria and a prior history of bladder cancer and completely avoided in individuals with active bladder cancer. Because of their ability to induce osmotic diuresis, SGLT2i, especially when used at the same time as diuretics, may pose a risk of postural hypotension, a minor decrease in blood pressure, and dizziness, symptoms caused by the contraction of the intravascular volume. Thus, a dose adjustment for the diuretic medication is to be taken into consideration, along with monitoring blood pressure and body weight every day, mainly in the first week of treatment initiation. Interestingly, SGLT2 inhibitors have also been linked to an increased risk of bone fractures, particularly for Canagliflozin. The mechanism behind this phenomenon may be related to increased serum concentrations of phosphate, due to increased reabsorption in the kidney tubules, which can interfere with mineral metabolism and affect bone density, and a slight increase in parathyroid hormone (PTH) concentrations, which would further promote bone resorption and increase the risk for fractures [15, 21, 22].

Glucagon-Like Peptide-1 Receptor Agonists (GLP-1 RAs)

Glucagon-like peptide-1 (GLP-1) receptor agonists, also known as incretin mimetics, are a class of drugs known for their ability to reduce serum glucose levels by enhancing insulin secretion in a glucose-dependent manner, thereby proving their utility in the treatment of T2DM. Moreover, they have demonstrated several cardiovascular protective effects by reducing blood pressure, improving the lipid panel, enhancing vascular endothelial function, and decreasing the incidence of MACE, with significant improvement in the prevention of CVD among patients suffering from T2DM [23].

GLP-1 is a naturally occurring peptide hormone produced by the enteroendocrine L-cells located in the mucosal layer of the distal jejunum, ileum, and colon, as a result of nutrient intake and stimulation of the neuroendocrine system. This incretin hormone is produced through the enzymatic degradation of proglucagon, a polypeptide precursor that further generates several bioactive peptides, including glucagon, GLP-1, and glucagon-like peptide-2 (GLP-2). GLP-1 plays a crucial role in the regulation of glucose homeostasis through its enhancement of glucose-induced insulin secretion ("insulinotropic incretin effect") and suppression of pancreatic glucagon secretion ("glucagonostatic incretin effect"). This phenomenon is revealed after oral glucose intake, which results in the release of GLP-1 and glucose-dependent insulinotropic polypeptide (GIP) from enteroendocrine cells (EECs). This leads to a more pronounced insulin secretory response in comparison to the secretory response of a potential intravenous glucose infusion, which is roughly one-third of that generated by oral glucose, both inducing similar plasma glucose levels. However, GLP-1's half-life is slightly short, with a duration of approximately

2–5 min, since it is further degraded and inactivated through enzymatic hydrolysis assisted by dipeptidyl-peptidase-4 (DPP-4), therefore losing its metabolic importance and being quickly eliminated through renal excretion [23, 24].

Glucagon-like peptide-1 receptor agonists (GLP-1 RAs) are synthetic compounds derived from GLP-1 after certain structural modifications, which replicate the biological properties of endogenous GLP-1 (Fig. 17.2). Their half-life is significantly prolonged due to their resistance to DPP-4's proteolytic activity, therefore reducing their excretion rate and ensuring increased biological potency. By demonstrating partial or complete homology with native GLP-1, GLP-1 RAs exhibit the same therapeutic effects, including increased insulin secretion, decreased glucagon secretion, suppressed appetite, and delayed gastric emptying. This incretin-based therapy can be classified into short-acting and long-acting agents. Short-acting medication includes Exenatide twice a day, Lixisenatide once a day, and oral Semaglutide once a day, whereas long-acting drugs, which should be administered once a week, include Semaglutide, Liraglutide, Exenatide, Albiglutide, and Dulaglutide [23].

The main differences between these two classes of agents are related to the ability of long-acting agonists to maintain more steady plasma levels of exogenous GLP-1 and their enhanced gastrointestinal tolerability due to a less pronounced effect on gastric evacuation. The first GLP-1 receptor agonist to ever be encountered was Exenatide (marketed as *Byetta*®), a synthetic compound based on exendin-4 and an exopeptide identified in the saliva of a venomous lizard found in the southwestern side of the United States, also known as *Heloderma suspectum* or the Gila monster. Exenatide presents nearly 50% homology to native GLP-1, with an

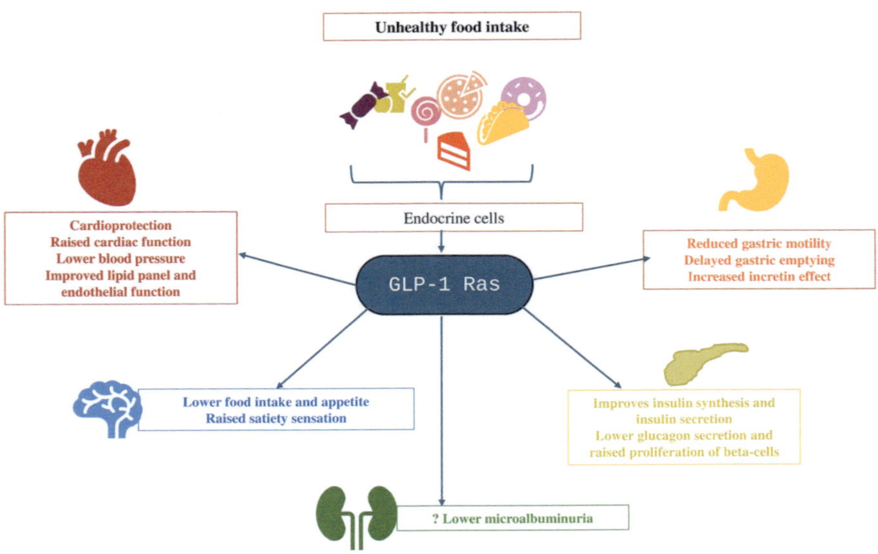

Fig. 17.2 Therapeutic effects of GLP-1 RAs

average half-life of approximately 3 hours, thus requiring 2–3 subcutaneous injections per day. Its major disadvantage is linked to low circulating plasma concentrations in the interval between the two injections, providing active circulating levels for only two important meals a day. This medication showed improved glycemic control and effective weight loss, demonstrating its safety profile when used in monotherapy or together with other glucose-lowering drugs [23, 25].

Liraglutide (marketed as *Victoza®* and *Saxenda®*) is a long-acting GLP-1 receptor agonist approved for the treatment of type 2 diabetes, while also demonstrating its effectiveness and long-term safety as a weight loss agent through delayed gastric evacuation and its appetite suppressant properties. Its resemblance to endogenous GLP-1 is quite remarkable, with a value of approximately 97% sequence homology. Since Liraglutide is connected to a free fatty acid side chain, this structural property promotes its binding to albumin, thus preventing its renal excretion and ensuring its safe use in case of renal dysfunction. Due to its half-life of nearly 13 hours, it is recommended that this compound be administered subcutaneously once a day. Apart from its efficiency as a glucose-reducing agent and its indication in weight management, due to its effect on reducing abdominal fat and visceral adipose tissue, Liraglutide has also demonstrated cardiovascular protective effects [23]. This GLP-1 RA has been shown to alleviate oxidative stress via diminishing ROS production and decreasing the number of small, dense LDL particles, thus reducing the substrate for LDL oxidation. Together with its ability to prevent the transformation of monocytes into foam cells, this therapeutic agent proves its beneficial effect on atherosclerotic plaque by significantly slowing its progression. Liraglutide has demonstrated its efficiency in decreasing the number of MACE events and reducing CV mortality, due to its ability to lower blood pressure, reduce HbA1c, and improve left-ventricular ejection fraction among HF patients. Moreover, Liraglutide could provide some substantial benefits regarding renal function, since recent studies have shown that it may have a positive impact on reducing early-onset macroalbuminuria. There are a series of possible risks associated with the initiation of Liraglutide, including nausea, vomiting, diarrhea, constipation, abdominal pain, acute pancreatitis, and increased lipase levels [23].

Semaglutide (marketed as *Ozempic®*) is the most effective GLP-1 RA in chronic weight management, besides other weight reduction measures, such as increased physical exercise and decreased calorie consumption. This agonist has a 94% homology to endogenous GLP-1, with a significant similarity to Liraglutide in terms of structure. However, it exhibits an even higher half-life of approximately 1 week, thus requiring administration of 2.4 mg Semaglutide once a week, by subcutaneous injection in the abdomen, the upper arm, or the thigh. Its binding to albumin is even stronger than the one with Liraglutide, thus exhibiting prolonged renal excretion, although Semaglutide can be eliminated to a lesser extent in the feces. This GLP-1 receptor agonist can also be administered in oral form, once a day, in tablets of 3, 7, and 14 mg, with relatively low bioavailability when it comes to gastrointestinal absorption. Regarding the mechanism of action, Semaglutide stimulates weight body reduction through its interaction with the GLP-1 receptors, primarily located at the surface of the pancreatic β-cells, in the central nervous system (CNS), and across the gastrointestinal tract. Its potential to traverse the blood–brain barrier more easily than Liraglutide makes it more effective in treating hypothalamic obesity through its interaction with the GLP-1 receptors located in the hypothalamus, thus enhancing the sensation of satiety and reducing the need for food intake [23]. Semaglutide 2.4 mg administered once a week subcutaneously exhibited a significant reduction in major adverse cardiovascular events by approximately 20%, possibly via its beneficial physiological effects, due to the decrease of excessive adipose tissue that might exert a direct influence on atherosclerosis and myocardial dysfunction. However, oral Semaglutide has not shown any cardiovascular benefits, hence it is not preferred for patients with preexisting cardiovascular disease. The most frequent adverse effects associated with the use of Semaglutide are gastrointestinal, and most patients who discontinue their treatment experience symptoms such as abdominal pain, nausea, vomiting, diarrhea, and constipation. The mechanism behind these manifestations may be related to the impaired gastric evacuation or the involvement of the centers in the brain that regulate the sensations of satiety, appetite, and nausea. Acute pancreatitis is a relatively rare adverse effect reported across patients treated with Semaglutide, with a 9-times higher risk in comparison with other weight reduction agents, especially in patients suffering from type 2 diabetes. The accompanying symptoms include nausea, vomiting, jaundice, severe upper abdominal pain, fever, and fatigue, with their severity varying from one case to another. The hypothetical mechanism behind this harmful side effect is related to an increase in pancreatic mass with enhanced exocrine cell proliferation, which can contribute to an obstruction in the outflow of pancreatic enzymes. Moreover, gallbladder-related disorders, such as cholelithiasis, could also pose serious health issues, potentially due to the suppression of cholecystokinin secretion and a diminished gallbladder evacuation [23, 26, 27].

Lixisenatide (marketed as *Adlyxin*® or *Lyxumia*®) is a short-acting GLP-1 RA based on the structure of exendin-4, which is also used in the treatment of type 2 diabetes, due to its effectiveness in reducing HbA1c levels, while also displaying a decrease in body weight and BMI. This oligopeptide exhibits a pronounced effect in reducing gastric emptying, but its efficacy in weight loss is significantly reduced compared to other GLP-1 RAs [27]. However, it appears that Lixisenatide is more successful in crossing the blood–brain barrier than Liraglutide and Semaglutide. It demonstrates a higher binding affinity for the GLP-1 receptors than the other two aforementioned. As for the effects on the cardiovascular system, Lixisenatide failed to demonstrate superiority in cardiovascular outcomes, hence exerting a neutral effect on the rate of cardiovascular events. The explanation regarding Lixisenatide's lack of effectiveness may be related to its short half-life compared to other agents from this class. Regarding pharmacokinetic properties, Lixisenatide is quickly absorbed after its subcutaneous administration, being removed from circulation through glomerular filtration. This agonist reaches its peak plasma concentration at 1–3.5 hours, with a half-life of approximately 3–4 hours. It should be administered once a day in the form of subcutaneous injection, within an hour before the first meal of the day, at the same time each day of the administration. More importantly, in case of missing a single shot, it is strongly recommended not to administer Lixisenatide after a meal. As well as other representatives from the GLP-1 RA's class, patients who were prescribed Lixisenatide exhibited similar adverse effects, including nausea, vomiting, dyspepsia, headaches, dizziness, fatigue, and pruritus at the site of the injection [23].

Renin-Angiotensin-Aldosterone System (RAAS) Inhibitors

The renin-angiotensin-aldosterone system is a crucial neurohormonal system that participates in the regulation of systemic blood pressure, fluid and electrolyte balance, and peripheral vascular resistance. Besides its physiological importance in controlling salt and water homeostasis, it also plays a significant role in some pathophysiological conditions, such as congestive heart failure, hypertension, acute myocardial infarction, chronic kidney disease, and T2DM. The blockade of this endocrine and paracrine system has demonstrated major improvements in renal and cardiovascular outcomes by lowering blood pressure and reducing renal and cardiac tissue remodeling [28].

The RAAS pathway starts when renin is secreted from the juxtaglomerular granular cells, located in the medial layer of the afferent arteriole. Prorenin, the biosynthetic precursor of renin produced in the liver, is activated via an irreversible proteolytic mechanism within the kidney by enzymes such as cathepsin B and proprotein convertase-1. The major stimuli, which contribute to the release of mature renin into the bloodstream, are represented by reduced renal perfusion, perceived by the mechanoreceptors located in the wall of the afferent arterioles, decreased sodium chloride (NaCl) flow to the distal convoluted tubule detected by macula densa, and increased sympathetic activity. Thus, renin is considered the rate-limiting enzyme, even though its half-life is about 10–15 min. Renin further converts angiotensinogen, an $\alpha 2$-globulin produced in the liver, to angiotensin I, a polypeptide lacking any biological activity [28]. Through the activity of angiotensin-converting enzyme (ACE), a zinc metalloproteinase typically expressed in the capillary blood vessels from the pulmonary circulation, angiotensin I is hydrolyzed and converted to angiotensin II (Ang II), the most important effector of RAAS and a potent vasoconstrictor, which regulates blood pressure and fluid homeostasis. Ang II's systemic effects include constriction of blood vessels by vascular smooth muscle contraction within the arterioles, with an increase in systemic vascular resistance and blood pressure, enhanced sodium reabsorption in the proximal convoluted tubule, thus increasing sodium and water retention, aldosterone secretion through the stimulation of the adrenal gland cortex, and stimulation of thirst centers in the brain, with subsequent secretion of vasopressin from the hypothalamus, which further increases water retention. ACE is also responsible for the degradation of bradykinin, a powerful endothelium-dependent vasodilator, to inactive fragments, thus lowering the circulating levels of endogenous molecules responsible for vasodilation. Furthermore,

Ang II is involved in the development of oxidative stress, fibrosis, and endothelial dysfunction, besides exerting pro-inflammatory and pro-fibrotic effects, thus demonstrating its involvement in the pathogenesis of atherosclerosis, hypertension, heart failure, and chronic kidney disease [29, 30].

The effects of this biologically active octapeptide are mediated by the interaction with two different G-protein-coupled receptors, namely, angiotensin type 1 (AT1-R) and type 2 (AT2-R) receptors, with counter-regulatory properties manifested in both cardiovascular and renal systems. AT1-R is a key part of the process of sodium and water reabsorption, as well as vasoconstriction, fibrosis, inflammation, oxidative stress, and tissue remodeling, whereas by stimulating AT2-R, Ang II promotes vasodilatation and natriuresis, while also exerting anti-inflammatory and anti-fibrotic effects. AT1-R can be found in the heart, kidney, vascular smooth muscle cells, platelets, brain, adipocytes, and adrenal gland, while AT2-R is located in the central nervous system, cardiomyocytes, kidney, uterus, and adrenal gland [31].

ACE inhibitors (ACEi) are a class of effective drugs that interfere with the renin-angiotensin-aldosterone system by competitively blocking the enzyme responsible for the conversion of Ang I to Ang II, thereby leading to decreased blood pressure, reduced preload and afterload, and diminished tissue remodeling [31]. These agents are used as first-line therapy in the treatment of hypertension, demonstrating their usefulness in improving renal and cardiovascular outcomes, reducing the number of cardiovascular-related hospitalizations, lowering albuminuria, and delaying the progression of CKD. ACE inhibitors demonstrate efficiency in decreasing systolic and diastolic blood pressure via vasodilation resulting from the inhibition of Ang II, thus proving useful in arterial hypertension treatment. As for the benefits of ACEi in the treatment of heart failure, ACEi have proven to reduce preload, afterload, and systolic wall stress, resulting in a significant increase in cardiac output without determining an increase in heart rate. Furthermore, by decreasing cardiac myocyte hypertrophy and by reducing left-ventricular mass, they exert beneficial effects in preventing cardiac remodeling and slowing the progression of this disease. These drugs have shown a reduction in deaths caused by heart failure, alongside a significant decrease in the incidence of deaths by arrhythmias, myocardial infarction, and fatal stroke. ACEi have also demonstrated nephroprotective effects by reducing microalbuminuria, through the decrease of glomerular capillary pressure, and by delaying the progression of CKD. Moreover, the effect of lowering blood pressure exerted by ACEi confirms the renoprotection assured by these drugs via reducing intraglomerular pressure, in this way preventing the development of ischemia within the renal system and blocking the fibrotic process that may occur in the interstitial tissue, due to the release of collagen and extracellular matrix from cells located in the tubules and mesangium [32].

According to their chemical structure, ACE inhibitors can be classified into three distinct groups: sulfhydryl-containing ACE inhibitors (Captopril, Zofenopril, Fentiapril), phosphorus-containing ACE inhibitors (Fosinopril), and dicarboxylic-containing ACE inhibitors (Enalapril, Ramipril, Benazepril, Perindopril, Lisinopril, Moexipril). Most ACE inhibitors are prescribed in oral form, apart from Enalapril, which can also be administered intravenously. The majority of ACEi are prodrugs, thus requiring hepatic activation, except for Lisinopril and Captopril, which do not require in vivo conversion to active metabolites to exert their therapeutic effects. Therefore, in case of hepatic impairment, a non-prodrug form, such as the two drugs aforementioned, is desired, as it exhibits acceptable oral availability and does not require hepatic activation [33].

Despite their numerous beneficial impacts on the renal and cardiovascular systems, these drugs exhibit several side effects, some of which can even pose a life-threatening risk (Fig. 17.3). Angioneurotic edema is the most important, yet rare, adverse effect, involving edema of the tongue, glottis, larynx, upper airways, and sometimes of the intestine. The pathogenesis of this dangerous side effect involves elevated levels of bradykinin, whose degradation is impeded, thus contributing to enhanced vascular permeability, with subsequent fluid extravasation and the development of edema. The symptoms commonly include swelling of the face, lips, tongue, and upper airways, without associated urticaria, dysphagia, dyspnea, dizziness, and fainting due to changes in blood pressure. Intestinal angioedema, which is more frequent in women, can present with diarrhea, vomiting, and severe abdominal pain due to a partial bowel obstruction caused by edema of the intestinal wall. Another significant adverse effect of these inhibitors is represented by an irritating, dry, nonproductive, persistent cough, which occurs predominantly in women, due to the accumulation of bradykinin in the upper respiratory tract, which further induces bronchoconstriction. Other adverse effects of ACEi include hypotension, which could appear as a first-dose effect or at any time during long-term treatment, hyperkaliemia, anemia caused by the suppression of erythropoietin production, skin rash, usually caused by using Captopril, nephrotic syndrome, and neutropenia [32, 34, 35].

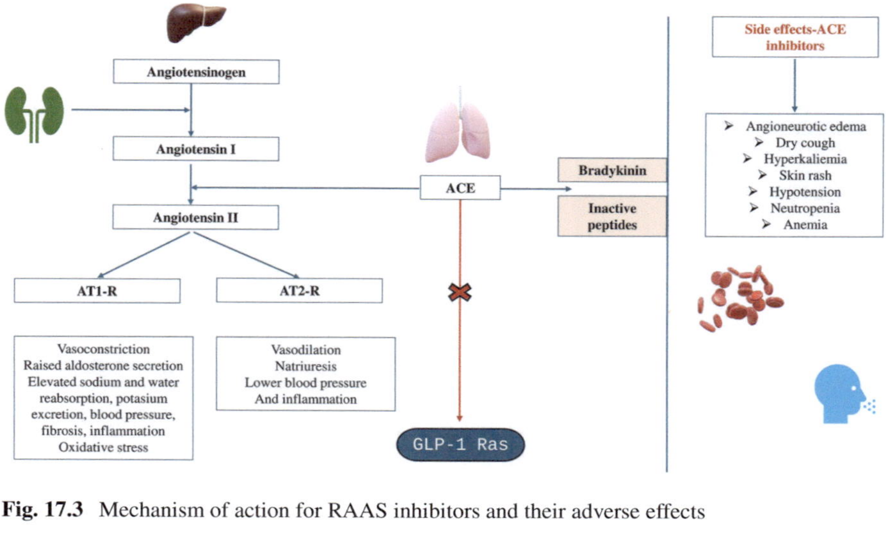

Fig. 17.3 Mechanism of action for RAAS inhibitors and their adverse effects

Angiotensin II Receptor Blockers (ARBs)

The angiotensin II receptor blockers (ARBs) are a class of antihypertensive agents that also interfere with the renin-angiotensin-aldosterone system, successfully used in the treatment of congestive heart failure and chronic kidney disease. These drugs have been developed as a potent alternative for ACE inhibitors, demonstrating fewer adverse effects, such as dry cough and angioedema, and more efficient Ang II inhibition through competitive antagonism of the AT1-R preventing Ang II from binding to its receptor, thereby reducing its biological effects. Their major advantage is related to the selectivity they demonstrate toward AT1-R, therefore allowing hyperstimulation of the AT2-R [34, 36]. These blood pressure-lowering agents exhibited beneficial nephroprotective and cardioprotective effects including reduced left-ventricular hypertrophy, decreased microalbuminuria, enhanced diastolic function, reduced incidence of ventricular arrhythmias, and improved renal function. Reduced blood pressure occurs as a result of decreased resistance in the peripheral vasculature, without potentially causing an increased heart rate. Most agents of this class can control blood pressure for 24 hours after one dose is administered per day. However, long-term effectiveness is associated with the prescription of these drugs for an extended period of time, with no worries regarding tachyphylaxis. Furthermore, ARBs have also demonstrated an increase in insulin sensitivity, and it has also been proven that Losartan could potentially reduce serum uric acid levels by increasing uric acid excretion, with a subsequent reduced risk of heart attack and stroke (Fig. 17.4) [36].

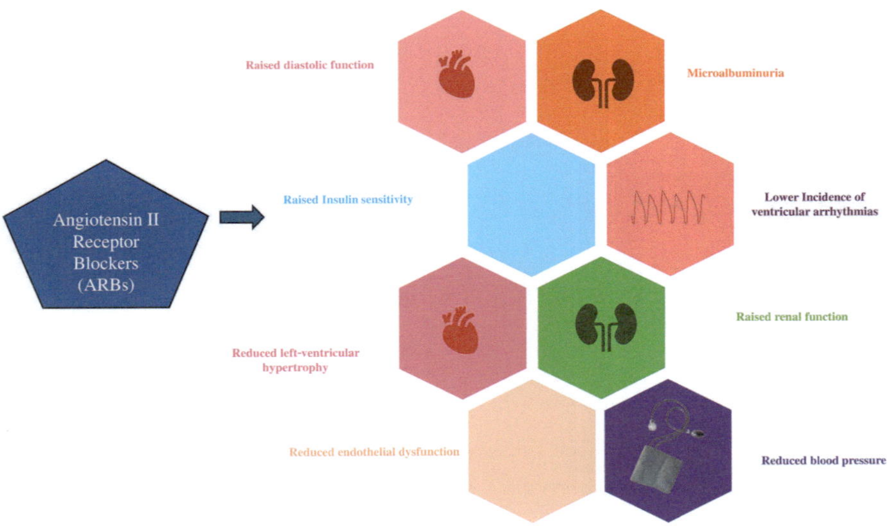

Fig. 17.4 Beneficial systemic effects of ARBs

Their pharmacokinetic properties exhibit powerful protein binding and slow dissociation once attached to the receptor. Some of these agents are prodrugs (e.g., Candesartan cilexetil) that need to be converted to an active metabolite, as in the case of Losartan. Its major active metabolite is represented by EXP 3174, which is 10 to 40 times more potent than Losartan and displays a longer duration of action, despite its reduced oral availability. Losartan is quickly absorbed after its oral administration, later being excreted through urine and feces, like most representatives from this class. Regarding their half-life, it can be short for Losartan and Candesartan cilexetil (1–4 hours), intermediate for Valsartan and Eprosartan (5–10 hours), and extended for Telmisartan, Candesartan, and Irbesartan (11–38 hours). In comparison to ACE inhibitors, angiotensin II receptor blockers exhibit fewer adverse effects, including dizziness, headaches, fatigue, and diarrhea, with a reduced incidence of cough, the main side effect of ACEi, and even fewer reported cases of angioedema [36].

New Perspectives and Treatments for CKM Syndrome

Angiotensin Receptor-Neprilysin Inhibitors (ARNi)

Angiotensin receptor-neprilysin inhibitors (ARNi) represent a class of drugs that have proven their effectiveness in the treatment of chronic heart failure with reduced ejection fraction (HFrEF). The most recent discovery of this category is Sacubitril/Valsartan (marketed as *Entresto*®), which brings together an angiotensin II receptor blocker (Valsartan) with a neprilysin inhibitor (Sacubitril). Sacubitril is a prodrug that requires activation in order to exert its effects as a neprilysin inhibitor, which include preventing the degradation of natriuretic peptides mediated by neprilysin. Since the natriuretic peptide (NP) system has beneficial effects on the pathogenesis of heart failure, such as vasodilation, diuresis, and natriuresis, the inhibition of neprilysin extends the duration of NPs and allows them to antagonize the unfavorable effects of RAAS. Moreover, as neprilysin is also responsible for the breakdown of angiotensin II, the use of a neprilysin inhibitor leads to the accumulation of Ang II, thereby additionally requiring an angiotensin II receptor blocker to suppress the harmful effects induced by a notable excess of Ang II. Since bradykinin is another substance that can be degraded by neprilysin, Sacubitril leads to bradykinin accumulation, which promotes histamine release, inflammation, bronchospasm, and increased vascular permeability, thus enhancing the risk of developing dry cough and angioedema. Therefore, it is strongly recommended that ACEi and Sacubitril/Valsartan be administered at a time interval of approximately 36 hours to prevent the occurrence of this life-threatening risk [37, 38].

HFrEF, Sacubitril/Valsartan has also demonstrated potential benefits in the management of systemic hypertension. Through enhanced diuresis and natriuresis, along with systemic vasodilation, Sacubitril/Valsartan leads to reduced peripheral vascular resistance and volume contraction, finally resulting in a decrease in systemic blood pressure. It is also suggested that ARNi could possess antiarrhythmic properties, possibly by limiting cardiac remodeling or via direct effects on cardiomyocytes, consequently reducing the incidence of sudden cardiac death [37]. Several factors are incriminated in the reduced incidence of arrhythmia-related deaths, including improvement of left-ventricular function, reduction of fibrosis within the myocardial tissue, improvement in hemodynamic parameters, and decreased sympathetic activity. Regarding glycemic control, there is some evidence that Sacubitril/Valsartan could potentially improve insulin sensitivity, due to the accumulation of bradykinin caused by neprilysin inhibition, while also being responsible for an increase in GLP-1, which further leads to an increased release of insulin and reduced secretion of glucagon. Although further research is needed to investigate the potential benefits of Sacubitril/Valsartan on the development of CKD, its use has been associated with a delay in CKD progression and a decrease in the number of cardiovascular events (Fig. 17.5) [37, 38]. After oral administration, this combination, which includes an equimolar ratio (1:1) of the ARB and the neprilysin inhibitor, is broken down into Sacubitril and Valsartan. Sacubitril/Valsartan can be administered with or without food, as it does not interfere with nutrient absorption. Upon ingestion, Sacubitril is further hydrolyzed by carboxyl esterases, thus being converted to Sacubitrilat, also known as LBQ657, the active form of this compound, which also exhibits elevated plasma protein binding. Regarding adverse effects, several have been reported after the use of Sacubitril/Valsartan, including hypotension, dizziness, hyperkaliemia, renal impairment, and possibly cerebral amyloid angiopathy, in association with special polymorphisms, in individuals who have received chronic treatment with ARNi [37–39].

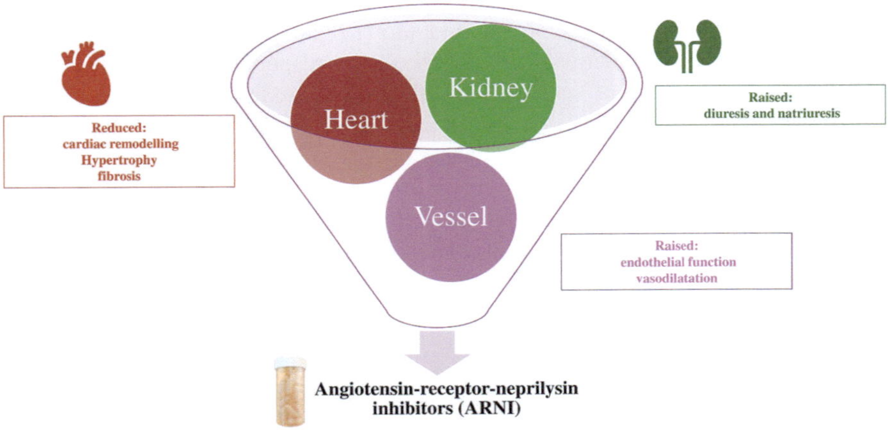

Fig. 17.5 The main beneficial effects of ARNi

Pentoxifylline—Potential Effects on Proteinuria

Pentoxifylline (PTX) is a nonselective phosphodiesterase (PDE) inhibitor that displays significant anti-fibrotic, anti-inflammatory, and antiproliferative effects, being a well-known therapeutic strategy in the treatment of intermittent claudication, associated with chronic occlusive peripheral vascular diseases of the limbs [40]. This methylxanthine derivative exerts its beneficial hemorheologic effects by increasing blood flow via reducing blood viscosity and improving the flexibility of red blood cells. In recent years, the effect of pentoxifylline on the renal system has been thoroughly investigated. Patients treated with PTX exhibited a significant reduction in urinary protein excretion, thus potentially demonstrating its properties as an antiproteinuric agent. PTX has been shown to reduce tumor necrosis factor-α (TNF-α) levels through the inhibition of TNF mRNA transcription, hence exerting its anti-inflammatory effect. Chronic kidney disease involves a pro-inflammatory state and concomitant increased glomerular permeability; thus, the use of PTX could supposedly diminish proteinuria and postpone the reduction in eGFR. By inhibiting PDE, PTX prevents the inactivation of cyclic adenosine-3,5-monophosphate (cAMP), thus leading to elevated levels of cAMP, which results in the activation of protein kinase A (PKA), with subsequent diminished synthesis of pro-inflammatory cytokines, such as TNF-α, IL-1, and IL-6 [40]. Therefore, it is suggested that pentoxifylline could be an attractive therapeutic agent in delaying CKD progression, with significant improvements in alleviating the inflammatory and fibrotic processes [41]. Concerning its pharmacokinetics, this compound is quickly absorbed in the gastrointestinal tract upon its ingestion. Yet, it is recommended to be accompanied by food intake to diminish gastrointestinal irritation. Pentoxifylline is later metabolized by erythrocytes and hepatic cells, is further eliminated through urine and feces, and its half-life is between 0.4 and 0.8 hours. Its key metabolites have a half-life of approximately 1–1.5 hours, and they can be secreted in breast milk, thus emphasizing the need for caution when prescribing this drug to breastfeeding mothers. This therapeutic approach is also accompanied by several side effects, including nausea, vomiting, abdominal discomfort, diarrhea, chest pains, arrhythmias, dyspnea, tachycardia, dizziness, and headaches. Concerning drug–drug interactions, Pentoxifylline's concomitant use with antihypertensive and antidiabetic drugs has shown minor reductions in blood pressure and an enhancement of the anti-glycemic action of glucose-lowering agents. Therefore, upon the prescription of Pentoxifylline, the monitoring of blood pressure and glucose levels is strongly recommended to prevent the occurrence of hypoglycemia, hypotension, and fainting. Moreover, hemoglobin, hematocrit, and Prothrombin Time (PT) and International Normalized Ratio (INR) (PT/INR) should also be observed, especially in patients receiving antiplatelet agents, who have a history of ischemic stroke, thus being at risk of potential bleeding [40, 41].

As seen, CKM should be investigated and prevented as much as possible firstly through lifestyle modifications. Proper medication treatment elected via an interdisciplinary team may benefit the patients when discussing disease prevention, disease onset, evolution, and cardiovascular adverse events.

Learning Objectives

- The intricate interplay between cardiovascular, renal, and metabolic systems is perceived as a significant challenge by healthcare professionals, due to the complex pathophysiology of CKM.
- Current guidelines focus on preventive strategies including lifestyle changes, and newer drugs such as iSGLT2 that are indicated not only in CVD but also in CKD and metabolic diseases such as diabetes.

Key Reading

- Lifestyle modification is a pivotal factor in managing CKM syndrome, represented by weight loss, dietary changes, increased moderate physical activity, smoking cessation, moderate alcohol consumption, and reduced salt intake.
- Besides lifestyle changes, cognitive–behavioral therapy has emerged as an adjuvant therapeutic approach in obese patients.
- Current therapeutic options are represented by SGLT2 inhibitors, GLP-1 Ras, RAAS inhibitors, ARBs, ARNIs, and even Pentoxifylline.
- These medications have pleiotropic effects beneficial in CKM; the treatment should be individualized by an interdisciplinary team for better management and improved quality of patients' health.

References

1. Ndumele CE, Rangaswami J, Chow SL, Neeland IJ, Tuttle KR, Khan SS, et al. Cardiovascular-kidney-metabolic health: a presidential advisory from the American Heart Association. Circulation. 2023;148(20):1606–35. https://doi.org/10.1161/cir.0000000000001184. Epub 20231009. PubMed PMID: 37807924
2. Kim HL, Chung J, Kim KJ, Kim HJ, Seo WW, Jeon KH, et al. Lifestyle modification in the Management of Metabolic Syndrome: statement from Korean Society of CardioMetabolic syndrome (KSCMS). Korean Circ J. 2022;52(2):93–109. https://doi.org/10.4070/kcj.2021.0328. PubMed PMID: 35128848; PubMed Central PMCID: PMC8819565
3. Dresen E, Notz Q, Menger J, Homayr AL, Lindner M, Radke DI, et al. What the clinician needs to know about medical nutrition therapy in critically ill patients in 2023: a narrative review. Nutr Clin Pract. 2023;38(3):479–98. https://doi.org/10.1002/ncp.10984. Epub 20230405. PubMed PMID: 37021324
4. Li Z, Liu X, Ma X, Xiao M, Zhang X, Deng Y, et al. The potential of dietary strategies: the impact of low-carbohydrate diet on cardiovascular-kidney-metabolic syndrome. medRxiv. 2025:2025.01.03.25319951. https://doi.org/10.1101/2025.01.03.25319951.
5. Mooradian AD. The merits and the pitfalls of low carbohydrate diet: a concise review. J Nutr Health Aging. 2020;24(7):805–8. https://doi.org/10.1007/s12603-020-1417-1. PubMed PMID: 32744579

6. Norwitz NG, Loh V. A standard lipid panel is insufficient for the care of a patient on a high-fat, low-carbohydrate ketogenic diet. Front Med (Lausanne). 2020;7:97. Epub 20200415. doi: https://doi.org/10.3389/fmed.2020.00097. PubMed PMID: 32351962; PubMed Central PMCID: PMC7174731.
7. Plata C, Cruz C, Cervantes LG, Ramírez V. The gut microbiota and its relationship with chronic kidney disease. Int Urol Nephrol. 2019;51(12):2209–26. https://doi.org/10.1007/s11255-019-02291-2. Epub 20191001. PubMed PMID: 31576489
8. Rossi M, Johnson DW, Campbell KL. The kidney-gut axis: implications for nutrition care. J Ren Nutr. 2015;25(5):399–403. https://doi.org/10.1053/j.jrn.2015.01.017. Epub 20150323. PubMed PMID: 25812908
9. Dowis K, Banga S. The potential health benefits of the ketogenic diet: a narrative review. Nutrients. 2021;13(5) https://doi.org/10.3390/nu13051654. Epub 20210513. PubMed PMID: 34068325; PubMed Central PMCID: PMC8153354
10. Bostock ECS, Kirkby KC, Taylor BV, Hawrelak JA. Consumer reports of "Keto Flu" associated with the ketogenic diet. Front Nutr. 2020;7:20. https://doi.org/10.3389/fnut.2020.00020. Epub 20200313. PubMed PMID: 32232045; PubMed Central PMCID: PMC7082414
11. O'Neill B, Raggi P. The ketogenic diet: pros and cons. Atherosclerosis. 2020;292:119–26. https://doi.org/10.1016/j.atherosclerosis.2019.11.021. Epub 20191128. PubMed PMID: 31805451
12. Lavie CJ, Ozemek C, Carbone S, Katzmarzyk PT, Blair SN. Sedentary behavior, exercise, and cardiovascular health. Circ Res. 2019;124(5):799–815. https://doi.org/10.1161/circresaha.118.312669. PubMed PMID: 30817262
13. Sebastian SA, Padda I, Johal G. Cardiovascular-kidney-metabolic (CKM) syndrome: a state-of-the-art review. Curr Probl Cardiol. 2024;49(2):102344. https://doi.org/10.1016/j.cpcardiol.2023.102344. Epub 20231214. PubMed PMID: 38103820
14. Garcia-Silva J, Borrego IRS, Navarrete NN, Peralta-Ramirez MI, Águila FJ, Caballo VE. Efficacy of cognitive-behavioural therapy for lifestyle modification in metabolic syndrome: a randomised controlled trial with a 18-months follow-up. Psychol Health. 2024;39(2):195–215. https://doi.org/10.1080/08870446.2022.2055023. Epub 20220328. PubMed PMID: 35345950
15. Tentolouris A, Vlachakis P, Tzeravini E, Eleftheriadou I, Tentolouris N. SGLT2 inhibitors: a review of their antidiabetic and cardioprotective effects. Int J Environ Res Public Health. 2019;16(16) https://doi.org/10.3390/ijerph16162965. Epub 20190817. PubMed PMID: 31426529; PubMed Central PMCID: PMC6720282
16. Vallon V, Verma S. Effects of SGLT2 inhibitors on kidney and cardiovascular function. Annu Rev Physiol. 2021;83:503–28. https://doi.org/10.1146/annurev-physiol-031620-095920. Epub 20201116. PubMed PMID: 33197224; PubMed Central PMCID: PMC8017904
17. Thomas MC, Cherney DZI. The actions of SGLT2 inhibitors on metabolism, renal function and blood pressure. Diabetologia. 2018;61(10):2098–107. https://doi.org/10.1007/s00125-018-4669-0. Epub 20180822. PubMed PMID: 30132034
18. Heerspink HJ, Perkins BA, Fitchett DH, Husain M, Cherney DZ. Sodium glucose cotransporter 2 inhibitors in the treatment of diabetes mellitus: cardiovascular and kidney effects, potential mechanisms, and clinical applications. Circulation. 2016;134(10):752–72. https://doi.org/10.1161/circulationaha.116.021887. Epub 20160728. PubMed PMID: 27470878
19. Manolis AS, Manolis TA, Manolis AA. Ketone bodies and cardiovascular disease: an alternate fuel source to the rescue. Int J Mol Sci. 2023;24(4) https://doi.org/10.3390/ijms24043534. Epub 20230210. PubMed PMID: 36834946; PubMed Central PMCID: PMC9962558
20. Garcia-Ropero A, Badimon JJ, Santos-Gallego CG. The pharmacokinetics and pharmacodynamics of SGLT2 inhibitors for type 2 diabetes mellitus: the latest developments. Expert Opin Drug Metab Toxicol. 2018;14(12):1287–302. https://doi.org/10.1080/17425255.2018.155187 7. Epub 20181129. PubMed PMID: 30463454

21. Bailey CJ, Day C, Bellary S. Renal protection with SGLT2 inhibitors: effects in acute and chronic kidney disease. Curr Diab Rep. 2022;22(1):39–52. https://doi.org/10.1007/s11892-021-01442-z. Epub 20220203. PubMed PMID: 35113333; PubMed Central PMCID: PMC8888485
22. Salvatore T, Galiero R, Caturano A, Rinaldi L, Di Martino A, Albanese G, et al. An overview of the cardiorenal protective mechanisms of SGLT2 inhibitors. Int J Mol Sci. 2022;23(7) https://doi.org/10.3390/ijms23073651. Epub 20220326. PubMed PMID: 35409011; PubMed Central PMCID: PMC8998569
23. Zheng Z, Zong Y, Ma Y, Tian Y, Pang Y, Zhang C, et al. Glucagon-like peptide-1 receptor: mechanisms and advances in therapy. Signal Transduct Target Ther. 2024;9(1):234. https://doi.org/10.1038/s41392-024-01931-z. Epub 20240918. PubMed PMID: 39289339; PubMed Central PMCID: PMC11408715
24. Nauck MA, Meier JJ. Incretin hormones: their role in health and disease. Diabetes Obes Metab. 2018;20(Suppl 1):5–21. https://doi.org/10.1111/dom.13129. PubMed PMID: 29364588
25. Ma X, Liu Z, Ilyas I, Little PJ, Kamato D, Sahebka A, et al. GLP-1 receptor agonists (GLP-1RAs): cardiovascular actions and therapeutic potential. Int J Biol Sci. 2021;17(8):2050–68. https://doi.org/10.7150/ijbs.59965. Epub 20210511. PubMed PMID: 34131405; PubMed Central PMCID: PMC8193264
26. Rizzo M, Nikolic D, Patti AM, Mannina C, Montalto G, McAdams BS, et al. GLP-1 receptor agonists and reduction of cardiometabolic risk: potential underlying mechanisms. Biochimica et Biophysica Acta (BBA). 2018;1864(9 Pt B):2814–21. https://doi.org/10.1016/j.bbadis.2018.05.012. Epub 20180518. PubMed PMID: 29778663
27. Trujillo JM, Nuffer W, Ellis SL. GLP-1 receptor agonists: a review of head-to-head clinical studies. Ther Adv Endocrinol Metab. 2015;6(1):19–28. https://doi.org/10.1177/2042018814559725. PubMed PMID: 25678953; PubMed Central PMCID: PMC4321870
28. Harrison-Bernard LM. The renal renin-angiotensin system. Adv Physiol Educ. 2009;33(4):270–4. https://doi.org/10.1152/advan.00049.2009. PubMed PMID: 19948673
29. Nádasy GL, Balla A, Dörnyei G, Hunyady L, Szekeres M. Direct vascular effects of angiotensin II (a systematic short review). Int J Mol Sci. 2024;26(1) https://doi.org/10.3390/ijms26010113. Epub 20241226. PubMed PMID: 39795971; PubMed Central PMCID: PMC11719566
30. Patel S, Rauf A, Khan H, Abu-Izneid T. Renin-angiotensin-aldosterone (RAAS): the ubiquitous system for homeostasis and pathologies. Biomed Pharmacother. 2017;94:317–25. https://doi.org/10.1016/j.biopha.2017.07.091. Epub 20170731. PubMed PMID: 28772209
31. Kanugula AK, Kaur J, Batra J, Ankireddypalli AR, Velagapudi R. Renin-angiotensin system: updated understanding and role in physiological and pathophysiological states. Cureus. 2023;15(6):e40725. https://doi.org/10.7759/cureus.40725. Epub 20230621. PubMed PMID: 37350982; PubMed Central PMCID: PMC10283427
32. Messerli FH, Bangalore S, Bavishi C, Rimoldi SF. Angiotensin-converting enzyme inhibitors in hypertension: to use or not to use? J Am Coll Cardiol. 2018;71(13):1474–82. https://doi.org/10.1016/j.jacc.2018.01.058. PubMed PMID: 29598869
33. Brown NJ, Vaughan DE. Angiotensin-converting enzyme inhibitors. Circulation. 1998;97(14):1411–20. https://doi.org/10.1161/01.cir.97.14.1411. PubMed PMID: 9577953
34. Turner JM, Kodali R. Should angiotensin-converting enzyme inhibitors ever be used for the management of hypertension? Curr Cardiol Rep. 2020;22(9):95. https://doi.org/10.1007/s11886-020-01352-8. Epub 20200709. PubMed PMID: 32648000; PubMed Central PMCID: PMC7344347
35. Na Takuathung M, Sakuludomkan W, Khatsri R, Dukaew N, Kraivisitkul N, Ahmadmusa B, et al. Adverse effects of angiotensin-converting enzyme inhibitors in humans: a systematic review and meta-analysis of 378 randomized controlled trials. Int J Environ Res Public Health. 2022;19(14) https://doi.org/10.3390/ijerph19148373. Epub 20220708. PubMed PMID: 35886227; PubMed Central PMCID: PMC9324875

36. Israili ZH. Clinical pharmacokinetics of angiotensin II (AT1) receptor blockers in hypertension. J Hum Hypertens. 2000;14(Suppl 1):S73–86. https://doi.org/10.1038/sj.jhh.1000991. PubMed PMID: 10854085
37. Kuchulakanti PK. ARNI in cardiovascular disease: current evidence and future perspectives. Future Cardiol. 2020;16(5):505–15. https://doi.org/10.2217/fca-2019-0089. Epub 20200422. PubMed PMID: 32319309
38. Volpe M, Rubattu S, Battistoni A. ARNi: a novel approach to counteract cardiovascular diseases. Int J Mol Sci. 2019;20(9) https://doi.org/10.3390/ijms20092092. Epub 20190428. PubMed PMID: 31035359; PubMed Central PMCID: PMC6539682
39. Chrysant SG. Pharmacokinetic, pharmacodynamic, and antihypertensive effects of the neprilysin inhibitor LCZ-696: sacubitril/valsartan. J Am Soc Hypertens. 2017;11(7):461–8. https://doi.org/10.1016/j.jash.2017.04.012. Epub 20170525. PubMed PMID: 28652105
40. Badri S, Dashti-Khavidaki S, Lessan-Pezeshki M, Abdollahi M. A review of the potential benefits of pentoxifylline in diabetic and non-diabetic proteinuria. J Pharm Pharm Sci. 2011;14(1):128–37. https://doi.org/10.18433/j3bp4g. PubMed PMID: 21501559
41. Chen YM, Chiang WC, Lin SL, Tsai TJ. Therapeutic efficacy of pentoxifylline on proteinuria and renal progression: an update. J Biomed Sci. 2017;24(1):84. https://doi.org/10.1186/s12929-017-0390-4. Epub 20171113. PubMed PMID: 29132351; PubMed Central PMCID: PMC5683556

Chapter 18
Comprehensive Management Strategies for Cardiovascular–Kidney–Metabolic Syndrome

Anca Ouatu and Oana Nicoleta Buliga-Finiş

Introduction

Heart failure, chronic kidney disease (CKD), and type 2 diabetes (T2D) are the main components of the cardiovascular–kidney–metabolic syndrome, also known as cardio–renal–metabolic (CRM) syndrome. This condition is a complex and interdependent interaction between the cardiovascular, renal, and metabolic systems [1].

Based on available data, CKM syndrome is a progressive disorder that typically starts early in life when biological, social, and environmental stressors or exposures cause excess and dysfunctional adipose tissue to accumulate, which in turn causes inflammation, oxidative stress, and insulin resistance [2, 3].

Type 2 diabetes, hypertension, hypertriglyceridemia, metabolic syndrome (MetS), and other metabolic risk factors are often preceded by excess and dysfunctional adipose tissue and chronic kidney disease (CKD) [4]. These frequently coexisting comorbidities lead to progressive declines in kidney function, subclinical abnormalities of myocardial structure and function, and subclinical coronary atherosclerosis (represented by coronary artery calcification) over time. These conditions increase the risk of developing clinical cardiovascular disease (CVD), kidney failure, disability, and death. Identifying windows for preventive action in the early stages of CKM syndrome, when patients are often asymptomatic, is crucial.

A. Ouatu · O. N. Buliga-Finiş (✉)
Grigore T. Popa University of Medicine and Pharmacy, Iasi, Romania
e-mail: oana-nicoleta.buliga-finis@umfiasi.ro

M. Floria, D. M. Tanase (eds.), *Cardiovascular-Kidney-Metabolic Syndrome*,
https://doi.org/10.1007/978-3-032-11445-7_18

Additionally, the aggressiveness of preventive measures should be tailored to the absolute risk of CVD and the projected net benefit [5].

There are five stages of CKM syndrome:

- *Stage 0*: Absence of CKM risk factors.
- *Stage 1*: Excess body fat, dysfunctional body fat, or both; hyperglycemia or prediabetes are examples of dysfunctional body fat.
- *Stage 2*: CKD at moderate to high risk, metabolic risk factors, or both.
- *Stage 3*: High projected CVD risk, very high-risk CKD, or subclinical CVD that overlaps with CKM risk factors.
- *Stage 4*: Overlap of risk factors for CKM with clinical CVD. There are two substages under this stage, namely 4a (without renal failure) and 4b (with kidney failure) [6].

Screening

From conception to later adulthood, CVD develops over the course of a person's life, and exposure to risk factors for disease development starts even before conception [2]. Due to the process of genomic imprinting, child cardiometabolic risk factors are impacted by maternal obesity and hypertension during pregnancy [7, 8]. Risk factor reduction, especially the control of hypertension, is associated with slower progression of chronic kidney disease (CKD); in pediatric populations, CKD is associated with the development of CVD risk factors and with increased CVD mortality [9, 10].

Between the ages of 9 and 11 and again between the ages of 17 and 21, a lipid panel should be examined. In addition, individuals who are overweight or obese and at a higher risk of type 2 diabetes or metabolic dysfunction-associated steatotic liver disease should have their impaired glucose tolerance (as measured by hemoglobin A1c (HbA1c), oral glucose tolerance test, or fasting glucose) and alanine aminotransferase evaluated.

According to studies, maintaining optimal cardiovascular health throughout middle age requires continuing healthy lifestyle choices from childhood through young adulthood [11]. Children who participate in school-based programs that encourage physical activity and healthy eating by focusing on students, staff, and families or improving the school environment have been demonstrated to lose weight and have a higher chance of reaching optimal cardiovascular health [12, 13]. Young adults are less likely to develop CKM risk factors, including MetS and prediabetes/diabetes, over time if they avoid gaining weight as they age [14].

Preventing the development of metabolic risk factors in individuals with excess or disordered adiposity is the main goal of the stage 1 approach [15]. Intentional weight loss lowers the risk of metabolic risk factors in people who are overweight in a dose–response manner; benefits are clinically meaningful at ≥5% weight loss [16]. Both bariatric surgery and obesity medications are useful supplements to lifestyle modification; in matched observational studies, bariatric surgery was associated with reduced incidence of cardiovascular disease and death [17, 18]. It is crucial to consider both anthropometric and glycemic measures when evaluating metabolic risk and the need for changing one's lifestyle in order to identify individuals with dysfunctional adiposity even in the absence of elevated anthropometric measures [19].

Preventive Measures

The prevention of obesity by lifestyle adjustment, which includes behavioral and nutritional education as well as the recruitment of the main societal stakeholders, is essential for preventing the great majority of metabolic illnesses [20]. Obesity may be prevented or regressed by a variety of childhood and teenage interventions, such as lifestyle changes imposed through education [21].

It may be possible to further preserve normoglycemia and prevent the emergence of future complications by detecting diabetes early and treating it promptly to keep it stable for as long as possible [22].

Early identification and screening for complications such as CVD, HF, and CKD may allow for the prompt administration of new medications that have been demonstrated to impact the course of the disease and lower mortality, such as glucagon-like peptide-receptor agonists 1 (GLP1-RA) and sodium-glucose co-transporter-2 inhibitors (SGLT2i) [23].

Higher HbA1c levels have been linked to an increased risk of morbidity and mortality in individuals with HF and type 2 diabetes who are not taking glucose-lowering drugs. However, this association might not hold valid once glucose-lowering pharmaceutical treatment has begun. It is important to provide lifestyle guidance on food, exercise, and lowering saturated fat to all individuals with lipid disorders. People with markedly elevated triglyceride levels should also reduce their intake of alcohol and carbohydrates [24].

The implementation of lifestyle adjustments is recommended, including quitting smoking, eating a diet high in fiber and low in saturated fat, engaging in aerobic physical activity, strength training, and getting better sleep [25].

There are various dietary patterns that can be followed, but it is crucial to prioritize fruits, vegetables, whole-grain cereals, and low-fat protein sources. Limiting salt consumption is advised. There are specific recommendations to increase dietary fiber, control carbohydrate intake, and restrict alcohol and saturated and trans fats [26]. Exercise training that combines resistance and aerobic components is useful for controlling glucose levels and preventing the onset of type 2 diabetes. In those with type 2 diabetes, regular moderate-to-intense physical activity improves metabolic management and cardiovascular risk factors [27, 28].

Reaching low-density lipoprotein-cholesterol (LDL-C) and blood-pressure goals is very crucial. Long-term, lifestyle changes reduce mortality and future microvascular and macrovascular hazards. Healthcare professionals and patients should communicate in a personalized way to enhance knowledge and promote lifestyle management and support adherence to medication therapy, thereby optimizing target goals and achieving high levels of adherence [24].

Early Diagnosis

Additionally, the American Heart Association (AHA) CKM framework suggests measuring the albumin–creatinine ratio (ACR) and estimated glomerular filtration rate (eGFR) in the urine of people, who are at risk [29].

The Kidney Disease: Improving Global Outcomes (KDIGO) CKD staging approach states that a wide risk estimate for CKD progression, CVD events, and total death can be obtained by combining the evaluation of albuminuria and eGFR, both of which are associated with changes in pulse pressure (PP) [30].

Furthermore, a higher risk of morbidities including cardiovascular events, renal dysfunction, or metabolic damage may be indicated by an elevated PP (a marker of arterial stiffness) [31, 32]. Age, body mass index (BMI), raised cholesterol, and elevated mean arterial pressure are all highly associated with higher PP. Arterial wall stiffness may be the cause of a rising PP with age. One way to calculate PP, a marker for atherosclerotic diseases, is by subtracting the diastolic blood pressure (DBP) from the systolic blood pressure. The Framingham study shows that PP is a more powerful indicator of coronary heart disease than blood pressure, and a rising PP is also linked to type 2 diabetes [30].

Additionally, according to a study conducted in Japan, PP may be a risk indicator for the progression of CKD [33].

People in *stage 0* have no metabolic, cardiovascular, or renal risk factors, as well as no indications of organ damage. Maintaining a healthy lifestyle is crucial at this stage to prevent the development of risk factors and to halt disease progression.

Patients in *stage 1* have early metabolic risk factors such as dyslipidemia, hypertension, or abdominal obesity. Early identification of these risk factors permits prompt therapies through weight control and lifestyle changes, which eventually decrease renal and cardiovascular disorders.

In *stage 2*, patients may present with resistant hypertension, newly diagnosed diabetes, impaired glucose tolerance, or chronic kidney disease (CKD) with an eGFR of more than 45 mL/min/1.73 m^2. Moreover, metabolic disorders such as hypertriglyceridemia and persistent albuminuria may manifest. At this point, it is recommended to implement comprehensive therapies that focus on blood pressure optimization, cholesterol management, glycemic control, and antialbuminuric treatments.

The hallmark of *stage 3* is subclinical organ dysfunction. eGFR 30–45 mL/min/1.73 m^2, coronary calcification, elevated hs-troponin, elevated brain natriuretic peptide (BNP) and N-terminal proBNP (NT-proBNP) (BNP/NT-proBNP), moderate-to-severe diastolic dysfunction, ejection fraction (EF) $< 50\%$ are among the main findings. A comprehensive approach requires addressing renal, cardiac, and metabolic complications.

The most severe stage of the CKM syndrome is known as *stage 4,* during which patients display overt clinical signs and significant organ damage, such as acute cardiovascular events, end-stage renal disease, or advanced heart failure. The management of this stage requires a complex approach in which the specialist is chosen depending on the patient's main comorbidity [1].

Coordinated Care

According to the advisory, interdisciplinary care can be strengthened by collaborative and comprehensive care strategies, such as value-based and volume-based models, which can help to improve treatment and clinical outcomes for patients with multiple comorbid conditions within CKM syndrome and lessen the fragmentation of current healthcare based on subspecialty "silos." [34, 35].

In order to develop a strategy to address the CKM syndrome that encompasses prevention initiatives, early diagnosis, and treatment along the entire spectrum of the CKM syndrome, coordination between the various scientific societies (primary care, nephrology, cardiology, and endocrinology) as well as patient associations and health authorities is mandatory [36].

By helping patients navigate between various specialists, CKM coordinators can improve primary care physician support and teamwork. The capacity to depend more on telemedicine or the CKM coordinator and interdisciplinary team in health facilities or regions with fewer subspecialists will help address the current disparities in access to subspecialists and lengthy wait times [37]. A synthetic overview of clinical and biological parameters in CKM is presented in Table 18.1.

Table 18.1 Clinical and biological parameters in CKM

CKM stage	Parameters
Stage 0 Stage 1	Blood pressure, waist circumference, ECG, urine tests, creatinine and transaminases, in addition to blood glucose, HbA1c, and lipid profile assessments (HDL included),
Stage 2	eGFR or increased UACR kidney ultrasound, ECG, echocardiography, and BNP/NT proBNP levels; monitoring HbA1c, assessing glucose intolerance, and performing Doppler ultrasound of the lower limbs
Stage 3	Elevated BNP/NT-proBNP or Hs-troponin, carotid atheromas, and ECG abnormalities. N eGFR 30–45 mL/min/1.73 m^2 and/or UACR >300 mg/g.
Stage 4	Advanced renal and cardiovascular disease Frequent monitoring

Treatment

In order to support a value-based approach to guaranteeing high-quality and timely access to CKM care, it is recommended that a multidisciplinary CKM team work with primary care clinicians to provide protocolized guidance for the care of patients with ≥2 overlapping CKM conditions (diabetes, CKD, and advanced subclinical/clinical CVD) (Table 18.2) [5].

Glucose-Reducing Medications

Given the comparable pathophysiologic backgrounds and frequent co-occurrence of T2D, HF, and CKD, treating CMR comorbidities with a holistic therapeutic approach will improve patient outcomes and improve patient health. Numerous clinical trials demonstrate the beneficial effects of new glucose-lowering medications, including glucagon-like peptide 1 receptor agonists (GLP-1 RA) and sodium–glucose cotransporter 2 inhibitors (SGLT2i) [38].

In the context of type 2 diabetes, SGLT2 inhibitors have been demonstrated to lower the risk of significant adverse cardiovascular events and progression of renal disease. Regardless of their glucose-lowering effects, SGLT2i have demonstrated notable blood pressure-lowering effects in patients with type 2 diabetes mellitus (T2DM) and hypertension. According to a recent meta-analysis, SGLT2i lowers DBP by 2.39 mmHg (95% confidence interval (CI): −4.11 to −0.67) and 24-h ambulatory systolic blood pressure (SBP) by 5.06 mmHg (95% CI, −7.10 to −3.01) [39]. Significant SBP reductions of about 12 mmHg were attained in nonobese patients with T2DM and CKD, indicating that baseline renal function and BMI may affect effectiveness [40].

Table 18.2 Medication recommendation across specific population in CKM syndrome

T2D	SGLT2 inhibitor
T2D + ASCVD	SGLT2 inhibitor GLP-1RA PCSK9 inhibitor statin therapy
CKD + T2D	SGLT2 inhibitors nonsteroidal MRA GLP-1 RA RAS inhibitor
HF + T2D	ACE inhibitors/ARBs β-blockers SGLT2 inhibitor
CKD + HF	SGLT2 inhibitor Angiotensin receptor/neprilysin inhibitor nonsteroidal MRA GLP-1 RA

ASCVD atherosclerotic cardiovascular disease, *CKD* chronic kidney disease, *T2D* type 2 diabetes mellitus, *HF* heart failure

An SGLT2 inhibitor or GLP-1RA is recommended for individuals with diabetes and established atherosclerotic cardiovascular disease (ASCVD) to reduce the risk of major adverse cardiovascular events and cardiovascular death. The SGLT2 inhibitor also lowers their chance of hospitalization for heart failure. When deciding between these medications for patients with diabetes and ASCVD, a comorbidity-based strategy is recommended. For people with CKD or concurrent HF, an SGLT2 inhibitor is recommended, and for those with a BMI of 35 kg/m^2, an HbA1c of 9%, or high insulin dosages, a GLP-1RA is advised [41].

Regardless of ejection fraction, diabetes, or baseline urine albumin-to-creatinine ratio (UACR), SGLT2 inhibitors are also advised for all patients with CKD and HF [42, 43].

Given the moderate glucose-lowering benefits of SGLT2 inhibitors, additional antihyperglycemic medications may be required for patients with CKD and diabetes, particularly in the presence of HF, to establish glycemic control [44].

Across the eGFR range, the use of angiotensin receptor/neprilysin inhibitors is likewise linked to a slower deterioration in kidney function and fewer adverse renal events, as well as an incremental improvement in blood pressure control [5].

When compared to placebo, a meta-analysis that investigated how GLP-1RAs affected blood pressure in people with and without type 2 diabetes found that they reduced SBP modestly. The mean difference (MD) for semaglutide was −3.40 mmHg, for liraglutide it was −2.61 mmHg, for dulaglutide it was −1.46 mmHg, and for exenatide it was −3.36 mmHg. Lower glycated hemoglobin levels and BMI were closely associated with lower SBP for semaglutide [45]. Likewise, in patients with T2D and CKD, the selective, nonsteroidal mineralocorticoid receptor antagonist finerenone has demonstrated cardiorenal benefits (Table 18.3) [46, 47]. Finerenone is approved for the treatment of T2D-related CKD (stages 3 and 4 with albuminuria) and has been shown to delay the course of CKD and lower the cardiovascular risk for those with T2D and CKD [48]. Regardless of baseline BMI, finerenone's positive effects on clinical events and symptoms were constant in patients with HF, who had a modestly reduced or preserved ejection fraction. Patients with higher BMI may have a bigger influence on the primary outcome, as suggested by the FINEARTS-HF trial [49]. The combination of finerenone and empagliflozin was associated with decreases in blood pressure and proteinuria in an animal model of organ damage linked to hypertension, indicating a potential extra benefit with both medications [50]. Additionally, the addition of SGLT2 inhibitors may reduce the incidence of finerenone-induced hyperkalemia. Since mineralocorticoid receptor (MR) antagonists have a lower risk of hyperkalemia, the FIDELIO investigation found that no patient receiving concurrent treatment with finerenone and an SGLT2 inhibitor had serum potassium levels greater than 6.0 mmol/L [51]. Balcinrenone, a novel nsMRA, has recently been developed and has demonstrated positive effects on surrogate kidney and heart failure markers [52].

It has been demonstrated that several pharmacological and non-pharmacological strategies provide concurrent metabolic, cardioprotective, and renoprotective advantages, improving patient outcomes along the CaReMe spectrum.

Table 18.3 Main effects of CKM syndrome medications

SGLT2i	Reduces oxidative stress Reduces cardiovascular mortality and morbidity Improves endothelial function Reduces kidney fibrosis
PCSK9i	Reduces MACE No renal toxicity Provides cardiovascular protection
sGCa	Improves renal perfusion Prevents progression of CKD Reduces the accumulation of ROS
GLP-1 RAs	Lowers intraglomerular pressure Promotes weight loss Reduces ROS accumulation Reduces the risk of atherosclerosis Reduces the incidence of MACE
Finerenone	Reduces CKD progression and cardiovascular events in diabetic patients

MACE major adverse cardiovascular events, *ROS* reactive oxigen species, *SGLT2i* sodium–glucose cotransporter 2 inhibitors, *PCSK9i* proprotein convertase Subtilisin/Kexin Type 9 inhibitors, *sGCa* soluble guanylate cyclase activators, *CKD* chronic kidney disease

Weight-Reducing Medications

Losing weight steadily raises the chance of acquiring normoglycemia [53]. Depending on the underlying comorbidities and body mass index (BMI), pharmaceutical and surgical procedures should be considered if lifestyle changes alone are unable to achieve a weight loss of at least 7% [54].

For those with obesity and common CVD, purposeful weight loss ought to be a treatment objective. To improve metabolic risk factor control in patients with CVD and to enhance functional status and quality of life in patients with HF, moderately purposeful weight loss (5–10%) should be the goal [55].

Anti-obesity drugs based on glucagon-like peptide 1 (GLP-1) have transformed obesity treatment due to their capacity to reduce body weight by a significant 15–25% and enhance clinical results, such as lowering cardiovascular events in individuals with obesity and preexisting CVD [56]. GLP-1 RAs and a combined glucose-dependent insulinotropic polypeptide (GIP)/GLP-1 RA reduced A1C levels in obese individuals without diabetes [57, 58].

Phentermine/topiramate does not reduce weight as effectively as GLP-1 RA-based medicines, but it does improve cardiovascular risk factors such as blood pressure and cholesterol. It is possible to experience elevated creatinine, elevated heart rate, and an increased risk of sleep disturbances. In patients with untreated closed-angle glaucoma, phentermine/topiramate should not be used [59].

Blood Pressure-Reducing Medications

There may be a common thread among the elements of metabolic syndrome, as the renin–angiotensin–aldosterone system plays a significant role in the development of high blood pressure and has been linked to the etiology of obesity, dyslipidemia, and insulin resistance [60]. Renin–angiotensin system inhibitors (RASis) lower blood pressure and lower the risk of kidney failure in people with diabetes and albuminuria. They also show some renoprotection in patients with nondiabetic renal disorders that are proteinuric [61].

Managing hypertension should adhere to recognized protocols, which include changing one's lifestyle, implementing a low-sodium, balanced diet, and using medication when necessary [62]. The target blood pressure for both those with and without diabetes is less than 130/80 mm Hg. For added kidney function protection, individuals with CKD and diabetes, who have albuminuria, should take RAAS inhibitors as part of their antihypertensive medication prescription [5]. In order to lower the lifetime risk of ASCVD, HF, and CKD, the goal blood pressure for most individuals with diabetes and cardiorenal risk is less than 130/80 mm Hg, according to several outcome trials. A target blood pressure of less than 120/80 mm Hg is advised for those with chronic kidney disease (CKD), stroke risk, and many elderly patients [63].

LDL-C-Reducing Medications

To further reduce LDL-C, ezetimibe, a cholesterol absorption inhibitor, is frequently used in combination with statins or other non-statin medications. The cardiovascular benefit of baseline statin medication was additive in the Improved Reduction of Outcomes: Vytorin Efficacy International Trial (IMPROVE-IT), particularly for individuals with type 2 diabetes [64–66].

In the case of LDL-C ≥70 mg/dL on maximally tolerated statin therapy, ezetimibe with a PCSK9 inhibitor or another drug may be considered for intensive LDL-lowering therapy. Many people with diabetes and ASCVD fall into the subgroup with very high-risk ASCVD [67].

A class of monoclonal antibodies (such as alirocumab and evolocumab) or small interfering RNA (siRNA) treatments (such as inclisiran) known as proprotein convertase subtilisin/kexin type 9 inhibitors (PCSK9i) lowers LDL-C levels by blocking PCSK9-mediated degradation of LDL receptors [68]. Because CKM patients frequently have a high or extremely high risk of ASCVD, intensive lipid-lowering medication is required [69].

In individuals with severe CKD, statin intolerance, or those who need further LDL-C lowering, PCSK9i provides a well-tolerated and effective alternative [70].

Fibrate therapy (fenofibrate combined with statin therapy) is indicated for marked hypertriglyceridemia (≥500 mg/dL), whereas icosapent ethyl should be considered for moderate hypertriglyceridemia (135–499 mg/dL) [5].

Niacin lowers triglycerides and may lower LDL-C to a moderate extent. When taken with statins, side effects include flushing, pruritus, nausea, rising blood sugar, and perhaps worsened myopathy. Hepatotoxicity can happen, especially in people who use over-the-counter niacin supplements [65].

For patients with CKM syndrome, soluble guanylate cyclase activators (sGCa) offer a potentially effective treatment approach for cardiovascular and renal impairment [71]. sGC activators preserve cellular components such as lipids, proteins, and DNA by lowering the buildup of ROS. These components are essential for preserving the integrity of the kidney and heart tissues. Apart from reducing oxidative stress, sGC activators also control inflammatory reactions by inhibiting the production of pro-inflammatory cytokines such as TNF-α, G-CSF, IL-1α, IL-1β, IL-6, IL-12, IL-17α, and CCL-2. Because patients with CKM have very high levels of these cytokines in their plasma, sGC activators help to minimize the negative consequences of chronic inflammation, including organ failure, fibrosis, and endothelial damage, by reducing inflammatory signaling [72].

Patients with CKM benefit most from sGC activators because they enhance heart function and lessen the burden on the cardiovascular system. Renal perfusion and tubulointerstitial fibrosis are two important pathways linked to kidney disease that are improved by sGC activators [73, 74].

Converging Therapies in CKM Syndrome Stages

Choosing the best therapy for patients with metabolic risk factors, CKD, and CVD requires careful consideration of the disease phenotype, the existence of comorbid disorders, and the anticipated net benefit of treatments, particularly in cases of advanced CKD. The interaction of concomitant diseases, particularly chronic kidney disease (CKD), complicates the treatment of heart failure and necessitates close observation for hyperkalemia [75, 76].

A personalized therapy for each stage of the CKM syndrome is presented in Figs. 18.1, 18.2, 18.3, and 18.4.

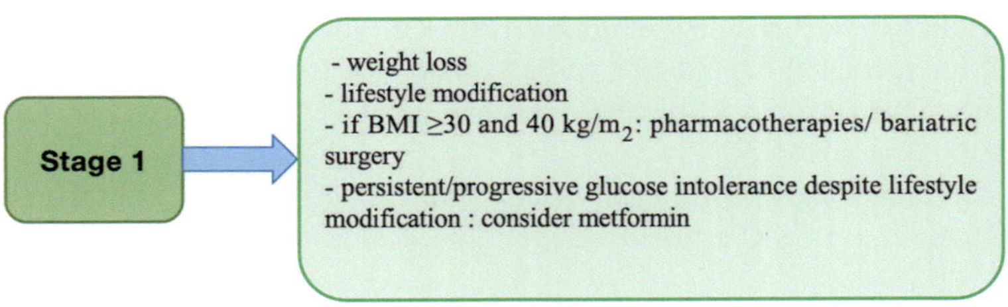

Fig. 18.1 Personalized therapy strategy in stage 1 of CKM

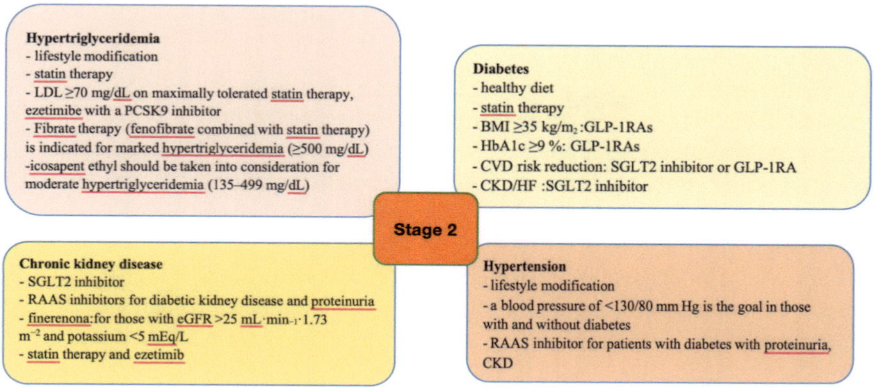

Fig. 18.2 Personalized therapy strategy in stage 2 of CKM

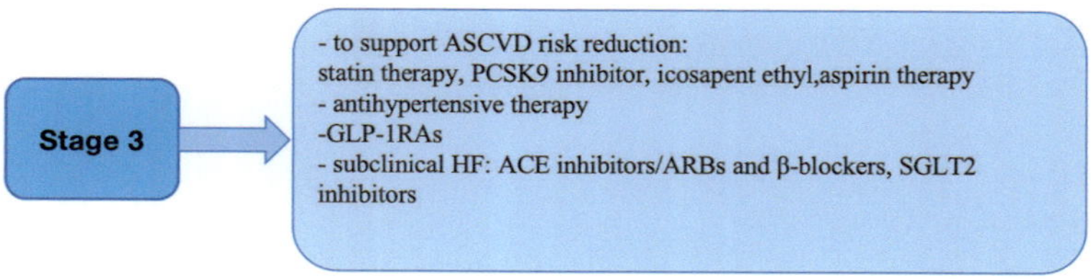

Fig. 18.3 Personalized therapy strategy in stage 3 of CKM

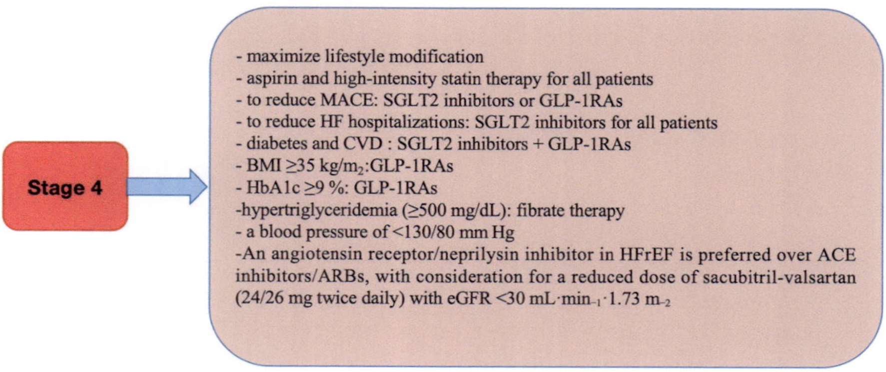

Fig. 18.4 Personalized therapy strategy in stage 4 of CKM

Conclusion

A comprehensive, multidisciplinary strategy that incorporates cardiology, nephrology, and diabetology is mandatory for the effective care of the CKM syndrome, to address the complex interactions between organ dysfunctions. Clinical results can be improved by better coordination between specialists and primary care through a structured, multidisciplinary paradigm backed by shared protocols, telemedicine, and dynamic referral routes.

Improving clinical results and lowering healthcare costs require a shift in the way that we treat cardiorenal metabolic illnesses from fragmented to patient-centered, holistic methods.

Learning Objectives

- Understanding the interaction between cardiorenal syndrome and metabolic disorders in order to maximize treatment modalities.
- Focus on CKM management by adopting a comprehensive and personalized approach, *reducing care fragmentation, and considering interdisciplinary care.*
- Develop strategies for applying combination therapies based on the stages of the CKM syndrome.
- It is essential to *comprehend the relationships between CVD and CKD medications as well as the risk-based application of protective therapeutics* such as SGLT2 inhibitors, GLP-1RAs, and RAAS inhibitors based on CKM.
- Implement strategies that address risk factors identification, screening tools, and lifestyle changes for patients with CKM.

Key Learning

- *A comprehensive strategy for prevention, screening, and management of the CKM syndrome* is necessary to enhance results and lower long-term morbidity and death.
- *New treatments that address the complex characteristics of CKM include* nonsteroidal mineralocorticoid receptor antagonists, SGLT2 inhibitors paired with GLP-1 receptor agonists, and combined GLP-1/GIP receptor agonists.
- *Improving obesity prevention and control* is a clinical and public health goal since obesity is a major contributor to the CKM syndrome.

- Clinical results can be improved by better coordination between specialists and primary care through a structured, *multidisciplinary paradigm backed by shared protocols, telemedicine, and dynamic referral routes.*
- The disease phenotype, the presence of concomitant conditions, and the expected net benefit of treatments must all be carefully considered when *selecting the appropriate course of treatment for patients with metabolic risk factors, CKD, and CVD, especially in cases of advanced CKD.*

References

1. Iacoviello M, Gori M, Grandaliano G, Minutolo R, Pitocco D, Trevisan R. A holistic approach to managing cardio-kidney metabolic syndrome: insights and recommendations from the Italian perspective. Front Cardiovasc Med. 2025;12:1583702. https://doi.org/10.3389/fcvm.2025.1583702.
2. Larque E, Labayen I, Flodmark CE, Lissau I, Czernin S, Moreno LA, Pietrobelli A, Widhalm K. From conception to infancy: early risk factors for childhood obesity. Nat Rev Endocrinol. 2019;15:456–78. https://doi.org/10.1038/s41574-019-0219-1.
3. Brown CL, Halvorson EE, Cohen GM, Lazorick S, Skelton JA. Addressing childhood obesity: opportunities for prevention. Pediatr Clin N Am. 2015;62:1241–61. https://doi.org/10.1016/j.pcl.2015.05.013.
4. Longo M, Zatterale F, Naderi J, Parrillo L, Formisano P, Raciti GA, Beguinot F, Miele C. Adipose tissue dysfunction as determinant of obesity-associated metabolic complications. Int J Mol Sci. 2019;20:2358. https://doi.org/10.3390/ijms20092358.
5. Ndumele CE, et al. A synopsis of the evidence for the science and clinical management of Cardiovascular-Kidney-Metabolic (CKM) syndrome: a scientific statement from the American Heart Association. Circulation. 2023;148(20):1606–35. https://doi.org/10.1161/CIR.0000000000001186.
6. Eknoyan G, Lameire N, Eckardt K, Kasiske B, Wheeler D, Levin A, Stevens PE, Bilous RW, Lamb EJ, Coresh J. KDIGO 2012 clinical practice guideline for the evaluation and management of chronic kidney disease. Kidney Int. 2013;3:5–14. https://doi.org/10.7326/0003-4819-158-11-201306040-00007.
7. Page KA, Luo S, Wang X, Chow T, Alves J, Buchanan TA, Xiang AH. Children exposed to maternal obesity or gestational diabetes mellitus during early fetal development have hypothalamic alterations that predict future weight gain. Diabetes Care. 2019;42:1473–80. https://doi.org/10.2337/dc18-2581.
8. Kang J, Lee CN, Li HY, Hsu KH, Lin SY. Genome-wide DNA methylation variation in maternal and cord blood of gestational diabetes population. Diabetes Res Clin Pract. 2017;132:127–36. https://doi.org/10.1016/j.diabres.2017.07.034.
9. Mitsnefes MM. Cardiovascular disease in children with chronic kidney disease. J Am Soc Nephrol. 2012;23:578–85. https://doi.org/10.1681/ASN.2011111115.
10. ESCAPE Trial Group, Wuhl E, Trivelli A, Picca S, Litwin M, Peco-Antic A, Zurowska A, Testa S, Jankauskiene A, Emre S, Caldas-Afonso A, et al. Strict blood-pressure control and progression of renal failure in children. N Engl J Med. 2009;361:1639–50. https://doi.org/10.1056/NEJMoa0902066.
11. Lloyd-Jones DM, Allen NB, Anderson CAM, Black T, brewer LC, Foraker RE, Grandner MA, Lavretsky H, Perak AM, Sharma G, On behalf of the American Heart Association, et al. Life's essential 8: updating and enhancing the American Heart Association's construct of car-

diovascular health: a presidential advisory from the American Heart Association. Circulation. 2022;146:e18–43. https://doi.org/10.1161/CIR.0000000000001078.

12. Guo P, Zhou Y, Zhu Y. Effects of a school-based lifestyle intervention on ideal cardiovascular health in Chinese children and adolescents: a national, multicentre, cluster-randomised controlled trial. Lancet Glob Health. 2023;11:S14. https://doi.org/10.1016/S2214-109X(23)00097-9.
13. Waters E, de Silva-Sanigorski A, Hall BJ, Brown T, Campbell KJ, Gao Y, Armstrong R, Prosser L, Summerbell CD. Interventions for preventing obesity in children. Cochrane Database Syst Rev. 2011;7(7):CD001871. https://doi.org/10.1002/14651858.CD001871.pub3.
14. Lloyd-Jones DM, Liu K, Colangelo LA, Yan LL, Klein L, Loria CM, Lewis CE, Savage P. Consistently stable or decreased body mass index in young adulthood and longitudinal changes in metabolic syndrome components: the coronary artery risk development in young adults study. Circulation. 2007;115:1004–11. https://doi.org/10.1161/CIRCULATIONAHA.106.648642.
15. Gudzune KA, Bennett WL, Cooper LA, Bleich SN. Perceived judgment about weight can negatively influence weight loss: a cross-sectional study of overweight and obese patients. Prev Med. 2014;62:103–7. https://doi.org/10.1016/j.ypmed.2014.02.001.
16. Look AHEAD Research Group, pi-Sunyer X, Blackburn G, Brancati FL, bray GA, bright R, Clark JM, Curtis JM, Espeland MA, Foreyt JP, graves K, et al. reduction in weight and cardiovascular disease risk factors in individuals with type 2 diabetes: one-year results of the Look AHEAD trial. Diabetes Care. 2007;30:1374–83. https://doi.org/10.2337/dc07-0048.
17. Sjostrom L, Peltonen M, Jacobson P, Sjostrom CD, Karason K, Wedel H, Ahlin S, Anveden A, Bengtsson C, Bergmark G, et al. Bariatric surgery and long-term cardiovascular events. JAMA. 2012;307:56–65. https://doi.org/10.1001/jama.2011.1914.
18. Bethel MA, Patel RA, Merrill P, Lokhnygina Y, Buse JB, Mentz RJ, Pagidipati NJ, Chan JC, Gustavson SM, Iqbal N, et al. Cardiovascular outcomes with glucagon-like peptide-1 receptor agonists in patients with type 2 diabetes: a meta-analysis. Lancet Diabetes Endocrinol. 2018;6:105–13. https://doi.org/10.1016/S2213-8587(17)30412-6.
19. Ross R, Neeland IJ, Yamashita S, Shai I, Seidell J, Magni P, Santos RD, Arsenault B, Cuevas A, Hu FB, et al. Waist circumference as a vital sign in clinical practice: a consensus statement from the IAS and ICCR working group on visceral obesity. Nat Rev Endocrinol. 2020;16:177–89. https://doi.org/10.1038/s41574-019-0310-7.
20. Kristensen SL, Rørth R, Jhund PS, et al. Cardiovascular, mortality, and kidney outcomes with GLP-1 receptor agonists in patients with type 2 diabetes: a systematic review and meta-analysis of cardiovascular outcome trials. Lancet Diabetes Endocrinol. 2019. Oct;7(10):776–85. https://doi.org/10.1016/S2213-8587(19)30249-9.
21. Lancet Diabetes Endocrinol. 2022;10(7):488–8.
22. Laiteerapong N, Ham SA, Gao Y, et al. The legacy effect in type 2 diabetes: impact of early control on future complications (The Diabetes & Aging Study). Diabetes Care. 2019;42(3):416–26. https://doi.org/10.2337/dc17-1144.
23. Mosenzon O, Del Prato S, Schechter M, et al. From glucose lowering agents to disease/diabetes modifying drugs: a "SIMPLE" approach for the treatment of type 2 diabetes. Cardiovasc Diabetol. 2021;20(1):92. https://doi.org/10.1186/s12933-021-01281-y.
24. Ibrahim M, et al. Cardio-renal-metabolic disease in primary care setting. Diabetes Metab Res Rev. 2024;40(3):e3755. https://doi.org/10.1002/dmrr.3755.
25. Marx N, Federici M, Schütt K, ESC Scientific Document Group, et al. 2023 ESC Guidelines for the management of cardiovascular disease in patients with diabetes. Eur Heart J. 2023;44:ehad192. https://doi.org/10.1093/eurheartj/ehad192.
26. Estruch R, Ros E, Salas-Salvadó J, PREDIMED Study Investigators, et al. Primary prevention of cardiovascular disease with a Mediterranean diet. N Engl J Med. 2013;368(14):1279–90. https://doi.org/10.1056/NEJMoa1200303. Epub 2013. Feb 25. Retraction in: N Engl J Med. 2018 Jun 21;378(25):2441–2442. Erratum in: N Engl J Med. 2014 Feb 27;370(9):886. Corrected and republished in: N Engl J Med. 2018 Jun 21;378(25):e34

27. Sluik D, Buijsse B, Muckelbauer R, et al. Physical activity and mortality in individuals with diabetes mellitus: a prospective study and meta-analysis. Arch Intern Med. 2012;172(17):1285–95. https://doi.org/10.1001/archinternmed.2012.3130.
28. Wahid A, Manek N, Nichols M, et al. Quantifying the association between physical activity and cardiovascular disease and diabetes: a systematic review and meta-analysis. J Am Heart Assoc. 2016;5(9):e002495. https://doi.org/10.1161/JAHA.115.002495.
29. Bansal N, Weiner D, Sarnak M. Cardiovascular-kidney-metabolic health syndrome: what does the American Heart Association framework mean for nephrology? J Am Soc Nephrol. 2024;35:649–52. https://doi.org/10.1681/ASN.0000000000000323.
30. Ahmed MJ, Ali O, Ahmed A, Omar W, Ahmed K. The effect of cardiovascular–kidney–metabolic disease on pulse pressure in patients with type II diabetes. J Curr Cardiol. 2025;3(1):25–31. https://doi.org/10.4103/JCC.JCC_2_25.
31. Geng TT, Talaei M, Jafar TH, Yuan JM, Koh WP. Pulse pressure and the risk of end-stage renal disease among Chinese adults in Singapore: the Singapore Chinese Health Study. J Am Heart Assoc. 2019;8:e013282. https://doi.org/10.1161/JAHA.119.013282.
32. Domanski M, Norman J, Wolz M, Mitchell G, Pfeffer M. Cardiovascular risk assessment using pulse pressure in the first national health and nutrition examination survey (NHANES I). Hypertension. 2001;38:793–7. https://doi.org/10.1161/hy1001.092966.
33. Maeda T, Yokota S, Nishi T, Funakoshi S, Tsuji M, Satoh A, et al. Association between pulse pressure and progression of chronic kidney disease. Sci Rep. 2021;11:23275. https://doi.org/10.1038/s41598-021-02809-8.
34. Porter ME, Teisberg EO. How physicians can change the future of health care. JAMA. 2007;297:1103–11. https://doi.org/10.1001/jama.297.10.1103.
35. Handelsman Y, Anderson JE, Bakris GL, Ballantyne CM, Beckman JA, Bhatt DL, et al. DCRM multispecialty practice recommendations for the management of diabetes, cardiorenal, and metabolic diseases. J Diabetes Complicat. 2022;36:155931. https://doi.org/10.1016/j.jdiacomp.2021.108101.
36. Cases A, Broseta JJ, Marquésc M, Cigarráne S, Julián JC, Alcázar R, Ortiz A. Cardiovascular-kidney-metabolic syndrome definition and its role in the prevention, risk staging, and treatment. An opportunity for the Nephrology. Nefrologia. 2024;44(6):771–83. https://doi.org/10.1016/j.nefroe.2024.11.011.
37. Patel RB, Al Rifai M, McEvoy JW, Vaduganathan M. Implications of specialist density for diabetes care in the United States. JAMA Cardiol. 2019;4:1174–5. https://doi.org/10.1001/jamacardio.2019.3796.
38. Marassi M, Fadini GP. The cardio-renal-metabolic connection: a review of the evidence. Cardiovasc Diabetol. 2023;22:195. https://doi.org/10.1186/s12933-023-01937-x.
39. Wilding JPH, Batterham RL, Davies M, Van Gaal LF, Kandler K, Konakli K, Lingvay I, McGowan BM, Oral TK, Rosenstock J, et al. Weight regain and cardiometabolic effects after withdrawal of Semaglutide: the STEP 1 trial extension. Diabetes Obes Metab. 2022;24:1553–64. https://doi.org/10.1111/dom.14725.
40. Shiina K. Who benefits from the blood pressure-lowering effects of SGLT2 inhibitors in patients with type 2 diabetes mellitus and chronic kidney disease?—obese or non-obese? Hypertens Res. 2024;47:681–2. https://doi.org/10.1038/s41440-023-01543-0.
41. ElSayed NA, Aleppo G, Aroda VR, Bannuru RR, Brown FM, Bruemmer D, Collins BS, Das SR, Hilliard ME, Isaacs D, et al. 10: cardiovascular disease and risk management: standards of care in diabetes–2023. Diabetes Care. 2023;46:S158–90. https://doi.org/10.2337/dc23-S010.
42. Nuffield Department of Population Health Renal Studies Group; SGLT2 inhibitor Meta-Analysis Cardio-Renal Trialists' Consortium. Impact of diabetes on the effects of sodium glucose co-transporter-2 inhibitors on kidney outcomes: collaborative meta-analysis of large placebo-controlled trials. Lancet. 2022;400:1788–801. https://doi.org/10.1016/S0140-6736(22)02074-8.

43. Vaduganathan M, Docherty KF, Claggett BL, Jhund PS, de Boer RA, Hernandez AF, Inzucchi SE, Kosiborod MN, Lam CSP, Martinez F, et al. SGLT-2 inhibitors in patients with heart failure: a comprehensive meta-analysis of five randomised controlled trials. Lancet. 2022;400:757–67. https://doi.org/10.1016/S0140-6736(22)01429-5.
44. Tuttle KR, Lakshmanan MC, Rayner B, Busch RS, Zimmermann AG, Woodward DB, Botros FT. Dulaglutide versus insulin glargine in patients with type 2 diabetes and moderate-to-severe chronic kidney disease (AWARD-7): a multicentre, open-label, randomised trial. Lancet Diabetes Endocrinol. 2018;6:605–17. https://doi.org/10.1016/S2213-8587(18)30104-9.
45. Rivera FB, Lumbang GNO, Gaid DRM, Cruz LLA, Magalong JV, Bantayan NRB, Lara-Breitinger KM, Gulati M, Bakris G. Glucagon-like Peptide-1 receptor agonists modestly reduced blood pressure among patients with and without diabetes mellitus: a meta-analysis and meta-regression. Diabetes Obes Metab. 2024;26:2209–28. https://doi.org/10.1111/dom.15529.
46. Bakris GL, Agarwal R, Anker SD, Pitt B, Ruilope LM, Rossing P, et al. Effect of finerenone on chronic kidney disease outcomes in type 2 diabetes. N Engl J Med. 2020;383:2219–29. https://doi.org/10.1056/NEJMoa2025845.
47. Pitt B, Filippatos G, Agarwal R, Anker SD, Bakris GL, Rossing P, et al. Cardiovascular events with Finerenone in kidney disease and type 2 diabetes. N Engl J Med. 2021;385:2252–63. https://doi.org/10.1056/NEJMoa2110956.
48. González-Juanatey JR, Górriz JL, Ortiz A, Valle A, Soler MJ, Facila L. Cardiorenal benefits of finerenone: protecting kidney and heart. Ann Med. 2023 Dec;55(1):502–13. https://doi.org/10.1080/07853890.2023.2171110.
49. Butt JH, Henderson AD, Jhund PS, Claggett BL, Desai AS, Lay-Flurrie J, Viswanathan P, Lage A, Scheerer MF, Lam CSP, Senni M, Shah SJ, Voors AA, Bauersachs J, Fonseca C, Kosiborod MN, Linssen GCM, Petrie MC, Schou M, Verma S, Zannad F, Pitt B, Vaduganathan M, Solomon SD, McMurray JJV. Finerenone, obesity, and heart failure with mildly reduced/preserved ejection fraction: prespecified analysis of FINEARTS-HF. J Am Coll Cardiol. 2025;85(2):140–55. https://doi.org/10.1016/j.jacc.2024.10.111.
50. Kolkhof P, Hartmann E, Freyberger A, Pavkovic M, Mathar I, Sandner P, et al. Effects of finerenone combined with empagliflozin in a model of hypertension-induced end-organ damage. Am J Nephrol. 2021;52:642–52. https://doi.org/10.1159/000516213.
51. Jose Luis G, José Ramón G-J, Lorenzo F, Maria Jose S, Alfonso V, Alberto O. Finerenone: towards a holistic therapeutic approach to patients with diabetic kidney disease. Nefrologia. 2023;43(4):386–98. https://doi.org/10.1016/j.nefroe.2023.09.002.
52. Lam CSP, Køber L, Kuwahara K, Lund LH, Mark PB, Mellbin LG, et al. Balcinrenone plus dapaglifozin in patients with heart failure and chronic kidney disease: results from the phase 2b MIRACLE trial. Eur J Heart Fail. 2024;26(8):1727–35. https://doi.org/10.1002/ejhf.3294.
53. Sallar A, Dagogo-Jack S. Regression from prediabetes to normal glucose regulation: state of the science. Exp Biol Med (Maywood). 2020;245(10):889–96. https://doi.org/10.1177/1535370220915644.
54. American Diabetes Association Professional Practice Committee. Obesity and weight management for the prevention and treatment of type 2 diabetes: standards of care in diabetes—2024. Diabetes Care. 2024;47:S145–s57. https://doi.org/10.2337/dc24-S008.
55. McDowell K, Petrie MC, Raihan NA, Logue J. Effects of intentional weight loss in patients with obesity and heart failure: a systematic review. Obes Rev. 2018;19:1189–204. https://doi.org/10.1111/obr.12707.
56. Lincoff AM, Brown-Frandsen K, Colhoun HM, Deanfield J, Emerson SS, Esbjerg S, et al. Semaglutide and cardiovascular outcomes in obesity without diabetes. N Engl J Med. 2023;389:2221–32. https://doi.org/10.1056/NEJMoa2307563.
57. Jastreboff AM, Aronne LJ, Ahmad NN, Wharton S, Connery L, Alves B, et al. Tirzepatide once weekly for the treatment of obesity. N Engl J Med. 2022;387:205–16. https://doi.org/10.1056/NEJMoa2206038.

58. Perreault L, Davies M, Frias JP, Laursen PN, Lingvay I, Machineni S, et al. Changes in glucose metabolism and glycemic status with once-weekly subcutaneous semaglutide 2.4 mg among participants with prediabetes in the STEP program. Diabetes Care. 2022;45:2396–405. https://doi.org/10.1016/j.metabol.2024.155931.
59. Chakhtoura M, Haber R, Ghezzawi M, Rhayem C, Tcheroyan R, Mantzoros CS. Pharmacotherapy of obesity: an update on the available medications and drugs under investigation. EClinicalMedicine. 2023;58:101882. https://doi.org/10.1016/j.eclinm.2023.101882.
60. Putnam K, Shoemaker R, Yiannikouris F. The renin-angiotensin system: a target of and contributor to dyslipidemias, altered glucose homeostasis, and hypertension of the metabolic syndrome. Am J Physiol Heart Circ Physiol. 2012;302:H1219–30. https://doi.org/10.1152/ajpheart.00796.2011.
61. Zhu D, Judge PK, Wanner C, Haynes R, Herrington WG. The prevention and management of chronic kidney disease among patients with metabolic syndrome. Kidney Int. 2025;107:816–24. https://doi.org/10.1016/j.kint.2024.12.021.
62. Whelton PK, Carey RM, Aronow WS, Casey DE, Collins KJ, Dennison Himmelfarb C, DePalma SM, Gidding S, Jamerson KA, Jones DW, et al. 2017 ACC/AHA/AAPA/ABC/ACPM/AGS/APhA/ASH/ASPC/NMA/PCNA guideline for the prevention, detection, evaluation, and management of high blood pressure in adults: a report of the American College of Cardiology/American Heart Association Task Force on Clinical Practice Guidelines. Circulation. 2018;138:e484–594. https://doi.org/10.1161/HYP.0000000000000066.
63. Handelsman Y, et al. Early intervention and intensive management of patients with diabetes, cardiorenal, and metabolic diseases. J Diabetes Complications. 2023;37:108389. https://doi.org/10.1016/j.jdiacomp.2022.108389.
64. Grundy SM, Stone NJ, Bailey AL, Beam C, Birtcher KK, Blumenthal RS, et al. 2018 AHA/ACC/AACVPR/AAPA/ABC/ACPM/ADA/AGS/APhA/ASPC/NLA/PCNA guideline on the management of blood cholesterol: a report of the American College of Cardiology/American Heart Association task force on clinical practice guidelines. J Am Coll Cardiol. 2019;73(24):e285–350. https://doi.org/10.1016/j.jacc.2018.11.002.
65. Handelsman Y, Jellinger PS, Guerin CK, Bloomgarden ZT, Brinton EA, Budoff MJ, et al. Consensus statement by the American Association of Clinical Endocrinologists and American College of endocrinology on the management of dyslipidemia and prevention of cardiovascular disease algorithm—2020 executive summary. Endocr Pract. 2020;26:1196–224. https://doi.org/10.1016/j.jdiacomp.2021.108101.
66. Cannon CP, Blazing MA, Giugliano RP, McCagg A, White JA, Theroux P, et al. Ezetimibe added to statin therapy after acute coronary syndromes. N Engl J Med. 2015;372:2387–97. https://doi.org/10.1016/j.dib.2016.04.059.
67. Visseren FLJ, Mach F, Smulders YM, Carballo D, Koskinas KC, Back M, Benetos A, Biffi A, Boavida JM, Capodanno D, et al. 2021 ESC guidelines on cardiovascular disease prevention in clinical practice. Eur Heart J. 2021;42:3227–337. https://doi.org/10.1093/eurheartj/ehab484.
68. Kheirkhah A, Lamina C, Kollerits B, Schachtl-Riess JF, Schultheiss UT, Forer L, Sekula P, Kotsis F, Eckardt KU, Kronenberg F, et al. PCSK9 and cardiovascular disease in individuals with moderately decreased kidney function. Clin J Am Soc Nephrol. 2022;17:809–18. https://doi.org/10.2215/CJN.01230122.
69. Quagliariello V, Bisceglia I, Berretta M, Iovine M, Canale ML, Maurea C, Giordano V, Paccone A, Inno A, Maurea N. PCSK9 inhibitors in cancer patients treated with immune-checkpoint inhibitors to reduce cardiovascular events: new frontiers in cardioncology. Cancers. 2023;15:1397. https://doi.org/10.3390/cancers15051397.
70. Amaro JM, Villanego F, Naranjo J, Orellana C, Vigara LA, Narváez CE, Torrado J, Cazorla JM, Rodríguez C, Mazuecos A. Treatment with PCSK9 inhibitors in patients with chronic kidney disease at very high cardiovascular risk. Nefrologia. 2023;43(Suppl. S2):133–5. https://doi.org/10.1016/j.nefroe.2024.01.015.

71. Liu R, Kang Y, Chen L. Activation mechanism of human soluble guanylate cyclase by stimulators and activators. Nat Commun. 2021;12:5492. https://doi.org/10.1038/s41467-021-25617-0.
72. Quagliariello V, Berretta M, Bisceglia I, Giacobbe I, Iovine M, Barbato M, Maurea C, Canale ML, Paccone A, Inno A, et al. In the era of cardiovascular–kidney–metabolic syndrome in cardio-oncology: from pathogenesis to prevention and therapy. Cancer. 2025;17(7):1169. https://doi.org/10.3390/cancers17071169.
73. Viswanathan T, Lang CC, Petty RD, Baxter MA. Cardiotoxicity and chemotherapy-the role of precision medicine. Diseases. 2021;9:90. https://doi.org/10.3390/diseases9040090.
74. Reinhart GA, Harrison PC, Lincoln K, Chen H, Sun P, Hill J, Qian HS, McHugh MC, Clifford H, Ng KJ, et al. The novel, clinical-stage soluble guanylate cyclase activator BI 685509 protects from disease progression in models of renal injury and disease. J Pharmacol Exp Ther. 2023;384:382–92. https://doi.org/10.1124/jpet.122.001423.
75. de Boer IH, Khunti K, Sadusky T, Tuttle KR, Neumiller JJ, Rhee CM, Rosas SE, Rossing P, Bakris G. Diabetes management in chronic kidney disease: a consensus report by the American Diabetes Association (ADA) and Kidney Disease: Improving Global outcomes (KDIGO). Diabetes Care. 2022;45:3075–90. https://doi.org/10.2337/dci22-0027.
76. Mullens W, Martens P, Testani JM, Tang WHW, Skouri H, Verbrugge FH, Fudim M, Iacoviello M, Franke J, Flammer AJ, et al. Renal effects of guideline-directed medical therapies in heart failure: a consensus document from the heart failure Association of the European Society of cardiology. Eur J Heart Fail. 2022;24:603–19. https://doi.org/10.1002/ejhf.2471.

Chapter 19
Multidisciplinary Team Approaches and Future Perspectives for Cardiovascular–Kidney–Metabolic Syndrome

Anca Ouatu and Oana Nicoleta Buliga-Finiş

Introduction

The cardiovascular-kidney-metabolic (CKM) syndrome is a growing, complex disorder characterized by the interaction of chronic heart disease, chronic kidney disease, and metabolic disorders, most notably diabetes mellitus (DM) and obesity, which often coexist and mutually potentiate each other [1].

This continuum of related conditions has a steadily increasing prevalence that is closely related to the global rise in type 2 DM and CVD risk factors. Recent reports indicate that up to 50% of patients with type 2 diabetes mellitus present with three or more components of the cardiovascular-kidney-metabolic syndrome, underlining both the clinical magnitude and the heterogeneity of this pathophysiological condition [2].

The presence of cardiovascular comorbidities (e.g., ischemic heart disease, heart failure, arterial hypertension), and/or chronic kidney disease, and concomitantly presented metabolic disturbances (i.e., hyperglycemia, dyslipidemia), forms a vicious pathogenic interplay. It exhibits a vicious cycle of positive mutual amplification: metabolic dysfunction accelerates atherosclerosis and renal impairment, but the damage to the heart and kidney aggravates metabolic disorder and the risk of cardiovascular disease [3].

Without targeted intervention, this heterogeneous clinical condition leads to significant morbidity and mortality. Hence, an inclusive model of close collaboration across disciplines needs to be established, one that represents the CKM syndrome in all its diversity and allows both preventive measures and treatment concepts to be realized [4].

A. Ouatu · O. N. Buliga-Finiş (✉)
Grigore T. Popa University of Medicine and Pharmacy, Iasi, Romania
e-mail: oana-nicoleta.buliga-finis@umfiasi.ro

M. Floria, D. M. Tanase (eds.), *Cardiovascular-Kidney-Metabolic Syndrome*,
https://doi.org/10.1007/978-3-032-11445-7_19

The Role of the Multidisciplinary Team in CKM Syndrome

The complex profile of patients with the CKM syndrome, which presents with simultaneous cardiac, renal, and metabolic disorders, requires a close team effort between the different medical specialties. According to the available guidelines, the multidisciplinary team consists of a cardiologist, nephrologist, endocrinologist/diabetologist, nutritionist/dietitian, general practitioner, specialized nurse, clinical pharmacist, and other healthcare professionals (e.g., physiotherapist, psychologist) [5].

The individual role of each member in the multidisciplinary team is unique within the integrated approach to the CKM syndrome. The cardiologist directs management of systolic or diastolic dysfunction, coronary artery disease, and hypertension to ensure that hemodynamics are improved and major cardiovascular events are avoided. The nephrologist follows the renal function, adjusts pharmacotherapy according to the estimated GFR (eGFR), treats albuminuria, and intervenes to prevent progression to advanced stages of chronic kidney disease (CKD) and avoid the need for renal replacement therapy. The diabetologist/endocrinologist considers the optimal management of glycemia, weight, and lipids with therapy tailored to include medications with established cardiovascular and renal benefits. The nutritionist adjusts personalized diet plans taking into account the disease stage and associated illnesses, while the general practitioner secures the continuity of care, periodically monitors risk factors, and integrates both primary and secondary prevention. This combined approach allows therapeutic decisions that take into account potential effects on individual target organs [3].

In CKM syndrome management, there have been many cases where patient-oriented comprehensive care, in a variety of fields, has been recommended by clinical guidelines; however, integrating this type of care has been difficult to accomplish. This multidisciplinary approach is especially important for the advanced-stage patients, where the risk of complications is significantly higher. In contrast, the traditional model of care, where specializations operate independently, results in treatment lags, gaps, omissions, and underuse of evidence-based services. For instance, the cardiovascular and renal benefits of SGLT2 inhibitors and GLP-1 receptor agonists are convincingly established; yet, fewer than 20% of individuals with type 2 diabetes and atherosclerotic cardiovascular disease are treated with these agents in usual care. Such an unwarranted gap, at least in part, reflects the absence of successful inter-specialty collaborations and emphasizes the requirement for a "unified-care" model for addressing all CKM elements [6].

Multi-institutional care paradigms for the CKM syndrome differ in international practice depending on clinical and organizational conditions. Some centers have developed specialized units in which patients are seen by several specialists in a single clinical visit and therapeutic decisions are made through joint decision-making. Other facilities have interdisciplinary clinical committees that meet to discuss difficult cases and develop comprehensive treatment plans. In certain healthcare organizations, care coordination is managed by navigational personnel, who follow patient trajectories and facilitate inter-specialty cooperation [5].

Regardless of the model, good communication between specialists and a patient-centered approach that includes biological, psychosocial, and functional dimensions is crucial. This approach has demonstrated benefits in clinical outcomes and quality of care, while also optimizing costs for health institutions by lowering complications and readmissions. Accordingly, the multidisciplinary team assumes a central role in current CKM syndrome care, determining a comprehensive, individualized, and sustainable care model for complex patients [7].

Prevention and Risk Stratification in CKM Syndrome

As the CKM syndrome is progressive and cumulative, interventions need to be implemented as early as possible and sustained over the individual's lifetime. Prevention should, ideally, start in childhood and adolescence because a healthy lifestyle adopted during these periods can substantially reduce the risk of obesity and, consequently, minimize the future burden of diabetes and cardiovascular disease [8].

Healthy nutrition education in schools and encouragement of physical activity during childhood and adolescence with the involvement of families and communities is a fundamental aspect of primary prevention for obesity and metabolic syndrome in the general population. The available data indicate that primordial prevention (prevention of the development of risk factors) even has the potential to reverse early obesity among young people, with beneficial long-term effects. Hence, lifestyle preventive activities may be focused on the young population and may have a crucial effect not only on the incidence of the CKM syndrome, but also on the burden it will place on society in the coming decades [8].

Among young and middle-aged adults, prevention emphasizes the early detection of cardio-metabolic risk factors and presymptomatic phases of disease. In primary care, blood pressure monitoring and measurement of glycemic and lipid profiles, together with body mass index (BMI) review will lead to the early diagnosis of hypertension, prediabetes, dyslipidemia, and obesity, all of which represent factors associated to an increased chance of developing a CKM syndrome. All patients with DM should have annual renal evaluation using the estimated glomerular filtration rate (eGFR) and urinary albumin–creatinine ratio (UACR), according to international guidelines. However, the application of these guidelines is modest at best [9].

Recent research results show that only approximately 58% of the diabetic population in the United States are screened for their renal function every year, with similar figures reported for Europe (57% in the Netherlands and at levels as low as 29% in France) [10, 11]. This low rate of screening simply highlights the importance of strengthening the secondary prevention by facilitating early detection of subclinical complications. Even mild renal dysfunction is associated with an elevated risk of death and major cardiovascular events. In patients with DM, the early onset of CKD is linked to a reduction in life expectancy by up to 16 years—an impact that may exceed that of myocardial infarction. Thus, the early recognition of target organ impairment, particularly heart and kidney damage in individuals with high metabolic risk, is a pivotal point in the clinical care of the CKM syndrome [11].

After the determination of risk profiles or the presence of early-stage disease, patient stratification based on the intensity of CKM components is critical for matching the intensity of therapeutic interventions. Four phases of CKM syndrome progression can be recognized that may help in guiding clinical practice:

- **Stage 1** (initial stage): Early accumulation of metabolic risk factors (e.g., metabolic syndrome, prediabetes) without evidence of target organ damage.
- **Stage 2** (subclinical stage): It refers to early evidence of organ damage, which includes microalbuminuria, mildly decreased eGFR, left-ventricular hypertrophy, or subclinical atherosclerosis.
- **Stage 3** (clinical-stage): This stage involves the presence of established cardiometabolic disease, such as diagnosed type 2 diabetes, persisting hypertension, stage 3 chronic kidney disease, and stable coronary artery disease.
- **Stage 4** (end stage): This represents major multiorgan failure, including end-stage heart failure, stage 4–5 CKD, the requirement for dialysis, and concurrent multiple macrovascular and microvascular complications.

This staging system allows individualized treatment (Table 19.1).

Early care is focused on aggressive lifestyle modification and tight risk factor management. As the disease progresses, multimodal therapy, including specific pharmacologic treatments as well as interventional procedures, is required in specific patients [12]. In this context, European guidelines suggest that patients at very high cardiovascular risk, including those with concomitant established atherosclerotic cardiovascular disease, diabetics, and those with chronic kidney disease, should reach a target of LDL-cholesterol level <55 mg/dL (~1.4 mmol/L) with at least a 50% decrease from baseline LDL-cholesterol levels. For those with frequent cardiovascular events within a short period of time, an LDL goal of <40 mg/dL might be appropriate [13]. Similarly, blood pressure management in patients with diabetes and renal insufficiency should target blood pressure levels <130/80 mmHg, and the therapeutic goal for HbA1c should be ~7%, individualized according to patient characteristics and hypoglycemia risk. These examples illustrate the importance of CKM syndrome stratification in the clinical setting because the degree of intervention invasiveness and complexity should be placed in relation to the overall severity of cardio-renal and metabolic impairment [14].

After the first diagnosis, such patients require life-long surveillance by established protocols as they refer to third prevention in order to stop further progression of the disease or avoid any further complications. CKM syndrome patients should have regular clinical and laboratory assessments, depending on the stage of the disease and the patient's risk. For example, a patient with diabetes and early nephropathy should have blood pressure, glucose/HbA1c, lipid profile, and renal function

Table 19.1 Suggested treatment approaches for cardiovascular-kidney-metabolic syndrome based on disease progression

CKM Stage	Clinical description	Pharmacological treatment	Nutritional therapy	Microbiota-targeted therapies
Stage 1 (incipient)	Metabolic risk factors present (metabolic syndrome, prediabetes), without organ involvement	Possibly statins at high risk	Mediterranean, DASH, Nordic, plant-based diet Promoting a healthy lifestyle from childhood	Diet rich in prebiotic fibers (fruits, vegetables, whole grains) Preventing dysbiosis by avoiding dietary imbalances
Stage 2 (subclinic)	Early-stage structural lesions (microalbuminuria, eGFR ↓, LVH, subclinical atherosclerosis)	Statins Blood pressure and HbA1c control ACEi/ARB (with nephroprotective role)	Cardio-metabolic validated diets Monitoring salt, saturated fat and sugar intake	Diet rich in fermentable fibers Stimulating the growth of beneficial bacteria (e.g., Lactobacillus, Bifidobacterium) through a diet rich in plant-based fiber
Stage 3 (manifest)	Established clinical condition (T2DM, HTN, stage 3 CKD, stable coronary artery disease)	SGLT2 inhibitors GLP-1 agonists Statins ± ezetimibe/PCSK9i ACEi/ARBs Finerenone (nonsteroidal MRA)	Adapted diets (e.g. Mediterranean with adjustments) Adjusting potassium intake in CKD	Plant-based diet to reduce uremic toxins Promoting eubiosis and reducing dysbiosis Avoiding excess animal protein
Stage 4 (advanced)	Advanced heart failure, CKD stages 4–5, dialysis, multiple complications	Complex regimens with: SGLT2i (if eGFR allows), GLP-1 RA, ACEi/ARBs, MRAs, diuretics, beta-blockers, statins Careful monitoring of adverse effects (hyperkalemia, hypotension) Multifaceted treatment planes in selected cases or in clinical trials, RNA therapies (e.g. zilebesiran, vupanorsen) are being explored for specific molecular targets (dyslipidemia, HTN, renal impairment)	Mediterranean or plant-based diet with restrictions (e.g., potassium) Adjusting protein intake Involving a dietitian	Reducing uremic toxins through: High-fiber plant-based diet Use of probiotics/nutritional support Maintaining a healthy intestinal barrier

SGLT2i sodium–glucose cotransporter 2 inhibitors, *GLP-1 RA* glucagon-like peptide-1 receptor agonists, *ACEi* angiotensin-converting enzyme inhibitors, *ARB* angiotensin receptor blockers, *HTN* arterial hypertension, *PCSK9i* Proprotein Convertase Subtilisin/Kexin Type 9 inhibitors, *MRA* mineralocorticoid receptor antagonists, *eGFR* estimated glomerular filtration rate, *LVH* left ventricular hypertrophy, *HbA1c* hemoglobin A1c, *CKD* chronic kidney disease, *T2DM* type 2 diabetes mellitus, *CV* cardiovascular

measurement every 3–6 months. The therapeutic regimen should be adjusted to keep these parameters within the recommended range.

Follow-up programs should consist, in addition, of complementary tests for screening and progression of the disease: measurement of microalbuminuria and eGFR annually or more frequently, if necessary; early evidence of cardiac dysfunction by electrocardiography and echocardiography; evaluation of atherosclerosis by ankle-brachial index or carotid Doppler ultrasound; and regular ophthalmologist visits for diabetic retinopathy [15].

In such an integrated care model, findings of these surveillance concepts are equally shared with the caregivers in multidisciplinary teams, ensuring a unified and coordinated perspective on the patient's clinical course. This integration facilitates early identification of signs of decompensation, leading to early intervention and better prognosis and avoiding emergency hospitalizations [3]. A relevant example of such proactive monitoring is the screening of obese and cardiovascular patients for sleep apnea. A significant number of individuals (60% estimated) suffer from obstructive sleep apnea (OSA) in this population, and OSA has a negative impact on diabetes and blood pressure control; therefore, screening and treatment of this comorbid condition should be included in multidisciplinary cardio-metabolic clinics [16].

This comprehensive approach of care, with addressing all important comorbidities for the patient, not just only one organ dysfunction, is in line with the holistic and systemic approach and need for tertiary prevention in the CKM syndrome [3]. Therefore, prevention must be considered an ongoing continuum, from primary prevention (e.g., health education, pursuit of healthy lifestyles in childhood) to secondary and tertiary prevention, through proper risk stratification and close monitoring of the clinical course of diagnosed subjects. This proactive, "stepwise," and "patient-tailored" attitude actually represents the cornerstone for the large clinical benefits in terms of delayed disease progression, reduced incidence of major complications, and prolonged survival, achievable within an integrated, multimodality "therapeutic approach," which suits the complexity of the CKM syndrome [3].

Therapeutic Approaches to the Cardio–Kidney–Metabolic Syndrome

The management of the cardio–kidney–metabolic syndrome requires tailored therapy that combines effective pharmacological therapies exhibiting multiorgan benefit and durable lifestyle changes. The main goals of treatment are to manage metabolic disturbances, lower cardiovascular risk, and preserve long-term renal function. These objectives may be met by the use of therapeutic agents, which address the basic elements of the syndrome, such as hyperglycemia, hypertension, dyslipidemia, and progression of chronic kidney disease [4].

Pharmacological Treatment of CKM Syndrome

Some drugs have shown effectiveness in current CKM syndrome therapeutic regimens.

Notable among these, SGLT2 inhibitors (e.g., dapagliflozin, empagliflozin) have been shown to decrease the risk of hospitalization for heart failure and to also slow the loss of renal function—whether patients have diabetes or not. Current international guidelines advocate their trial as first-line therapy for proteinuric chronic kidney disease and heart failure with reduced ejection fraction [17].

In addition, glucagon-like peptide-1 (GLP-1) receptor agonists (e.g., liraglutide and semaglutide) provide glycemic and weight management benefit and have shown a reduction in major adverse cardiovascular events in patients with diabetes and established atherosclerotic cardiovascular disease (ACVD) [6].

In high-risk patients with kidney disease—especially if accompanied by diabetes and chronic albuminuria—nonsteroidal mineralocorticoid receptor antagonists (MRAs), such as finerenone, could provide supplementary protection to the kidney and the heart on top of inhibition of the classical renin–angiotensin–aldosterone system (RAAS) [18].

The management of dyslipidemia is also an essential part of CKM therapy. High-intensity or max-tolerated statins are still the first-line drugs. For very high-risk patients who do not reach the LDL-cholesterol goals, the addition of ezetimibe or proprotein convertase subtilisin/kexin type 9 (PCSK9) inhibitors may be required. Concurrently, antihypertensive therapies have to reach target blood pressure levels (<130/80 mmHg) using drugs with a reno- and cardioprotective action [19].

Patients treated in clinical practice for advanced CKM syndrome, including T2DM, coronary artery disease, and renal dysfunction, require more complex treatment regimens. This means SGLT2 inhibitors, GLP-1 receptor agonists, RAAS blocking agents, MRAs, statins, beta-blockers, diuretics, and antithrombotic treatment. These regimens require frequent monitoring and dosage adjustments, based on renal function, as well as the risk of adverse effects such as hyperkalemia or hypotension, highlighting the critical importance of inter-specialty cooperation [6].

Nutritional Therapy in CKM Syndrome

Since lifestyle change is an important therapy in early CKM syndrome, it is an important therapeutic method apart from pharmacological treatment. International guidelines underscore the importance of dietary changes and regular physical activity as effective measures against diabetes, obesity, and hypertension [4]. The adoption of diets or diet patterns like Mediterranean, DASH, Nordic, or a plant-based dietary pattern has been associated with better metabolic control and cardiovascular risk. In obesity, a combination of lifestyle modification and drug treatment is better than each in monotherapy. Nevertheless, long-term behavioral changes are difficult to sustain, and dropout is common [20]. This is to emphasize the importance of the multidisciplinary team of care, including the medical team, dietitians, psychologists, and health education coordinators.

The **Mediterranean diet** is one of the most widely studied dietary models for the prevention of cardiovascular, metabolic, and, lately, renal diseases. This diet is adhered to in a larger or smaller proportion as Mediterranean-type diet in Mediterranean countries and is distinctive by a high consumption of vegetables, fruits, legumes, greens, whole grains, nuts and seeds, frequent consumption of fish and seafood, the most part of fat being olive oil (extra-virgin) and fat sources, moderate intake of fermented dairy and red wine. Intake of red meat, saturated fat, ultra-processed foods, and refined sugar is restricted [21]. Even though the dietary fat content (35–40% of total calorific value) is moderate-to-high, these are mainly good fats, as the monounsaturated fat (oleic acid from olive oil, as an example) and the polyunsaturated fat, in particular the omega-3 fatty acids from oily fish (such as salmon, sardines, and mackerel). This lipid profile, along with a high content of fiber, polyphenols, vitamins, and minerals, gives the Mediterranean diet antiatherogenic, antioxidant, and anti-inflammatory properties [21].

The cardiovascular effects of the Mediterranean diet are widely described in observational and interventional studies. The PREDIMED randomized clinical trial found a ~30% relative risk reduction in major cardiovascular events (myocardial infarction, stroke, cardiovascular death) in those following a Mediterranean diet supplemented with either olive oil or nuts compared with a low-fat control diet [22]. Postulated mechanisms for benefits include better lipid panel (lower triglycerides and higher HDL-cholesterol), lower blood pressure, better insulin sensitivity, and reduced oxidative stress. These effects are of interest not only for primary and secondary cardiovascular prevention but also for the prevention of type 2 diabetes and for the treatment of hyperglycemia in established diabetes.

For obesity, the Mediterranean diet appears to be effective in achieving short-term weight loss and weight loss maintenance over a period of longer than 1 year, particularly in combination with caloric restriction, although this effect is comparable to other hypocaloric diets. Nephroprotective effects have also been suggested, mainly due to reduction of systolic and diastolic blood pressures, enhancement of the lipid profile, reduction of systemic inflammation and oxidative stress, and moderate protein intake, mostly of plant and fish origin.

Potassium intake should be monitored, as quite a bit of fruit and vegetables are consumed in this diet type [23] in advanced CKD stages. The Mediterranean diet is considered to be easily applicable in the medium and long term, due to its neutral character. In the setting of the CKM syndrome, this diet attenuates inflammatory markers, improves endothelial function to decrease global cardio-reno-metabolic risk. International guidelines unanimously advocate it as the preferred nutritional strategy for patients who are at cardiovascular and metabolic risk, as well as for those who simultaneously receive antiatherogenic drug treatment and act in synergy with its long-term benefits [23].

The Nordic, DASH, and Plant-Based Diets in the CKM Syndrome

A **Nordic diet** is a modern diet that promotes locally sourced and sustainably produced foods, typical of the Nordic countries such as Denmark, Finland, Iceland, Norway, and Sweden. It had been created as what was thought to be a more regionally adaptive and sustainable version of the Mediterranean diet. From a nutritional perspective, it is a balanced macronutrient spread and is abundant with bioactive compounds that can promote cardio-metabolic health [24]. Major components include: frequent consumption of local whole-grain products (rye, oats, barley), carrots, beets, cabbage, and broccoli were typically eaten often and in large quantities, polyphenol-rich berries (blueberries, cranberries, raspberries), fatty cold-water fish (salmon, herring, and mackerel), rapeseed (canola) oil as the principal fat source (rapeseed oil is rich in monounsaturated fats and alpha-linolenic acid omega-3-fatty acid), as well as (in Norway) low-fat milk products ("skim milk"), and traditional lean meat (especially in Sweden) were consumed in low to moderate amounts, including game meats and low-fat fermented milk. It promotes reducing consumption of red meat, saturated fats, added sugars, and highly processed foods [24].

This diet has been related to similar clinical benefits of the Mediterranean diet, especially regarding lipid profile improvement and systemic inflammation reduction. Randomized clinical trials have shown significant reductions in total and LDL cholesterol, elevation in HDL cholesterol and lowering of the apolipoprotein B/A1 ratio, without formal caloric restriction. In the SYSDIET trial that was performed in patients with metabolic syndrome, the Nordic diet resulted in decreases in inflammatory markers and better metabolic profile, whereas there were no major effects of the diet on body weight or blood pressure [25]. Its beneficial effects are, in fact, due to the combined action of several components: rapeseed and fish unsaturated fats (cardioprotective), whole grain and vegetable (soluble and insoluble) fibers (glycemic control, satiety), polyphenol antioxidants (anti-inflammatory and insulin-sensitizing), and low amounts of simple sugar intake (postprandial glycemic control) [26].

Epidemiological data indicate that high adherence to the Nordic diet has been associated with lower risk of type 2 diabetes and cardiovascular disease, although the evidence level is lower than that for the Mediterranean diet [26]. In patients with the CKM syndrome, the Nordic diet is an acceptable and effective alternative, particularly in areas where access to Mediterranean foods is limited. It uses local nutrient-rich ingredients suited to the climate and culture. Rapeseed oil can replace olive oil, and locally produced low-glycemic index fruits and vegetables substitute other carbohydrate sources [27]. Its metabolic benefits are particularly evident, without substantial weight loss, which means nutrient quality has an impact independent of weight reduction [25].

The **DASH (Dietary Approaches to Stop Hypertension) diet** was initially developed to prevent and treat hypertension, but it has since shown efficacy to prevent cardiovascular and metabolic disorders. This approach focuses on consuming generous amounts of vegetables, fruits, whole grains, low-fat dairy, lean meats (fish, poultry), legumes, nuts, and healthy vegetable fats, while limiting saturated and trans fats (e.g., fried foods, fatty red meat, processed meats), added sugars, and sodium [28]. The DASH diet has been demonstrated to lower BP, even in the absence of very low sodium intake, with mean decreases between 5 and 6 mmHg for systolic BP among hypertensive subjects in clinical trials. Benefits go beyond blood pressure lowering. Several meta-analyses have linked adherence to the DASH diet with reduced risks of cardiovascular disease (myocardial infarction and stroke), type 2 diabetes, specific cancers, and all-cause mortality [28].

Among individuals with metabolic syndrome, it has been found that adherence to the DASH diet was associated with decreased waist circumference and blood pressure, as well as triglyceride levels and increased HDL cholesterol, which would improve core features of the CKM syndrome [28]. The DASH diet is high in antioxidants and micronutrients and is also potentially beneficial for endothelial function, reducing systemic inflammation, and enhancing insulin sensitivity. Moderate salt reduction and optimum potassium: natrium ratio favor vascular health, while optimal protein intake and a moderate glycemic index support in weight and glucose control [29]. The DASH diet is the most recommended healthy model and often prescribed as the primary form of dietary therapy for hypertension, DM, early heart failure, and early CKD. The DASH principles are endorsed by International guidelines (American Heart Association and the American College of Cardiology (AHA/ACC), Kidney Disease: Improving Global Outcomes (KDIGO)), as a standard preventive and therapeutic approach to these diseases [29]. One additional benefit is its practical flexibility; it does not rely exclusively on "exotic" foods, being adaptable to cultures [28].

Plant-based diets encompass a wide variety of specific foods and food groups that are characterized by a predominant intake of plant-derived foods. These vary from lacto-ovo-vegetarian to completely vegan diets. In the CKM syndrome, these diets offer numerous documented benefits in controlling metabolic and cardiovascular risk factors [20]. Food of plant origin (vegetables, fruits, legumes, whole grains, nuts, seeds) provides soluble and insoluble fiber that reduces intestinal cholesterol absorption, impacts blood glucose, and enhances satiety. They are also low in saturated fat and dietary cholesterol, which can help lower LDL cholesterol. A relatively low energy density contributes to weight control, and a high content of micronutrients (vitamin C, potassium, magnesium, and natural antioxidants) contributes to the reduction of blood pressure and systemic inflammation [30].

Epidemiological findings suggest an association between a largely plant-based diet and lower prevalence of obesity, type 2 diabetes, and cardiovascular disease. The beneficial effects can be attributed to both the high-quality nutritional profile and the bioactive phytochemicals (flavonoids, lignans, carotenoids) that exert systemic antioxidant and anti-inflammatory effects [30]. From a nephrological point of view, plant-based diets have been linked to the reduced risk of incident CKD. Proposed mechanisms include a lower dietary acid load, reduced consumption of high bioavailable phosphorus from animal and processed sources, and decreased glomerular hyperfiltration, a compensatory but deleterious mechanism in the progression of CKD. The metabolic load of plant proteins is lower than that of animal proteins, a factor that assumes special importance in the early-to-moderate stages of CKD [31].

It is possible to consume the ideal amount of protein on a vegan diet, but it requires careful nutrition planning. Sufficient quantities of essential amino acids must be provided by using the right amino acid sources (legumes, cereals, nuts). Additives of vitamin B12 are obligatory in vegan diets. Consideration should be given to measuring iron, vitamin D, and omega-3 fatty acid status in some cases, although plant sources of alpha-linolenic acid (e.g., flaxseed, chia, walnuts) can make a considerable contribution to daily needs [20].

Plant-based diets can be used effectively for advanced CKD patients with close assessment of potassium intake. Selection of low- or moderate-potassium fruits and vegetables and the use of cooking methods (e.g., boiling) to diminish potassium content are suggested [31]. Clinical trials have demonstrated that patients with type 2 diabetes, who adhere to a vegetarian or vegan diet, can achieve a substantial improvement in glycemic control and reduction in lipids—or even reduce medication use. The plant-based diets have also been linked to weight loss, lower blood pressure, and reduced inflammation [32].

An experienced dietitian must be an integral part of the multidisciplinary team to ensure successful and safe application. Their role includes direct food selection, preventing nutrient deficiencies, and maintaining energy and macronutrient intakes. In reality, many people tend toward an approach that draws upon features of vegetarian and omnivorous diets, like semi-vegetarianism or flexitarianism, where the diet is mostly plants with small portions of animal products. These may be easier to sustain and confer similar benefits in CKM-risk reduction [33].

Gut Microbiome, a Potential New Therapeutic Target in CKM Syndrome: Influence on Uremic Toxins and Systemic Inflammation

Over the past few years, dysbiosis of the gut microbiota has been recognized as an important player in the pathogenesis and treatment of a number of chronic diseases, including cardio–renal–metabolic (CKM) syndrome. The structure and functional metabolism of the gut microbiome coordinate metabolic homeostasis, systemic inflammation, and the production of uremic toxins, particularly in advanced stages of chronic kidney disease (CKD) [34].

Gut dysbiosis, which causes an imbalance between the beneficial and the pathogenic bacteria in the gut, has been frequently reported in CKD patients. It is favored by high-protein diets, long-term medication use to manage symptoms (especially antibiotics or proton pump inhibitors), and the accumulation of nitrogenous waste products that change the intestinal environment. Dysbiosis results in an overgrowth of proteinolytic bacteria with the formation of toxic metabolites. These are not only retained in the bloodstream due to the impaired glomerular filtration, but also are involved in disease progression, as they can cause oxidative stress, endothelial dysfunction, and systemic inflammation [34].

Conversely, a saccharolytic-enriched microbiota consisting of butyrate-, propionate-, and acetate-producing bacteria such as *Bifidobacterium* and *Lactobacillus* can ferment dietary fibers into short-chain fatty acids (SCFAs) such as butyrate, propionate, and acetate. These metabolites have systemic anti-inflammatory activities, help maintain the overall integrity of the gut barrier, and regulate immune response by limiting endotoxin translocation, thereby reducing the chronic inflammation characteristic of the CKM syndrome [35].

Dietary modifications, especially plant-based interventions, are a promising avenue to reestablish eubiosis. These diets are rich in prebiotic fibers (e.g., inulin, fructo-oligosaccharides, resistant starch) that support the growth of beneficial bacteria, at the expense of reducing the availability of protein substrates that fuel the production of toxic metabolites [36].

Among diet-based interventions, other therapeutic strategies have also been investigated, such as the use of prebiotics, probiotics, and synbiotics. These approaches aim to target the microbiome through selective modulation, offering potential benefits for individuals with cardiovascular-kidney-metabolic syndrome. For instance, administration of *Lactobacillus casei* Shirota or *Bifidobacterium longum* has demonstrated to decrease serum concentrations of indoxyl sulfate and inflammation status in CKD subjects. In addition, intestinal adsorbents, such as AST-120, are being studied as binding agents for uremic toxins in the gastrointestinal tract to reduce their systemic absorbtion [35].

RNA-Based Therapeutics and Emerging Horizons in CKM Syndrome

RNA-based according to therapies emerge as a challenge for the management of the cardiovascular-kidney-metabolic syndrome, targeting basic molecular mechanisms of the diseases. Antisense oligonucleotides (ASOs) and small interfering RNA (siRNAs) have demonstrated potent effects in decreasing dyslipidemia and cardiovascular risk [37]. For example, therapies directed against apolipoprotein C-III (ApoC-III, e.g., volanesorsen) and angiopoietin-like protein-3 (ANGPTL3, e.g., vupanorsen) (reducing apoB-containing particles, triglycerides, and low-density lipoprotein (LDL) cholesterol) in patients with severely elevated dyslipidaemia will thereby tackle a fundamental aspect of the CKM syndrome.

Concurrently, siRNAs targeting the renin–angiotensin–aldosterone system, including zilebesiran, are under development to achieve long-term blood pressure control with nephroprotective and cardioprotective properties [37, 38]. For metabolic applications, experimental RNA-based therapeutic strategies are being designed to target the gene expression implicated in obesity and energy balance to enhance insulin sensitivity and body weight loss. In addition, in the early stages of CKD, RNA interference (RNAi)-based techniques, which are directed against oxidative stress and fibrosis, are being investigated for the purpose of stopping or decelerating the course of the disease.

While these efforts remain for clinical validation, they provide evidence of principles underlying the reversal of the treatment paradigm from symptomatic to molecular targeted therapy in CKM syndrome. Future integration of these treatments will depend on demonstration of long-term efficacy, as well as characterization of a safety profile and development of fair-access policies [37, 38].

Future Perspectives in the Management of Cardio-Kidney-Metabolic Syndrome

Firm synergy between therapeutic advance and systemic healthcare reform will be part of the recipe for successful management of the cardio- renal-metabolic syndrome in the future. The burden of the CKM syndrome can be decreased thanks to three main factors:

- Properly organized interdepartmental teams
- Broader availability of novel therapies
- Cost-effective population approaches to prevention [3]

Barriers to the setup of specialized cardiovascular-kidney-metabolic clinics include limited financial resources, high patient volume, and a shortage of healthcare specialists. Overcoming these barriers will necessitate health policies that encourage the broad implementation of proven integrated care models, target funding to multidisciplinary clinics, and transform medical education to prioritize cardio-metabolic medicine. In this context, the training and credentialing of board-certified cardiovascular-kidney-metabolic physicians, whose expertise spans cardiology, nephrology, and endocrinology/diabetology, could represent a critical strategy to develop a care system that is positioned to serve this complex population of patients [39].

Digital health technologies will play a central role in empowering the transformation of care delivery for CKM patients. Interlinkable health records and telemedicine, including remote patient monitoring, support better cross-specialty coordination and allow constant monitoring of key clinical signs and early identification of decompensation.

Yet, access to innovative treatments remains a major challenge [40]. Although medications including SGLT2 inhibitors, GLP-1 receptor agonists, and finerenone have been found to convey significant cardiovascular and renal benefits, availability in routine practice has been variable. Health policy should now be incorporating these therapies into reimbursement, with cost-effectiveness studies justifying this on the basis of reductions in hospitalization and delays in progression to end-stage kidney disease. Equitable access to such therapies, in particular for patients in socioeconomically underprivileged or resource-limited environments, needs to be a paramount priority.

At the same time, healthcare payment models need to change. Transition from a fee-for-service model to bundled payments for an integrated care model may encourage the development of multidisciplinary clinics and centers of excellence in cardiovascular-kidney-metabolic care, promoting holistic, coordinated patient care [2].

Future research into the CKM syndrome must reflect the true complexity of these patients. Multidisciplinary clinical trials with patients with multimorbidity are necessary to confirm the interventions in high-risk populations. Concurrently, translational research ought to investigate the pathogenic processes of the CKM syndrome (e.g., chronic inflammation, oxidative stress, and intestinal dysbiosis) to search for new therapeutic targets. Prospects for research on microbiome-directed interventions, anti-inflammatory and anti-fibrotic drugs, as well as gene therapy, are all potentially promising. In summary, up-to-date care of the CKM syndrome requires a multidimensional approach, including therapeutic innovation, structural organization of health services, and strong disease prevention public health activities—with a focus on prevention and personalization of care.

Conclusions

Cardio–kidney–metabolic (CKM) syndrome is one of the most important challenges in modern internal medicine, not only because of its increasing prevalence, complicated pathogenesis, and poor prognosis in terms of survival. There is an interplay between the metabolic, cardiovascular, and renal dysfunctions that contributes to the ongoing synergistic disease progression; therefore, a combined, interdisciplinary therapeutic strategy is warranted.

To optimize patient care, a change from the current model of care to a predictive approach based on risk assessment linked to prevention as a constant, across the continuum of life, early identification of complications, cardiovascular-kidney-metabolic risk stratification, and personalized intervention on the basis of the stage of disease and associated conditions is needed.

Current therapy combines pharmaceutical agents with demonstrated multisystem effects (e.g., SGLT2 inhibitors, GLP-1 receptor agonists, finerenone) and evidence-based nutritional interventions. Future directions also include the increasing availability of newer molecular therapies (RNA-based and gene therapies), as well as interventions targeting the gut microbiome.

Efforts to reduce the burden of the CKM syndrome should be focused on these three strategic areas: creating multidisciplinary clinics, reorganizing healthcare systems to ensure equitable accessibility to effective therapies, and emphasizing population-based prevention. Only a unified, collaborative, and truly patient-centered strategy can alter the trajectory of this complex condition and prevent its severe complications.

Learning Objectives

- **Define the rationale and structure of a multidisciplinary care model** in the management of the CKM syndrome, including the roles of various healthcare professionals
- **Identify key strategies for prevention and risk assessment**, from primary to tertiary prevention, in individuals at risk or diagnosed with the CKM syndrome
- **Understand the role of evidence-based nutritional approaches** (Mediterranean, Dietary Approaches to Stop Hypertension (DASH), Nordic, and plant-based diets) and be able to integrate into an individualized care plan
- **Recognize the importance of gut microbiome modulation** and its therapeutic role in reducing systemic inflammation and uremic toxin burden in the CKM syndrome
- **Identify and remember the promise and challenges of RNA-based therapeutic**s in targeting molecular mechanisms of cardiovascular, renal, and metabolic diseases
- **Assess future directions** in CKM care, including digital health tools

Key Learning

- **A multidisciplinary team approach**—including cardiologists, nephrologists, endocrinologists, nutritionists, general practitioners, pharmacists, and nurses—is essential for the effective and coordinated care of patients with CKM.
- **Early prevention and risk stratification** are essential to mitigate the lifelong progression and burden of the CKM syndrome.
- **Stage-based therapeutic planning** enables personalized treatment from lifestyle interventions in early stages, such as nutritional therapy that plays a central role in metabolic and cardiovascular risk reduction, and probiotic interventions that reduce inflammation to complex pharmacological treatments
- **Contemporary pharmacologic agents** that provide organ-protective benefits are underused in the CKM syndrome, and **RNA-based therapies** that target molecular drivers of dyslipidemia, hypertension, and renal damage require further validation
- **Future care** for the CKM syndrome will depend on health system reforms, integration of digital health, access to innovative treatments, and training of physicians specializing in CKM.

References

1. Kittelson KS, Junior AG, Fillmore N, Da Silva GR. Cardiovascular-kidney-metabolic syndrome – an integrative review. Prog Cardiovasc Dis. 2024;87:26–36. https://doi.org/10.1016/j.pcad.2024.10.012.
2. Belay KE, Feleke Y, Alemneh TA, Haile AM, Abebe DG. Social determinants of health for cardiovascular-kidney-metabolic syndrome among patients with diabetes. J Endocr Soc. 2024;9(1):bvae208. https://doi.org/10.1210/jendso/bvae208.
3. Iacoviello M, Gori M, Grandaliano G, Minutolo R, Pitocco D, Trevisan R. A holistic approach to managing cardio-kidney metabolic syndrome: insights and recommendations from the Italian perspective. Front Cardiovasc Med. 2025;12:1583702. https://doi.org/10.3389/fcvm.2025.1583702.
4. Ndumele CE, Rangaswami J, Chow SL, Neeland IJ, Tuttle KR, Khan SS, et al. Cardiovascular-kidney-metabolic health: a presidential advisory from the American Heart Association. Circulation. 2023;148(20):1606–35. https://doi.org/10.1161/CIR.0000000000001184.
5. Rangaswami J, Tuttle K, Vaduganathan M. Cardio-kidney-metabolic care models: toward achieving effective interdisciplinary care. Circ: Cardiovasc Qual Outcomes. 2020;13(11):e007264. https://doi.org/10.1161/CIRCOUTCOMES.120.007264.
6. Krentz A, Jacob S, Heiss C, Sattar N, Lim S, Khunti K, et al. Rising to the challenge of cardio-kidney-metabolic disease in the 21st century: translating evidence into best clinical practice to prevent and manage atherosclerosis. Atherosclerosis. 2024;396:118528. https://doi.org/10.1016/j.atherosclerosis.2024.118528.
7. Reducing Care Fragmentation to Boost CKM Disease Outcomes. Am J Manag Care. 2025;31(Spec. 3):SP157–61. https://doi.org/10.37765/ajmc.2025.89711.

8. Van Buren DJ, Tibbs TL. Lifestyle interventions to reduce diabetes and cardiovascular disease risk among children. Curr Diabetes Rep. 2014;14(12):557. https://doi.org/10.1007/s11892-014-0557-2.
9. Ibrahim M, Ba-Essa EM, Baker J, Cahn A, Ceriello A, Cosentino F, et al. Cardio-renal-metabolic disease in primary care setting. Diabetes Metab Res. 2024;40(3):e3755. https://doi.org/10.1002/dmrr.3755.
10. Assogba F, Couchoud C, Roudier C, Pornet C, Fosse-Edorh S, Romon I, et al. Prevalence, screening and treatment of chronic kidney disease in people with type 2 diabetes in France: the ENTRED surveys (2001 and 2007). Diabetes Metab. 2012:38. https://doi.org/10.1016/j.diabet.2012.08.004.
11. Van Der Meer V, Nielen MM, Drenthen AJ, Van Vliet M, Assendelft WJ, Schellevis FG. Cardiometabolic prevention consultation in the Netherlands: screening uptake and detection of cardiometabolic risk factors and diseases – a pilot study. BMC Fam Pract. 2013;14(1):29. https://doi.org/10.1186/1471-2296-14-29.
12. Javaid A, Hariri E, Ozkan B, Lang K, Khan SS, Rangaswami J, et al. Cardiovascular-Kidney-Metabolic (CKM) Syndrome: a case-based narrative review. Am J Med Open. 2025;13:100089. https://doi.org/10.1016/j.ajmo.2025.100089.
13. Mach F, Baigent C, Catapano AL, Koskinas KC, Casula M, Badimon L, et al. 2019 ESC/EAS Guidelines for the management of dyslipidaemias: lipid modification to reduce cardiovascular risk. Eur Heart J. 2020;41(1):111–88. https://doi.org/10.1093/eurheartj/ehz455.
14. Marx N, Federici M, Schütt K, Müller-Wieland D, Ajjan RA, Antunes MJ, et al. 2023 ESC Guidelines for the management of cardiovascular disease in patients with diabetes. Eur Heart J. 2023;44(39):4043–140. https://doi.org/10.1093/eurheartj/ehad192.
15. American Diabetes Association Professional Practice Committee, ElSayed NA, Aleppo G, Bannuru RR, Bruemmer D, Collins BS, et al. 11. Chronic Kidney Disease and Risk Management: standards of care in diabetes – 2024. Diabetes Care. 2024;47(Supplement_1):S219–30. https://doi.org/10.2337/dc24-S011.
16. Yeghiazarians Y, Jneid H, Tietjens JR, Redline S, Brown DL, El-Sherif N, et al. Obstructive sleep apnea and cardiovascular disease: a scientific statement from the American Heart Association. Circulation. 2021;144(3) https://doi.org/10.1161/CIR.0000000000000988.
17. Krishnan A, Shankar M, Lerma EV, Wiegley N. Sodium Glucose Cotransporter 2 (SGLT2) inhibitors and CKD: are you a #Flozinator? Kidney Med. 2023;5(4):100608. https://doi.org/10.1016/j.xkme.2023.100608.
18. Lerma E, White WB, Bakris G. Effectiveness of nonsteroidal mineralocorticoid receptor antagonists in patients with diabetic kidney disease. Postgrad Med. 2023;135(3):224–33. https://doi.org/10.1080/00325481.2022.2060598.
19. Choi JY, Na JO. Pharmacological strategies beyond statins: ezetimibe and PCSK9 inhibitors. J Lipid Atheroscler. 2019;8(2):183. https://doi.org/10.12997/jla.2019.8.2.183.
20. Shi R, Mendoza-Sanchez M, Qadir M, Joshi S. A plant-based diet for cardiovascular risk reduction in kidney disease with a focus on cardiovascular-kidney-metabolic syndrome. Cardiol Clin. 2025:S0733865124001164. https://doi.org/10.1016/j.ccl.2024.12.006.
21. Finicelli M, Di Salle A, Galderisi U, Peluso G. The mediterranean diet: an update of the clinical trials. Nutrients. 2022;14(14):2956. https://doi.org/10.3390/nu14142956.
22. Ros E, Martínez-González MA, Estruch R, Salas-Salvadó J, Fitó M, Martínez JA, et al. Mediterranean diet and cardiovascular health: teachings of the PREDIMED study. Adv Nutr. 2014;5(3):330S–6S. https://doi.org/10.3945/an.113.005389.
23. Zheng X, Zhang W, Wan X, Lv X, Lin P, Si S, et al. The effects of Mediterranean diet on cardiovascular risk factors, glycemic control and weight loss in patients with type 2 diabetes: a meta-analysis. BMC Nutr. 2024;10(1):59. https://doi.org/10.1186/s40795-024-00836-y.
24. Nouripour F, Hejazi N. Nordic diet and cardio-metabolic diseases: a review. Int J Nutr Sci. 2019;4(3) https://doi.org/10.30476/IJNS.2019.82686.1025.

25. Gürdeniz G, Uusitupa M, Hermansen K, Savolainen MJ, Schwab U, Kolehmainen M, et al. Analysis of the SYSDIET Healthy Nordic Diet randomized trial based on metabolic profiling reveal beneficial effects on glucose metabolism and blood lipids. Clin Nutr. 2022;41(2):441–51. https://doi.org/10.1016/j.clnu.2021.12.031.
26. Lankinen M, Uusitupa M, Schwab U. Nordic diet and inflammation – a review of observational and intervention studies. Nutrients. 2019;11(6):1369. https://doi.org/10.3390/nu11061369.
27. Galbete C, Kröger J, Jannasch F, Iqbal K, Schwingshackl L, Schwedhelm C, et al. Nordic diet, Mediterranean diet, and the risk of chronic diseases: the EPIC-Potsdam study. BMC Med. 2018;16(1):99. https://doi.org/10.1186/s12916-018-1082-y.
28. Onwuzo C, Olukorode JO, Omokore OA, Odunaike OS, Omiko R, Osaghae OW, et al. DASH Diet: a review of its scientifically proven hypertension reduction and health benefits. Cureus. 2023; https://doi.org/10.7759/cureus.44692.
29. Campbell AP. DASH eating plan: an eating pattern for diabetes management. Diabetes Spectr. 2017;30(2):76–81. https://doi.org/10.2337/ds16-0084.
30. Koch CA, Kjeldsen EW, Frikke-Schmidt R. Vegetarian or vegan diets and blood lipids: a meta-analysis of randomized trials. Eur Heart J. 2023;44(28):2609–22. https://doi.org/10.1093/eurheartj/ehad211.
31. Gunadhar P. Preventing progression of chronic kidney disease with plant-based diet. Clin Med Rev Case Rep. 2021;8(9) https://doi.org/10.23937/2378-3656/1410365.
32. Kim H, Lee K, Rebholz CM, Kim J. Plant-based diets and incident metabolic syndrome: results from a South Korean prospective cohort study. Jia W, editor. PLoS Med. 2020;17(11):e1003371. https://doi.org/10.1371/journal.pmed.1003371.
33. Bruns A, Greupner T, Nebl J, Hahn A. Plant-based diets and cardiovascular risk factors: a comparison of flexitarians, vegans and omnivores in a cross-sectional study. BMC Nutr. 2024;10(1):29. https://doi.org/10.1186/s40795-024-00839-9.
34. He M, Wei W, Zhang Y, Xiang Z, Peng D, Kasimumali A, et al. Gut microbial metabolites SCFAs and chronic kidney disease. J Transl Med. 2024;22(1):172. https://doi.org/10.1186/s12967-024-04974-6.
35. Koppe L, Mafra D, Fouque D. Probiotics and chronic kidney disease. Kidney Int. 2015;88(5):958–66. https://doi.org/10.1038/ki.2015.255.
36. Sidhu SRK, Kok CW, Kunasegaran T, Ramadas A. Effect of plant-based diets on gut microbiota: a systematic review of interventional studies. Nutrients. 2023;15(6):1510. https://doi.org/10.3390/nu15061510.
37. Mohammadi A, Karimian A, Shokri K, Mohammadi A, Hazhir-Karzar N, Bahar R, et al. RNA therapies in cardio-kidney-metabolic syndrome: advancing disease management. J Cardiovasc Transl Res. 2025; https://doi.org/10.1007/s12265-025-10603-4.
38. Blom DJ, Marais AD, Moodley R, Van Der Merwe N, Van Tonder A, Raal FJ. RNA-based therapy in the management of lipid disorders: a review. Lipids Health Dis. 2022;21(1):41. https://doi.org/10.1186/s12944-022-01649-3.
39. Cases A, Broseta JJ, Marqués M, Cigarrán S, Julián JC, Alcázar R, et al. La definición del síndrome cardiovascular-reno-metabólico (cardiovascular-kidney-metabolic syndrome) y su papel en la prevención, estatificación del riesgo y tratamiento. Una oportunidad para la Nefrología. Nefrología. 2024;44(6):771–83. https://doi.org/10.1016/j.nefro.2024.05.001.
40. Liang F, Yang X, Peng W, Zhen S, Cao W, Li Q, et al. Applications of digital health approaches for cardiometabolic diseases prevention and management in the Western Pacific region. Lancet Regional Health West Pac. 2024;43:100817. https://doi.org/10.1016/j.lanwpc.2023.100817.

Index

M. Floria, D. M. Tanase (eds.), *Cardiovascular-Kidney-Metabolic Syndrome*, https://doi.org/10.1007/978-3-032-11445-7

D

E

G

H

I

K

MIX
Papier aus verantwortungsvollen Quellen
Paper from responsible sources
FSC® C105338

If you have any concerns about our products,
you can contact us on
ProductSafety@springernature.com

In case Publisher is established outside the EU,
the EU authorized representative is:
Springer Nature Customer Service Center GmbH
Europaplatz 3, 69115 Heidelberg, Germany

Printed by Libri Plureos GmbH
in Hamburg, Germany